Improving the Quality of Health Care for Mental and Substance-Use Conditions

Committee on Crossing the Quality Chasm: Adaptation to
Mental Health and Addictive Disorders

Board on Health Care Services

INSTITUTE OF MEDICINE
OF THE NATIONAL ACADEMIES

THE NATIONAL ACADEMIES PRESS
Washington, DC
www.nap.edu

THE NATIONAL ACADEMIES PRESS • 500 Fifth Street, N.W. • Washington, DC 20001

NOTICE: The project that is the subject of this report was approved by the Governing Board of the National Research Council, whose members are drawn from the councils of the National Academy of Sciences, the National Academy of Engineering, and the Institute of Medicine. The members of the committee responsible for the report were chosen for their special competences and with regard for appropriate balance.

This study was supported by multiple contracts and grants between the National Academy of Sciences and the Substance Abuse and Mental Health Services Administration (SAMHSA) of the Department of Health and Human Services (Contract No. 282-99-0045), the Robert Wood Johnson Foundation (Grant No. 048021), the Annie E. Casey Foundation (Grant No. 204.0236), the National Institute on Drug Abuse and the National Institute on Alcohol Abuse and Alcoholism (Contract No. N01-OD-4-2139), the Veterans Health Administration (Contract No. DHHS 223-01-2460/TO21), and through a grant from the CIGNA Foundation. Any opinions, findings, conclusions, or recommendations expressed in this publication are those of the authors and do not necessarily reflect the view of the organizations and agencies that provided support for this project.

Library of Congress Cataloging-in-Publication Data

Institute of Medicine (U.S.). Committee on Crossing the Quality Chasm:
  Adaptation to Mental Health and Addictive Disorders.
  Improving the quality of health care for mental and substance-use
conditions / Committee on Crossing the Quality Chasm: Adaptation to
Mental Health and Addictive Disorders, Board on Health Care Services.
    p. ; cm. — (Quality chasm series)
  Includes bibliographical references and index.
  ISBN 0-309-10044-5 (full book)
  1. Substance abuse—Treatment. 2. Community mental health services.
3. Substance abuse—Patients—Services for.   I. Title. II. Series.
  [DNLM: 1. Mental Disorders—therapy. 2. Substance-Related Disorders—therapy. 3. Patient-Centered Care. 4. Quality of Health Care.
WM 400 I59i 2006]
  RC564.I47 2006
  362.29—dc22

2005036202

Additional copies of this report are available from the National Academies Press, 500 Fifth Street, N.W., Lockbox 285, Washington, DC 20055; (800) 624-6242 or (202) 334-3313 (in the Washington metropolitan area); Internet, http://www.nap.edu.

For more information about the Institute of Medicine, visit the IOM home page at: **www.iom.edu.**

The serpent has been a symbol of long life, healing, and knowledge among almost all cultures and religions since the beginning of recorded history. The serpent adopted as a logotype by the Institute of Medicine is a relief carving from ancient Greece, now held by the Staatliche Museen in Berlin.

*"Knowing is not enough; we must apply.
Willing is not enough; we must do."*
—Goethe

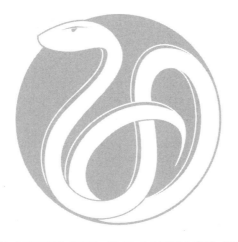

INSTITUTE OF MEDICINE
OF THE NATIONAL ACADEMIES

Advising the Nation. Improving Health.

THE NATIONAL ACADEMIES
Advisers to the Nation on Science, Engineering, and Medicine

The **National Academy of Sciences** is a private, nonprofit, self-perpetuating society of distinguished scholars engaged in scientific and engineering research, dedicated to the furtherance of science and technology and to their use for the general welfare. Upon the authority of the charter granted to it by the Congress in 1863, the Academy has a mandate that requires it to advise the federal government on scientific and technical matters. Dr. Ralph J. Cicerone is president of the National Academy of Sciences.

The **National Academy of Engineering** was established in 1964, under the charter of the National Academy of Sciences, as a parallel organization of outstanding engineers. It is autonomous in its administration and in the selection of its members, sharing with the National Academy of Sciences the responsibility for advising the federal government. The National Academy of Engineering also sponsors engineering programs aimed at meeting national needs, encourages education and research, and recognizes the superior achievements of engineers. Dr. Wm. A. Wulf is president of the National Academy of Engineering.

The **Institute of Medicine** was established in 1970 by the National Academy of Sciences to secure the services of eminent members of appropriate professions in the examination of policy matters pertaining to the health of the public. The Institute acts under the responsibility given to the National Academy of Sciences by its congressional charter to be an adviser to the federal government and, upon its own initiative, to identify issues of medical care, research, and education. Dr. Harvey V. Fineberg is president of the Institute of Medicine.

The **National Research Council** was organized by the National Academy of Sciences in 1916 to associate the broad community of science and technology with the Academy's purposes of furthering knowledge and advising the federal government. Functioning in accordance with general policies determined by the Academy, the Council has become the principal operating agency of both the National Academy of Sciences and the National Academy of Engineering in providing services to the government, the public, and the scientific and engineering communities. The Council is administered jointly by both Academies and the Institute of Medicine. Dr. Ralph J. Cicerone and Dr. Wm. A. Wulf are chair and vice chair, respectively, of the National Research Council.

www.national-academies.org

JEFFREY H. SAMET, Professor of Medicine and Social and Behavioral Sciences and Vice Chair for Public Health, Boston University Schools of Medicine and Public Health and Chief, General Internal Medicine at Boston Medical Center

TOM TRABIN, Consultant in behavioral health care and informatics, El Cerrito, CA

MARK D. TRAIL, Chief of the Medical Assistance Plans, Georgia Department of Community Health, Atlanta

ANN CATHERINE VEIERSTAHLER, Nurse, advocate, and person with bipolar illness, Milwaukee, WI

CYNTHIA WAINSCOTT, Chair, National Mental Health Association, Cartersville, GA

CONSTANCE WEISNER, Professor, Department of Psychiatry, University of California, San Francisco, and Investigator, Division of Research, Northern California Kaiser Permanente

Study Staff

ANN E. K. PAGE, Study Director and Senior Program Officer, Board on Health Care Services

REBECCA BENSON, Senior Project Assistant (11/03–11/04)

RYAN PALUGOD, Senior Project Assistant (11/04–1/06)

Board on Health Care Services

JANET M. CORRIGAN, Director (11/03–5/05)

CLYDE BEHNEY, Acting Director (6/05–12/05)

JOHN RING, Director (12/05–)

ANTHONY BURTON, Administrative Assistant

TERESA REDD, Financial Associate

Reviewers

This report has been reviewed in draft form by individuals chosen for their diverse perspectives and technical expertise, in accordance with procedures approved by the NRC's Report Review Committee. The purpose of this independent review is to provide candid and critical comments that will assist the institution in making its published report as sound as possible and to ensure that the report meets institutional standards for objectivity, evidence, and responsiveness to the study charge. The review comments and draft manuscript remain confidential to protect the integrity of the deliberative process. We wish to thank the following individuals for their review of this report:

ALLEN DIETRICH, Dartmouth Medical School, Hanover, New Hampshire

MICHAEL FITZPATRICK, National Alliance for the Mentally Ill, Arlington, Virginia

HOWARD GOLDMAN, University of Maryland at Baltimore School of Medicine

MICHAEL HOGAN, Ohio Department of Mental Health, Columbus

TEH-WEI HU, University of California, Berkeley School of Public Health

EDWARD JONES, PacifiCare Behavioral Health, Van Nuys, California

DAVID LEWIS, Brown University Center for Alcohol and Addiction Studies, Providence, Rhode Island

JOHN MONAHAN, University of Virginia School of Law, Charlottesville

GAIL STUART, Medical University of South Carolina College of Nursing, Charleston

MICHAEL TRUJILLO, University of New Mexico School of Medicine, Albuquerque

WILLIAM WHITE, Port Charlotte, Florida

Although the reviewers listed above have provided many constructive comments and suggestions, they were not asked to endorse the conclusions or recommendations nor did they see the final draft of the report before its release. The review of this report was overseen by FLOYD BLOOM, The Scripps Research Institute and Neurome, Inc., La Jolla, California, and JUDITH R. LAVE, University of Pittsburgh, Pennsylvania. Appointed by the National Research Council and Institute of Medicine, they were responsible for making certain that an independent examination of this report was carried out in accordance with institutional procedures and that all review comments were carefully considered. Responsibility for the final content of this report rests entirely with the authoring committee and the institution.

Foreword

Improving the Quality of Health Care for Mental and Substance-Use Conditions represents the intersection of two key developments now taking place in health care. One is the increasing attention to improving the quality of health care in ways that take account of patients' preferences and values along with scientific findings about effective care. The second important development comes from scientific research that enables us to better understand and treat mental and substance-use conditions. New technologies such as neuroimaging and genomics, for example, enable us to observe the brain in action and examine the interplay of genetic and environmental factors in mental and substance-use illnesses. These advances are potentially valuable to the more than 10 percent of the U.S. population receiving health care for mental and substance-use conditions; the many millions more who need but do not receive such care; and their families and friends, employers, teachers, and policy makers who encounter the effects of these illnesses in their personal lives, in the workplace, in schools, and in society at large.

This report puts forth an agenda for capitalizing on these two developments. Using the quality improvement framework contained in the predecessor Institute of Medicine report *Crossing the Quality Chasm: A New Health System for the 21st Century,* it calls for action from clinicians, health care organizations, purchasers, health plans, quality oversight organizations, researchers, public policy makers, and others to ensure that individuals with mental and substance-use health conditions receive the care that they need to recover. Importantly, the report's recommendations are not directed solely to clinicians and organizations that specialize in the delivery of health care for mental and substance-use conditions. As the report notes, the link between mental and substance-use problems and illnesses and general health and health care is very strong. This is especially true with respect to chronic illnesses, which now are the leading cause of illness, disability, and death in the United States. As the committee that conducted this study concluded, improving our nation's general health and the quality problems of our general health care system depends upon equally attending to the quality problems in health care for mental and substance-use conditions. The committee calls on primary care providers, other specialty health care providers, and all components of our general health care system to attend to the mental and substance-use health care needs of those they serve.

Dealing equally with health care for mental, substance-use, and general health conditions requires a fundamental change in how we as a society and health care system think about and respond to these problems and illnesses. Mental and substance-use problems and illnesses should not be viewed as separate from and unrelated to overall health and general health care. Building on this integrated concept, this report offers valuable guidance on how all can help to achieve higher-quality health care for people with mental or substance-use problems and illnesses. To this end, the Institute of Medicine will itself seek to incorporate attention to issues in health care for mental and substance-use problems and illnesses into its program of general health studies.

Harvey V. Fineberg, MD, PhD
President, Institute of Medicine

Preface

The charge to the Committee on Crossing the Quality Chasm: Adaptation to Mental Health and Addictive Disorders was broad, encompassing health care for both mental and substance-use conditions, the public and private sectors, and the comprehensive range of issues addressed in the 2001 Institute of Medicine report *Crossing the Quality Chasm: A New Health System for the 21st Century*. The committee was pleased to be asked to address this breadth of issues. Despite the frequent co-occurrence of mental and substance-use conditions, studies and reports that address both are unusual, as are those that cut across both the public and private sectors. We are grateful to our sponsors for having the vision to recognize the need for this study. Although the committee at times found the different histories, vocabularies, and other characteristics of these groups of illnesses and delivery systems challenging, we also acknowledged the unique strengths that each brought to the study, respected each others' positions, and reached consensus on issues that have traditionally been characterized by great disharmony. Having expertise in both mental and substance-use health care and the perspectives of the public and private sectors at the table was essential to the committee's efforts to craft a strategic agenda for improving the quality of health care for mental and substance-use conditions for all. The committee hopes that joint mental and substance-use studies and public–private partnership initiatives will become routine.

Although the focus of this study was on solving the *problems* of health care for mental and substance-use conditions—some of which are more complex than those associated with general health care—the committee also recognized its *strengths*. Health care for mental and substance-use conditions has led the way in promoting patient-centered care (a key quality aim set forth in the *Quality Chasm* report) in a number of ways: through the strong voice of consumers, their families, and consumer advocacy organizations in shaping mental health care; the long-standing use of peer support programs in facilitating recovery from substance-use illnesses; and research on how to enable decision making in the face of cognitive impairment. Moreover, the commitment and strength of the workforce delivering health care for mental and substance-use conditions are remarkable. This workforce has persevered in the face of limited attention to mental and substance-use illnesses by health professions schools, constrained resources at care delivery sites, stigma and discrimination, and an inadequate overall infrastructure to support the delivery of high-quality treatment services. This report identifies what it will take to build the needed infrastructure and fully support the workforce in delivering quality care.

This report also identifies gaps in our knowledge of how to effectively prevent and treat mental and substance-use illnesses. While science has developed a strong armamentarium of effective psychosocial therapies and medications for treating mental and substance-use problems and illnesses, research is still needed to identify how best to meet the special needs of children; older adults; individuals who are members of cultural or ethnic minorities; and those with complex and co-occurring mental, substance-use, and general health care illnesses. Moreover, translational research is needed to determine how to apply existing knowledge in usual settings of care.

The agenda and road map the committee has outlined for building the infrastructure needed to improve the quality of health care for mental and substance-use conditions is comprehensive, demanding, and critically important. It is our hope that the government agencies, purchasers, health plans, health care organizations, and other public- and private-sector leaders called upon to act on these recommendations will do so quickly so that we, our loved ones, friends, coworkers—indeed all Americans—can receive the high quality care for mental and substance-use conditions that is crucial to overall good health.

Mary Jane England
Chair

Acknowledgments

The Committee on Crossing the Quality Chasm: Adaptation to Mental Health and Addictive Disorders thanks the many individuals and organizations who so generously contributed their time, expertise, and sometimes personal experiences to the development of this report. Foremost we thank the consumers and their families who so eloquently testified to the committee about the power of good-quality health care to enable recovery from mental and substance-use problems and illnesses. Nancy Fudge, participant in the Florida Self-Directed Care Program; Michael M. Faenza, President and CEO of the National Mental Health Association; Eileen White, on behalf of the National Alliance for the Mentally Ill; Jane A. Walker, Executive Director of the Maryland Coalition of Families for Children's Mental Health; Johnny W. Allem, President of the Johnson Institute; Tom Leibfried, Program Director at the National Mental Health Consumers' Self-Help Clearinghouse; E. Clark Ross, Chief Executive Officer of CHADD (Children and Adults with Attention-Deficit/Hyperactivity Disorder); and Sue Bergeson, Vice President of the Depression and Bipolar Support Alliance generously shared their knowledge of mental and substance-use problems and illnesses, health care for these conditions, and pathways to improvement based on their own experiences and those of the individuals they represent.

Many other individuals and organizations provided testimony and other assistance to the committee. We thank John Oldham, Chairman of the Council on Quality Care at the American Psychiatric Association; Jalie A. Tucker, Chair of the Board of Professional Affairs at the American Psychological Association; Wilma Townsend, on behalf of the National Alliance of Multiethnic Behavioral Health Organizations; Allen J. Dietrich, representing the American Academy of Family Physicians; Gerry Schmidt, Clinical Affairs Consultant to NAADAC (the Association for Addiction Professionals); Ruth Hughes from the Substance Abuse and Mental Health Services Administration's (SAMHSA) Center for Mental Health Services Human Resources Work Group Alliance; Carolyn Russell, Director of the Florida Self-Directed Care Program; Jonathan Stanley, Assistant Director of the Treatment Advocacy Center; Linda Rosenberg, President and CEO of the National Council for Community Behavioral Healthcare; Frank Ghinassi, representing the National Association of Psychiatric Health Systems; Robert Sheehan, President of the National Association for Children's Behavioral Health; Michael B. Harle, representing Therapeutic Communities of America; Ronald J. Hunsicker, President and CEO of the National Association of Addiction Treatment Providers, Inc.; Marvin D. Seppala, representing the Partnership for Recovery; Wesley Sowers, President of the American Association of Community Psychiatrists; Robert Booth, Executive Director of the American Board of Examiners in Clinical Social Work; Mara Shrek, also representing the American Board of Examiners in Clinical Social Work; Elizabeth J. Clark, Executive Director, and Mickey J. W. Smith, Senior Policy Associate, both of the National Association of Social Workers; William F. Northey, Professional Development and Research Specialist at the American Association for Marriage and Family Therapy; Sandra Talley, President of the American Psychiatric Nurses Association; Thomas W. Nolan, Senior Fellow at the Institute for Healthcare Improvement; David H. Gustafson, Principal Investigator, Network for the Improvement of Addiction Treatment, University of Wisconsin-Madison; Vijay Ganju, Director of the Center for Mental Health Quality and Accountability at the National Association of State Mental Health Program Directors Research Institute, Inc.; Robert Johnson, representing the National Association of State Alcohol and Drug Abuse Directors; Howard B. Shapiro, Executive Director of the State Associations of Addiction Services; Pamela Greenberg, Executive Director of the American Managed Behavioral Healthcare Association; Melissa M. Staats, Executive Director of the National Association of County Behavioral Health Directors; Mark Willenbring, Director of the Division of Treatment and Recovery Research at the National Institute on Alcohol Abuse and Alcoholism; John A. Paton, representing the Software and Technology Vendor's Association; Lisa Teems, representing the Employee Assistance Programs Alliance; Joan M. Pearson, Principal, Towers Perrin; Dale A. Masi, President and CEO of Masi Research Consultants, Inc.; Neal Adams, Medical Director for Adult Services, California Department of Mental Health; Pamela S. Hyde, Secretary of the New Mexico Human Services Department; Joy M. Grossman at the Center for Studying Health System Change; Patricia A. Taylor, Executive Director of Faces & Voices of Recovery; Kevin D. Hennessey, Science to Service Coordinator at SAMHSA;

Sarah A. Wattenberg, Public Health Advisor at SAMHSA; and staff of the Greater Los Angeles Veterans Healthcare Center EQUIP project and their sponsors at the Veterans Administration Health Services Research & Development Service and Quality Enhancement Research Initiative.

Several national experts on topics relevant to the committee's work also provided invaluable assistance by preparing commissioned papers on the issues under study. We thank Scott Y. H. Kim, MD, PhD, from the University of Michigan Medical School, for his paper on "Impact of Mental Illness and Substance-Related Disorders on Decision-Making Capacity and Its Implications for Patient-Centered Mental Health Care Delivery"; Elyn R. Saks, JD, from the University of Southern California Law School, and Dilip V. Jeste, MD, from the University of California-San Diego, for their papers on "Capacity to Consent to or Refuse Treatment and/or Research: Theoretical Considerations" and "Decisional Capacity in Mental Illness and Substance Use Disorders: Empirical Database and Policy Considerations"; Judith Cook, PhD, from the University of Illinois-Chicago, for her paper on "'Patient-Centered' and 'Consumer-Directed' Mental Health Services"; Ellen Harris, JD, and Chris Koyanagi of the Judge David L. Bazelon Center for Mental Health Law, for their paper on "Obstacles to Choice: Statutory, Regulatory, Administrative and Other Barriers That Impede Consumer-Directed Care in Mental Health"; Constance M. Horgan, ScD, and Deborah W. Garnick, ScD, both of Brandeis University, for their paper on "The Quality of Care for Adults with Mental and Addictive Disorders: Issues in Performance Measurement"; Christina Bethell, PhD, of the Oregon Health and Science University School of Medicine, for her paper on "Taking the Next Step to Improve the Quality of Child and Adolescent Mental and Behavioral Health Care Services: Current Status and Promising Strategies for Quality Measurement;" Robert Rosenheck, MD, of the Veterans Administration Northeast Program Evaluation Center, for his paper "Mental Health and Substance Abuse Services for Veterans: Experience with Performance Evaluation in the Department of Veterans Affairs"; Benjamin C. Grasso, MD, Executive Director of the Institute for Self-Directed Care, for his paper on "The Safety of Health Care for Individuals with Mental Illness and Substance Use Disorders"; Susan Stefan, JD, from the Center for Public Representation, for her paper on "Patient-Centered Care/Self-Directed Care: Legal, Policy and Programmatic Considerations"; Mark D. Weist, of the University of Maryland School of Medicine, Carl E. Paternite, PhD, of Miami University (Ohio), and Steven Adelsheim, MD, of the University of New Mexico Health Sciences Center, for their paper "School-Based Mental Health Services"; John Landsverk, PhD, of the Child and Adolescent Services Research Center at Children's Hospital-San Diego, for his paper "Improving the Quality of Mental Health and Substance Abuse Treatment Services for Children Involved in Child Welfare"; Nancy Wolff, PhD, of Rutgers

University, for her paper "Law and Disorder: The Case Against Diminished Responsibility"; Joseph J. Cocozza, PhD, of the National Center for Mental Health and Juvenile Justice and Policy Research Associates, Inc., for his paper "Juvenile Justice Systems: Improving Mental Health Treatment Services for Children and Adolescents"; John A. Morris, MSW, of Comprehensive NeuroScience, Inc. and the University of South Carolina School of Medicine, Eric N. Goplerud, PhD, of George Washington University Medical Center, and Michael A. Hoge, PhD, of Yale University School of Medicine, for their paper "Workforce Issues in Behavioral Health"; and Timothy S. Jost, JD, of Washington and Lee University School of Law, for his paper on "Constraints on Sharing Mental Health Treatment Information Imposed by Federal and State Medical Records Privacy Laws." In addition, Jennifer Kraszewski, graduate student at The George Washington University, and Craig Bremmer, Senior Research Associate at the Institute for Health Policy and Health Services Research at the University of Cincinnati Medical Center, collected and analyzed information pertaining to accreditation and performance measurement in health care for mental and substance-use conditions, respectively.

At the Institute of Medicine, Karen Adams, PhD, provided expert consultation and advice on self-efficacy, patient activation, and other aspects of patient-centered care. Danitza Valdivia once again provided ever-ready and gracious assistance regardless of the task or timeline, and Bill McLeod and the staff of the George E. Brown Library provided sustained professional support in the location and retrieval of voluminous reference materials.

Rona Briere of Briere Associates, Inc. provided expert copy editing, and Alisa Decatur excellent proofreading and manuscript preparation assistance.

Finally, we thank the Annie E. Casey Foundation, CIGNA Foundation, the National Institute on Alcohol Abuse and Alcoholism (NIAAA), the National Institute on Drug Abuse (NIDA), The Robert Wood Johnson Foundation, SAMHSA within the U.S. Department of Health and Human Services, and the Veterans Health Administration (VHA) of the Department of Veterans Affairs for their support for the application of the *Quality Chasm* framework as a tool for improving the quality of health care for mental and substance-use conditions, for their leadership in calling for a study to address the intertwined issues of mental health and substance use, and for their financial support for this study. We also are especially grateful to key personnel within these agencies and organizations who spearheaded efforts to get this study under way and provided ongoing data, information, and support and encouragement throughout the committee's efforts. We especially thank Ronald W. Manderscheid, PhD, Chief of the Survey and Analysis Branch in the Center for Mental Health Services, and Mady Chalk, PhD, Director of the Division of Services Improvement in the Center for Substance Abuse Treatment, both within SAMHSA; Constance Pechura, PhD, and Victor A. Capoccia, PhD, both Senior Program Officers at The Robert Wood Johnson Foundation; Rhonda Robinson Beale, MD, Senior Vice President and Chief Medical Officer at CIGNA Behavioral Health; Frances M. Murphy MD, MPH, Deputy Under Secretary for Health, Department of Veterans Affairs; Stephen W. Long, Executive Officer, NIAAA; Wilson M. Compton, Director, Division of Epidemiology, Services and Prevention Research, and Jerry P. Flanzer, PhD, Senior Health Science Administrator, both of NIDA; and Patrick McCarthy, PhD, Vice President, Systems and Service Reform, the Annie E. Casey Foundation.

Contents

Tables, Figures, and Boxes

TABLES

FIGURES

BOXES

Summary

ABSTRACT

Millions of Americans today receive health care for mental or substance-use problems and illnesses. These conditions are the leading cause of combined disability and death among women and the second highest among men.

Effective treatments exist and continually improve. However, as with general health care, deficiencies in care delivery prevent many from receiving appropriate treatments. That situation has serious consequences—for people who have the conditions; for their loved ones; for the workplace; for the education, welfare, and justice systems; and for the nation as a whole.

A previous Institute of Medicine report, Crossing the Quality Chasm: A New Health System for the 21st Century *(IOM, 2001), put forth a strategy for improving health care overall—a strategy that has attained considerable traction in the United States and other countries. However, health care for mental and substance-use conditions has a number of distinctive characteristics, such as the greater use of coercion into treatment, separate care delivery systems, a less developed quality measurement infrastructure, and a differently structured marketplace. These and other differences raised questions about whether the* Quality Chasm *approach is applicable to health care for mental and substance-use conditions and, if so, how it should be applied.*

1

This new report examines those differences, finds that the Quality Chasm *framework can be applied to health care for mental and substance-use conditions, and describes a multifaceted and comprehensive strategy for doing so and thereby ensuring that:*

- *Individual patient preferences, needs, and values prevail in the face of residual stigma, discrimination, and coercion into treatment.*
- *The necessary infrastructure exists to produce scientific evidence more quickly and promote its application in patient care.*
- *Multiple providers' care of the same patient is coordinated.*
- *Emerging information technology related to health care benefits people with mental or substance-use problems and illnesses.*
- *The health care workforce has the education, training, and capacity to deliver high-quality care for mental and substance-use conditions.*
- *Government programs, employers, and other group purchasers of health care for mental and substance-use conditions use their dollars in ways that support the delivery of high-quality care.*
- *Research funds are used to support studies that have direct clinical and policy relevance and that are focused on discovering and testing therapeutic advances.*

The strategy addresses issues pertaining to health care for both mental and substance-use conditions and the essential role of health care for both conditions in improving overall health and health care. In so doing, it details the actions required to achieve those ends—actions required of clinicians; health care organizations; health plans; purchasers; state, local, and federal governments; and all parties involved in health care for mental and substance-use conditions.

MILLIONS OF AMERICANS USE HEALTH CARE FOR MENTAL OR SUBSTANCE-USE CONDITIONS

Each year, more than 33 million Americans use health care services for their mental problems and illnesses[1] or conditions resulting from their use

---

[1]Whenever possible, this report uses the words "problems" and illnesses," as opposed to "disorders," for reasons explained in the full report. Nonetheless, the word "disorder" appears often in this report because it is used so frequently in the literature. Collectively, this report refers to problems and illnesses as "conditions."

of alcohol, inappropriate use of prescription medications, or illegal drugs. About 28 million Americans aged 18 or older (13 percent of this population) received mental health treatment in an inpatient or outpatient setting in 2003[2] (SAMHSA, 2004a), and more than 6 percent of American children and adolescents aged 5–17 had contact with a mental health professional in a 12-month period according to the 1998–1999 National Health Interview survey (Simpson et al., 2004). The rates are higher still for adolescents and working-age adults: 5 million (20.6 percent) of those aged 12–17 received treatment or counseling for emotional or behavioral problems in 2003 (SAMHSA, 2004a), and a nearly identical proportion (20.1 percent) of those aged 18–54 received treatment for mental and/or substance-use (M/SU)[3] problems and illnesses in 2001–2003 (Kessler et al., 2005). More than 3 million (1.4 percent) of those aged 12 or older reported receiving some kind of treatment during 2003 for a problem related to alcohol or drug use (SAMHSA, 2004a). Millions more reported that they needed treatment for M/SU conditions but did not receive it (Mechanic and Bilder, 2004; SAMHSA, 2004a; Wu et al., 2003). From 2001 to 2003, only 40.5 percent of those aged 18–54 who met a specific definition of severe mental illness received any treatment (Kessler et al., 2005). And, in contrast with the more than 3 million Americans aged 12 or older who received treatment during 2003 for a problem related to alcohol or drug use, more than six times that number (9.1 percent of this age group) reported abusing or being physiologically dependent on alcohol; illicit drugs, such as marijuana, cocaine, heroin, hallucinogens, or stimulants; prescription drugs used for nonmedical purposes; or a combination of these (SAMHSA, 2004a).

We know these people, and we know why they contact health care providers for M/SU treatment. We do so ourselves—for our own M/SU problems and illnesses and for those of our parents, our children, our spouses, our loved ones. We know about these conditions from other family members and from our neighbors, friends, teachers, and coworkers—and from the homeless people we pass on the street. What we can see for ourselves—our teenager's friend battling anorexia, our friend's spouse with a drinking problem, our own family member recovering from depression, or our child with attention deficit hyperactivity disorder (ADHD)—is reflected daily in the first-person accounts of public figures about their own M/SU illnesses and recovery. We hear of newswoman Jane Pauley's treatment for and recovery from bipolar illness; astronaut Buzz Aldrin's recovery from alcoholism and depression; former First Lady Betty Ford's recovery from alcoholism; actress Drew Barrymore's recovery from depression,

---

[2]This figure does not include treatment solely for substance use.

[3]Throughout this report, the committee uses the acronym M/SU to refer to "mental and/or substance use."

alcoholism, and other substance-use problems; former National Football League running back Earl Campbell's recovery from panic and anxiety disorder; "60 Minutes" host Mike Wallace's, interviewer Larry King's, and columnist Art Buchwald's recovery from depression; country music singer Charlie Pride's recovery from bipolar illness and alcoholism; Hall of Fame jockey Julie Krone's recovery from posttraumatic stress disorder; television news (ABC's "20/20," "Nightline," and "World News Tonight") producer Bill Lichtenstein's recovery from bipolar illness; CNN founder Ted Turner's recovery from bipolar illness; Nobel prize-winning mathematician and economist John Nash's recovery from schizophrenia; and many other such cases. As articulated in the 1999 surgeon general's report on mental health (Anthony, 1993 cited in DHHS, 1999:98):

> a person with mental illness can recover even though the illness is not "cured". . . . [Recovery] is a way of living a satisfying, hopeful, and contributing life even with the limitations caused by illness.

TREATMENT CAN BE EFFECTIVE

M/SU problems and illnesses occur with a wide array of diagnoses and varied severity. Many people with these conditions require only a short-term intervention to help them cope successfully with a less severe M/SU problem, such as anxiety or distress caused by loss of a loved one, loss of a job, or some other life-changing event; to help them change their unhealthy behaviors, such as heavy drinking or drug experimentation; or to prevent their condition from worsening. People with mental illnesses—such as severe anxiety, depression, posttraumatic stress disorder, or a physiologic dependence on alcohol or some other drug—require treatments of longer duration. Sometimes the illnesses become chronic, as is the case with such diseases as diabetes, asthma, and heart disease. Regardless of the nature of their conditions, what all people with M/SU problems and illnesses have in common is the hope that when they seek help for their condition, they will receive care that enables them either to eliminate it or to manage it successfully so that they can live happy, productive, and satisfying lives—care that enables them to recover.

Research on the interplay among genetic, environmental, biologic, and psychosocial factors in brain function and M/SU illnesses provides the means to accomplish that goal. The results of research to date have revealed our lifelong ability to influence the structure and functioning of our brains through manipulation of environmental and behavioral factors (our brains' "plasticity") and have enabled the development of improved psychotherapies ("talk" therapies), drug therapies, and psychosocial services. Effective mental health interventions range from the use of specific medications (such as clozapine) to treat schizophrenia better in some people (Essock et al., 2000; Rosenheck et al., 1999) to the application of specific models for treating depression in primary care (Pirraglia et al., 2004) and providing supported housing for homeless persons with mental illness (Rosenheck et al., 2003). Those and other mental health interventions have been demonstrated to be cost-effective.

Similarly, advances in understanding the behavioral and social factors that lead to substance use and dependence, in identifying key neuropathways and chemical changes that generate the cravings characteristic of dependence, and in developing means to block these cravings have resulted in a spectrum of evidence-based pharmacologic and psychosocial treatments for people who have problems with or are dependent on substances—treatments that produce results similar to or better than those obtained with treatments for other chronic illnesses (McLellan et al., 2000). New medications, such as buprenorphine, are effective in reducing opioid use (Johnson et al., 2000) and can be prescribed routinely in physicians' offices. Naltrexone and acamprosate show efficacy in treating alcohol dependence (Kranzler and Van Kirk, 2001; O'Malley et al., 2003). The efficacy of nonpharmacologic treatments for drug dependence—such as cognitive behavioral therapy, motivational enhancement treatment, and contingency management—has been demonstrated (Higgins and Petry, 1999). Also effective are 12-step mutual-support groups, such as Alcoholics Anonymous, particularly as an adjunct to treatment and as a form of long-term aftercare (Emrick et al., 1993; Tonigan et al., 2003; Weisner et al., 2003). Brief advice from a physician and office-based counseling interventions can reduce the use of alcohol in problem drinkers (Fleming et al., 1997; Ockene et al., 1999). As a result of these and other advances, patients who remain in treatment for use of alcohol, opioids, or cocaine are less likely to relapse or resume their harmful substance use (Gossop et al., 1999; Miller and Wilbourne, 2002; Miller et al., 2001; Prendergast et al., 2002). Overall, research is increasingly demonstrating that care for M/SU problems and illnesses is both effective (it works) and cost-effective (it is a good value).

QUALITY PROBLEMS HINDER EFFECTIVE TREATMENT AND RECOVERY

As in the case of general health care, despite what is known about effective care for M/SU conditions, numerous studies have documented a discrepancy between M/SU care that is known to be effective and care that is actually delivered. A review of studies published from 1992 through 2000 assessing the quality of care for many different M/SU illnesses (including alcohol withdrawal, bipolar disorder, depression, panic disorder, psychosis, schizophrenia, and substance use) found that only 27 percent of the studies reported adequate rates of adherence to established clinical practice guidelines (Bauer, 2002). Later studies have continued to document departures from evidence-based practice guidelines for illnesses as varied as ADHD (Rushton et al., 2004), anxiety disorders (Stein et al., 2004), comorbid mental and substance-use illnesses (Watkins et al., 2001), depression in adults (Simon et al., 2001) and children (Richardson et al., 2004), opioid dependence (D'Aunno and Pollack, 2002), and schizophrenia (Buchanan et al., 2002). In a landmark study of the quality of a wide variety of health care received by U.S. citizens, people with alcohol dependence were found to receive care consistent with scientific knowledge only about 10.5 percent of the time (McGlynn et al., 2003).

Poor care has serious consequences for the people seeking treatment, especially the most severely ill. One review of the charts of 31 randomly selected patients in a state psychiatric hospital detected 2,194 medication errors during the patients' collective 1,448 inpatient days. Of those errors, 58 percent were judged to have the potential to cause severe harm (Grasso et al., 2003). The use of seclusion and restraints in inpatient mental health facilities is estimated to cause 150 deaths in the United States each year (SAMHSA, 2004b). Moreover, a continuing failure of the health care system in some cases to provide *any* treatment for M/SU illness has been documented (Kessler et al., 2005), even when people are receiving other types of health care and have financial and geographic access to treatment (Jaycox et al., 2003; SAMHSA, 2004a; Watkins et al., 2001). Diagnostic failures and failures to treat can be lethal; M/SU illnesses are leading risk factors for suicide (Maris, 2002).

DEFICIENCIES IN CARE HAVE CONSEQUENCES FOR THE NATION

In addition to the personal consequences of ineffective, unsafe, or no treatment for M/SU illnesses, consequences are felt directly in the workplace; in the education, welfare, and justice systems; and in the nation's economy as a whole. Together, unipolar major depression and drug and alcohol use and dependence are the leading cause of death and disability among American women and the second highest among men (behind heart disease) (Michaud et al., 2001). M/SU problems and illnesses also co-occur with a substantial number of general medical illnesses, such as heart disease and cancer (Katon, 2003; Mertens et al., 2003), and adversely affect the results of treatment for these conditions. About one-fifth of patients hospitalized for a heart attack, for example, suffer from major depression, and evidence from multiple studies makes clear that post–heart attack depression roughly triples one's risk of dying from a future attack or other heart condition (Bush et al., 2005).

Evidence is mounting that M/SU problems and illnesses result in a considerable burden on the workplace and cost to employers owing to absenteeism, "presenteeism" (attending work with symptoms that impair performance), days of disability, and "critical incidents," such as on-the-job accidents (Burton et al., 2004; Goetzel et al., 2002; Kessler et al., 2001).

M/SU problems and illnesses lead to poor educational achievement by children (Green and Goldwyn, 2002; Weinfield et al., 1999; Zeanah et al., 2003), which itself breeds emotional and behavioral problems. Children with poor school achievement are at risk for delinquent and antisocial behavior (Yoshikawa, 1995) and for dropping out of school and rapid, repeated adolescent pregnancies (Linares et al., 1991).

M/SU problems and illnesses also shape the nation's child welfare system. Almost 48 percent of a nationally representative sample of children aged 2–14 who were investigated by child welfare services in 1999–2000 had a clinically significant need for mental health care (Burns et al., 2004). Because of limitations of insurance for mental health care, some families resort to placing their severely mentally ill children in the child welfare system, even though the children are not neglected or abused, to secure mental health services otherwise unavailable (GAO, 2003); parents who take this step must sometimes give up custody of their children (Giliberti and Schulzinger, 2000).

Similarly, children who are not guilty of any offense are often placed in local juvenile justice systems or incarcerated for the same purpose. The U.S. Government Accountability Office counted about 9,000 children who entered state and local juvenile justice systems under those circumstances in 2001 but estimated that the number of such children was likely to be higher (GAO, 2003). The emotional toll on the children is high. Some 48 percent of facilities that hold youths awaiting community mental health services report suicide attempts among them (U.S. House of Representatives, 2004).

The proportion of adult U.S. residents incarcerated has been increasing annually—from a rate of 601 persons in custody per 100,000 U.S. residents in 1995 to 715 per 100,000 in 2003. In the middle of 2003, the nation's prisons and jails held 2,078,570 persons—one in every 140 residents (Harrison and Karberg, 2004). The U.S. Bureau of Justice Statistics estimates that about 16 percent of all persons in jails and prisons report either having a mental disorder or staying overnight in a psychiatric facility (Mumola, 1999). Overall, the costs of providing no or ineffective treatment—as well as the costs of treatment—impose a sizable burden on the nation.

A STRATEGY HAS BEEN DEVELOPED TO
IMPROVE OVERALL HEALTH CARE

The inadequacy of M/SU health care is a dimension of the poor quality of *all* health care. The quality problems of overall health care received substantial attention among the health care community and the public at large as a result of two previous Institute of Medicine (IOM) reports: *To Err Is Human: Building a Safer Health System* (IOM, 2000) and *Crossing the Quality Chasm: A New Health System for the 21st Century* (IOM, 2001). The *Quality Chasm* report also garnered consensus around a framework and strategies for achieving substantial improvements in quality. The framework identifies six aims for high-quality health care (see Box S-1) and 10 rules for redesigning the nation's health care system (see Box S-2).

Crossing the Quality Chasm's framework and recommendations have attracted the attention of many health care leaders, including those addressing health care for mental and substance-use conditions. As a result, the Annie E. Casey Foundation, the CIGNA Foundation, the National Institute on Alcohol Abuse and Alcoholism, the National Institute on Drug Abuse, The Robert Wood Johnson Foundation, the Substance Abuse and Mental Health Services Administration (SAMHSA) in the U.S. Department of

---

BOX S-1 The Six Aims of High-Quality Health Care

Safe—avoiding injuries to patients from the care that is intended to help them.

Effective—providing services based on scientific knowledge to all who could benefit and refraining from providing services to those not likely to benefit (avoiding underuse and overuse, respectively).

Patient-centered—providing care that is respectful of and responsive to individual patient preferences, needs, and values and ensuring that patient values guide all clinical decisions.

Timely—reducing waits and sometimes harmful delays for both those who receive and those who give care.

Efficient—avoiding waste, including waste of equipment, supplies, ideas, and energy.

Equitable—providing care that does not vary in quality because of personal characteristics such as gender, ethnicity, geographic location, and socioeconomic status.

SOURCE: IOM, 2001:5–6.

BOX S-2 The *Quality Chasm's* Ten Rules to Guide the Redesign of Health Care

1. Care based on continuous healing relationships. Patients should receive care whenever they need it and in many forms, not just face-to-face visits. This rule implies that the health care system should be responsive at all times (24 hours a day, every day) and that access to care should be provided over the Internet, by telephone, and by other means in addition to face-to-face visits.

2. Customization based on patient needs and values. The system of care should be designed to meet the most common types of needs but have the capability to respond to individual patient choices and preferences.

3. The patient as the source of control. Patients should be given the necessary information and the opportunity to exercise the degree of control they choose over health care decisions that affect them. The health system should be able to accommodate differences in patient preferences and encourage shared decision making.

4. Shared knowledge and the free flow of information. Patients should have unfettered access to their own medical information and to clinical knowledge. Clinicians and patients should communicate effectively and share information.

5. Evidence-based decision making. Patients should receive care based on the best available scientific knowledge. Care should not vary illogically from clinician to clinician or from place to place.

6. Safety as a system property. Patients should be safe from injury caused by the care system. Reducing risk and ensuring safety require greater attention to systems that help prevent and mitigate errors.

7. The need for transparency. The health care system should make information available to patients and their families that allows them to make informed decisions when selecting a health plan, hospital, or clinical practice, or choosing among alternative treatments. This should include information describing the system's performance on safety, evidence-based practice, and patient satisfaction.

8. Anticipation of needs. The health system should anticipate patient needs, rather than simply reacting to events.

9. Continuous decrease in waste. The health system should not waste resources or patient time.

10. Cooperation among clinicians. Clinicians and institutions should actively collaborate and communicate to ensure an appropriate exchange of information and coordination of care.

SOURCE: IOM, 2001:8.

Health and Human Services, and the Veterans Health Administration of the U.S. Department of Veterans Affairs charged the IOM as follows:

> *Crossing the Quality Chasm: A New Health System for the 21st Century* identified six dimensions in which the United States health system functions at far lower levels than it should (i.e., safety, effectiveness, patient-centeredness, timeliness, efficiency and equity) and concluded that the current health care system is in need of fundamental change. The IOM is to explore the implications of that conclusion for the field of mental health and addictive disorders, and identify the barriers and facilitators to achieving significant improvements along all six of these dimensions. The committee will examine both environmental factors such as payment, benefits coverage and regulatory issues, as well as health care organization and delivery issues. Based on a review of the evidence, the committee will develop an "agenda for change."

To respond to this charge, IOM convened the Committee on Crossing the Quality Chasm: Adaptation to Mental Health and Addictive Disorders. This report presents the committee's analysis of the issues and of how the distinctive features of M/SU health care should be addressed in quality improvement initiatives.

THE *QUALITY CHASM* STRATEGY IS APPLICABLE TO HEALTH CARE FOR MENTAL AND SUBSTANCE-USE CONDITIONS

Despite the quality problems shared with health care generally, M/SU health care is distinctive in significant ways. Those distinctive features include the greater stigma attached to M/SU diagnoses; more frequent coercion of patients into treatment, especially for substance-use problems and conditions; a less developed infrastructure for measuring and improving the quality of care; the need for a greater number of linkages among the multiple clinicians, organizations, and systems providing care to patients with M/SU conditions; less widespread use of information technology; a more educationally diverse workforce; and a differently structured marketplace for the purchase of M/SU health care.

Despite these and other differences, the committee found that M/SU health care and general health care share many characteristics. Moreover, evidence of a link between M/SU illnesses and general health (and health care) is very strong, especially with respect to chronic illnesses and injury (Katon, 2003; Kroenke, 2003). The committee concludes that improving the nation's *general* health and resolving the quality problems of the overall health care system will require attending equally to the quality problems of M/SU health care. Accordingly, the committee offers two overarching recommendations.

Overarching Recommendation 1. Health care for general, mental, and substance-use problems and illnesses must be delivered with an understanding of the inherent interactions between the mind/brain and the rest of the body.

With respect to the quality of M/SU health care, the committee's analysis shows that the recommendations set forth in *Crossing the Quality Chasm* for the redesign of health care are as applicable to M/SU as to general health care. Because of its distinctive features, however, the application of those aims, rules, and redesign strategies to M/SU health care must be specially tailored.

Overarching Recommendation 2. The aims, rules, and strategies for redesign set forth in *Crossing the Quality Chasm* should be applied throughout M/SU health care on a day-to-day operational basis, but tailored to reflect the characteristics that distinguish care for these problems and illnesses from general health care.

To implement this overarching recommendation and achieve success in quality improvement, the committee proposes that the agenda for change embodied in recommendations 3.1 through 9.2 below be undertaken by clinicians; organizations; health plans; purchasers; state, local, and federal governments; and all other parties involved in M/SU health care.

Foremost, consumers of health care for M/SU conditions face a number of obstacles to patient-centered care that generally are not encountered by consumers of general health care. As mentioned above, the shame, stigma, and discrimination still experienced by some consumers of M/SU services can prevent them from seeking care (Peter D. Hart Research Associates Inc., 1998; SAMHSA, 2004a) and inappropriately nourish doubts about their competence to make decisions on their own behalf (Bergeson, 2004; Leibfried, 2004; Markowitz, 1998; Wright et al., 2000). Moreover, insurance coverage for M/SU treatment is more limited than that for general health care, so it is more difficult to obtain and continue the care needed. Finally, more M/SU than general health care patients are coerced into treatment and subject to questions about whether they should be allowed to make decisions about their care. To address those issues, the committee makes two recommendations:[4]

Recommendation 3-1. To promote patient-centered care, all parties involved in health care for mental or substance-use conditions should

---

[4]The committee's recommendations for improving the quality of M/SU health care are numbered according to the chapter of the main report in which they appear; for example, recommendation 3-1 is the first recommendation in Chapter 3.

support the decision-making abilities and preferences for treatment and recovery of persons with M/SU problems and illnesses.

- Clinicians and organizations providing M/SU treatment services should:
    - Incorporate informed, patient-centered decision making throughout their practices, including active patient participation in the design and revision of patient treatment and recovery plans, the use of psychiatric advance directives, and (for children) informed family decision making. To ensure informed decision making, information on the availability and effectiveness of M/SU treatment options should be provided.
    - Adopt recovery-oriented and illness self-management practices that support patient preferences for treatment (including medications), peer support, and other elements of the wellness recovery plan.
    - Maintain effective, formal linkages with community resources to support patient illness self-management and recovery.
- Organizations providing M/SU treatment should also:
    - Have in place policies that implement informed, patient-centered participation and decision making in treatment, illness self-management, and recovery plans.
    - Involve patients and their families in the design, administration, and delivery of treatment and recovery services.
- Accrediting bodies should adopt accreditation standards that require the implementation of these practices.
- Health plans and direct payers of M/SU treatment services should:
    - For persons with chronic mental illnesses or substance-use dependence, pay for peer support and illness self-management programs that meet evidence-based standards.
    - Provide consumers with comparative information on the quality of care provided by practitioners and organizations, and use this information themselves when making their purchasing decisions.
    - Remove barriers to and restrictions on effective and appropriate treatment that may be created by copayments, service exclusions, benefit limits, and other coverage policies.

Recommendation 3-2. Coercion should be avoided whenever possible. When coercion is legally authorized, patient-centered care is still applicable and should be undertaken by:

- Making the policies and practices used for determining dangerousness and decision-making capacity transparent to patients and their caregivers.

- Obtaining the best available comparative information on safety, effectiveness, and availability of care and providers, and using that information to guide treatment decisions.
- Maximizing patient decision making and involvement in the selection of treatments and providers.

The infrastructure needed to measure, analyze, publicly report, and improve the quality of M/SU health care is less well developed than that for general health care. As a result, there has been less measurement and improvement of M/SU health care than of general health care (AHRQ, 2003; Garnick et al., 2002). A related issue is that methods used to disseminate evidence-based practice to providers have not always been evidence-based themselves. To build a stronger infrastructure to support the delivery of high-quality care, the committee recommends a five-part strategy: (1) more coordination in filling gaps in the evidence base; (2) a stronger, more coordinated, and evidence-based approach to disseminating evidence to clinicians; (3) improved diagnosis and assessment strategies; (4) a stronger infrastructure for measuring and reporting the quality of M/SU health care; and (5) support for quality improvement practices at the sites of M/SU health care.

Recommendation 4-1. To better build and disseminate the evidence base, the Department of Health and Human Services (DHHS) should strengthen, coordinate, and consolidate the synthesis and dissemination of evidence on effective M/SU treatments and services by the Substance Abuse and Mental Health Services Administration; the National Institute of Mental Health; the National Institute on Drug Abuse; the National Institute on Alcohol Abuse and Alcoholism; the National Institute of Child Health and Human Development; the Agency for Healthcare Research and Quality; the Department of Justice; the Department of Veterans Affairs; the Department of Defense; the Department of Education; the Centers for Disease Control and Prevention; the Centers for Medicare and Medicaid Services; the Administration for Children, Youth, and Families; states; professional associations; and other private-sector entities.

To implement this recommendation, DHHS should charge or create one or more entities to:

- Describe and categorize available M/SU preventive, diagnostic, and therapeutic interventions (including screening, diagnostic, and symptom-monitoring tools), and develop individual procedure codes and definitions for these interventions and tools for their use in administrative datasets approved under the Health Insurance Portability and Accountability Act.

- Assemble the scientific evidence on the efficacy and effectiveness of these interventions, including their use in varied age and ethnic groups; use a well-established approach to rate the strength of this evidence, and categorize the interventions accordingly; and recommend or endorse guidelines for the use of the evidence-based interventions for specific M/SU problems and illnesses.
- Substantially expand efforts to attain widespread adoption of evidence-based practices through the use of evidence-based approaches to knowledge dissemination and uptake. Dissemination strategies should always include entities that are commonly viewed as knowledge experts by general health care providers and makers of public policy, including the Centers for Disease Control and Prevention, the Agency for Healthcare Research and Quality, the Centers for Medicare and Medicaid Services, the Office of Minority Health, and professional associations and health care organizations.

Recommendation 4-2. Clinicians and organizations providing M/SU services should:

- Increase their use of valid and reliable patient questionnaires or other patient-assessment instruments that are feasible for routine use to assess the progress and outcomes of treatment systematically and reliably.
- Use measures of the processes and outcomes of care to continuously improve the quality of the care provided.

Recommendation 4-3. To measure quality better, DHHS, in partnership with the private sector, should charge and financially support an entity similar to the National Quality Forum to convene government regulators, accrediting organizations, consumer representatives, providers, and purchasers exercising leadership in quality-based purchasing for the purpose of reaching consensus on and implementing a common, continuously improving set of M/SU health care quality measures for providers, organizations, and systems of care. Participants in this consortium should commit to:

- Requiring the reporting and submission of the quality measures to a performance measure repository or repositories.
- Requiring validation of the measures for accuracy and adherence to specifications.
- Ensuring the analysis and display of measurement results in formats understandable by multiple audiences, including consumers,

those reporting the measures, purchasers, and quality oversight organizations.

- Establishing models for the use of the measures for benchmarking and quality improvement purposes at sites of care delivery.
- Performing continuing review of the measures' effectiveness in improving care.

Recommendation 4-4. To increase quality improvement capacity, DHHS, in collaboration with other government agencies, states, philanthropic organizations, and professional associations, should create or charge one or more entities as national or regional resources to test, disseminate knowledge about, and provide technical assistance and leadership on quality improvement practices for M/SU health care in public- and private-sector settings.

Recommendation 4-5. Public and private sponsors of research on M/SU and general health care should include the following in their research funding priorities:

- Development of reliable screening, diagnostic, and monitoring instruments that can validly assess response to treatment and that are practicable for routine use. These instruments should include a set of M/SU "vital signs": a brief set of indicators—measurable at the patient level and suitable for screening and early identification of problems and illnesses and for repeated administration during and following treatment—to monitor symptoms and functional status. The indicators should be accompanied by a specified standardized approach for routine collection and reporting as part of regular health care. Instruments should be age- and culture-appropriate.
- Refinement and improvement of these instruments, procedures for categorizing M/SU interventions, and methods for providing public information on the effectiveness of those interventions.
- Development of strategies to reduce the administrative burden of quality monitoring systems and to increase their effectiveness in improving quality.

In numerous and complex ways, M/SU care is separated both structurally and functionally from other components of the health care system. Not only is M/SU care separated from general health care, but health care services for mental and substance-use conditions are separated from each other despite these conditions' high rate of co-occurrence. In addition, people with severe M/SU illnesses often must receive care from separate public programs. These disconnected care-delivery arrangements require multiple provider "handoffs" of patients for different services and the transmission of information to and joint planning by all these providers, organizations, and agencies if coordination is to occur. The situation is exacerbated by special legal and organizational prohibitions on sharing M/SU information. To address this situation, the committee makes the following recommendations:

Recommendation 5-1. To make collaboration and coordination of patients' M/SU health care services the norm, providers of the services should establish clinically effective linkages within their own organizations and between providers of mental health and substance-use treatment. The necessary communications and interactions should take place with the patient's knowledge and consent and be fostered by:

- Routine sharing of information on patients' problems and pharmacologic and nonpharmacologic treatments among providers of M/SU treatment.
- Valid, age-appropriate screening of patients for comorbid mental, substance-use, and general medical problems in these clinical settings and reliable monitoring of their progress.

Recommendation 5-2. To facilitate the delivery of coordinated care by primary care, mental health, and substance-use treatment providers, government agencies, purchasers, health plans, and accreditation organizations should implement policies and incentives to continually increase collaboration among these providers to achieve evidence-based screening and care of their patients with general, mental, and/or substance-use health conditions. The following specific measures should be undertaken to carry out this recommendation:

- Primary care and specialty M/SU health care providers should transition along a continuum of evidence-based coordination models from (1) formal agreements among mental, substance-use, and primary health care providers; to (2) case management of mental, substance-use, and primary health care; to (3) collocation of mental, substance-use, and primary health care services; and then to (4) delivery of mental, substance-use, and primary health care through clinically integrated practices of primary and M/SU care providers. Organizations should adopt models to which they can most easily transition from their current structure, that best meet the needs of their patient populations, and that ensure accountability.

- DHHS should fund demonstration programs to offer incentives for the transition of multiple primary care and M/SU practices along this continuum of coordination models.
- Purchasers should modify policies and practices that preclude paying for evidence-based screening, treatment, and coordination of M/SU care and require (with patients' knowledge and consent) all health care organizations with which they contract to ensure appropriate sharing of clinical information essential for coordination of care with other providers treating their patients.
- Organizations that accredit mental, substance-use, or primary health care organizations should use accrediting practices that assess, for all providers, the use of evidence-based approaches to coordinating mental, substance-use, and primary health care.
- Federal and state governments should revise laws, regulations, and administrative practices that create inappropriate barriers to the communication of information between providers of health care for mental and substance-use conditions and between those providers and providers of general care.

Recommendation 5-3. To ensure the health of persons for whom they are responsible, M/SU providers should:

- Coordinate their services with those of other human services and education agencies, such as schools, housing and vocational rehabilitation agencies, and providers of services for older adults.
- Establish referral arrangements for needed services.

Providers of services to high-risk populations—such as child welfare agencies, criminal and juvenile justice agencies, and long-term care facilities for older adults—should use valid, age-appropriate, and culturally appropriate techniques to screen all entrants into their systems to detect M/SU problems and illnesses.

Recommendation 5-4. To provide leadership in coordination, DHHS should create a high-level, continuing entity reporting directly to the secretary to improve collaboration and coordination across its mental, substance-use, and general health care agencies, including the Substance Abuse and Mental Health Services Administration; the Agency for Healthcare Research and Quality; the Centers for Disease Control and Prevention; and the Administration for Children, Youth, and Families. DHHS also should implement performance measures to monitor its progress toward achieving internal interagency collaboration and publicly report its performance on these measures annually. State governments should create analogous linkages across state agencies.

Health care providers' ability to obtain information on a patient's health, health care, and potential treatments quickly and to share this information in a timely manner with other providers caring for the patient is essential to effective and coordinated care. To that end, major public- and private-sector collaborations are under way to develop the essential components of a National Health Information Infrastructure (NHII). However, M/SU health care currently is not well addressed by NHII initiatives, nor are NHII initiatives well incorporated into other public-sector information technology efforts for M/SU health care. M/SU health care also lags behind general health care in its use of information technology. To realize the potential of the NHII for consumers of M/SU health care, the committee makes the following recommendations:

Recommendation 6-1. To realize the benefits of the emerging National Health Information Infrastructure (NHII) for consumers of M/SU health care services, the secretaries of DHHS and the Department of Veterans Affairs should charge the Office of the National Coordinator of Health Information Technology and the Substance Abuse and Mental Health Services Administration to jointly develop and implement a plan for ensuring that the various components of the emerging NHII— including data and privacy standards, electronic health records, and community and regional health networks—address M/SU health care as fully as general health care. As part of this strategy:

- **DHHS should create and support a continuing mechanism to engage M/SU health care stakeholders in the public and private sectors in developing consensus-based recommendations for the data elements, standards, and processes needed to address unique aspects of information management related to M/SU health care. These recommendations should be provided to the appropriate standards-setting entities and initiatives working with the Office of the National Coordinator of Health Information Technology.**
- **Federal grants and contracts for the development of components of the NHII should require and use as a criterion for making awards the involvement and inclusion of M/SU health care.**
- **The Substance Abuse and Mental Health Services Administration should increase its work with public and private stakeholders to support the building of information infrastructure components that address M/SU health care and coordinate these information initiatives with the NHII.**
- **Policies and information technology infrastructure should be used to create linkages (consistent with all privacy requirements) among patient records and other data sources pertaining to M/SU ser-**

vices received from health care providers and from education, social, criminal justice, and other agencies.

Recommendation 6-2. Public- and private-sector individuals, including organizational leaders in M/SU health care, should become involved in, and provide for staff involvement in, major national committees and initiatives working to set health care data and information technology standards to ensure that the unique needs of M/SU health care are designed into these initiatives at their earliest stages.

Recommendation 6-3. National associations of purchasers—such as the National Association of State Mental Health Program Directors, the National Association of State Alcohol and Drug Abuse Directors, the National Association of State Medicaid Directors, the National Association of County Behavioral Health Directors, the American Managed Behavioral Healthcare Association, and the national Blue Cross and Blue Shield Association—should decrease the burden of variable reporting and billing requirements by standardizing requirements at the national, state, and local levels.

Recommendation 6-4. Federal and state governments, public- and private-sector purchasers of M/SU health care, and private foundations should encourage the widespread adoption of electronic health records, computer-based clinical decision-support systems, computerized provider order entry, and other forms of information technology for M/SU care by:

- Offering financial incentives to individual M/SU clinicians and organizations for investments in information technology needed to participate fully in the emerging NHII.
- Providing capital and other incentives for the development of virtual networks to give individual and small-group providers standard access to software, clinical and population data and health records, and billing and clinical decision-support systems.
- Providing financial support for continuing technical assistance, training, and information technology maintenance.
- Including in purchasing decisions an assessment of the use of information technology by clinicians and health care organizations for clinical decision support, electronic health records, and other quality improvement applications.

A much greater variety of providers is licensed to diagnose and treat M/SU illnesses than is the case for general medical conditions. Physicians, certain advanced practice nurses, and physician assistants are generally licensed to diagnose and treat general health conditions. By contrast, clinicians licensed to diagnose and treat M/SU conditions include psychologists, psychiatrists, other specialty or primary care physicians, social workers, psychiatric nurses, marriage and family therapists, addiction therapists, and a variety of counselors (such as school counselors, pastoral counselors, guidance counselors, and drug and alcohol counselors). These various types of clinicians are likely to have differing education, training, and therapeutic approaches. As a result, the M/SU workforce is not uniformly equipped with respect to the knowledge and skills needed to provide high-quality services. This situation is compounded by other deficiencies in education that exist across all types of clinicians, as well as long-standing problems in achieving cultural diversity in the workforce and an adequate supply of clinicians for all geographic areas. These problems have persisted despite recurring, short-lived initiatives to address them. The committee recommends a long-term, sustained commitment to developing the M/SU workforce by following a model that provides sustained attention to the nation's physician and nursing workforce.

Recommendation 7-1. To ensure sustained attention to the development of a stronger M/SU health care workforce, Congress should authorize and appropriate funds to create and maintain a Council on the Mental and Substance-Use Health Care Workforce as a public–private partnership. Recognizing that the quality of M/SU services is dependent upon a highly competent professional workforce, the council should develop and implement a comprehensive plan for strengthening the quality and capacity of the workforce to improve the quality of M/SU services substantially by:

- Identifying the specific clinical competencies that all M/SU professionals must possess to be licensed or certified and the competencies that must be maintained over time.
- Developing national standards for the credentialing and licensure of M/SU providers to eliminate differences in the standards now used by the states. Such standards should be based on core competencies and should be included in curriculums and education programs across all the M/SU disciplines.
- Proposing programs to be funded by government and the private sector to address and resolve such long-standing M/SU workforce issues as diversity, cultural relevance, faculty development, and continuing shortages of the well-trained clinicians and consumer providers needed to work with children and the elderly; and programs for training competent clinician administrators.

- Providing a continuing assessment of M/SU workforce trends, issues, and financing policies.
- Measuring the extent to which the plan's objectives have been met and reporting annually to the nation on the status of the M/SU workforce.
- Soliciting technical assistance from public–private partnerships to facilitate the work of the council and the efforts of educational and accreditation bodies to implement its recommendations.

Recommendation 7-2. Licensing boards, accrediting bodies, and purchasers should incorporate the competencies and national standards established by the Council on the Mental and Substance-Use Health Care Workforce in discharging their regulatory and contracting responsibilities.

Recommendation 7-3. The federal government should support the development of M/SU faculty leaders in health professions schools, such as schools of nursing and medicine, and in schools and programs that educate M/SU professionals, such as psychologists and social workers. The aim should be to narrow the gaps among what is known through research, what is taught, and what is done by those who provide M/SU services.

Recommendation 7-4. To facilitate the development and implementation of core competencies across all M/SU disciplines, institutions of higher education should place much greater emphasis on interdisciplinary didactic and experiential learning and should bring together faculty and trainees from their various education programs.

The ease with which several of the above recommendations can be carried out depends on how accommodating the marketplace is to their implementation. The M/SU health care marketplace is distinguished from the general health care marketplace in several ways, including the dominance of government (state and local) purchasers, the frequent purchase of insurance for M/SU health care separately from that for other health care (the use of "carve-out" arrangements), the tendency of the private insurance marketplace to avoid covering or to offer more limited coverage to persons with M/SU illnesses, and government purchasers' greater use of direct provision and purchase of care rather than insurance arrangements. Attending to those differences is essential if the marketplace is to promote quality improvement in M/SU health care. The committee recommends four ways of strengthening the marketplace to that end.

Recommendation 8-1. Health care purchasers that offer enrollees a choice of health plans should evaluate and select one or more available tools for use in reducing selection-related incentives to limit the coverage and quality of M/SU health care. Risk adjustment, payer "carveouts," risk-sharing or mixed-payment contracts, and benefit standardization across the health plans offered can partially address selection-related incentives. Congress and state legislatures should improve coverage by enacting a form of benefit standardization known as parity for coverage of M/SU treatment.

Recommendation 8-2. State government procurement processes should be reoriented so that the greatest weight is given to the quality of care to be provided by vendors.

Recommendation 8-3. Government and private purchasers should use M/SU health care quality measures (including measures of the coordination of health care for mental, substance-use, and general health conditions) in procurement and accountability processes.

Recommendation 8-4. State and local governments should reduce the emphasis on the grant-based systems of financing that currently dominate public M/SU treatment systems and should increase the use of funding mechanisms that link some funds to measures of quality.

Finally, despite how much is known about ways to improve the quality of M/SU health care, knowledge gaps remain. In particular, there has been much less research to identify how to make treatments effective when given in usual settings of care and in the presence of common confounding problems (such as comorbid conditions and social stressors) than research to determine the efficacy of specific treatments under rigorously controlled conditions. In addition, there are many gaps in knowledge about effective treatment, especially for children and adolescents, and there is a paucity of information about the most effective ways to ensure the consistent application of research findings in routine clinical practice. To fill these knowledge gaps, the committee recommends the formulation of a coordinated research agenda for quality improvement in M/SU health care and the use of more-diverse research approaches.

Recommendation 9-1. The secretary of DHHS should provide leadership, strategic development support, and additional funding for research and demonstrations aimed at improving the quality of M/SU health care. This initiative should coordinate the existing quality improvement research efforts of the National Institute of Mental Health, National Institute on Drug Abuse, National Institute on Alcohol Abuse and Alcoholism, Department of Veterans Affairs, Substance Abuse and Mental Health Services Administration, Agency for Healthcare Research and Quality, and Centers for Medicare and Medicaid Services, and it should develop and fund cross-agency efforts in necessary new research. To that end, the initiative should address the full range of research needed to reduce gaps in knowledge at the clinical, services, systems, and policy levels and should establish links to and encourage expanded efforts by foundations, states, and other nonfederal organizations.

Recommendation 9-2. Federal and state agencies and private foundations should create health services research strategies and innovative approaches that address treatment effectiveness and quality improvement in usual settings of care delivery. To that end, they should develop new research and demonstration funding models that encourage local innovation, that include research designs in addition to randomized controlled trials, that are committed to partnerships between researchers and stakeholders, and that create a critical mass of interdisciplinary research partnerships involving usual settings of care. Stakeholders should include consumers/patients, parents or guardians of children, clinicians and clinical teams, organization managers, purchasers, and policy makers.

REFERENCES

AHRQ (Agency for Healthcare Research and Quality). 2003. *National Healthcare Quality Report*. Rockville, MD: U.S. Department of Health and Human Services.

Anthony WA. 1993. Recovery from mental illness: The guiding vision of the mental health service system in the 1990s. *Psychological Rehabilitation Journal* 16(4):11–24.

Bauer MS. 2002. A review of quantitative studies of adherence to mental health clinical practice guidelines. *Harvard Review of Psychiatry* 10(3):138–153.

Bergeson S. 2004. Testimony before the Institute of Medicine Workshop on Crossing the Quality Chasm: An Adaptation to Mental Health and Addictive Disorders. Washington, DC, July 14. Available from Institute of Medicine.

Buchanan RW, Kreyenbuhl J, Zito JM, Lehman A. 2002. The schizophrenia PORT pharmacological treatment recommendations: Conformance and implications for symptoms and functional outcome. *Schizophrenia Bulletin* 28(1):63–73.

Burns BJ, Phillips SD, Wagner R, Barth RP, Kolko DJ, Campbel Y, Landsverk J. 2004. Mental health need and access to mental health services by youths involved with child welfare: A national survey. *Journal of the American Academy of Child and Adolescent Psychiatry* 43(8):960–970.

Burton WN, Pransky G, Conti DJ, Chen C-Y, Edington DW. 2004. The association of medical conditions and presenteeism. *Journal of Occupational and Environmental Medicine* 46(6), Supplement:S38–S45.

Bush DE, Ziegeldtein RC, Patel UV, Tghombs BD, Ford DE, Fauerbach JA, McCann UD, Stewart KJ, Tsilidis KK, Patel AL, Feuerstein CJ, Bass EB. 2005. *Post-Myocardial Infarction Depression. Summary.* AHRQ Publication Number 05-E018-1. Evidence Report/Technology Assessment Number 123. Rockville, MD: Agency for Healthcare Research and Quality.

D'Aunno T, Pollack HA. 2002. Changes in methadone treatment practices: Results from a national panel study, 1988–2000. *Journal of the American Medical Association* 288(7): 850–856.

DHHS (Department of Health and Human Services). 1999. *Mental Health: A Report of the Surgeon General.* Rockville, MD: DHHS.

Emrick CD, Tonigan JS, Montgomery H, Little L. 1993. Alcoholics Anonymous: What is currently known? In: McCrady BS, Miller WR, eds. *Research on Alcoholics Anonymous: Opportunities and Alternatives.* New Brunswick, NJ: Rutgers Center of Alcohol Studies. Pp. 41–78.

Essock SM, Frisman LK, Covell NH, Hargreaves WA. 2000. Cost-effectiveness of clozapine compared with conventional antipsychotic medication for patients in state hospitals. *Archives of General Psychiatry* 57(10):987–994.

Fleming M, Barry K, Manwell L, Johnson K, London R. 1997. Brief physician advice for problem alcohol drinkers: A randomized controlled trial in community-based primary care practices. *Journal of the American Medical Association* 277(13):1039–1045.

GAO (General Accounting Office). 2003. *Child Welfare and Juvenile Justice: Federal Agencies Could Play a Stronger Role in Helping States Reduce the Number of Children Placed Solely to Obtain Mental Health Services.* GAO-03-397. [Online]. Available: http://www.gao.gov/new.items/d03397.pdf [accessed October 25, 2004].

Garnick DW, Lee MT, Chalk M, Gastfriend D, Horgan CM, McCorry F, McLellan AT, Merrick EL. 2002. Establishing the feasibility of performance measures for alcohol and other drugs. *Journal of Substance Abuse Treatment* 23(4):375–385.

Giliberti M, Schulzinger R. 2000. *Relinquishing Custody: The Tragic Result of Failure to Meet Children's Mental Health Needs.* Washington, DC: Bazelon Center for Mental Health Law.

Goetzel RZ, Ozminkowski RJ, Sederer LI, Mark TL. 2002. The business case for quality mental health services: Why employers should care about the mental health and well-being of their employees. *Journal of Occupational and Environmental Medicine* 44(4): 320–330.

Gossop M, Marsden J, Stewart D, Rolfe A. 1999. Treatment retention and one year outcomes for residential programmes in England. *Drug and Alcohol Dependence* 57(2):89–98.

Grasso BC, Genest R, Jordan CW, Bates DW. 2003. Use of chart and record reviews to detect medication errors in a state psychiatric hospital. *Psychiatric Services* 54(5): 677–681.

Green J, Goldwyn R. 2002. Annotation: attachment disorganization and psychopathology: New findings in attachment research and their potential implications for developmental psychopathology in childhood. *Journal of Child Psychology and Psychiatry* 43(7): 835–846.

Harrison PM, Karberg JC. 2004. *Prison and Jail Inmates at Midyear 2003.* Bureau of Justice Statistics Bulletin. Office of Justice Programs, U.S. Department of Justice (NCJ 203947). [Online]. Available: http://www.ojp.usdoj.gov/bjs/pub/pdf/pjim03.pdf [accessed August 4, 2004].

Higgins S, Petry N. 1999. Contingency management: Incentives for sobriety. *Alcohol Research Health* 23(2):122–127.

IOM (Institute of Medicine). 2000. *To Err Is Human: Building a Safer Health System.* Washington, DC: National Academy Press.

IOM. 2001. *Crossing the Quality Chasm: A New Health System for the 21st Century*. Washington, DC: National Academy Press.

Jaycox LH, Morral AR, Juvonen J. 2003. Mental health and medical problems and service use among adolescent substance users. *Journal of the American Academy of Child & Adolescent Psychiatry* 42(6):701–709.

Johnson R, Chatuape M, Strain E, Walsh S, Stitzer M, Bigelow G. 2000. A comparison of levomethadyl acetate, buprenorphine, and methadone for opioid dependence. *New England Journal of Medicine* 343(18):1290–1297.

Katon W. 2003. Clinical and health services relationships between major depression, depressive symptoms, and general medical illness. *Biological Psychiatry* 54(3):216–226.

Kessler RC, Greenberg PE, Mickelson KD, Meneades LM, Wang PS. 2001. The effects of chronic medical conditions on work loss and work cutback. *Journal of Occupational and Environmental Medicine* 43:218–225.

Kessler RC, Demler O, Frank RG, Olfson M, Pincus HA, Walters EE, Wang P, Wells KB, Zaslavsky AM. 2005. Prevalence and treatment of mental disorders, 1990 to 2003. *The New England Journal of Medicine* 352(24):2515–2523.

Kranzler H, Van Kirk J. 2001. Efficacy of naltrexone and acamprosate for alcoholism treatment: A meta-analysis. *Alcoholism: Clinical and Experimental Research* 25(9):1335–1341.

Kroenke K. 2003. Patients presenting with somatic complaints: Epidemiology, psychiatric comorbidity and management. *International Journal of Methods in Psychiatric Research* 12(1):34–43.

Leibfried T. 2004. Testimony before the Institute of Medicine Committee on Crossing the Quality Chasm: Adaptation to Mental Health and Addictive Disorders. Washington, DC, July 14. Available from the Institute of Medicine.

Linares LO, Leadbetter BJ, Kato PM, Jaffe L. 1991. Predicting school outcomes for minority group adolescent mothers: Can subgroups be identified? *Journal of Research on Adolescence* 1(4):379–400.

Maris RW. 2002. Suicide. *The Lancet* 360(9329):319–326.

Markowitz FE. 1998. The effects of stigma on the psychological well-being and life satisfaction of persons with mental illness. *Journal of Health and Social Behavior* 39(4):335–347.

McGlynn EA, Asch SM, Adams J, Keesey J, Hicks J, DeCristofaro A, Kerr EA. 2003. The quality of health care delivered to adults in the United States. *New England Journal of Medicine* 348(26):2635–2645.

McLellan AT, Lewis DC, O'Brien CP, Kleber HD. 2000. Drug dependence, a chronic medical illness: Implications for treatment, insurance, and outcomes evaluation. *Journal of the American Medical Association* 284(13): 1689–1695.

Mechanic D, Bilder S. 2004. Treatment of people with mental illness: A decade-long perspective. *Health Affairs* 23(4):84–95.

Mertens JR, Lu YW, Parthasarathy S, Moore C, Weisner CM. 2003. Medical and psychiatric conditions of alcohol and drug treatment patients in an HMO: Comparison with matched controls. *Archives of Internal Medicine* 163(20):2511–2517.

Michaud CM, Murray CJL, Bloom BR. 2001. Burden of disease: Implications for future research. *Journal of the American Medical Association* 285(5):535–539.

Miller WR, Wilbourne P. 2002. Mesa Grande: A methodological analysis of clinical trials of treatments for alcohol use disorders. *Addiction* 97(3):265–277.

Miller WR, Walters ST, Bennett ME. 2001. How effective is alcoholism treatment? *Journal of Studies on Alcohol* 62:211–220.

Mumola CJ. 1999. *Substance Abuse and Treatment, State and Federal Prisoners, 1997*. NCJ 172871. Washington, DC: Bureau of Justice Statistics, Department of Justice.

Ockene J, Adams A, Hurley T, Wheler E, Hebert J. 1999. Brief physician- and nurse practitioner-delivered counseling for high-risk drinkers: Does it work? *Archives of Internal Medicine* 159(18):2198–2205.

O'Malley S, Rounsaville B, Farren C, Namkoong K, Wu R, Robinson J, O'Connor P. 2003. Initial and maintenance naltrexone treatment for alcohol dependence using primary care vs. specialty care: A nested sequence of three randomized trials. *Archives of Internal Medicine* 163(14):1695–1704.

Peter D. Hart Research Associates Inc. 1998. *The Road to Recovery: A Landmark National Study on Public Perceptions of Alcoholism and Barriers to Treatment.* Washington DC: Peter D. Hart Research Associates Inc. and The Recovery Institute.

Pirraglia PA, Rosen AB, Hermann RC, Olchanski NV, Neumann P. 2004. Cross-utility analysis studies of depression management: A systematic review. *American Journal of Psychiatry* 161(12):2155–2162.

Prendergast M, Podus D, Chang E, Urada D. 2002. The effectiveness of drug abuse treatment: A meta-analysis of comparison group studies. *Drug and Alcohol Dependence* 67(1): 53–72.

Richardson LP, Di Giuseppe D, Christakis DA, McCauley E, Katon W. 2004. Quality of care for Medicaid-covered youth treated with antidepressant therapy. *Archives of General Psychiatry* 61(5):475–480.

Rosenheck R, Cramer J, Allen E, Erdos J, Frisman LK, Xu W, Thomas J, Henderson W, Charney D. 1999. Cost-effectiveness of clozapine in patients with high and low levels of hospital use. Department of Veterans Affairs Cooperative Study Group on Clozapine in Refractory Schizophrenia. *Archives of General Psychiatry* 56(6):565–572.

Rosenheck R, Kasprow W, Frisman L, Liu-Mares W. 2003. Cost-effectiveness of supported housing for homeless persons with mental illness. *Archives of General Psychiatry* 60(9): 940–951.

Rushton JL, Fant K, Clark SJ. 2004. Use of practice guidelines in the primary care of children with Attention-Deficit Hyperactivity Disorder. *Pediatrics* 114(1):e23–e28. [Online]. Available: http://www.pediatrics.aappublications.org.cgi/reprint/114/1/e23 [accessed September 1, 2005].

SAMHSA (Substance Abuse and Mental Health Services Administration). 2004a. *Results from the 2003 National Survey on Drug Use and Health: National Findings.* DHHS Publication Number SMA 04-3964. NSDUH Series H-25. Rockville, MD: SAMHSA.

SAMHSA. 2004b. *SAMHSA Action Plan: Seclusion and Restraint—Fiscal Years 2004 and 2005.* [Online]. Available: http://www.samhsa.gov/Matrix/SAP_seclusion.aspx [accessed February 20, 2005].

Simon GE, Von Korff M, Rutter CM, Peterson DA. 2001. Treatment processes and outcomes for managed care patients receiving new antidepressant prescriptions from psychiatrists and primary care physicians. *Archives of General Psychiatry* 58(4):395–401.

Simpson GA, Scott G, Henderson MJ, Manderscheid RW. 2004. Estimates of attention, cognitive, and emotional problems, and health services use by U.S. school-age children. In: Manderscheid RW, Henderson MJ, eds. *Mental Health, United States, 2002.* DHHS Publication number: (SMA) 3938. Rockville, MD: Substance Abuse and Mental Health Services Administration. Pp. 105–119.

Stein MB, Sherbourne CD, Craske MG, Means-Christensen A, Bystritsky A, Katon W, Sullivan G, Roy-Byrne PP. 2004. Quality of care for primary care patients with anxiety disorders. *American Journal of Psychiatry* 161(12):2230–2237.

Tonigan JS, Connors GJ, Miller WR. 2003. Participation and involvement in Alcoholics Anonymous. In: Babor TF, Del Boca FK, eds. *Treatment Matching in Alcoholism.* Cambridge, UK, and New York: Cambridge University Press. pp 184–204.

U.S. House of Representatives. 2004. *Incarceration of Youth Who Are Waiting for Community Mental Health Services in the United States.* Committee on Government Reform, Minority staff. Special Investigations Division. [Online]. Available: http://www.house.gov/reform/min/pdfs_108_2/pdfs_inves/pdf_health_mental_health_youth_incarceration_july_2004_rep.pdf [accessed September 1, 2005].

Watkins KE, Burnam A, Kung F-Y, Paddock S. 2001. A national survey of care for persons with co-occurring mental and substance use disorders. *Psychiatric Services* 52(8):1062–1068.

Weinfield N, Stroufe LA, Egeland B, Carlson EA. 1999. The nature of individual differences in infant -caregiver attachment. In: Cassidy J, Shaver PR, eds. *Handbook of Attachment.* New York, NY: Guilford Press.

Weisner C, Ray GT, Mertens J, Satre D, Moore C. 2003. Short-term alcohol and drug treatment outcomes predict long-term outcome. *Drug and Alcohol Dependence* 71(3): 281–294.

Wright ER, Gronfein WP, Owens TJ. 2000. Deinstitutionalization, social rejection, and the self-esteem of former mental patients. *Journal of Health and Social Behavior* 41(1): 68–90.

Wu L-T, Ringwalt CL, Williams CE. 2003. Use of substance abuse treatment services by persons with mental health and substance use problems. *Psychiatric Services* 54(3):363–369.

Yoshikawa H. 1995. Long-term effects of early childhood programs on social outcomes and delinquency. *The Future of Children* 5(3):51–75.

Zeanah CH, Keyes A, Settles L. 2003. Attachment relationship experiences and childhood psychopathology. *Annals of the New York Academy of Sciences* 1008:22–30.

1

The *Quality Chasm* in Health Care for Mental and Substance-Use[1] Conditions

Summary

Each year more than 33 million Americans use mental health services or services to treat their problems and illnesses resulting from alcohol, inappropriate use of prescription medications, or illegal drugs. Together, mental and substance-use illnesses are the leading cause of combined death and disability for women of all ages and for men aged 15–44, and the second highest for all men. When appropriately treated, individuals with these conditions can recover and lead satisfying and productive lives. Conversely, when treatment is not provided or is of poor quality, these conditions can have serious consequences for individuals, their loved ones, their workplaces, and the nation as a whole.

---

[1]In this report, whenever possible, we use the phrasing "substance-use problems and illnesses" rather than the terms "addiction" or substance "abuse." We do not use the term "addiction" because some consider it pejorative; because it is not a formal diagnostic term; and because many of the conditions, problems, and policies discussed in this report pertain to people with much less severe alcohol and other drug-use conditions. We chose not to use the term substance "abuse," both because it is diagnostically imprecise in the context of this report and because outside of strict diagnostic nomenclature, it too can be considered pejorative. We instead use the phrases "substance-use *illnesses*" when discussing the diagnostic family of alcohol and other drug-use illnesses and "substance-use *problems*" when discussing the problems associated with the unhealthy use of alcohol and other drugs. Nonetheless, these words appear in some places in the report because they are used so often in the literature, and it is not always possible to interpret the meaning of the word "abuse."

Although science continues to advance our knowledge about the etiology of mental and substance-use problems and illnesses and how to treat them effectively, health care for these conditions— like general health care—frequently is not delivered in ways that are consistent with science, ways that enable improvement and recovery. Moreover, care is sometimes unsafe; more often, it is not delivered at all. This gap between what can and should be and what exists is so large that, as with general health care, it constitutes a "chasm" as defined in the 2001 Institute of Medicine report, Crossing the Quality Chasm: A New Health System for the 21st Century. *Using that report as its template, this report puts forth an agenda for improving the quality of health care for mental and substance-use conditions.*

MORE THAN 33 MILLION AMERICANS ANNUALLY RECEIVE CARE

Each year more than 33 million Americans use mental health services or services to treat their problems and illnesses[2] resulting from alcohol, inappropriate use of prescription medications, or illegal drugs. Approximately 28 million Americans aged 18 or older (13 percent of this population) received mental health treatment in an inpatient or outpatient setting in 2003[3] (SAMHSA, 2004a), and more than 6 percent of American children and adolescents aged 5–17 had contact with a mental health professional in a 2-month period according to the 1998–1999 National Health Interview Survey (Simpson et al., 2004). The rates are higher still for adolescents: 20.6 percent of those aged 12–17 (5 million youths) received treatment or counseling for emotional or behavioral problems in 2003 (SAMHSA, 2004a); in addition, more than 3 million Americans aged 12 or older (1.4 percent of this group) reported receiving some kind of treatment during 2003 for a problem related to alcohol or other drug use (SAMHSA,

---

[2]Whenever possible, this report uses the words "problems" and "illnesses" (as opposed to "disorders") because "disorder," as defined in the American Psychiatric Association's *Diagnostic and Statistical Manual of Mental Disorders* (DSM-IV-TR), refers to "a *clinically significant* behavioral or psychological syndrome or pattern that occurs in an individual and that is associated with present distress (e.g., a painful symptom) or disability (i.e., impairment in one or more important areas of functioning) or with a significantly increased risk of suffering death, pain, disability, or an important loss of freedom" (emphasis added) (American Psychiatric Association, 2000:xxxi). The committee's use of the word "problem" acknowledges that not everyone with a need for mental health care has such significant impairment that it qualifies as a "disorder." Nonetheless, the word "disorder" appears often in this report because it is used so frequently in the literature.

[3]This figure does not include treatment solely for substance use.

2004a). Combining mental and substance-use problems and illnesses, more than 20 percent of U.S. adults aged 18–54 received care for these conditions during a 12-month period between 2001 and 2003 (Kessler et al., 2005). Millions more reported that they needed treatment for their mental and/or substance-use (M/SU)[4] problems or illnesses but did not receive it (Mechanic and Bilder, 2004; SAMHSA, 2004a; Wu et al., 2003). Fewer than half of adults aged 18–54 who met a definition of severe mental illness received treatment for the condition during a 12-month period between 2001 and 2003 (Kessler et al., 2005). And in contrast to the more than 3 million Americans aged 12 or older who received treatment during 2003 for a problem related to alcohol or other drug use, more than six times that number (approximately 21.6 million, or 9.1 percent of this age group) reported abusing or being physiologically dependent upon alcohol; illicit drugs such as marijuana, cocaine, heroin, hallucinogens, or stimulants; prescription drugs used for nonmedical purposes; or a combination of these (SAMHSA, 2004a).

Many individuals using services to address their mental or substance-use problems require only a short-term intervention to address their condition (Bernstein et al., 2005; Fleming et al., 1997; Ockene et al., 1999). They may be experiencing, for example, anxiety or other distress over the loss of a loved one or a job or some other life-changing event. They may be engaging in occasional heavy drinking or be teenagers experimenting with drugs. These and other less severe problems that many individuals encounter at some point in their lives are not considered mental illnesses or drug dependence but are occasions during which an individual might need assistance to cope with a stressful situation, change unhealthy behaviors, and prevent the condition from worsening. Mental illnesses and substance dependence, in contrast, involve significantly more distress, disability, chronicity, and physical risk and interfere with performing routine activities such as working, attending school, or participating fully in relationships.

Individuals with M/SU problems and illnesses represent a wide range of diagnoses, severity of illness, and disability. What they all have in common, however, is the hope that when they seek help for their condition, they will receive care that is safe, effective, and of good overall quality. They expect that such care will enable them either to recover completely from an acute mental or substance-use illness or manage the illness successfully so they can live happy, productive, and satisfying lives. As articulated in the 1999 Surgeon General's report on mental health (Anthony, 1993 as cited in DHHS, 1999:98):

---

[4]Throughout this report we use the acronym M/SU to refer to "mental and/or substance use."

... a person with mental illness can recover even though the illness is not "cured".... [Recovery] is a way of living a satisfying, hopeful, and contributing life even with the limitations caused by illness.

Although a conceptual model of recovery from chronic M/SU illnesses is not yet fully developed (Onken et al., 2004), recovery as articulated in the Surgeon General's report has been an accepted concept in use for over a century for individuals with alcohol-use problems and illnesses (White, 1998). More recently, recovery has become a widely accepted goal not just of mental health care (NAMI, 2005; New Freedom Commission on Mental Health, 2003), but of treatment for all individuals with M/SU problems and illnesses.

CONTINUING ADVANCES IN CARE AND TREATMENT ENABLE RECOVERY

The U.S. Surgeon General, the National Institutes of Health (NIH), the Substance Abuse and Mental Health Services Administration (SAMHSA), the Institute of Medicine (IOM), and many others (DHHS, 1999; IOM, 1997) continue to document ongoing advances in our understanding of M/SU problems and illnesses. These advances include the development of efficacious psychotherapies, drug therapies, and psychosocial services, as well as strategies for delivering these treatments effectively. Dissemination of information on brain functioning—the interplay of genetic, environmental, biological, and psychosocial factors in brain function and M/SU illnesses; our ability throughout our lives to influence the structure and functioning of our brains through environmental and behavioral factors (our brains' "plasticity"); and improved treatments—has helped educate consumers,[5] the health care community, and the public at large about M/SU problems and illnesses and the effectiveness of care for these conditions. Now that NIH has made translation of bench science to clinical applications a high priority in its strategic plans for the coming years (NIMH, 2005; Zerhouni, 2003), society is poised to reap even greater returns from developments in such basic science fields as genetics, proteomics, neuro-

---

[5]The committee notes that many different words are used to refer to individuals who are in need of or receive M/SU health care, including "patient," "client," "consumer," "survivor," "recipient," "beneficiary," and others. The committee respects the different perspectives represented by proponents of each of these terms. For convenience, we use the terms "patients," "consumers," and "clients" interchangeably in this report because of their widespread use by the public at large and within general and specialty health care systems. The use of these words is not intended to exclude the families of adults who, with the consent of the individual patient, can play an essential therapeutic role. With respect to children and adolescents, we always intend these words to include families and other informal caregivers.

imaging, and animal models of behavior (Gould and Manji, 2004; Sarver et al., 2002; Tecott, 2003).

The past decade also has seen rapid growth in the science of evaluating the costs and effectiveness of health interventions. These approaches increasingly demonstrate that care for many M/SU problems and illnesses can be both effective (i.e., it can work) and cost-effective (i.e., it can represent a good value). Recent studies have used these approaches to evaluate a variety of mental health interventions, ranging from use of a specific medication (clozapine) in populations with schizophrenia (Essock et al., 2000; Rosenheck et al., 1999), to using specific models for treating depression in primary care (Pirraglia et al., 2004), to providing supported housing for homeless persons with mental illness (Rosenheck et al., 2003). These and other mental health interventions have been found to be as or more cost-effective than many treatments currently provided in general medical practice. Consistent with these findings, more than half of adults who received treatment for mental health problems in 2003 reported that their treatment improved their ability to manage daily activities "a great deal" or "a lot" (SAMHSA, 2004a).

A large body of research shows likewise that treatment for alcohol and other drug problems and illnesses is effective. Many people who enter treatment decrease their substance use and have fewer problems (Finney and Moos, 1991; McLellan et al., 2000; Miller et al., 2001). Recent years have seen many scientific advances in understanding the behavioral and social factors that lead to substance use and dependence, in identifying key neuropathways and chemical changes that create the cravings characteristic of alcohol or drug dependence, and in developing mechanisms to block these effects. These advances have resulted in a spectrum of evidence-based pharmacological and psychosocial treatments for individuals who misuse or are dependent on substances—treatments that produce results similar to or better than those obtained with treatments for other chronic illnesses (McLellan et al., 2000). New medications, such as buprenorphine, are effective in significantly reducing opioid use (Johnson et al., 2000). In contrast to the first medication for opiate dependence (methadone), buprenorphine can be prescribed routinely in physicians' offices. Naltrexone and acamprosate also show efficacy in treating alcohol dependence (Kranzler and Van Kirk, 2001; O'Malley et al., 2003) and may be more acceptable to patients than disulfiram, the first medication approved for treating that condition.[6]

Nonpharmacological treatments for drug dependence, such as cognitive behavioral therapy and motivational enhancement treatment, have also

---

[6]Disulfiram produces a very uncomfortable physiological reaction in the individual when alcohol is consumed, and does not reduce craving.

demonstrated efficacy. Twelve-step mutual support groups such as Alcoholics Anonymous are effective as well, particularly as an adjunct to treatment and as a form of long-term aftercare (Emrick et al., 1993; Tonigan et al., 2003; Weisner et al., 2003). Contingency management, a treatment modality that employs positive reinforcement for desired behaviors and withholding of reinforcement or punitive measures for undesired behaviors has shown efficacy for treatment of the use of alcohol, cocaine, and other psychostimulants (Higgins and Petry, 1999). Brief advice from a physician and office-based alcohol counseling interventions have been shown to reduce episodes of binge drinking as well as alcohol use in problem drinkers (Fleming et al., 1997; Ockene et al., 1999). Organizing care to address co-occurring conditions, such as by integrating alcohol and drug treatment with medical services (Weisner et al., 2001) and combining substance-use and mental health services, also optimizes outcomes (Moggi et al., 1999), as well as cost (Parthasarathy et al., 2003). The latter approach is particularly effective for adolescents, in whom co-occurring substance-use and mental health problems are very common (Clark et al., 1997; Sterling and Weisner, 2005). As a result of these advances, patients who enter and remain in treatment for use of alcohol, opioids, or cocaine are less likely to relapse or resume use (Gossop et al., 1999; Miller and Wilbourne, 2002; Prendergast et al., 2002).

Additional good news is found in recent studies showing some improvements in access to and receipt of care. Over the past decade, although the prevalence of M/SU problems and illnesses has remained the same, a greater proportion of adults aged 18–54 with these conditions has received treatment (Kessler et al., 2005). This has been especially true of those with the most severe mental illnesses (Kessler et al., 2005; Mechanic and Bilder, 2004). The rate of treatment for depression appears to have more than tripled between 1987 and 1997 (Olfson et al., 2002), and improvements have been seen in access to care and treatment for children (Glied and Cuellar, 2003).

On the other hand, the same reports showing improved access to care for people with the most severe mental illnesses show declining access for those with less severe mental illnesses (Mechanic and Bilder, 2004) and ethnic minorities (Kessler et al., 2005), and many people who need treatment for M/SU illnesses still do not receive it (Kessler et al., 2005; Mechanic and Bilder, 2004; SAMHSA, 2004a). Moreover, M/SU health care, like general health care, is frequently delivered in ways that are not consistent with scientific evidence. Sometimes care also is unsafe. When untreated or poorly treated, M/SU problems and illnesses can have serious consequences for the afflicted individuals, their loved ones, and society as a whole.

POOR CARE HINDERS IMPROVEMENT
AND RECOVERY FOR MANY

Numerous studies document the discrepancy between the M/SU care that is known to be effective and the care that is actually delivered. A review of all peer-reviewed studies published from 1992 through 2000 assessing the quality of care for many different M/SU clinical conditions (including alcohol withdrawal, bipolar illness, depression, panic disorder, psychosis, schizophrenia, and substance abuse) found that only 27 percent of the studies reported adequate rates of adherence to established clinical practice guidelines (Bauer, 2002). Subsequent studies have continued to document clinicians' departures from evidence-based practice guidelines for conditions as varied as attention deficit hyperactivity disorder (ADHD) (Rushton et al., 2004), anxiety disorders (Stein et al., 2004), comorbid mental and substance-use illnesses (Watkins et al., 2001), depression in adults (Simon et al., 2001a) and children (Richardson et al., 2004), opioid dependence (D'Aunno and Pollack, 2002), and schizophrenia (Buchanan et al., 2002). In a landmark study of the quality of a wide variety of health care received by U.S. citizens, individuals with alcohol dependence were found to receive care consistent with scientific knowledge only about 10.5 percent of the time (McGlynn et al., 2003).

In other clinical care situations, the absence of clinical practice guidelines further contributes to worrisome variation in the care individuals receive. One 1999–2000 study of the care received by children and adolescents at residential treatment centers in four states found that 42.9 percent were receiving antipsychotic medications without having any history of or current psychosis and were thus receiving such medications for "off-label" purposes (Rawal et al., 2004). Seclusion and restraints continue to be used in inpatient mental health facilities despite their resulting in substantial psychological and physical harm to patients (GAO, 1999), including an estimated 150 deaths in the United States annually (SAMHSA, 2004b), and despite a Cochrane Collaboration finding that "few other forms of treatment which are applied to patients with various psychiatric diagnoses are so lacking in basic information about their proper use and efficacy" (Sailas and Fenton, 2005).

Moreover, recent studies reaffirm that the health care system sometimes fails to provide *any* treatment for M/SU illnesses (Kessler et al., 2005; Mechanic and Bilder, 2004), even when afflicted individuals are receiving other types of health care and have financial and geographic access to care. A 1997–1998 national survey found that among persons with probable co-occurring M/SU conditions who received treatment for one condition, fewer than a third (28.6 percent) received treatment for the other (Watkins et al.,

2001). A later longitudinal study of 1,088 youths in residential or outpatient treatment for drug use showed that although 67 percent reported having severe mental health problems upon admission, only 24 percent reported receiving mental health services within the 3 months following their admission (Jaycox et al., 2003). The 2003 National Survey on Drug Use and Health documents similar failure to treat adults (SAMHSA, 2004a). And despite the very frequent co-occurrence of M/SU and general health care problems and illnesses, coordination among providers of M/SU care and the other sectors of care delivery is highly inadequate (New Freedom Commission on Mental Health, 2003).

Departures from known standards of care, variations in care in the absence of care standards, failure to treat M/SU problems and illnesses, and lack of coordination are of concern for many reasons. While they may often represent ineffective care, there is evidence that they can also threaten patient safety. In addition to the substantial psychological and physical harm to patients caused by the use of seclusion and restraints noted above, injuries from drug errors are common. A retrospective, multidisciplinary review of the charts of 31 randomly selected patients in a state psychiatric hospital discharged during a 4$1/2$-month study period detected 2,194 medication errors during these patients' collective 1,448 inpatient days.[7] Of these errors, 19 percent were rated as having the potential to cause minor harm, 23 percent the potential to cause moderate harm, and 58 percent the potential to cause severe harm (Grasso et al., 2003). Moreover, because M/SU illnesses are leading risk factors for suicide (Maris, 2002), failures to diagnose and treat them effectively can be lethal.

The receipt of ineffective and unsafe care by large numbers of people with M/SU illnesses is of particular concern because some of the unique features of these illnesses—such as the symptoms of major depression or schizophrenia—and their treatments could render patients less able to detect and avoid errors and more vulnerable to the consequences of errors that occur. The residual stigma attached to some M/SU illnesses also may make individuals with these diagnoses less willing to report errors and adverse events, and less likely to be believed when they do so. Most significant, the delivery of ineffective or unsafe care, or the failure to deliver any care, has serious consequences for individuals, their loved ones, and the nation as a whole.

---

[7]These medication error rates are consistent with rates reported in studies involving general medical hospitals, but the distribution of the types of errors is markedly different: a much higher proportion of the errors (66 percent) occurred during the administration of a medication as opposed to its prescription, transcription, or dispensing. The authors note that at the time the study was conducted, medication administration was performed by medical technicians, as opposed to licensed nurses—a practice discontinued after the study (Grasso et al., 2003).

FAILURE TO PROVIDE EFFECTIVE CARE HAS SERIOUS PERSONAL AND SOCIETAL CONSEQUENCES

A Leading Cause of Disability and Death in the United States

A 1996 study of the global burden of diseases, injuries, and risk factors conducted by the World Health Organization and the World Bank assessed for the first time the relative burden of 107 of the world's most common diseases as of 1990. Using the metric of disability-adjusted life years (DALYs), representing the combined effect of years of life lost to premature death and years of life lived with a disability, the study assessed fatal and nonfatal health outcomes and objectively calculated the relative burden of major diseases and injuries. The results documented for the first time the profound effect of M/SU illnesses on death and disability worldwide and in the United States. In developed regions of the world, unipolar major depression was the second leading cause of death and disability (next to heart disease) for all ages,[8] and the leading cause for individuals aged 15–44. Alcohol use ranked highest for males aged 15–44 and fifth across all ages. Alcohol use also was an underlying factor in a substantial portion of traffic accidents (which were ranked fourth for all ages and sexes and second only to alcohol for males aged 15–44). Schizophrenia and bipolar disorder ranked thirteenth and fifteenth for all ages in developed regions. Other drug use ranked twenty-second. In developed regions of the world and in countries with established market economies such as the United States, when all neuropsychiatric conditions were combined, they were responsible for more death and disability than any other category of health conditions, outranking cardiovascular diseases; cancers; and a combined category of communicable, maternal, perinatal, and nutritional illnesses (Murray and Lopez, 1996).

The major causes of DALYs differ somewhat for the United States, but M/SU illnesses remain prominent. In 1996, unipolar major depression was second only to ischemic heart disease for American women as the cause of DALYs. For men, traffic accidents ranked second; alcohol abuse and dependence ranked fifth; and depression and drug use ranked tenth and eleventh, respectively. Combined, unipolar major depression, drug use, and alcohol abuse and dependence are the leading cause of death and disability for American women and the second highest for men (behind heart disease) (Michaud et al., 2001). If mental illness diagnoses other than unipolar major depression were included, the DALYs would be even higher.

Moreover, mental or substance-use problems and illnesses seldom occur in isolation; approximately 15–43 percent of the time they co-occur

---

[8]Predominantly because of the disability (rather than mortality) it produces.

(Kessler et al., 1996; Kessler, 2004).[9] They also accompany a substantial number of general medical illnesses, such as diabetes, heart disease, neurological illnesses, and cancers (Katon, 2003); sometimes masquerade as separate somatic problems (Katon, 2003); and often go undetected (Kroenke et al., 2000; Saitz et al., 1997). M/SU illnesses significantly compromise the treatment outcomes for general health conditions, increase the use and cost of general health care (Katon, 2003), and have adverse consequences for workplace productivity and costs (as discussed below). Mental illness also is a major risk factor for the development of adverse health behaviors such as smoking, overeating, and a sedentary lifestyle (Katon, 2003).

Great Cost to the Nation

The disabilities and other adverse effects resulting from M/SU illnesses impose a sizable cost on the nation (Frank and McGuire, 2000). Considering health care spending alone, M/SU problems and illnesses represent the fifth most expensive category of health care conditions[10] in the United States among individuals not residing in nursing homes or other institutions (Thorpe et al., 2004). Direct spending[11] for M/SU health care by all health care purchasers in the United States totaled an estimated $104 billion in 2001 (82 percent for mental and 18 percent for substance-use illnesses), representing 7.6 percent of all health care spending (Mark et al., 2005). Additional costs attributable to M/SU illnesses (e.g., secondary health problems, loss of productivity in the workplace, and social problems requiring the involvement of the welfare and criminal and juvenile justice systems) are even higher. Nationally, the estimated direct and indirect costs for alcohol-related illnesses, injuries, and other consequences, excluding those associated with the use of other drugs, were estimated at $185 billion in 1998. More than 70 percent of these costs were due to lost productivity resulting from alcohol-related illness and premature death (NIAAA, 2000). These direct and indirect costs affect employers, the child welfare system, the juvenile and criminal justice systems, education systems, and other sectors of society.

---

[9]Among some treatment groups, rates of co-occurrence can be even higher. Among those with a nonalcohol drug-use disorder who sought treatment for that disorder, for example, 60.3 percent had at least one independent mood disorder, and 55.2 percent had a comorbid alcohol-use disorder (Grant et al., 2004a).

[10]Next to heart disease, trauma, cancer, and lung diseases.

[11]Includes only spending for health care in which M/SU illnesses are listed as the primary illness being treated. Thus, for example, costs of treating cirrhosis secondary to alcohol dependence are not captured; nor, for example, are other health problems brought on by substance use if the substance-use illness is not being treated, and other indirect costs of these illnesses, such as costs to the juvenile and criminal justice systems. Also not captured is care that is coded as another illness (e.g., back pain).

Decreased Productivity in the Workplace

Evidence is mounting that M/SU illnesses result in a considerable burden on the workplace and cost to employers due to absenteeism, "presenteeism" (i.e., attending work with symptoms that impair performance), days of disability, and "critical incidents" such as significant task failures and accidents. All cause a decrease in workplace productivity. Depression is the most frequently studied M/SU illness with respect to the workplace because it is highly prevalent among working-age adults and associated with substantial work impairment (Burton et al., 2004; Kessler et al., 2001a; Stewart et al., 2003); however, substance dependence and generalized anxiety disorders also are very common and associated with high levels of work impairment (Kessler et al., 2001a).

As part of a 2001–2002 national survey of American workers designed to better understand the relationship between health and productivity, interviews were conducted to determine the effect of depression on worker productivity. "Lost productive time" (LPT) was measured by summing employee self-reports of the hours per week absent from work for health-related reasons and hours of health-related reduced performance on workdays. Workers with depression reported significantly more total health-related LPT than workers without depression—on average, a loss of 5.6 hours per week compared with 1.5 hours per week for those without depression. Fully 81 percent of LPT was attributable not to absenteeism, but to reduced performance while at work—the component of reduced performance often invisible to employers because it is not captured in routine administrative data as are absenteeism, use of leave, and disability (Stewart et al., 2003). Indeed, there is evidence that improving care for depression can increase worker productivity and decrease absenteeism (Rost et al., 2004).

The accuracy of retrospective data self-reported by individuals with depression has been questioned (because the symptoms of depression may predispose individuals to appraise their productivity negatively). Yet when worker performance is measured by other valid and reliable means (Kessler et al., 2004), major depression continues to be associated with poor work performance more consistently than is the case for other high-prevalence conditions (allergies, arthritis, back pain, headaches, high blood pressure, and asthma) (Wang et al., 2004).

Decreased Achievement by Children in School

Emotional and behavioral problems of children and the M/SU problems and illnesses of their parents also are important predictors of poor school outcomes. Risk factors for early school failure include maternal depression; parental substance-use problems and illnesses; early behavior problems, particularly aggression; and maltreatment. Several M/SU-related risk factors, including parental trauma, maternal depression, maternal alcoholism, and other substance-use problems and illnesses also are associated with disorganized attachment behaviors in infants (i.e., insecure and inconsistent patterns of attachment to key caregivers) (Ainsworth and Eichberg, 1992; Carlson et al., 1989; Green and Goldwyn, 2002; O'Connor et al., 1987; Teti et al., 1995; van Ijzendoorn et al., 1999). Those behaviors in turn lead to lower IQ and poorer school performance (van Izjendoorn and van Vliet-Vissers, 1988; Zeanah et al., 2003). Children of untreated depressed mothers, for example, have significantly more behavior and school achievement problems than children of nondepressed mothers (Greenberg et al., 1999; Gross et al., 1995; Sinclair and Murray, 1998). Children who experience trauma also have higher rates of school problems than children who are not maltreated, including lower IQ scores, lower test scores in math and English, less social acceptance as perceived by the child, increased absence from class, and more grade repetitions (Eckenrode et al., 1995; Wodarski et al., 1990).

Although risk factors often associated with substance-use problems and illnesses (such as poor maternal nutrition, health, and prenatal care) make it difficult to attribute school problems solely to in utero drug exposure, it is clear that maternal substance-use problems and illnesses are strongly associated with adverse effects on children's cognitive, physical, and social development. Maternal alcohol consumption during pregnancy is associated with intrauterine growth retardation and low birth weight, which affect later cognitive and social development (Streissguth et al., 1994). Children exposed to alcohol in utero also have been found to have behavioral and social difficulties, such as trouble cooperating and paying attention and problems with impulsivity (Spohr et al., 1994). Findings of studies of prenatal exposure to other drugs, such as cocaine, heroin, and amphetamines, suggest that such exposure results in lower general intelligence and impairs school functioning (Eriksson and Zeterstrom, 1994; van Baar and de Graaff, 1994; van Baar et al., 1994). Other studies have found that although prenatal exposure to cocaine does not affect intellectual ability or academic achievement, it does affect the ability to sustain attention (Richardson et al., 1996).

These risks that place children on a dangerous trajectory toward school failure are compounded by the fact that academic failure itself breeds emotional and behavioral problems. Repeating a grade in school is associated with several specific behavioral problems and illnesses, such as ADHD, obsessive-compulsive disorder and other specific anxiety disorders, and major depressive disorder (Velez et al., 1989). Grade retention also predicts school dropout and rapid, repeated adolescent pregnancies (Linares et al., 1991). This is not a minor problem. According to one national study, 7.6 percent of children repeat kindergarten or first grade (Byrd and Weitzman, 1994). Children who are unable to achieve mastery on standard measures of school achievement also are at risk for delinquent and antisocial behavior (Yoshikawa, 1995), and children with early reading difficulties have increased rates of conduct problems up to the age of 16 (Fergusson et al., 1997).

Increased Burden on the Child Welfare System

The nation's child welfare system also is greatly affected by the high prevalence of and disability associated with M/SU illnesses. Foremost, children who are reported to and investigated by the child welfare system for maltreatment typically have experienced a number of known risk factors for the development of emotional and behavioral problems, including abuse, neglect, poverty, parental substance-use problems and illnesses, and domestic violence. As a result, almost half (47.9 percent) of a nationally representative, random sample of children aged 2–14 who were investigated by child welfare services in 1999–2000 had a clinically significant need for mental health care (Burns et al., 2004).

In addition, the U.S. Government Accountability Office (GAO) has found that, because of limitations on insurance coverage, some families resort to placing their children (most often adolescents with severe mental illness) in the child welfare system even though the family is not neglectful or abusive of the child. Because the child welfare system often is able to secure mental health services otherwise unavailable to them, parents use the system for this purpose even though they are placing their children in systems not designed to care for children who have not been abused or neglected (GAO, 2003). Doing so sometimes requires parents to give up legal custody of their children and place them in an out-of-home residential or foster care setting (Giliberti and Schulzinger, 2000). In Virginia, for example, a 2004 study of the use of the state's foster care program for mental health services found that 2,008 children in foster care as of June 1, 2004—approximately 1 of every 4 children in the system at that time— were there either because their parents wanted them to have mental health care not fully covered by their insurance or because the family did not have access to any insurance (Jenkins, 2004).

Finally, the stresses involved with child protective services investigation and judicial decision making, and for those who are placed in foster care the stress of removal from home, also constitute risk factors for maladaptive outcomes, including emotional, social, behavioral, and psychiatric problems warranting mental health treatment (Landsverk, 2005).

Demands on the Juvenile and Criminal Justice Systems

Juvenile justice Between 60 and 75 percent of youth in the juvenile justice system have a diagnosable mental disorder (Otto et al., 1992; Teplin et al., 2002; Wierson et al., 1992), and it is conservatively estimated, although the evidence is less clear, that approximately 20 percent have a severe mental illness (Cocozza and Skowyra, 2000; Grisso, 2004). Many youths in the juvenile justice system with mental illness also have a co-occurring substance-use problem or illness. Although the research on this issue is limited, a recent study of juvenile detainees in Cook County, Illinois, found that nearly 30 percent of females and more than 20 percent of males with substance-use disorders had major mental disorders as well (Abram et al., 2003).

Moreover, like youths who are not abused or neglected but are placed in child welfare solely to obtain mental health services, many children who are not guilty of any offence are placed in local juvenile justice systems and incarcerated solely to obtain such services not otherwise available. Although no formal counting and tracking of such children takes place, juvenile justice officials in 33 counties in the 17 states with the largest populations of children under age 18 estimated that approximately 9,000 such children entered their systems under these circumstances in 2001; county estimates ranged from 0 to 1,750, with a median of 140. Nationwide the number of children placed in juvenile justice systems is likely to be higher; 11 states reported to GAO that they could not provide estimates even though they were aware that such placements occur (GAO, 2003).

In a subsequent 2003 survey of all (698) secure juvenile detention facilities in the United States,[12] two-thirds of such facilities reported holding youths (prior to, after, or absent any pending adjudication) because they were awaiting community mental health services. In addition, seventy-one facilities in 33 states reported holding youths with mental problems or illnesses who had charges against them. As one detention facility administrator explained, "We are receiving juveniles that five years ago would have been in an inpatient mental health facility. . .we have had a number of juveniles who should no more be in our institution than I should be able to fly" (U.S. House of Representatives, 2004:8). A majority of detention facilities reported holding children under age 13; 117 reported holding children aged 10 and under; and 1 facility reported holding a 7-year-old child. Moreover, 27 percent of facilities holding children awaiting services rated the mental health treatment in their facility as "poor," "very poor," or "none." The emotional toll on these children is high. Fully 48 percent of facilities that hold juveniles waiting for community mental health services report suicide attempts among these youths (U.S. House of Representatives, 2004).

---

[12]Response rate = 75 percent.

Criminal justice In mid-2003, the nation's prisons and jails held 2,078,570 persons—1 in every 140 U.S. residents[13]—and this rate has been increasing annually, from 601 persons in custody per 100,000 U.S. residents in 1995 to 715 persons in custody per 100,000 residents in 2003 (Harrison and Karberg, 2004). Although a rigorous epidemiological study of the prevalence of M/SU illnesses in correctional settings has not taken place,[14] the U.S. Bureau of Justice estimates that approximately 16 percent of all persons in jails and state prisons report either having a mental disorder or staying overnight in a psychiatric facility, as do 7 percent of those in federal prisons (Ditton, 1999). Substance-use problems and illnesses play a larger role in incarceration. Approximately two-thirds of incarcerated individuals were under the influence of alcohol or drugs at the time of their offense, and nearly 60 percent of all state prisoners report using substances other than alcohol in the month prior to offending (Mumola, 1999). Moreover, in an average year, approximately one-third of new admissions to prisons result from parole violations, nearly 16 percent of which are drug-related (Hughes et al., 2001).

Because prisons and jails are legally required to provide medical treatment to inmates with medical needs (Haney and Specter, 2003; Metzner, 2002), approximately 95 percent of state correctional facilities report providing some form of mental health treatment to prisoners. The treatment provided includes screening for mental illness at intake (78 percent), assessing psychiatric problems (79 percent), delivering round-the-clock mental health care (63 percent), providing therapy or counseling (84 percent), prescribing psychotropic medications (83 percent), and providing reentry assistance (72 percent). On average, 1 in 8 prisoners in state prisons is engaged in structured counseling, and 1 in 10 is receiving psychotropic medication (Beck and Maruschak, 2001). The majority of jails also report providing some type of mental health treatment—most often screening at intake (78 percent), followed by psychotropic medication (66 percent), 24-hour care (47 percent), routine therapy or counseling (46 percent), and psychiatric evaluation (38 percent) (Stephan, 2001). Yet on average, mental health services are being provided at a level that is roughly half the estimated need (Wolff, 2004).

Although substance-use problems and illnesses play a larger role in incarceration than do mental illnesses, they receive less treatment (Wolff,

---

[13]The majority (66 percent) of these were in state or federal prisons, the remainder in local jails.

[14]A more rigorous study of the prevalence of M/SU illnesses in correctional settings, modeled on the prevalence studies of the general population in the United States (Kessler et al., 2001) and the correctional and general population in the United Kingdom (ONS, 1998), has been called for (Wolff, 2004).

2004). One study found that roughly one in four state prisoners received any treatment for substance-use problems, with a higher percentage (40 percent) receiving such treatment if they reported drug use at the time of their offense. The most common treatment received was self-help group/ peer counseling (Mumola, 1999). Similarly, although substance-use treatment or other programs, such as education or self-help, were provided by the majority of jails (73 percent) in 1998, only 20 percent of convicted jail inmates who were actively involved with drugs prior to their admission to jail had participated in substance-use treatment or program subsequent to their incarceration. Treatment (i.e., detoxification units, group/individual counseling, and residential programs) was provided by approximately 43 percent of jail facilities. Nearly two-thirds of jails reported providing access to drug or alcohol education or self-help groups (Wilson, 2000).

How These Adverse Consequences Can Be Mitigated

The delivery of effective treatment for M/SU problems and illnesses could mitigate many of the serious individual and societal consequences discussed above. Findings of observational studies and some controlled trials indicate that effective treatment for depression, for example, can result in improved productivity in the workplace, and this might substantially offset the cost of the treatment (Goetzel et al., 2002; Simon et al., 2001b; Wang et al., 2003). Treatment for this and other M/SU illnesses also might help ameliorate the adverse effects of emotional or behavioral problems and illnesses on children's educational achievement, as well as reduce the burden on the child welfare and juvenile justice systems. At a minimum, provision of effective treatment ensures that funds spent for treatment will not be wasted.

A CHARGE TO CROSS THE QUALITY CHASM

The high prevalence and adverse consequences of M/SU problems and illnesses, the availability of many efficacious treatments, and the widespread delivery of poor-quality care are increasingly being recognized by consumers, purchasers, care providers, and policy makers. Similar concerns about the safety, ineffectiveness, and poor quality of U.S. health care overall have previously received substantial attention among the health care community, the lay press, and the public at large as a result of two IOM reports—*To Err Is Human: Building a Safer Health System* (IOM, 2000) and *Crossing the Quality Chasm: A New Health System for the 21st Century* (IOM, 2001). These reports have played a key role in focusing national attention on problems in the quality of the nation's health care, while garnering consensus on strategies for achieving significant quality improvements. Both reports underscore that the vast majority of problems in the quality of health care are not the result of poorly motivated, uncaring, or unintelligent health care personnel but instead result from numerous barriers to high-quality health care imposed by the delivery systems in which clinicians work. Some of these barriers occur at the level of the patient's interaction with the clinician (e.g., not having sufficient time during the patient visit to talk with the clinician); some at the level of interactions among different clinicians serving the patient (e.g., poor communication, collaboration, and coordination of care); some within the organization in which care is delivered (e.g., poor decision support for clinicians); and some in the environment external to the delivery of care (e.g., the arenas of policy, payment, and regulation) (Berwick, 2002).

Crossing the Quality Chasm speaks to all of these barriers to quality health care[15] and has gained considerable traction in the health care community since its publication. As the subject of more than 50 peer-reviewed articles in the medical literature and hundreds of lay publications and coverage in other media, it has attracted the attention of many health care leaders. In the M/SU sector, the American College of Mental Health Administration (ACMHA), for example, focused on the report at its 2002 summit meeting of leaders from public and private behavioral health care systems. Summit meeting participants reached strong consensus that the *Quality Chasm* framework is immediately relevant and applicable to the concerns of behavioral health systems of care and policy. Attendees also endorsed the IOM paradigm as a strategic planning blueprint for the redesign of the behavioral health care system. However, because the *Quality Chasm* report did not separately address the unique characteristics of health care for mental and substance-use conditions (e.g., the use of coercion into treatment; the delivery of care through non-health care sectors, such as schools), attendees also agreed on the need to develop a strategy for applying the framework and recommendations of the *Quality Chasm* to address the unique characteristics of M/SU health care (ACMHA, undated).

---

[15] *Crossing the Quality Chasm* identifies four different levels for intervening in the delivery of health care: (1) the experience of patients; (2) the functioning of small units of care delivery ("microsystems"), such as surgical teams or nursing units; (3) the functioning of organizations that house the microsystems; and (4) the environment of policy, payment, regulation, accreditation, and similar external factors that shape the context in which health care organizations deliver care. Whereas *To Err Is Human* speaks mainly to the fourth level, *Crossing the Quality Chasm* addresses primarily the first and second levels—how the experiences of patients and the work of microsystems of care, such as health care teams, nursing units, or individual health care workers delivering care to patients, should be changed (Berwick, 2002). Both of these reports direct less attention to the third level above—the organizations that house the microsystems.

As a result of ACMHA leadership, there was a convergence of support from many sectors for adapting the *Quality Chasm* framework to M/SU health care. With support from the Annie E. Casey Foundation, the CIGNA Foundation, the National Institute on Alcohol Abuse and Alcoholism, the National Institute on Drug Abuse, The Robert Wood Johnson Foundation, SAMHSA within the U.S. Department of Health and Human Services, and the Veterans Health Administration of the U.S. Department of Veterans Affairs, the IOM was given the following charge:

> *Crossing the Quality Chasm: A New Health System for the 21st Century* identified six dimensions in which the United States health system functions at far lower levels than it should (i.e., safety, effectiveness, patient-centeredness, timeliness, efficiency and equity) and concluded that the current health care system in is in need of fundamental change. The IOM is to explore the implications of that conclusion for the field of mental health and addictive disorders, and identify the barriers and facilitators to achieving significant improvements along all six of these dimensions. The committee will examine both environmental factors such as payment, benefits coverage and regulatory issues, as well as health care organization and delivery issues. Based on a review of the evidence, the committee will develop an "agenda for change."

To carry out this charge, in 2004 the IOM convened a multidisciplinary committee of experts in mental, substance-use, and general health care; public- and private-sector M/SU health care delivery; primary care; consumer issues; integration of service; ethics; economics; Medicaid; racial and ethnic disparities in care; veterans' health and health care; child M/SU health care; geriatrics; informatics; and systems engineering (see Appendix A for the biographical sketches of committee members). This report is the result of their efforts.

As the committee's charge and expertise indicate, the scope of this study was large, encompassing both public and private sectors, children and adults, and health care for mental and substance-use problems and illnesses. In particular, addressing health care for both mental and substance-use conditions in a single report was challenging; major public- and private-sector initiatives and reports have nearly always addressed only one or the other (DHHS, 1999; New Freedom Commission on Mental Health, 2003). Nonetheless, the committee found this dual focus to be appropriate and invaluable to its analysis of the evidence and formulation of policy recommendations, given the interconnected nature of these conditions and the resulting need for coordinated policy and care delivery. Indeed, the committee believes that in future initiatives to improve the quality of M/SU health care, expertise in health care for both mental and substance-use conditions should always be at the table.

SCOPE OF THE STUDY

At the beginning of its deliberations, the committee identified several issues that it decided should be excluded from this study to best focus its efforts. The special considerations involved in delivering care in rural areas consistent with the *Quality Chasm* recommendations are addressed in a separate IOM report (IOM, 2005), and thus are not addressed here. Similarly, a separate study on emergency care was under way at the same time as this study. Readers are directed to the reports of the IOM Committee on the Future of Emergency Care in the U.S. Health System, which will include discussion of the impact of M/SU illnesses on emergency departments and the quality of M/SU health care these facilities provide. Moreover, although touched on briefly in this report, difficulties in achieving diversity in the health care workforce and addressing disparities in health care likewise have been the subject two recent IOM reports (IOM, 2003, 2004). Also, because of the committee's expansive charge, it was not able to attend to the unique issues related to dementia and the mental health care needs of older adults in long-term care facilities; the committee calls attention to the need for further study and resources focused on this population. Finally, *Crossing the Quality Chasm* sets forth a "patient-centered, treatment-focused" approach to improving *individual* health care, as opposed to a "population-centered, prevention-focused" approach to improving *public* health. The committee recognizes that much work is needed to apply public health interventions to M/SU problems and illnesses and briefly touches on a few of these issues in this report. However, resource limitations and the scope of the committee's charge and expertise made it infeasible to address more fully this very important aspect of improving M/SU health care.

ORGANIZATION OF THE REPORT

In carrying out its charge, the committee focused on those characteristics of M/SU health care that distinguish it from non-M/SU health care (what is referred to throughout this report as "general" health care). These characteristics are briefly described in Chapter 2, along with the *Quality Chasm* framework. The report then examines how the *Quality Chasm* framework can be applied to achieve high-quality M/SU care, focusing first on patient-centered care (Chapter 3) and then on safe and effective care (Chapter 4). Approaches to implementing the *Quality Chasm* rule of coordinating health care across general, mental, and substance-use health conditions are discussed in Chapter 5. Chapter 6 mirrors the original *Quality Chasm* report by addressing the application of information technology to facilitate changes needed to improve the quality of care. This report also parallels the *Quality Chasm* report by reviewing in a separate chapter

(Chapter 7) changes needed in the M/SU health care workforce to implement the committee's recommendations. New approaches to purchasing M/SU health care to create incentives for these changes are discussed in Chapter 8. Finally, Chapter 9 identifies areas in need of additional research. Appendix A contains further discussion of the *Quality Chasm* aims and rules and the organization of this report.

The report also contains overarching recommendations (in Chapter 2) as well as more specific recommendations for quality improvement. These latter recommendations, organized topically in Chapters 3–9, are collected and grouped according to the entities charged with their implementation in a series of tables at the end of Chapter 9.

REFERENCES

Abram K, Teplin L, McClelland G, Dulcan M. 2003. Comorbid psychiatric disorders in youth in juvenile detention. *Archives of General Psychiatry* 60(11):1097–1108.

ACMHA (American College of Mental Health Administration), undated. Summit 2002. Crossing the Quality Chasm: Translating the Institute of Medicine Report for Behavioral Health. March 13-16, 2002. Santa Fe, New Mexico [Online] Available: http://www.acmha.org/summit/summit_2002.cfm [accessed November 29, 2005].

Ainsworth M, Eichberg C. 1992. Effects on infant-mother attachment of unresolved loss of an attachment figure or other traumatic experience. In: Parkes C, Stevenson-Hinde J, Marris P, eds. *Attachment across the Life-Cycle*. New York: Routledge. Pp. 160–183.

American Psychiatric Association. 2000. *Diagnostic and Statistical Manual of Mental Disorders*. Fourth Edition, Text Revision, DSM-IV-TR ed. Washington, DC: American Psychiatric Association.

Anthony WA. 1993. Recovery from mental illness: The guiding vision of the mental health service system in the 1990s. *Psychological Rehabilitation Journal* 16(4):11–24.

Bauer MS. 2002. A review of quantitative studies of adherence to mental health clinical practice guidelines. *Harvard Review of Psychiatry* 10(3):138–153.

Beck AJ, Maruschak LM. 2001. *Mental Health Treatment in State Prisons, 2000*. NCJ 188215. Washington, DC: Bureau of Justice Statistics, U.S. Department of Justice.

Bernstein J, Bernstein E, Tassiopoulos K, Heeren T, Levenson S, Hingson R. 2005. Brief motivational intervention at a clinic visit reduces cocaine and heroin use. *Drug and Alcohol Dependence* 77(1):49–59.

Berwick D. 2002. A user's manual for the IOM's "Quality Chasm" report. *Health Affairs* 21(3):80–90.

Buchanan RW, Kreyenbuhl J, Zito JM, Lehman A. 2002. The schizophrenia PORT pharmacological treatment recommendations: Conformance and implications for symptoms and functional outcome. *Schizophrenia Bulletin* 28(1):63–73.

Burns BJ, Phillips SD, Wagner R, Barth RP, Kolko DJ, Campbel Y, Landsverk J. 2004. Mental health need and access to mental health services by youths involved with child welfare: A national survey. *Journal of the American Academy of Child and Adolescent Psychiatry* 43(8):960–970.

Burton WN, Pransky G, Conti DJ, Chen C-Y, Edington DW. 2004. The association of medical conditions and presenteeism. *Journal of Occupational and Environmental Medicine* 46(6):S38–S45.

Byrd RS, Weitzman ML. 1994. Predictors of early grade retention among children in the United States. *Pediatrics* 93(3):481–487.

Carlson V, Cicchettti D, Barnett D, Braunwald K. 1989. Finding order in disorganization: Lessons from maltreated infant's attachments to their caregivers. In: Cicchetti D, Carlson V, eds. *Child Maltreatment: Theory and Research on the Causes and Consequences of Child Abuse and Neglect.* New York: Cambridge University Press. Pp. 494–528.

Clark DB, Pollock N, Bukstein OG, Mezzich AC, Bromberger JT, Donovan JE. 1997. Gender and comorbid psychopathology in adolescents with alcohol dependence. *Journal of the American Academy of Child and Adolescent Psychiatry* 36(9):1195–1203.

Cocozza J, Skowyra K. 2000. Youth with mental disorders: Issues and emerging responses. *Juvenile Justice* VII(1) [Online]. Available: http://www.ncjrs.org/html/ojjnl_2000_4/contents.html [accessed January 19, 2006].

D'Aunno T, Pollack HA. 2002. Changes in methadone treatment practices: Results from a national panel study, 1988–2000. *Journal of the American Medical Association* 288(7):850–856.

DHHS (U.S. Department of Health and Human Services). 1999. *Mental Health: A Report of the Surgeon General.* Rockville, MD: DHHS.

Ditton P. 1999. *Mental Health and Treatment of Inmates and Probationers.* NCJ 174463. Washington DC: Bureau of Justice Statistics, Department of Justice.

Eckenrode J, Rowe E, Laird M, Brathwaite J. 1995. Mobility as a mediator of the effects of child maltreatment on academic performance. *Child Development* 66(4):1130–1142.

Emrick CD, Tonigan JS, Montgomery H, Little L. 1993. Alcoholics Anonymous: What is currently known? In: McCrady BS, Miller WR, eds. *Research on Alcoholics Anonymous: Opportunities and Alternatives.* New Brunswick, NJ: Rutgers Center of Alcohol Studies. Pp. 41–78.

Eriksson M, Zeterstrom R. 1994. Amphetamine addiction during pregnancy: 10-year follow-up. *Acta Pediatrica,* Supplement 404:27–31.

Essock SM, Frisman LK, Covell NH, Hargreaves WA. 2000. Cost-effectiveness of clozapine compared with conventional antipsychotic medication for patients in state hospitals. *Archives of General Psychiatry* 57(10):987–994.

Fergusson DM, Horwood LJ, Lynskey MT. 1997. Attentional difficulties in middle childhood and psychosocial outcomes in young adulthood. *Journal of Child Psychology and Psychiatry* 38(6):633–644.

Finney JW, Moos RH. 1991. The long-term course of treated alcoholism: I. Mortality, relapse, and remission rates and comparisons with community controls. *Journal of Studies on Alcohol* 52(1):44–54.

Fleming M, Barry K, Manwell L, Johnson K, London R. 1997. Brief physician advice for problem alcohol drinkers: A randomized controlled trial in community-based primary care practices. *Journal of the American Medical Association* 277(13):1039–1045.

Frank RG, McGuire TG. 2000. Economics and mental health. In: Cuyler AJ, Newhouse JP, eds. *Handbook of Health Economics.* Vol. 1B, No. 17. Amsterdam, The Netherlands: Elsevier Science B.V. Pp. 893–954.

GAO (Government Accountability Office). 1999. *Mental Health: Improper Restraint or Seclusion Use Places People at Risk.* GAO/HEHS-99-176. Washington, DC: GAO. [Online]. Available: http://www.gao.gov/archive/1999/he99176.pdf [accessed September 2, 2005].

GAO. 2003. *Child Welfare and Juvenile Justice: Federal Agencies Could Play a Stronger Role in Helping States Reduce the Number of Children Placed Solely to Obtain Mental Health Services.* GAO-03-397. Washington, DC: GAO. [Online]. Available: http://www.gao.gov/new.items/d03397.pdf [accessed October 25, 2004].

Giliberti M, Schulzinger R. 2000. *Relinquishing Custody: The Tragic Result of Failure to Meet Children's Mental Health Needs.* Washington, DC: Bazelon Center for Mental Health Law.

Glied S, Cuellar AE. 2003. Trends and issues in child and adolescent mental health. *Health Affairs* 22(5):39–50.

Goetzel RZ, Ozminkowski RJ, Sederer LI, Mark TL. 2002. The business case for quality mental health services: Why employers should care about the mental health and well-being of their employees. *Journal of Occupational and Environmental Medicine* 44(4): 320–330.

Gossop M, Marsden J, Stewart D, Rolfe A. 1999. Treatment retention and one year outcomes for residential programmes in England. *Drug and Alcohol Dependence* 57(2):89–98.

Gould TD, Manji HK. 2004. The molecular medicine revolution and psychiatry: Bridging the gap between basic neuroscience research and clinical psychiatry. *Journal of Clinical Psychiatry* 65(5):598–604.

Grant BF, Stinson FS, Dawson DA, Chou P, Dufour MC, Compton W, Pickering RP, Kaplan K. 2004a. Prevalence and co-occurrence of substance use disorders and independent mood and anxiety disorders: Results from the National Epidemiologic Survey on Alcohol and Related Conditions. *Archives of General Psychiatry* 61(8):807–816.

Grant BF, Stinson FS, Dawson DA, Chou SP, Ruan WJ, Pickering RP. 2004b. Co-occurrence of 12-month alcohol and drug use disorders and personality disorders in the United States: results from the National Epidemiologic Survey on Alcohol and Related Conditions. *Archives of General Psychiatry* 61(4):361–368.

Grasso BC, Genest R, Jordan CW, Bates DW. 2003. Use of chart and record reviews to detect medication errors in a state psychiatric hospital. *Psychiatric Services* 54(5):677–681.

Green J, Goldwyn R. 2002. Annotation: attachment disorganization and psychopathology: New findings in attachment research and their potential implications for developmental psychopathology in childhood. *Journal of Child Psychology and Psychiatry* 43(7): 835–846.

Greenberg M, Lengua L, Coie J, Pinderhughes E. 1999. Predicting developmental outcomes at school entry using a multiple-risk model: Four American communities. The Conduct Problems Prevention Research Group. *Developmental Psychology* 35(2):403–417.

Grisso T. 2004. *Double Jeopardy: Adolescent Offenders with Mental Disorders*. Chicago, IL: University of Chicago Press.

Gross D, Conrad B, Fogg L, Willis L, Garvey C. 1995. A longitudinal study of maternal depression and preschool children's mental health. *Nursing Research* 44(2):96–101.

Haney C, Specter D. 2003. Treatment rights in uncertain legal times. In: Ashford JB, Sales BD, Reid WH, eds. *Treating Adult and Juvenile Offenders with Special Needs*. Washington, DC: American Psychological Association. Pp. 51–80.

Harrison PM, Karberg JC. 2004. *Prison and Jail Inmates at Midyear 2003*. Bureau of Justice Statistics Bulletin, Office of Justice Programs, NCJ 203947. Washington, DC: U.S. Department of Justice. [Online]. Available: http://www.ojp.usdoj.gov/bjs/pub/pdf/pjim03.pdf [accessed August 4, 2004].

Higgins S, Petry N. 1999. Contingency management. Incentives for sobriety. *Alcohol Research and Health* 23(2):122–127.

Hughes TA, Wilson DJ, Beck AJ. 2001. *Trends in State Parole, 1990–2000*. Bureau of Justice Statistics, NCJ 184735. Washington, DC: U.S. Department of Justice. [Online]. Available: http://www.Ojp.Usdoj.Gov/Bjs/Pub/Pdf/Tsp00.Pdf [accessed July 31, 2005].

IOM (Institute of Medicine). 1997. *Dispelling the Myths About Addiction: Strategies to Increase Understanding and Strengthen Research*. Washington, DC: National Academy Press.

IOM. 2000. *To Err Is Human: Building a Safer Health System*. Washington, DC: National Academy Press.

IOM. 2001. *Crossing the Quality Chasm: A New Health System for the 21st Century*. Washington, DC: National Academy Press.

IOM. 2003. *Unequal Treatment: Confronting Racial and Ethnic Disparities in Healthcare.* Washington, DC: The National Academies Press.

IOM. 2004. *In the Nation's Compelling Interest: Ensuring Diversity in the Health-Care Workforce.* Washington, DC: The National Academies Press.

IOM. 2005. *Quality through Collaboration: The Future of Rural Health.* Washington, DC: The National Academies Press.

Jaycox LH, Morral AR, Juvonen J. 2003. Mental health and medical problems and service use among adolescent substance users. *Journal of the American Academy of Child & Adolescent Psychiatry* 42(6):701–709.

Jenkins CL. 2004, November 29. Mental illness sends many to foster care. *The Washington Post.* Metro Section. Pp. B1 and B4, Column 1.

Johnson R, Chatuape M, Strain E, Walsh S, Stitzer M, Bigelow G. 2000. A comparison of levomethadyl acetate, buprenorphine, and methadone for opioid dependence. *New England Journal of Medicine* 343(18):1290–1297.

Katon W. 2003. Clinical and health services relationships between major depression, depressive symptoms, and general medical illness. *Biological Psychiatry* 54(3):216–226.

Kessler RC. 2004. Impact of substance abuse on the diagnosis, course, and treatment of mood disorders. The epidemiology of dual diagnosis. *Biological Psychiatry* 56(10):730–737.

Kessler RC, Nelson CB, McGonagle KA, Edlund MJ, Frank, RG, Leaf PJ. 1996. The epidemiology of co-occurring addictive and mental disorders: Implications for prevention and service utilization. *American Journal of Orthopsychiatry* 66(1):17–31.

Kessler RC, Greenberg PE, Mickelson KD, Meneades LM, Wang PS. 2001a. The effects of chronic medical conditions on work loss and work cutback. *Journal of Occupational and Environmental Medicine* 43(3):218–225.

Kessler RC, Costello EJ, Merikangas KR, Ustun TB. 2001b. Psychiatric epidemiology: Recent advances and future directions. In: Manderscheid RW, Henderson MJ, eds. *Mental Health, United States, 2000.* DHHS Publication Number: (SMA) 01-3537. Washington, DC: U.S. Government Printing Office. Pp. 29–42.

Kessler RC, Ames M, Hymel PA, Loeppke R, McKenas DK, Richling DE, Stang PE, Ustun TB. 2004. Using the World Health Organization Health and Work Performance Questionnaire (HPQ) to evaluate the indirect workplace costs of illness. *Journal of Occupational and Environmental Medicine* 46(Supplement 6):S23–S37.

Kessler RC, Demler O, Frank RG, Olfson M, Pincus HA, Walters EE, Wang P, Wells KB, Zaslavsky AM. 2005. Prevalence and treatment of mental disorders, 1990 to 2003. *New England Journal of Medicine* 352(24):2515–2523.

Kranzler H, Van Kirk J. 2001. Efficacy of naltrexone and acamprosate for alcoholism treatment: A meta-analysis. *Alcoholism: Clinical and Experimental Research* 25(9):1335–1341.

Kroenke K, Taylor-Vaisey A, Dietrich AJ, Oxman TE. 2000. Interventions to improve provider diagnosis and treatment of mental disorders in primary care: A critical review of the literature. *Psychosomatics* 41(1):39–52.

Landsverk J. 2005. *Improving the Quality of Mental Health and Substance Use Treatment Services for Children Involved in Child Welfare.* Notes: Paper commissioned by the Institute of Medicine Committee on Crossing the Quality Chasm: Adaptation to Mental Health and Addictive Disorders.

Linares LO, Leadbetter BJ, Kato PM, Jaffe L. 1991. Predicting school outcomes for minority group adolescent mothers: Can subgroups be identified? *Journal of Research on Adolescence* 1(4):379–400.

Maris RW. 2002. Suicide. *The Lancet* 360(9329):319–326.

Mark TL, Coffey RM, Vandivort-Warren R, Harwood HJ, King EC, the MHSA Spending Estimates Team. 2005. U.S. spending for mental health and substance abuse treatment, 1991–2001. *Health Affairs, Web Exclusive* W5-133–W5-142.

McGlynn EA, Asch SM, Adams J, Keesey J, Hicks J, DeCristofaro A, Kerr EA. 2003. The quality of health care delivered to adults in the United States. *New England Journal of Medicine* 348(26):2635–2645.

McLellan AT, Lewis DC, O'Brien CP, Kleber HD. 2000. Drug dependence, a chronic medical illness: Implications for treatment, insurance, and outcomes evaluation. *Journal of the American Medical Association* 284(13): 1689–1695.

Mechanic D, Bilder S. 2004. Treatment of people with mental illness: A decade-long perspective. *Health Affairs* 23(4):84–95.

Metzner JL. 2002. Class action litigation in correctional psychiatry. *Journal of the American Academy of Psychiatry and the Law* 30(1):19–29.

Michaud CM, Murray CJL, Bloom BR. 2001. Burden of disease: Implications for future research. *Journal of the American Medical Association* 285(5):535–539.

Miller WR, Walters ST, Bennett ME. 2001. How effective is alcoholism treatment? *Journal of Studies on Alcohol* 62:211–220.

Miller W, Wilbourne P. 2002. Mesa Grande: A methodological analysis of clinical trials of treatments for alcohol use disorders. *Addiction* 97(3):265–277.

Moggi F, Hirsbrunner HP, Brodbeck J, Bachmann KM. 1999. One-year outcome of an integrative inpatient treatment for dual diagnosis patients. *Addictive Behaviors* 24(4): 589–592.

Mumola CJ. 1999. *Substance Abuse and Treatment, State and Federal Prisoners, 1997.* NCJ 172871. Washington, DC: Bureau of Justice Statistics, U.S. Department of Justice.

Murray CJL, Lopez AD. 1996. The global burden of disease in 1990: Final results and their sensitivity to alternative epidemiological perspectives, discount rates, age-weights and disability weights. In: Murray CJL, Lopez AD, eds. *The Global Burden of Disease: A Comprehensive Assessment of Mortality and Disability from Diseases, Injuries, and Risk Factors in 1990 and Projected to 2020.* Cambridge, MA: The Harvard School of Public Health on behalf of the World Health Organization and the World Bank. Pp. 247–293.

NAMI (National Alliance for the Mentally Ill). 2005. *Consumer Support: Recovery.* [Online]. Available: http://www.nami.org/Content/NabigationMenuFind_Support/Consumer_Support/Recovery.htm [accessed May 3, 2005].

New Freedom Commission on Mental Health. 2003. *Achieving the Promise: Transforming Mental Health Care in America. Final Report.* DHHS Publication Number SMA-03-3832. Rockville, MD: U.S. Department of Health and Human Services.

NIAAA (National Institute on Alcohol Abuse and Alcoholism). 2000. *10th Special Report to the U.S. Congress on Alcohol and Health.* [Online]. Available: http://www.niaaa.nih.gov/publications/10 report [accessed May 6, 2005].

NIMH (National Institute of Mental Health). 2005. *NIMH Strategic Plans and Priorities.* [Online]. Available: www.nimh.nih.gov/strategic/strategicplanmenu.cfm [accessed September 1, 2005].

Ockene J, Adams A, Hurley T, Wheler E, Hebert J. 1999. Brief physician- and nurse practitioner-delivered counseling for high-risk drinkers: Does it work? *Archives of Internal Medicine* 159(18):2198–2205.

O'Connor M, Sigman M, Brill N. 1987. Disorganization of attachment in relation to maternal alcohol consumption. *Journal of Consulting and Clinical Psychology* 55(6):831–836.

Olfson M, Marcus SC, Druss B, Elinson L, Tanielian T, Pincus HA. 2002. National trends in the outpatient treatment of depression. *Journal of the American Medical Association* 287(2):203–209.

O'Malley S, Rounsaville B, Farren C, Namkoong K, Wu R, Robinson J, O'Connor P. 2003. Initial and maintenance naltrexone treatment for alcohol dependence using primary care vs. specialty care: A nested sequence of three randomized trials. *Archives of Internal Medicine* 163(14):1695–1704.

Onken SJ, Craig CM, Ridgway P, Ralph RO, Cook JA. 2004. *An Analysis of the Definitions and Elements of Recovery: A Review of the Literature.* Paper Prepared for the National Consensus Conference on Mental Health Recovery and Systems Transformation. Held in Rockville, MD on December 16, 2004: U.S. Department of Health and Human Services.

ONS (Office of National Statistics). 1998. *Psychiatric Morbidity among Prisoners in England and Wales.* London, UK: The Stationery Office.

Otto R, Greenstein J, Johnson M, Friedman K. 1992. Prevalence of mental disorders among youth in the juvenile justice system. In: Cocozza J, ed. *Responding to the Mental Health Needs of Youth in the Juvenile Justice System.* Seattle, WA: National Coalition for the Mentally Ill in the Criminal Justice System.

Parthasarathy S, Mertens J, Moore C, Weisner C. 2003. Utilization and cost impact of integrating substance abuse treatment and primary care. *Medical Care* 41(3):357–367.

Pirraglia PA, Rosen AB, Hermann RC, Olchanski NV, Neumann P. 2004. Cost-utility analysis studies of depression management: A systematic review. *American Journal of Psychiatry* 161(12):2155–2162.

Prendergast M, Podus D, Chang E, Urada D. 2002. The effectiveness of drug abuse treatment: A meta-analysis of comparison group studies. *Drug and Alcohol Dependence* 67(1):53–72.

Rawal PH, Lyons JS, MacIntyre II JC, Hunter JC. 2004. Regional variation and clinical indicators of antipsychotic use in residential treatment: A four state comparison. *Journal of Behavioral Health Services and Research* 31(2):178–188.

Richardson GA, Conroy ML, Day NL. 1996. Prenatal cocaine exposure: Effects on the development of school-age children. *Neurotoxicology Teratology* 18(6):627–634.

Richardson LP, Di Giuseppe D, Christakis DA, McCauley E, Katon W. 2004. Quality of care for Medicaid-covered youth treated with antidepressant therapy. *Archives of General Psychiatry* 61(5):475–480.

Rosenheck R, Cramer J, Allen E, Erdos J, Frisman LK, Xu W, Thomas J, Henderson W, Charney D. 1999. Cost-effectiveness of clozapine in patients with high and low levels of hospital use. Department of Veterans Affairs Cooperative Study Group on Clozapine in Refractory Schizophrenia. *Archives of General Psychiatry* 56(6):565–572.

Rosenheck R, Kasprow W, Frisman L, Liu-Mares W. 2003. Cost-effectiveness of supported housing for homeless persons with mental illness. *Archives of General Psychiatry* 60(9):940–951.

Rost K, Smith JL, Dickinson M. 2004. The effect of improving primary care depression management on employee absenteeism and productivity: A randomized trial. *Medical Care* 42(12):1202–1210.

Rushton JL, Fant K, Clark SJ. 2004. Use of practice guidelines in the primary care of children with Attention-Deficit Hyperactivity Disorder. *Pediatrics* 114(1):e23–e28. [Online]. Available: http:// www.pediatrics.aappublications.org.cgi/reprint/114/1/e23 [accessed September 1, 2005].

Sailas E, Fenton M. 2005. Seclusion and restraint for people with serious mental illness. *The Cochrane Database of Systematic Reviews* (2):CD001163. Date of most recent update: September 24, 2005. Date of most recent substantive update: October 26, 1999.

Saitz R, Mulvey KP, Plough A, Samet JH. 1997. Physician unawareness of serious substance abuse. *American Journal of Drug and Alcohol Abuse* 23(3):343–354.

SAMHSA (Substance Abuse and Mental Health Services Administration). 2004a. *Results from the 2003 National Survey on Drug Use and Health: National Findings.* DHHS Publication Number SMA 04-3964. NSDUH Series H-25. Rockville, MD: U.S. Department of Health and Human Services.

SAMHSA. 2004b. *SAMHSA Action Plan: Seclusion and Restraint—Fiscal Years 2004 and 2005.* [Online]. Available: http://www.samhsa.gov/Matrix/SAP_seclusion.aspx [accessed February 20, 2005].

Sarver JH, Cydulka RK, Baker DW. 2002. Magnetic resonance spectroscopy and its applications in psychiatry. *Australian and New Zealand Journal of Psychiatry* 36(1):31–43.

Simon GE, Von Korff M, Rutter CM, Peterson DA. 2001a. Treatment processes and outcomes for managed care patients receiving new antidepressant prescriptions from psychiatrists and primary care physicians. *Archives of General Psychiatry* 58(4):395–401.

Simon GE, Barber C, Birnbaum HG, Frank RG, Greenberg PE, Rose RM, Wang PS, Kessler RC. 2001b. Depression and work productivity: The comparative costs of treatment versus nontreatment. *Journal of Occupational and Environmental Medicine* 43(1):2–9.

Simpson GA, Scott G, Henderson MJ, Manderscheid RW. 2004. Estimates of attention, cognitive, and emotional problems, and health services use by U.S. school-age children. In: Manderscheid RW, Henderson MJ, eds. *Mental Health, United States, 2002.* DHHS Publication number: (SMA) 3938. Rockville, MD: SAMHSA. Pp. 105–119.

Sinclair D, Murray L. 1998. Effects of postnatal depression on children's adjustment to school. Teacher's Reports. *British Journal of Psychiatry* 172(1):58–63.

Spohr HL, Willms J, Steinhausen HC. 1994. The fetal alcohol syndrome in adolescence. *Acta Paediatricia* (Supplement 404):19–26.

Stein MB, Sherbourne CD, Craske MG, Means-Christensen A, Bystritsky A, Katon W, Sullivan G, Roy-Byrne PP. 2004. Quality of care for primary care patients with anxiety disorders. *American Journal of Psychiatry* 161(12):2230–2237.

Stephan JJ. 2001. *Census of Jails, 1999.* NCJ 196633. Washington, DC: Bureau of Justice Statistics, U.S. Department of Justice. Available: http://www.ojp.usdoj.gov/bjs/pub/pdf/cj99.pdf [accessed September 2, 2004].

Sterling S, Weisner C. 2005. Chemical dependency and psychiatric services for adolescents in private managed care: Implications for outcomes. *Alcoholism: Clinical and Experimental Research* 25(5):801–809.

Stewart WF, Ricci JA, Chee E, Hahn SR, Morganstein D. 2003. Cost of lost productive work time among U.S. workers with depression. *Journal of the American Medical Association* 289(23):3135–3144.

Streissguth AP, Barr HM, Sampson PD, Bookstein FL. 1994. Prenatal alcohol and offspring development: The first fourteen years. *Drug and Alcohol Dependence* 36(2):89–99.

Tecott LH. 2003. The genes and brains of mice and men. *American Journal of Psychiatry* 160(4):646–656.

Teplin L, Abram K, McClelland G, Dulcan M, Mericle A. 2002. Psychiatric disorders in youth in juvenile detention. *Archives of General Psychiatry* 59(12):1133–1143.

Teti D, Gelfand D, Messinger D, Isabella R. 1995. Maternal depression and the quality of early attachment. *Developmental Psychology* 31(3):364–376.

Thorpe KE, Florence CS, Joski P. 2004. Which medical conditions account for the rise in health care spending? *Health Affairs* Web exclusive (W4):437–445.

Tonigan JS, Connors GJ, Miller WR. 2003. Participation and involvement in Alcoholics Anonymous. In: Babor TF, Del Boca FK, eds. *Treatment Matching in Alcoholism.* Cambridge, UK, and New York: Cambridge University Press. Pp 184–204.

U.S. House of Representatives. 2004. *Incarceration of Youth Who Are Waiting for Community Mental Health Services in the United States.* [Online]. Available: http://www.house.gov/reform/min/pdfs_108_2/pdfs_inves/pdf_health_mental_health_youth_incarceration_july_2004_rep.pdf [accessed September 1, 2005].

van Baar A, de Graaff BM. 1994. Cognitive development at preschool-age of infants of drug-dependant mothers. *Developmental Medicine and Child Neurology* 36(12):1063–1075.

van Baar AL, Soepatmi S, Gunning WB, Akkerhuis GW. 1994. Development after prenatal exposure to cocaine, heroin, and methadone. *Acta Paediatrica,* Supplement 404:40–46.

van Ijzendoorn MH, Schuengel C, Bakermans-Karenenburg. 1999. Disorganized attachment in early childhood: Meta-analysis of precursors, concomitants, and sequelae. *Developmental Pscyhopathology* 11:225–249.

van Izjendoorn M, van Vliet-Vissers M. 1988. The relationship between quality of attachment in infancy and IQ in kindergarten. *Journal of Genetics and Psychology* 149(1): 23–28.

Velez CN, Johnson J, Cohen P. 1989. A longitudinal analysis of selected risk factors for childhood psychopathology. *Journal of the American Academy of Child & Adolescent Psychiatry* 28(6):861–864.

Wang P, Simon G, Kessler R. 2003. The economic burden of depression and the cost-effectiveness of treatment. *International Journal of Methods in Psychiatric Research* 12(1):22–33.

Wang PS, Beck AL, Berglund P, McKenas DK, Pronk NP, Simon GE, Kessler RC. 2004. Effects of major depression on moment-in-time work performance. *American Journal of Psychiatry* 161(10):1885–1891.

Watkins KE, Burnam A, Kung F-Y, Paddock S. 2001. A national survey of care for persons with co-occurring mental and substance use disorders. *Psychiatric Services* 52(8):1062–1068.

Weisner C, Mertens J, Parthsarathy S, Moore C. 2001. Integrating primary medical care with addiction treatment: A randomized controlled trial. *Journal of the American Medical Association* 286(14):1715–1723.

Weisner C, Ray GT, Mertens J, Satre D, Moore C. 2003. Short-term alcohol and drug treatment outcomes predict long-term outcome. *Drug and Alcohol Dependence* 71(3): 281–294.

White WL. 1998. *Slaying the Dragon: The History of Addiction Treatment and Recovery in America.* Bloomington, IL: Chestnut Health Systems/Lighthouse Institute.

Wierson M, Forehand R, Frame C. 1992. Epidemiology and treatment of mental health problems in juvenile delinquents. *Advances in Behavior Research and Therapy* 14, 93–120.

Wilson DJ. 2000. *Drug Use, Testing and Treatment in Jails.* NCJ 179999. Washington, DC: Bureau of Justice Statistics, U.S. Department of Justice. [Online]. Available: http://www.ojp.usdoj.gov/bjs/pub/pdf/duttj.pdf [accessed August 11, 2005].

Wodarski JS, Kurtz PD, Gaudin JM, Howing PT. 1990. Maltreatment and the school-age child: Major academic, socioemotional, and adaptive outcomes. *Social Work* 35(6): 506–513.

Wolff NP. 2004. *Law and Disorder: The Case against Diminished Responsibility.* Notes: Paper commissioned by the Institute of Medicine Committee on Crossing the Quality Chasm: Adaptation to Mental Health and Addictive Disorders.

Wu L-T, Ringwalt CL, Williams CE. 2003. Use of substance abuse treatment services by persons with mental health and substance use problems. *Psychiatric Services* 54(3): 363–369.

Yoshikawa H. 1995. Long-term effects of early childhood programs on social outcomes and delinquency. *The Future of Children* 5(3):51–75.

Zeanah CH, Keyes A, Settles L. 2003. Attachment relationship experiences and childhood psychopathology. *Annals of the New York Academy of Sciences* 1008:22–30.

Zerhouni E. 2003. Medicine: The NIH roadmap. *Science* 302(5642):63–72.

2

A Framework for
Improving Quality

Summary

Crossing the Quality Chasm *identifies six aims and ten rules for redesigning the nation's health care system to achieve better-quality care. However, health care for mental and/or substance-use (M/SU) conditions in the United States historically has been more separated from general health care relative to other specialties. In addition, there are some significant differences between M/SU and general health care, including the implications of a mental or substance-use diagnosis for patient decision making; the more common use of coerced treatment; greater variation in the types of providers licensed to diagnose and treat M/SU illnesses; the need for linkages with a greater number of health, social, and public welfare systems; a less developed quality measurement infrastructure; less widespread adoption of information technology; and a differently structured marketplace for consumers and purchasers of M/SU health care.*

In analyzing these differences, the state of M/SU health care, and the Quality Chasm *framework for health care quality improvement, the committee finds that:*

- *M/SU health care—like general health care—is often ineffective, not patient-centered, untimely, inefficient, inequitable, and at times unsafe. It, too, requires fundamental redesign.*
- *Mental, substance-use, and general illnesses are highly interrelated, especially with respect to chronicity. Improving care*

delivery and health outcomes for any one of the three depends upon improving care delivery and outcomes for the others.

• *The* Quality Chasm *recommendations for the redesign of health care are as applicable to M/SU health care as they are to general health care.*

AIMS AND RULES FOR REDESIGNING HEALTH CARE

Crossing the Quality Chasm (IOM, 2001:6) proposes the following statement of purpose for the U.S. health care system:

> ... to continually reduce the burden of illness, injury, and disability, and to improve the health and functioning of the people of the United States.

To help achieve this purpose, the *Quality Chasm* report identifies six dimensions in which the U.S. health care system functions at far lower levels than it could and should, and translates these dimensions into national aims to guide the quality improvement efforts of all health care organizations, professional groups, public and private purchasers, and individual clinicians (see Box 2-1).

To further assist quality improvement efforts, the *Quality Chasm* report specifies an accompanying set of ten rules to guide the redesign of health care so as to accomplish the six quality aims (see Box 2-2).

BOX 2-1   The Six Aims of High-Quality Health Care

Safe—avoiding injuries to patients from the care that is intended to help them.

Effective—providing services based on scientific knowledge to all who could benefit and refraining from providing services to those not likely to benefit.

Patient-centered—providing care that is respectful of and responsive to individual patient preferences, needs, and values and ensuring that patient values guide all clinical decisions.

Timely—reducing waits and sometimes harmful delays for both those who receive and those who give care.

Efficient—avoiding waste, in particular waste of equipment, supplies, ideas, and energy.

Equitable—providing care that does not vary in quality because of personal characteristics such as gender, ethnicity, geographic location, and socioeconomic status.

**BOX 2-2   The *Quality Chasm's* Ten Rules to
Guide the Redesign of Health Care**

1. Care based on continuous healing relationships. Patients should receive care whenever they need it and in many forms, not just face-to-face visits. This rule implies that the health care system should be responsive at all times (24 hours a day, every day) and that access to care should be provided over the Internet, by telephone, and by other means in addition to face-to-face visits.

2. Customization based on patient needs and values. The system of care should be designed to meet the most common types of needs but have the capability to respond to individual patient choices and preferences.

3. The patient as the source of control. Patients should be given the necessary information and the opportunity to exercise the degree of control they choose over health care decisions that affect them. The health system should be able to accommodate differences in patient preferences and encourage shared decision making.

4. Shared knowledge and the free flow of information. Patients should have unfettered access to their own medical information and to clinical knowledge. Clinicians and patients should communicate effectively and share information.

5. Evidence-based decision making. Patients should receive care based on the best available scientific knowledge. Care should not vary illogically from clinician to clinician or from place to place.

6. Safety as a system property. Patients should be safe from injury caused by the care system. Reducing risk and ensuring safety require greater attention to systems that help prevent and mitigate errors.

7. The need for transparency. The health care system should make information available to patients and their families that allows them to make informed decisions when selecting a health plan, hospital, or clinical practice, or choosing among alternative treatments. This should include information describing the system's performance on safety, evidence-based practice, and patient satisfaction.

8. Anticipation of needs. The health system should anticipate patient needs, rather than simply reacting to events.

9. Continuous decrease in waste. The health system should not waste resources or patient time.

10. Cooperation among clinicians. Clinicians and institutions should actively collaborate and communicate to ensure an appropriate exchange of information and coordination of care.

SOURCE: IOM, 2001:8.

Finally, *Crossing the Quality Chasm* describes how achieving the six aims and following the ten rules requires a fundamental redesign of health care by health care organizations and delivery systems. This health care redesign must include adopting new ways of delivering care; making effective use of information technologies; managing the clinical knowledge and skills of the workforce; developing effective teams and coordinating care across patient conditions, services, and settings; improving how health care quality is measured; and adopting payment methods that create incentives for and reward good quality—all of which require attention to how workers are educated and deployed. Such changes have implications for all four levels of the health care system: (1) the interactions between patients and their individual clinicians; (2) the functioning of small units of care delivery ("microsystems"), such as interdisciplinary teams or staff located on inpatient units; (3) the functioning of organizations that house the microsystems; and (4) the environment of policy, payment, regulation, accreditation, and similar external factors that shape the environment in which health care organizations deliver care (Berwick, 2002).

In many ways, the delivery of health care for mental and/or substance-use (M/SU) problems and illnesses in the United States has evolved so that these four levels of the system operate very differently from the way they function in general health care. Therefore, focused examination and some specialized efforts will be required to apply the *Quality Chasm* rules and achieve significant improvements on all six quality aims in the M/SU domain.

DISTINCTIVE CHARACTERISTICS OF HEALTH CARE FOR MENTAL/SUBSTANCE-USE CONDITIONS

Greater Separation from Other Components of the Health Care System

M/SU health care differs from other specialty and nonspecialty health care in many ways. One of these is its greater degree of separation, both structurally and functionally, from other components of the health care system. This separation is historical in origin. Because of poor understanding of the biological aspects of M/SU illnesses and the lack of any medical treatments, care for individuals with these illnesses initially was viewed as a social rather than a medical problem. Specific therapies for mental illnesses were rarely mentioned in the medical literature before 1800. Sick individuals were often treated by ministers and women, rather than by doctors (Grob, 1994). Substance-use "disorders" similarly were viewed as manifestations of intellectual weakness or moral inferiority. In the early nineteenth century, for example, when alcoholism was beginning to be understood as a disease, "drunkards, along with unwed mothers, and those suffering from venereal disease, were routinely denied admission to America's earliest hospitals on the grounds that they were unworthy of community care" (White, 1998:4). Even when alcohol and other substance-use illnesses began to be recognized as biological diseases, medical treatment initially had little to offer, and most recovery assistance came from "mutual support" societies that were not part of health care (White, 1998).

Although understanding of the biological aspects of these illnesses and effective treatments has since greatly improved, the greater separation of M/SU health care from the rest of the system persists. This is manifested in part by society's continuing reliance on public-sector delivery systems and funding for M/SU care (Hogan, 1999; Mark et al., 2005); the resulting existence of a separate administration for these illnesses within federal (the Substance Abuse and Mental Health Services Administration [SAMHSA]) and state governments; frequent calls for the integration of health care services for mental and substance-use conditions with each other and with primary health care (Bazelon Center for Mental Health Law, 2004; DHHS, 2001; Jenkins and Strathdee, 2000; Minkoff, 2001; Torrey et al., 2002), and the separate purchase of M/SU health care by public- and private-sector purchasers. The separate purchasing of M/SU health care in most individuals' health insurance plans is known as "carving out" these services (Grazier and Eselius, 1999). "Carved-out" M/SU health care plans can be provided by companies separate from the main insurer or by subsidiaries of the primary insurer. Mental health care is even more separated from general health care for children and adolescents; they frequently receive mental health care through their schools, not through their primary health care provider (Burns et al., 1995; Kessler et al., 2001).

Some of these separations can have salutary effects, for example, by fostering recognition of and support for specialized knowledge of M/SU problems and illnesses and treatment expertise, and attenuating problems related to the adverse selection of individuals with M/SU illnesses in insurance plans. Moreover, some M/SU health care organizations involve individuals recovering from M/SU illnesses in the administration and delivery of services, providing a strong source of recovery support for others with these illnesses. At the same time, however, separation of those with M/SU problems and illnesses from the mainstream population might nurture the residual stigma and discrimination faced by some of these individuals (Corrigan et al., 2001, 2002; Kolodziej and Johnson, 1996). It can also pose obstacles to the coordination of M/SU health care services with each other and with general health care (IOM, 1997). Individuals needing these services often must interact with separate delivery systems to receive health care for general, mental, and substance-use conditions. These multiple delivery arrangements frequently have unreliable or nonexistent linkages with each other, creating opportunities for discontinuity of care. Chapter 5 addresses in greater detail these separation issues and the resulting need for better coordination of care, while Chapter 8 contains a more detailed discussion of the benefits and difficulties of carve-outs.

Additional Differences

Beyond the structural and functional separation discussed above, there are many other ways in which M/SU health care is distinctive. These differences, briefly summarized in Table 2-1 and in the text that follows, can have significant implications for efforts to apply the *Quality Chasm* aims and rules and are discussed more fully in succeeding chapters.

Consumer Role

Consumers of M/SU health care face a number of obstacles not generally encountered by consumers of general health care. Shame, stigma, and discrimination still experienced by some consumers of M/SU services may prevent them from seeking care (Peter D. Hart Research Associates, Inc., 2001; SAMHSA, 2004) and nourish both their own and providers' doubts about their competence to make decisions on their own behalf (Bergeson, 2004; Leibfried, 2004; Markowitz, 1998; Wright et al., 2000). These attitudes create obstacles to consumers' exercising the control of which they are capable over health care decisions that affect them and to their managing their illnesses effectively. Moreover, coerced treatment, which is common in substance-use health care and also seen (though less frequently) in mental health care for those with more severe mental illnesses, raises the question of how patients subjected to such treatment can make decisions about their care. As the locus of most M/SU treatment has shifted to the community, new mechanisms for pressuring or compelling individuals with these illnesses to undergo treatment have evolved, including coercion from the criminal justice and welfare systems, schools, and workplaces (Monahan et al., 2003, 2005; Sterling et al., 2004; Weisner et al., 2002).

At the same time, the long-standing history of individuals in recovery from substance-use illnesses helping to teach others about their illness and recovery strategies and supporting them in the recovery process is an advantage that consumers of substance-use health care services have when attempting to make informed health care choices and manage their illnesses. Mental health care is following in these footsteps; peer support programs are an emerging component of public-sector mental health services. Evidence shows that seeing or visualizing those similar to oneself successfully performing activities typically increases one's belief in one's own ability to perform those activities successfully (Bandura, 1997) and facilitates successful management of one's own chronic illness (Lorig et al., 2001) (see Chapter 3).

TABLE 2-1   Differences Between General Health Care and Health Care for Mental and Substance-Use Conditions

Attribute	Type of Care	
	General Health Care	Mental/Substance-Use Health Care
Consumer role in treatment	• Stigma is less common.	• Residual stigma persists, especially for substance-use illnesses.
	• Expectations are rising for consumer decision making in the purchase of health care and selection of treatments.	• Decision-making ability often is not anticipated or supported and often is challenged.
	• Coercion into treatment is rare.	• Coercion is common (especially for substance-use treatment).
	• The role of consumers in managing their chronic illnesses has only recently been emphasized.	• There is a long history of peer support/mutual support groups/recovering consumers as providers of alcohol and other drug treatment services. There has recently been a movement to do the same in mental health care.
Diagnostic methods	• Laboratory and physical exam findings, biological tests, imaging technologies, and other objective methods are frequently available to supplement the patient history and patient reports of symptoms used in making a diagnosis and monitoring care.	• Diagnosis relies more on results of interview tools and the patient history and involves more professional interpretation, with resulting greater variation in diagnosis.
Mode of clinician practice	• The majority of physicians practice in groups of three or more.	• Psychiatrists more often practice in solo or two-clinician practices. • Children's mental health care is often secured through schools and the welfare and juvenile justice systems.
Care delivery arrangements	• Care for multiple acute, chronic, and severe illnesses is delivered through the same health plan.	• Care for M/SU illnesses is often provided by a separate health plan.

TABLE 2-1   continued

Attribute	Type of Care	
	General Health Care	Mental/Substance-Use Health Care
	• Care for all types of illnesses is available through private-sector programs. • Determination of the need for a specialist is generally made by the patient and primary care provider. Primary care providers can routinely be paid for treating illnesses of all types.	• Care for chronic and severe illnesses is delivered through public-sector programs. • When consumers are covered by a separate managed behavioral health care plan, determination of the need for an M/SU specialist is made by the group purchaser, and the consumer is generally expected to receive care from such a specialist rather than from a primary care provider. Receiving M/SU health care from the primary care provider is not well supported.
	• Employee assistance programs (EAPs) play a more limited role.	• EAPs play a significant role in detection, referral, and treatment.
Quality measurement	• Both public- and private-sector leadership is involved. • Consensus exists on some core quality measures and specifications across the public and private sectors. • Well-established clinical administrative databases exist. • Quality measurement mechanisms for health plans, hospitals, and nursing homes have been in operation for several years.	• Leadership is predominantly from the public sector. • Less consensus exists on core measures across the public and private sectors. • Fewer established clinical databases exist. • Quality measurement and improvement mechanisms are less well developed.
Information sharing and technology	• Uniform, federally prescribed rules (implementing the Health Insurance Portability and Accountability Act [HIPAA]) exist for the sharing of clinical information and for	• The situation is similar to that for general health care, but with a larger number of state laws and regulations restricting the sharing of information.

(continued on next page)

TABLE 2-1   continued

| Attribute | Type of Care | |
	General Health Care	Mental/Substance-Use Health Care
	patient privacy and confidentiality, but more-protective state statutes take precedence. • The use of electronic health records, decision support, and other information technology (IT) applications is growing.	• IT is less well developed and less commonly used for clinical care support.
Workforce	• Only physicians and certain advanced practice nurses generally are licensed to diagnose and treat.	• A more diverse workforce is licensed to diagnose and treat, including psychologists, psychiatrists, other physicians, social workers, psychiatric nurses, marriage and family therapists, addiction therapists, and a variety of counselors with different education and certification requirements.
Marketplace and insurance coverage	• Private insurance and Medicare dominate purchasing. • Care is typically covered by insurance. Copayments are lower, and more visits/days of care are covered. • Non-M/SU specialty care is purchased under the same contract as primary care.	• State and local governments (including Medicaid) dominate purchasing. • Insurance provides less coverage. Copayments are higher, and fewer visits/days of care and therapies are covered. • M/SU insurance coverage is purchased separately ("carved out") from general health care.

Diagnostic Methods

Compared with general health care, relatively few laboratory, imaging, or other physical findings can be used to diagnose mental illnesses or substance dependence.[1] Accurate diagnosis instead relies primarily on clinical

---

[1]Substance use, but not dependence, can be detected by laboratory tests.

interviews with patients or their caregivers regarding the patient's symptoms and a clinician's application of expert, but still subjective, judgment. Moreover, different types of clinicians vary in the breadth, depth, and theoretical basis of their training (see Chapter 7). As a result, individuals with the same symptoms presenting to different mental health clinicians can receive very different diagnoses (Eaton et al., 2000; Kramer et al., 2000; Lefever et al., 2003; Lewczyk et al., 2003; McClellan, 2005; Mojtabai, 2002). In children, diagnoses may have an even greater range of variability because clinicians are greatly dependent upon parents' perceptions of the nature of the presenting problem. Subjectivity in diagnosis is also manifest in the different diagnoses received by individuals who are members of ethnic minorities (Bell and Mehta, 1980, 1981; Mukherjee et al., 1983). Criteria for accurately diagnosing M/SU problems and illnesses are found in the American Psychiatric Association's *Diagnostic and Statistical Manual of Mental Disorders*, now in its revised fourth edition (DSM-IV-TR). However, adherence to these guidelines is not uniform (Rushton et al., 2004), nor is training on the appropriate use of this manual required for professional credentialing.

Mode of Clinician Practice

A substantial proportion of mental health clinicians report that "individual practice" is either their primary or secondary[2] employment setting (Duffy et al., 2004) (see Table 2-2).

Among primary care and specialist physicians who are self-employed or employees of physician-owned medical groups,[3] psychiatrists are most likely to work in solo practices or small groups. Fully 85 percent practice in groups of one to three clinicians, compared with 53 percent of physicians overall, 54.9 percent of pediatricians, and 62.7 percent of internists (Cunningham, 2004).

Individual practice may be an impediment to the delivery of high-quality M/SU health care for multiple reasons. As described in Chapter 6, the size of health care provider organizations is related to the uptake of information technologies. Use of electronic health records, for example, is typically found in larger health care organizations (Brailer and Terasawa, 2003). Moreover, as articulated in *Crossing the Quality Chasm*, "Today,

---

[2]Many mental health practitioners work in multiple settings. For example, 60 percent of full-time psychiatrists reported working in two or more settings in 1998, as did 50 percent of psychologists in 2002, 20 percent of full-time counselors, and 29 percent of marriage /family therapists. Rates were higher for part-time counselors (Duffy et al., 2004).

[3]Residents and employees of hospitals, universities, medical schools, government, and health maintenance organizations (HMOs) are excluded.

TABLE 2-2   Percentage of Clinically Trained Specialty Mental Health Personnel Reporting Solo Practice as Their Primary or Secondary Place of Employment

Discipline	Percentage Reporting Solo Practice		
	Primary Employment	Secondary Employment	Reporting Year
Psychiatry	37.0	18.0	1998
Psychology	38.0	28.0	2002
Social work	18.5	27.1	2000
Counseling	15.1	21.6	2002
Marriage/family therapy	34.9	28.5	2000

SOURCE: Duffy et al., 2004.

no one clinician can retain all the information necessary for sound, evidence-based practice. No unaided human being can read, recall, and act effectively on the volume of clinically relevant scientific literature" (IOM, 2001:25). Clinicians in solo practice must assume all the burden of investigating, analyzing, purchasing, and maintaining decision support technologies, which can be prohibitively expensive when there is no economy of scale to be achieved.

Need to Navigate a Greater Number of Care Delivery Arrangements

As discussed above, the ways in which M/SU and other health care providers are separated are more numerous and complex than is the case for other health care generally. Not only is M/SU care separated from general health care, but health care services for mental and substance-use conditions are separated from each other despite the high rate of co-occurrence of these conditions. Also distinctive are the location of services needed by individuals with more severe mental and substance-use illnesses in public-sector programs apart from private-sector health care, and reliance on the education, child welfare, and juvenile and criminal justice systems to deliver M/SU services for many children and adults. These disconnected care delivery arrangements necessitate numerous patient interactions with different providers, organizations, and government agencies. They also require multiple provider "handoffs" of patients for different services, and the transmittal of information to and joint planning by all these providers, organizations, and agencies if coordination is to occur. Yet effective structures and processes to ensure coordination of care across clinicians and organizations are not in place. This situation is exacerbated by the widespread failure of general medical, mental health, and substance-use health care providers to look for and respond to co-occurring conditions, as well as legal and organizational prohibitions on sharing M/SU information. These issues are discussed more fully in Chapter 5.

Quality Measurement Infrastructure

The infrastructure required to measure, analyze, publicly report on, and improve the quality of M/SU health care is less well developed than that for general health care. As a result, less measurement of the safety, effectiveness, and timeliness of M/SU health care has taken place (AHRQ, 2003; Garnick et al., 2002) (see Chapter 4). This situation exists for several reasons. For example, multiple organizations and initiatives have put forth different core measurement sets and different approaches to identifying aspects of M/SU health care delivery to be measured. This problem is due in part to the fact that conceptualizing a framework for M/SU health care is more complex than is the case for general health care. The larger number of disciplines licensed to diagnose and treat M/SU problems and illnesses can require the involvement of a greater number of stakeholder groups in a consensus process. Further, as noted above, consumers have been more active in shaping the delivery of M/SU health care than that of general health care, again with implications for the numbers and diversity of stakeholders involved in a consensus process. Moreover, although general health care is delivered in both the private and public sectors, M/SU health care in the public sector serves a population with a clinical profile much different from that of those treated in the private sector—more often those with severe and chronic illnesses. Measures that may be meaningful to private-sector stakeholders may be less useful to those in the public sector, and vice versa.

The separation of M/SU and general health care also has sometimes created confusion about which entity is accountable for the quality of care that can be delivered through multiple arrangements (primary or specialty care, a general or a "carved out" health plan, school-based programs, etc.). For example, measures of M/SU quality required of comprehensive managed care organizations seeking accreditation are often not required of managed behavioral health organizations (MBHOs) seeking accreditation from the same organization.[4] Moreover, to produce many performance measures, data about the patient's entire illness—from detection to ongoing treatment—is required. When M/SU patients are served by arrangements such as carved-out managed behavioral health plans or employee assistance programs separate from their general health care plan or from each other, difficulties in

---

[4]Personal communication, Philip Renner, MBA, Assistant Vice President for Quality Measurement, National Committee for Quality Assurance, March 22, 2005.

linking the necessary data produced by different organizations can make many performance measures infeasible (Garnick et al., 2002).

Information Sharing and Technology

The need to share patient information across providers so that care can be coordinated is widely acknowledged as necessary to effective and appropriate care. This need was acknowledged most recently in regulations governing the privacy of individually identifiable health information under the authority of the Health Insurance Portability and Accountability Act (HIPAA) of 1996. Under HIPAA regulations, the routine sharing of information for treatment, payment, or health care operations is permissible without requiring patient consent. These regulations have provided some consistency with respect to the sharing of information on general health conditions and care, but much less so for M/SU health care.

HIPAA itself requires that regulations promulgated to implement its privacy provisions not supersede any more stringent provisions of state law pertaining to patient privacy. Each of the 50 states (and the District of Columbia) has a number of statutes that specifically govern aspects of mental health records. Many of these statutes and regulations are more stringent than the HIPAA requirements, and the variation among them is great (see Appendix B). Moreover, separate federal laws govern the release of information pertaining to an individual's treatment for alcohol or drug use. These federal laws are also superseded by state laws, which are more stringent. The preamble to the HIPAA privacy regulations recognizes the constraints of substance-use confidentiality laws and states that wherever one is more protective of privacy than the other, the more restrictive should govern. This means that clinicians providing treatment to the many individuals with co-occurring mental, substance-use, and general health problems and illnesses need to comply with multiple regulations and laws governing the release of information, as well as policies prescribed by the organization or organizations under whose auspices they provide care. This situation inhibits or at least confounds communications between M/SU and general health care providers. The need for an appropriate balance between privacy concerns and sharing of clinically relevant information among providers is addressed in Chapters 5 and 6.

Finally, while use of electronic health records, decision support, and other information technology applications is growing in general health care, their use in M/SU health care is more limited.

Greater Diversity of Types of Providers

Although the diagnosis and treatment of general health conditions are typically limited to physicians, certain advanced practice nurses, and physician assistants,[5] M/SU health care clinicians include psychologists, psychiatrists, other specialty or primary care physicians, social workers, psychiatric nurses, marriage and family therapists, addiction therapists, psychosocial rehabilitation therapists, sociologists, and a variety of counselors (e.g., school counselors, pastoral counselors, guidance counselors, and drug and alcohol counselors) (see Chapter 7). In addition to having differing education, training, and therapeutic approaches, these clinicians may not be educated in clinical practice guidelines for evidence-based care, receive training in their use, understand them, or be motivated to apply them (Manderscheid et al., 2001). As a result, some clinicians may be more committed to "schools" of practice than to evidence-based eclecticism (Jackim, 2003). Also, differences in educational curriculums make it difficult to credential providers in the large number of therapies in current use.

Differences in the Marketplace

State and local governments play a larger role in purchasing and delivering M/SU health care compared with general health care (Hogan, 1999). In 2001, Medicaid (a state-administered program) and other state and local government programs together paid for 52 percent of all M/SU health care in the United States, with Medicaid, the largest payer, representing more than a quarter of all spending on mental health care (Mark et al., 2005). Medicaid funds pay primarily for mental health care; the major source of funds for substance-use health care is federal block grants to states, which states use to purchase or provide services directly. Moreover, M/SU spending accounts for approximately 30 percent of all state and local spending (excluding Medicaid) for health care but represents only 4 percent of health care spending in the private sector. Between 1991 and 2001, annual spending by private insurers for substance-use treatment did not keep pace with inflation and declined in real dollars. In 1991, private insurers paid for 24 percent of all substance-use health care; in 2001 they paid for 13 percent (Mark et al., 2005). In general health care, payers are more often private insurers or the Medicare program.

The greater financial attention to M/SU health care in the public sector has several ramifications. First, because of the larger role of state and local governments, there is greater variability in how M/SU health care can be accessed and how providers are selected and reimbursed, as well as in the reporting requirements associated with the various local and state programs. Second, the greater visibility and financial consequences of M/SU

---

[5]Dentists, chiropractors, and podiatrists also are licensed to diagnose and treat, but typically within proscribed domains.

health care in the public as compared with the private sector may explain why leadership on some quality improvement initiatives, such as reduction in the use of restraints, performance measurement, and consumer-oriented health care, is more often found in the public than the private sector.

Moreover, although access to M/SU health care for some individuals has improved over the past decade (Kessler et al., 2005; Mechanic and Bilder, 2004), there are still unique obstacles to accessing these services. Insurers continue to impose greater limits on M/SU health care coverage by requiring higher copayments and deductibles, limiting benefits (Bureau of Labor Statistics, 2003), and excluding coverage altogether if an injured individual was under the influence of alcohol or some other drug (Cimons, 2004). These cost and insurance issues are a leading reason reported by consumers for not receiving needed M/SU treatment (SAMHSA, 2004).

Further, individuals with substance-use illnesses themselves may impede their access to care in the marketplace. Individuals with substance-use problems and illnesses who do not experience recovery on their own typically do not seek treatment until their condition becomes so severe that they must do so, or they are compelled by workplace problems, criminal offenses, and the like (Weisner and Schmidt, 2001). In a 2001 national survey of individuals in recovery from alcohol or other drug illnesses and their families, 60 percent reported that denial of "addiction" or refusal to admit the severity of the problem was the greatest barrier to their recovery. Embarrassment or shame was the second most frequently cited obstacle (Peter D. Hart Research Associates, Inc., 2001). This is unfortunate because, as noted in Chapter 1, evidence shows that interventions delivered to patients with substance-use problems and illnesses can reduce substance use (Bernstein et al., 2005; Fleming et al., 1997).

APPLYING THE *QUALITY CHASM* APPROACH TO HEALTH CARE FOR MENTAL AND SUBSTANCE-USE CONDITIONS

More detailed analyses of the above issues are presented in the following chapters. As a result of these analyses, the committee made an overall finding and formulated an overarching recommendation concerning the relationship between M/SU and general health care. In addition, the committee made two overall findings and formulated a second overarching recommendation pertaining to the feasibility of applying the *Quality Chasm* framework to M/SU health care.

Relationship between M/SU and General Health Care

In conducting its work, the committee, like many expert panels before it, was confronted by the "destructive," "artificial, centuries old separation of mind and body" that was criticized in the 1999 Surgeon General's Report on Mental Health (DHHS, 1999:Preface and p. *x*). Since that report was released, evidence for the effects of mental and substance-use problems and illnesses on each other and on general health and health care continues to accumulate (Bush et al., 2005; Katon, 2003; Kroenke, 2003). Depression and anxiety disorders are strongly associated with somatic symptoms, such as headache, fatigue, dizziness, and pain, that are the leading cause of outpatient medical visits and often medically unexplained (Kroenke, 2003). Similarly, substance-use problems and illnesses contribute to the misdiagnosis, difficult management, and poor outcomes associated with many of the most pervasive medical illnesses in this country, such as chronic pain, sleep disorders, breast cancer, hypertension, diabetes, pneumonia, and asthma (Howard et al., 2004; Rehm et al., 2003; Saitz et al., 1997). A substantial portion of individuals with chronic physical illnesses also have a comorbid M/SU problem or illness. A nationally representative survey of Americans found that among respondents with the four most common chronic general illnesses (hypertension, arthritis, asthma, and ulcers), the loss of whole or partial work days was confined largely to those to those who had a co-occurring mental condition (Kessler et al., 2003).

Examining in detail the effect of just one type of mental illness (depression) on one general health care condition (heart attack), a recent Agency for Healthcare Research and Quality (AHRQ) Evidence Report/Technology Assessment found that approximately one in five patients hospitalized for a heart attack suffers from major depression, and that the evidence is "strikingly consistent" that post–heart attack depression significantly increases one's risk of death from heart-related or other causes. Patients with depression are about three times more likely to die from a future heart attack or other heart problem. Fully 60–70 percent of individuals who become depressed when hospitalized for a heart attack continue to suffer from depression for 1–4 or more months after discharge, and during the first year following a heart attack, those with major depression can experience a delay in returning to work, worse quality of life, and worse physical and psychological health (Bush et al., 2005:5).

Overall Finding. Mental, substance-use, and general illnesses are highly interrelated, especially with respect to chronic illness and injury. Improving care delivery and health outcomes for any one of the three depends upon improving care delivery and outcomes for the others.

Overarching Recommendation 1. Health care for general, mental, and substance-use problems and illnesses must be delivered with an under-

standing of the inherent interactions between the mind/brain and the rest of the body.

Applicability of the *Quality Chasm* Framework

As a result of its analyses (contained in the succeeding chapters), the committee made the following two overall findings:

Overall Finding. M/SU health care—like general health care—is often ineffective, not patient-centered, untimely, inefficient, inequitable, and at times unsafe. It, too, requires fundamental redesign.

Overall Finding. The Quality Chasm *recommendations for the redesign of health care are as applicable to M/SU health care as they are to general health care.*

In light of the above findings, the committee makes the following recommendation:

Overarching Recommendation 2. The aims, rules, and strategies for redesign set forth in *Crossing the Quality Chasm* should be applied throughout M/SU health care on a day-to-day operational basis, but tailored to reflect the characteristics that distinguish care for these problems and illnesses from general health care.

The following chapters describe how to implement these overarching recommendations.

REFERENCES

AHRQ (Agency for Healthcare Research and Quality). 2003. *National Healthcare Quality Report*. Rockville, MD: U.S. Department of Health and Human Services.

Bandura A. 1997. *Self-Efficacy: The Exercise of Control*. New York: W.H. Freeman.

Bazelon Center for Mental Health Law. 2004. *Get It Together: How to Integrate Physical and Mental Health Care for People With Serious Mental Disorders*. Washington, DC: Judge David L. Bazelon Center for Mental Health Law.

Bell C, Mehta H. 1980. The misdiagnosis of black patients with manic depressive illness. *Journal of the National Medical Association* 73(2):141–145.

Bell CC, Mehta H. 1981. Misdiagnosis of black patients with manic depressive illness: Second in a series. *Journal of the National Medical Association* 73(2):101–1071.

Bergeson S. 2004, July 14. Testimony before the Institute of Medicine Committee on "Crossing the Quality Chasm: An Adaptation to Mental Health and Addictive Disorders." Washington, DC.

Bernstein J, Bernstein E, Tassiopoulos K, Heeren T, Levenson S, Hingson R. 2005. Brief motivational intervention at a clinic visit reduces cocaine and heroin use. *Drug and Alcohol Dependence* 77(1):40–59.

Berwick D. 2002. A user's manual for the IOM's "Quality Chasm" report. *Health Affairs* 21(3):80–90.

Brailer DJ, Terasawa E. 2003. *Use and Adoption of Computer-Based Patient Records in the United States.* PowerPoint Presentation to IOM Committee on Data Standards for Patient Safety on January 23, 2003. [Online]. Available: http://www.iom.edu/file.asp?id= 10988 [accessed October 17, 2004].

Bureau of Labor Statistics. 2003. *National Compensation Survey: Employee Benefits in Private Industry in the United States, 2000.* Bulletin 2555. Washington, DC: U.S. Department of Labor. [Online]. Available: http://stats.bls.gov/ncs/ebs/sp/ebbl0019.pdf [accessed February 25, 2004].

Burns BJ, Costello EJ, Angold A, Tweed D, Stangl D, Farmer EM, Erkanli, A. 1995. Data watch: Children's mental health service use across service sectors. *Health Affairs* 14(3):147–159.

Bush DE, Ziegeldtein RC, Patel UV, Thombs BD, Ford DE, Fauerbach JA, McCann UD, Stewart KJ, Tsilidis KK, Patel AL, Feuerstein CJ, Bass EB. 2005. *Post-Myocardial Infarction Depression. Summary.* AHRQ Publication Number 05-E018-1. Evidence Report/ Technology Assessment Number 123. Rockville, MD: Agency for Healthcare Research and Quality.

Cimons M. 2004. Ensuring Solutions to Alcohol Problems. *Challenging a Hidden Obstacle to Alcohol Treatment: Little Known Insurance Laws Thwart Screening in Emergency Rooms.* Washington, DC: George Washington University Medical Center.

Corrigan PW, River LP, Lundin RK, Penn DL, Uphoff-Wasowski K, Campion J, Mathisen J, Gagnon C, Bargman M, Goldstein H, Kubiak MA. 2001. Three strategies for changing attributions about severe mental illness. *Schizophrenia Bulletin* 27(2):187–195.

Corrigan PW, Rowan D, Green A, Lunding R, River P, Uphoff-Wasowski K, White K, Kubiak MA. 2002. Challenging two mental illness stigmas: Personal responsibility and dangerousness. *Schizophrenia Bulletin* 28(2):293–309.

Cunningham R. 2004. Professionalism reconsidered: Physician payment in a small-practice environment. *Health Affairs* 23(6):36–47.

DHHS (U.S. Department of Health and Human Services). 1999. *Mental Health: A Report of the Surgeon General.* Rockville, MD: Substance Abuse and Mental Health Services Administration, Center for Mental Health Services, and National Institutes of Health, National Institute of Mental Health, DHHS.

DHHS. 2001. *Report of a Surgeon General's Working Meeting on the Integration of Mental Health Services and Primary Health Care; 2000 November 30–December 1; Atlanta, Georgia.* Rockville, MD: U.S. Department of Health and Human Services.

Duffy FF, West JC, Wilk J, Narrow WE, Hales D, Thompson J, Regier DA, Kohout J, Pion GM, Wicherski MM, Bateman N, Whitaker T, Merwin EI, Lyon D, Fox JC, Delaney KR, Hanrahan N, Stockton R, Garbelman J, Kaladow J, Clawson TW, Smith SC, Bergman DM, Northey WF, Blankertz L, Thomas A, Sullivan LD, Dwyer KP, Fleischer MS, Woodruff CR, Goldsmith HF, Henderson MJ, Atay JJ, Manderscheid RW. 2004. Mental health practitioners and trainees. In Manderscheid RW, Henderson MJ, eds. *Mental Health, United States, 2002.* DHHS publication Number: (SMA) 3938. Rockville, MD: U.S. DHHS Substance Abuse and Mental Health Services Administration. Pp. 327–368.

Eaton WW, Neufeld K, Chen L, Cai G. 2000. A comparison of self-report and clinical diagnostic interviews for depression: Diagnostic interview schedule and schedules for clinical assessment in neuropsychiatry in the Baltimore Epidemiologic Catchment Area Follow-up. *Archives of General Psychiatry* 57(3):217–222.

Fleming M, Barry K, Manwell L, Johnson K, London R. 1997. Brief physician advice for problem alcohol drinkers. A randomized controlled trial in community-based primary care practices. *Journal of the American Medical Association* 277(13):1039–1045.

Garnick DW, Lee MT, Chalk M, Gastfriend D, Horgan CM, McCorry F, McLellan AT, Merrick EL. 2002. Establishing the feasibility of performance measures for alcohol and other drugs. *Journal of Substance Abuse Treatment* 23(4):375–385.

Grazier KL, Eselius LL. 1999. Mental health carve-outs: Effects and implications. *Medical Care Research and Review* 56 (Supplement 2):37–59.

Grob G. 1994. *The Mad Among Us: A History of the Care of America's Mentally Ill.* New York: Free Press.

Hogan MF. 1999. Public-sector mental health care: New challenges. *Health Affairs* 18(5):106–111.

Howard AA, Arnsten JH, Gourevitch MN. 2004. Effect of alcohol consumption on diabetes mellitus: A systematic review. *Annals of Internal Medicine* 140(3):211–219.

IOM (Institute of Medicine). 1997. Edmunds M, Frank R, Hogan M, McCarty Dennis, Robinson-Beale R, Weisner C, eds. *Managing Managed Care: Quality Improvement in Behavioral Health.* Washington, DC: National Academy Press.

IOM. 2001. *Crossing the Quality Chasm: A New Health System for the 21st Century.* Washington, DC: National Academy Press.

Jackim LW. 2003. Is all the evidence in? Range of popular treatments subsist despite lack of science base. Is that damaging? *Behavioral Healthcare Tomorrow* 12(5):21–26.

Jenkins R, Strathdee G. 2000. The integration of mental health care with primary care. *International Journal of Law and Psychiatry* 23(3–4):277–291.

Katon W. 2003. Clinical and health services relationships between major depression, depressive symptoms, and general medical illness. *Biological Psychiatry* 54(3):216–226.

Kessler RC, Costello EJ, Merikangas KR, Ustun TB. 2001. Psychiatric epidemiology: Recent advances and future directions. In: Manderscheid RW, Henderson MJ, eds. *Mental Health, United States, 2000.* DHHS Publication Number: (SMA) 01-3537. Washington, DC: U.S. Government Printing Office. Pp. 29–42.

Kessler RC, Ormel J, Demler O, Stang PE. 2003. Comorbid mental disorders account for the role impairment of commonly occurring chronic physical disorders: Results from the National Comorbidity Survey. *Journal of Occupational and Environmental Medicine* 45(12):1257–1266.

Kessler RC, Demler O, Frank RG, Olfson M, Pincus HA, Walters EE, Wang P, Wells KB, Zaslavsky AM. 2005. Prevalence and treatment of mental disorders, 1990 to 2003. *New England Journal of Medicine* 352(24):2515–2523.

Kolodziej ME, Johnson BT. 1996. Interpersonal contact and acceptance of persons with psychiatric disorders: A research synthesis. *Journal of Consulting and Clinical Psychology* 64(6):1387–1396.

Kramer TL, Daniels AS, Zieman GL, Willimas C, Dewan N. 2000. Psychiatric practice variations in the diagnosis and treatment of major depression. *Psychiatric Services* 51(3):336–340.

Kroenke K. 2003. Patients presenting with somatic complaints: Epidemiology, psychiatric co-morbidity and management. *International Journal of Methods in Psychiatric Research* 12(1):34–43.

Lefever G, Arcona A, Antonuccio D. 2003. ADHD among American schoolchildren: Evidence of overdiagnosis and overuse of medication. *The Scientific Review of Mental Health Practice* 21(1). [Online]. Available: http://www.srmph.org/0201-adhd.html [accessed November 2, 2004].

Leibfried T. 2004. Testimony before the Institute of Medicine Committee on Crossing the Quality Chasm: Adaptation to Mental Health and Addictive Disorders. Notes: Testimony given in Washington, DC, July 14. Available from the Institute of Medicine.

Lewczyk CM, Garland AF, Hurlburt MS, Gearity J, Hough RL. 2003. Comparing DISC-IV and clinician diagnoses among youths receiving public mental health services. *Journal of the American Academy of Child and Adolescent Psychiatry* 42(3):349–356.

Lorig KR, Ritter P, Stewart AA, Sobel D, Brown BW, Bandura A, Gonzalez VM, Laurent DD, Holman HR. 2001. Chronic disease self-management program: 2-year health status and health care utilization outcomes. *Medical Care* 39(11):1217–1223.

Manderscheid RW, Henderson MJ, Brown DY. 2001. Status of national accountability efforts at the millenium. In: Manderscheid RW, Henderson MJ, eds. *Mental Health, United States, 2000.* DHHS Publication number: (SMA) 01-3537. Washington, DC: U.S. Government Printing Office. Pp. 43–52.

Mark TL, Coffey RM, Vandivort-Warren R, Harwood HJ, King EC, the MHSA Spending Estimates Team. 2005. U.S. spending for mental health and substance abuse treatment, 1991–2001. *Health Affairs, Web Exclusive* W5-133–W5-142.

Markowitz FE. 1998. The effects of stigma on the psychological well-being and life satisfaction of persons with mental illness. *Journal of Health and Social Behavior* 39(4):335–347.

McClellan J. 2005. Commentary: Treatment guidelines for child and adolescent bipolar disorder. *Journal of the American Academy of Child and Adolescent Psychiatry* 44(3): 236–239.

Mechanic D, Bilder S. 2004. Treatment of people with mental illness: A decade-long perspective. *Health Affairs* 23(4):84–95.

Minkoff K. 2001. Program components of a comprehensive integrated care system for seriously mentally ill patients with substance disorders. *New Directions for Mental Health Services* (91):17–30.

Mojtabai R. 2002. Diagnosing depression and prescribing antidepressants by primary care physicians: The impact of practice style variations. *Mental Health Services Research* 4(2):109–118.

Monahan J, Swartz M, Bonnie RJ. 2003. Mandated treatment in the community for people with mental disorders. *Health Affairs* 22(5):28–38.

Monahan J, Redlich AD, Swanson J, Robbins PC, Appelbaum PS, Petrilla J, Steadman HJ, Swartz M, Angell B, McNiel DE. 2005. Use of leverage to improve adherence to psychiatric treatment in the community. *Psychiatric Services* 56(1):37–44.

Mukherjee S, Shukla S, Woodle J, Rosen AM, Olarte S. 1983. Misdiagnosis of schizophrenia in bipolar patients: A multiethnic comparison. *American Journal of Psychiatry*, 140(12): 1571–1574.

Peter D. Hart Research Associates, Inc. 2001. *The Face of Recovery.* Washington, DC: Peter D. Hart Research Associates, Inc.

Rehm J, Room R, Graham K, Monteiro M, Gmel G, Sempos C. 2003. The relationship of average volume of alcohol consumption and patterns of drinking to burden of disease: An overview. *Addiction* 98(9):1209–1228.

Rushton JL, Fant K, Clark SJ. 2004. Use of practice guidelines in the primary care of children with Attention-Deficit Hyperactivity Disorder. *Pediatrics* 114(1):e23–e28. [Online]. Available: http:// www.pediatrics.org/cgi/content/full/114/1/e23 [accessed September 1, 2005].

Saitz R, Ghali WA, Moskowitz MA. 1997. The impact of alcohol-related diagnoses on pneumonia outcomes. *Archives of Internal Medicine* 157(13):1446–1452.

SAMHSA (Substance Abuse and Mental Health Services Administration). 2004. *Results from the 2003 National Survey on Drug Use and Health: National Findings.* DHHS Publication Number SMA 04-3964. NSDUH Series H-25. Rockville, MD: U.S. Department of Health and Human Services.

Sterling S, Kohn C, Lu Y, Weisner C. 2004. Pathways to substance abuse treatment for adolescents in an HMO. *Journal of Psychoactive Drugs* 36(4):439–453.

Torrey WC, Drake RE, Cohen M, Fox LB, Lynde D, Gorman P, Wyzik P. 2002. The challenge of implementing and sustaining integrated dual disorders treatment programs. *Community Mental Health Journal* 38(6):507–521.

Weisner C, Schmidt L. 2001. Rethinking access to alcohol treatment. In: Galanter M, ed. *Services Research in the Era of Managed Care.* New York: Kluwer Academic/Plenum Press. Pp. 107–136.

Weisner C, Matzger H, Tam T, Schmidt L. 2002. Who goes to alcohol and drug treatment? Understanding utilization within the context of insurance. *Journal of Studies on Alcohol* 63(6):673–682.

White WL. 1998. *Slaying the Dragon: The History of Addiction Treatment and Recovery in America.* Bloomington, IL: Chestnut Health Systems/Lighthouse Institute.

Wright ER, Gronfein WP, Owens TJ. 2000. Deinstitutionalization, social rejection, and the self-esteem of former mental patients. *Journal of Health and Social Behavior* 41(1): 68–90.

3

Supporting Patients' Decision-Making Abilities and Preferences

Summary

Residual stigma, discrimination, and the multiple types of coercion that sometimes bring individuals with mental and/or substance-use (M/SU) illnesses into treatment have substantial implications for their ability to receive care that is respectful of and responsive to their individual preferences, needs, and values—what the Quality Chasm *report refers to as "patient-centered care." Concerns about impaired decision making and the risk of violence are responsible for much of this stigma and the resulting discrimination. The failure of many to understand the biological and medical nature of drug dependence creates additional stigma for those individuals whose alcohol or other drug use has progressed to physiological dependence. Moreover, coerced treatment, common in substance-use health care though less so in mental health care, raises the question of how all patients with M/SU illnesses can be the source of control for their treatment decisions.*

However, there is great diversity in the decision-making abilities of individuals with M/SU illnesses—just as there is in the general population. Even when care is coerced, patients can and should have a voice in the options available within their care plan. Actively supporting these patients' decision making at the point of care delivery can preserve respect for patient preferences, needs, and values and improve patient outcomes. The committee recommends specific actions that all clinicians, organizations, accrediting bodies, health plans, and purchasers involved in M/SU health care should take to ensure patient-centered care for individuals with M/SU problems and illnesses. It further recommends actions to preserve patient-centered care when coercion into treatment is unavoidable.

RULES TO HELP ACHIEVE PATIENT-CENTERED CARE

Crossing the Quality Chasm defines "patient-centered care" as care that is "respectful of and responsive to *individual* patient preferences, needs, and values and ensur[es] that patient values guide all clinical decisions" (emphasis added) (IOM, 2001:40). A number of the rules for redesigning health care set forth in the *Quality Chasm* report (see Box 2-2 in Chapter 2) relate to achieving patient-centered care (see Box 3-1).

The aim of patient-centered care and its associated rules emphasize (1) clinical care that is based on individual patient preferences, needs, values, and decision making; and (2) patient access to and receipt of information that permits well-informed health care decisions. Yet consumers of all types of health care face substantial barriers to making such decisions. These

---

BOX 3-1 Rules for Patient-Centered Care

Customization based on patient needs and values. The system of care should be designed to meet the most common types of needs but have the capability to respond to individual patient choices and preferences.

The patient as the source of control. Patients should be given the necessary information and the opportunity to exercise the degree of control they choose over health care decisions that affect them. The health system should be able to accommodate differences in patient preferences and encourage shared decision making.

Shared knowledge and the free flow of information. Patients should have unfettered access to their own medical information and to clinical knowledge. Clinicians and patients should communicate effectively and share information.

The need for transparency. The health care system should make available to patients and their families information that allows them to make informed decisions when selecting a health plan, hospital, or clinical practice, or choosing among alternative treatments. This should include information describing the system's performance on safety, evidence-based practice, and patient satisfaction.

Anticipation of needs. The health system should anticipate patient needs, rather than simply reacting to events.

SOURCE: IOM, 2001:8.

barriers include inadequate comparative information and poorly structured mechanisms to enable meaningful choices of plans, providers, and treatments[1]; poor general and health literacy (IOM, 2004a); a tension that can sometimes occur between consumer-directed and evidence-based care (IOM, 2001); and providers' lack of understanding of cultural differences.

When one is diagnosed with a mental and/or substance-use (M/SU) illness (and sometimes an M/SU problem), additional obstacles to decision making arise from the lingering stigma attached to some of these illnesses and from the practice of coerced treatment. The effects of this stigma and coercion (especially as they relate to perceptions of patients as having impaired decision-making abilities and posing a danger) are complex and have substantial ramifications for the delivery of patient-centered care. These issues and related evidence are presented in the following four sections of this chapter, which address, respectively:

- Effects of stigma and discrimination in impairing patient decision making, patient-centered care, and patient outcomes. Understanding these effects points to actions that can counteract stigma and discrimination.
- Two stereotypes that uniquely stigmatize individuals with M/SU problems and illnesses—impaired decision making and dangerousness—as well as additional stigmatizing misperceptions about drug dependence.
- Coercion into treatment that results from concerns about impaired decision making and dangerousness.
- Actions clinicians, organizations, insurance plans, and governments (federal, state and local) can take to combat stigma and discrimination and support patient-centered care.

The committee's recommendations for achieving patient-centered M/SU care are presented in the final section.

HOW STIGMA AND DISCRIMINATION IMPEDE PATIENT-CENTERED CARE

"Stigma" is defined as the negative labeling and stereotyping of a group of individuals that is based on some observable trait they share and that

---

[1]Some consumer information needs and choices pertain to the patient's role as a consumer in the health care marketplace, that is, as a purchaser of health insurance and chooser of both health plan and individual providers. Other information needs and choices relate to consumers' role within the patient–health care provider treatment relationship, one that involves selecting among different treatments and being active partners in the management of their illness and recovery. This chapter addresses the individual's role as patient within the treatment relationship; the patient's role as informed consumer and purchaser in the health care marketplace is discussed in Chapter 8.

leads to discrimination against them by individuals or society at large (Corrigan and Penn, 1999; Link and Phelan, 2001). "Stigma" refers to the negative attitudes toward members of a group; "discrimination" refers to the behaviors that result from these attitudes.

Within a stigmatized group, different personal, social, and economic resources shape the lives and personal power of individual group members and produce substantial variation in the extent to which any given member personally experiences the effects of stigma (Link and Phelan, 2001). Nevertheless, American society as a whole—like that of most if not all countries—has for centuries stigmatized individuals with M/SU illnesses and discriminated against them socially, in employment, and in their efforts to secure such necessities of life as housing (Farina, 1998; Join Together, 2003; SAMHSA, 2000). Although understanding of the causes of mental illnesses has improved among the general population over the past 50 years, stigma continues (Hall et al., 2003; Pescosolido et al., undated) to varying degrees for individuals with different M/SU illnesses. In general, substance-use illnesses are more stigmatized than mental illnesses, and some mental illnesses (e.g., schizophrenia) more than others (e.g., major depression) (Mann and Himelein, 2004; Martin et al., 2000).

Two negative stereotypes in particular stigmatize individuals with M/SU illnesses and affect their ability to receive patient-centered care: (1) misperceptions about the extent to which individuals with various M/SU illnesses are capable of making decisions about their treatment, and (2) erroneous beliefs about the extent to which these individuals pose a danger to themselves or others (Martin et al., 2000).[2] Individuals who have developed physiological drug dependence may also suffer from the erroneous stereotype that their drug cravings and compulsion to continue using drugs in the face of serious adverse consequences are solely a matter of weak moral character or lack of willpower (SAMHSA, 2000). This failure to understand the biological mechanisms and consequences of drug dependence interferes with these individuals' ability to participate in and receive care that may be most effective in treating their chronic condition.

Evidence pertaining to the above stereotypes is presented in the next section. In this section, we examine three ways in which these stereotypes threaten the receipt of patient-centered care: (1) by lessening patients' ability to participate in the management of their illness and achieve desired treatment outcomes; (2) by encouraging pessimistic and non-therapeutic attitudes and behaviors among clinicians, making them less

---

[2]Individuals with mental illnesses also historically have been stereotyped as possessing a number of other negative attributes, such as lack of interpersonal skills; the display of alienating behaviors; and among the seriously mentally ill, unattractive appearance (Farina, 1998; Martin et al., 2000).

likely to foster and support patients' self-management efforts; and (3) by promoting discriminatory public policies that create barriers to patient-centered care and recovery. All three of these effects of stereotyping can contribute to poorer health outcomes (Link and Phelan, 2001). Understanding them can point to ways of remedying them and thereby promoting patient-centered care.

Adverse Effects on Patients' Ability to Manage Their Care and Achieve Desired Health Outcomes

As noted below, the adverse effects of stigma lead down a pathway to diminished health outcomes. The steps along this pathway are depicted in Figure 3.1 and described below.

Stigma → ↓ Self-Esteem → ↓ Self-Efficacy → ↓ Ability to Manage Chronic Illness → ↓ Health Outcomes/Recovery

FIGURE 3-1   The stigma pathway to diminished health outcomes.

Diminished Self-Esteem

Stigma influences not just how individuals with M/SU illnesses are perceived by others, but also how they perceive themselves (Farina, 1998; Link and Phelan, 2001; Wahl, 1999; Wright et al., 2000). Individuals with a mental illness who have greater concerns about or experiences with stigmatization[3] have lower self-esteem (Link et al., 2001; Wright et al., 2000), perform more poorly on tasks (Farina, 1998), and have weaker social and leisure relationships and interactions (Perlick et al., 2001), all of which are associated with a greater risk of relapse or no remission (Cronkite et al., 1998; Sherbourne et al., 1995). Among individuals with mental health problems, stigma also is associated with not taking prescribed medications (Sirey et al., 2001) and is a significant reason why some individuals do not seek treatment (SAMHSA, 2004b). Moreover, stigma leads to self-deprecation and compromised feelings of mastery over life circumstances (Wright et al., 2000), and thereby diminishes beliefs and expectations regarding self-determination and the ability to make decisions on one's own behalf. In short, diminished self-esteem correlates with decreased belief in "self-efficacy" (Markowitz, 1998).

---

[3]Evidence suggests that actual experiences with social rejection are likely to be a more powerful influence than the expectation of rejection (Wright et al., 2000).

Decreased Self-Efficacy

Perceived self-efficacy refers to a person's belief that that he or she is capable of carrying out a course of action to reach a desired goal. Self-efficacy beliefs touch every aspect of peoples' lives—whether they think productively, self-defeatedly, pessimistically, or optimistically; how well they motivate themselves and persevere in the face of adversity; their vulnerability to stress and depression; the life choices they make; the courses of action they pursue; how much effort they will make in pursuing a course of action; and their emotional reactions to the course of events. Self-efficacy also is a critical determinant of how well knowledge and skills are obtained (Pajares, 2002) and an excellent predictor of behavior. Unless people believe they can produce desired events through their actions, they have little incentive to act. Self-efficacy beliefs are constructed from four main sources of information: personal experience of mastery; vicarious experience through others with similar characteristics; verbal persuasion; and physiological capability, strength, and vulnerabilities (Bandura, 1997b).

There is evidence that self-efficacy is key to individuals' successful self-management of a variety of chronic illnesses and achievement of resulting improvements in health outcomes (Lorig and Holman, 2003; Lorig et al., 2001; Shoor and Lorig, 2002), as well as an important component of recovery from substance use (Samet et al., 1996). Self-efficacy is among the most powerful predictors of favorable posttreatment outcomes among treated alcohol patients (Project MATCH Research Group, 1998). It is also theorized to be a common mechanism in the effectiveness of psychosocial treatments for a variety of mental illnesses (Bandura, 1997a; Mueser et al., 2002).

Impaired Illness Self-Management

Illness self-management encompasses the day-to-day tasks an individual carries out to live successfully with chronic illness(es). Experts in the study of effective illness self-management interventions identify five core skills needed by patients: problem solving, decision making, resource utilization, formation of an effective patient–provider relationship, and taking action. These five skills are necessary to manage the effects of illness in three areas: medical or behavioral health practices, social and interpersonal role functioning, and emotional management (Lorig and Holman, 2003). These skills pertain, for example, to monitoring illness symptoms; using medications appropriately; practicing behaviors conducive to good health in such areas as nutrition, sleep, and exercise; employing stress reduction practices and managing negative emotions; using community resources appropriately; communicating effectively with health care providers; and practicing health-related problem solving and decision making. Self-management support programs for a variety of chronic illnesses, including heart disease, lung disease, stroke, and arthritis, have been shown to reduce pain and disability, lessen fatigue, decrease needed visits to physicians and emergency rooms, and increase self-reported energy and health. These improvements in health outcomes are strongly associated with increased self-efficacy (Bodenheimer et al., 2002a; Lorig and Holman, 2003; Lorig et al., 2001).[4]

Components of illness self-management for individuals with chronic mental illnesses such as schizophrenia and bipolar illness (i.e., psychoeducation, behavioral practices to support taking medications appropriately, relapse prevention, and teaching of coping skills and actions to alleviate symptoms) also have been developed, tested, and found effective in addressing many of the behaviors necessary for patient recovery (Mueser et al., 2002). A standardized approach for illness self-management has been developed and empirically validated by Stanford University (Stanford University School of Medicine, 2005). Illness self-management also is included as one of the six essential components of the Chronic Care Model (Bodenheimer et al., 2002b), which is discussed in Chapter 5 and is achieving improved health outcomes for a variety of physical and mental illnesses.

Weakened Patient Activation and Self-Determination

Self-efficacy and self-management also are related to the concepts of "patient activation" and "patient self-determination." "Patient activation" refers to the constellation of skills, knowledge, beliefs, and behaviors necessary for an individual to manage a chronic illness successfully (Von Korff et al., 1997). An "activated" patient also is one of the key elements of the Chronic Care Model (Bodenheimer et al., 2002a). Self-determination theory is concerned with individuals' innate inner resources for personality development and behavioral regulation and how these resources are influenced by social contexts so as to affect human motivation (Ryan and Deci, 2000). Research in this area has established the central importance to self-determination of three innate psychological needs: self-perceived competence (self-efficacy, discussed above), autonomy, and relatedness. This research also has shown that people must perceive themselves as competent

---

[4]A recent analysis of self-management education programs (Warsi et al., 2004) found a small to moderate effect on outcomes for some clinical conditions (diabetes and hypertension) but no significant consistent benefit for asthma programs. This same analysis noted wide variation in the methodologies used and inconsistent reporting of measures of self-efficacy in these programs. Experts caution that many programs calling themselves self-management programs do not teach all the core skills involved and fail to address the necessary scope of issues (Lorig and Holman, 2003).

(self-efficacious) and experience their behavior as volitional if they are to possess intrinsic motivation (Cook, 2004).

Whether one is discussing patient self-management, self-activation, or self-determination, the underlying theme is the same: patients' behaviors will be determined by how meaningful a given problem is to them and how capable of resolving the problem they perceive themselves to be. As described above, stigma can adversely affect individuals' self-efficacy beliefs, their ability to manage their M/SU illness, and thereby their recovery. Clinicians, through their clinical expertise and close relationship with their patients, should be vehicles for increasing their clients' beliefs in their self-efficacy. However, not all providers foster their patients' self-efficacy beliefs and support patient decision making—the second way in which stigma obstructs patient-centered care.

Stigma Affects Clinician Attitudes and Behaviors

Because of their scientific knowledge and special relationship with their patients, clinicians have a singular opportunity through their attitudes and practices to promote patient self-esteem, self-efficacy, decision making about treatment, illness self-management practices, and recovery. While many health care professionals exemplify these positive attitudes and related practices in their treatment relationships with their patients, some do not. Testimony to the committee from consumer groups (Bergeson, 2004; Leibfried, 2004) revealed that poor provider support for patients' decision making and illness self-management and pessimistic beliefs about their abilities were serious obstacles to their decision making and recovery. As articulated by one speaker (Bergeson, 2004):

> We believe that the majority of physicians and other health care providers must fundamentally change their approach toward their patients, an approach revealed through the use of that "special voice." Sadly, far too many professionals have a manner of speaking to us as if we are slightly stupid children.
>
> It's that voice that reminds us that we aren't really partners in care with our health care providers. No matter that we may know more about the latest efficacy data on specific medications than our doctors; no matter that we may be following rTMS and vagus nerve studies as treatment options and our nurses haven't even heard of them; no matter that we may be aware of the outcomes of CBT [cognitive behavioral therapy] with bipolar patients, and our talk therapist—who is most frequently a social worker—isn't schooled in the fundamentals of CBT.
>
> It's that voice that reminds us that health care providers still think of themselves as taking care of us, instead of working with us. It's the voice of learned helplessness.

Such negative and discouraging attitudes and practices are a serious problem. Experts in self-efficacy research note that it is usually easier to weaken self-efficacy beliefs through negative appraisals than to strengthen them through positive comments (Pajares, 2002).

With respect to treatment for substance dependence, some providers hold the stereotypical view discussed above that fails to understand the biological aspects of dependence and regards the illness simply as a matter of failed willpower or weak character. As a result, a treatment provider or program may not offer or support a patient's choice to use medications, such as methadone, to treat the illness.

Nontherapeutic clinician attitudes and behaviors may have several sources. First, health care providers, through general societal acculturation, initially can be expected to hold the same attitudes and beliefs about individuals with M/SU illnesses as society at large unless they have had substantial prior contact with such individuals (Corrigan et al., 2001; Kolodziej and Johnson, 1996) and/or been assimilated into a different culture that counteracts this misinformation. However, the clinical settings in which some graduate mental health students receive their training provide predominantly inpatient as opposed to outpatient care. Graduate education of medical residents, for example, has been slow to shift training away from inpatient settings (Hoge et al., 2002). Clinical training in inpatient settings, as opposed to the ambulatory settings in which most individuals receive treatment, provides experience with patients with mental illnesses during their most acutely ill phase and may thus reinforce a view of those with such illnesses as being more disabled than is the case. Moreover, most academic education and training programs for clinicians focus on the *cognitive* domain of learning, along with some *skill* development. Few programs have content or instructional strategies targeting the *affective* or attitudinal domain of learning. Thus it should not be a surprise that clinicians' attitudes may mirror those of society at large and be unchanged by their education (Stuart et al., 2004).

Also, as discussed in Chapter 7, education of the general health care workforce has addressed substance-use illnesses inadequately. To the extent that health care providers do not understand and have knowledge of alcohol and drug dependence as distinct diseases, their treatment of these illnesses will be ineffective. Unfortunately, evidence presented in Chapter 4 indicates that such poor understanding and limited knowledge may be widespread. In one study, treatment of alcohol problems and illnesses nationally ranked the lowest on measures of health care quality for a wide variety of illnesses (McGlynn et al., 2003).

Moreover, the terminology used by society to refer to M/SU health care is different from that used in general health care and may foster stigmatizing beliefs. For example, "mental illness" often is used as a singular noun instead of the plural "mental illnesses." Research indicates that some people attach different levels of stigma to different mental illnesses, based in part on the extent to which a given illness is perceived as treatable (Mann and Himelein, 2004). Consistent with this attitude, surveys of the public show a reluctance to label an individual as "mentally ill," but a greater willingness to use more-specific mental health labels, such as "schizophrenia," "major depression," or "alcohol dependence" (Link et al., 1999). A one-size-fits-all label of "mental illness" could foster a perception that all mental illnesses have equal consequences, disabilities, and handicaps, and perhaps contribute to stereotyping. In contrast, we no longer typically refer to individuals as having "cancer" as if it is a single disease; rather, we more often (and more accurately) refer to them as having leukemia, breast cancer, melanoma, lung cancer, colon cancer, prostate cancer, etc. A parallel can also be drawn with references to HIV, measles, tuberculosis, and so on instead of simply "infectious disease."

In addition, some terminology and phrasing used in M/SU health care is different from that commonly used in general health care and may encourage clinicians' nontherapeutic attitudes. For example, the terms mental "disorders" (as in the *Diagnostic and Statistical Manual of Mental Disorders* [DSM]) and emotional "disturbances"[5] are used to describe mental illnesses, problems, and symptoms. In general health care, the terms "disorders," "disordered" and "disturbance" are used less frequently. The International Classification of Diseases (ICD), the coding system used in the United States and worldwide for the collection and analysis of health care data, generally uses the terminology "diseases," "conditions," "symptoms," "problems," and "complaints" for most health conditions but, like the DSM, typically refers to mental illnesses and conditions as "disorders" (AMA, 2001). Calling mental and emotional problems and illnesses "disorders" and "disturbances" disinclines those so labeled and those applying the labels to think of individuals thus afflicted as having an illness, a condition, symptoms, or perhaps a "problem" that is amenable to short-term intervention. Rather, these labels could contribute to a perception that mental illnesses and problems should be viewed differently from most general health care illnesses, symptoms, and problems.

Moreover, the phrasing "serious and persistent," used in some federal laws to refer to a subset of mental illnesses, has no counterpart in general medical care, which describes general illnesses with similar consequences as "severe" and "chronic." The word "serious," for example, is not used in general health care terminology such as that in the ICD (e.g., it is not

---

[5]The term "serious emotional disturbance" is found in multiple federal statutes and regulations (e.g., the Individuals with Disabilities Education Act [IDEA], Public Law 101-476) and has thus pervaded the vocabulary of mental health care for children.

common to talk about "serious" cancers). The term "persistent" could connote a lack of belief in the ability to improve and recover. A less pejorative and clinically more meaningful way to categorize individuals with mental illnesses that are accompanied by chronic functional limitations might be to refer to them as having mild, moderate, or severe disability associated with a mental illness symptom or diagnosis, rather than referring to them as "seriously" mentally ill.

The use of the word "abuse" as opposed to substance "use" or "dependence" also has been identified as pejorative. It implies that alcohol or other drug dependence connotes a "willful commission of an abhorrent (wrong and sinful) act" and misstates the nature of alcohol or drug use and dependence (White, undated:4).

Recognizing the power of terminology to contribute to stigma, the Substance Abuse and Mental Health Services Administration's (SAMHSA) National Treatment Plan Initiative for improving substance abuse health care called for a language audit to identify problems inherent in the terminology used in the field and in public discussions, and for the development of a nonstigmatizing taxonomy to describe alcoholism, drug "addiction," and available treatments and services (SAMHSA, 2000). A similar process could be beneficial in reducing stigmatizing language used throughout the mental health field.

Finally, major factors in clinicians' beliefs and behaviors may be notions of M/SU patients' inability to make decisions competently and difficulties encountered when individuals are coerced into treatment—a common occurrence for those entering treatment for substance use. Evidence on both of these factors is discussed later in this chapter.

Relationship Between Stigma and Discriminatory Policies

The discrimination that results from stigma can be direct from person to person, such as that described above, or may involve an individual in a position of authority denying employment, housing, or a social relationship to an individual who is a member of a stigmatized group. More structurally imbedded societal discrimination can also occur, as when treatment settings are located in more disadvantaged neighborhoods or when society decides to expend fewer resources on a stigmatized group (Corrigan and Watson, 2003; Link and Phelan, 2001). Thus, the effects of stigma extend beyond the attitudes and practices of individual members of the public, patients, and clinicians to influence public policy as well—the third way in which stigma obstructs patient-centered care. The most visible manifestation of this level of discrimination is the more limited insurance coverage of M/SU health care compared with general health care. Such discrimination is also seen in public policies that impose additional penalties beyond those imposed by the judicial system on individuals convicted of some types of drug use.

Discrimination in Health Insurance Coverage

Coverage of mental health care Despite federal and state laws aimed at encouraging equal coverage of mental health and other health benefits offered by employers,[6] the National Compensation Survey of private employers, conducted in 2000 by the Department of Labor, documented that inpatient and outpatient mental health care is less often covered in employee health benefit plans than is general health care. Approximately 7 percent of employees with medical care benefits do not have inpatient or outpatient mental health care included in their benefit package. Of the 93 percent of employees with mental health benefits, 85 and 93 percent are subject to limitations on inpatient and outpatient mental health benefits, respectively, that are more restrictive than those on general medical benefits. The most common difference is more restrictions on inpatient days of care and outpatient visits, experienced by 76 and 72 percent of employees, respectively. Higher copayments or coinsurance for inpatient and outpatient care are also experienced by 16 and 50 percent, respectively (Bureau of Labor Statistics, 2003).[7]

Results of a 2002 survey of public employers indicate that limitations on inpatient and outpatient days of care may have increased over the past few years, while cost sharing has declined (Barry et al., 2003). In 2003, 27 percent of workers in public and private firms with three or more workers were restricted to 20 or fewer outpatient visits per year, and 37 percent were restricted to 21–30 inpatient days per year. An additional 13 percent were limited to 20 or fewer inpatient days per year (Claxton et al., 2003). These benefit limits most often are reached by individuals with some of the most severe mental illness diagnoses, including depression, bipolar illness, and psychoses. Moreover, some state laws narrowly define mental illness to include only specific diagnoses, such as schizophrenia,

---

[6]The Mental Health Parity Act, passed by Congress in 1996, prohibited annual or lifetime dollar limits on coverage in firms with 50 or more employees unless equal limits were placed on nonmental health care. However, the law did not prohibit other types of benefit coverage disparities, such as different copayment requirements and limits on outpatient visits or inpatient days. Also, although 34 states have enacted some form of parity legislation, these laws vary greatly in the population covered, types of limitations prohibited, and excluded diagnoses (Barry et al., 2003).

[7]The Medicare program similarly requires a 50 percent copayment for visits to a psychiatrist, in contrast to a 20 percent copayment for visits for other illnesses.

schizoaffective disorder, bipolar disorder, major depression, and obsessive-compulsive disorder (Health Policy Tracking Service, 2004).

There is also evidence that benefit limits are reached more often by children than adults (Peele et al., 1999). In addition, some specific diagnoses that are common in childhood, such as autism, attention deficit hyperactivity disorder (ADHD), and conduct disorders, are excluded from coverage under certain private health benefit plans (Peck and Scheffler, 2002; Peele et al., 2002). In other cases, benefits are constructed in ways that prevent effective treatment for some childhood conditions (Peck and Scheffler, 2002).

The U.S. Government Accountability Office (GAO) found that such limitations on insurance coverage contribute to the phenomenon whereby some families resort to placing their children (most often adolescents with severe mental illness) in the child welfare or juvenile justice system even though the family is not neglectful or abusive of the child, and the child has committed no criminal or delinquent act. Because the child welfare and juvenile justice systems often have ways of paying for mental health services, they are used by parents for this purpose even though they were not designed to care for children who have not been abused or neglected or committed a criminal or delinquent act (GAO, 2003). Doing so sometimes requires parents to give up legal custody of their children and place them in an out-of-home residential or foster care setting (Giliberti and Schulzinger, 2000). In 2001, 19 states and 30 counties estimated that 12,700 children in their jurisdictions were placed in the child welfare or juvenile justice system for the purpose of receiving mental health services. Because there is no systematic tracking of these children, the extent to which this phenomenon occurs nationally is unknown; however, GAO states that it is likely higher than the numbers reported by this limited number of states (GAO, 2003). In Virginia alone, for example, 2,008 children—approximately 1 of every 4 children in Virginia's foster care system as of June 1, 2004—were there either because mental health care was not fully covered by the parents' insurance or because the family did not have access to any insurance (Jenkins, 2004).

Coverage of substance-use health care Individuals with substance-use illnesses face even greater discrimination in insurance coverage than those with mental illnesses. Fewer employer-sponsored health plans cover substance-use treatment than cover either general or mental health care. Only 84 and 85 percent of employers providing medical care benefits, respectively, have coverage for outpatient drug or alcohol rehabilitation, compared with 100 percent who have coverage for general hospital and physician office visits and 93 percent who have coverage for inpatient and outpatient mental health care. When coverage for substance-use illnesses is available, it also is typically more restrictive than that for general illnesses (Bureau of Labor Statistics, 2003). For example, some policies provide for only two lifetime episodes of treatment for substance-use problems or illnesses.[8] Although as of 2000, 41 states and the District of Columbia either explicitly included substance-use treatment within the scope of their mental health benefit laws or had separate statutes addressing substance-use treatment coverage, 13 of these state laws covered only treatment for alcoholism, as opposed to treatment for other drug use (GAO, 2000).

Moreover, private insurers sometimes deny insurance claims for the care of an injury sustained by an individual if he or she was intoxicated or under the influence of any narcotic at the time of the injury. A late 1998 review of insurance statutes in all 50 states found that 38 states and the District of Columbia allowed policies that denied health insurance coverage for injuries due to alcohol use (Rivara et al., 2000). Representative data do not exist on the extent to which insurance plans exercise these provisions. However, provider perceptions that this may occur and result in denial of reimbursement discourage emergency departments and trauma centers from screening for alcohol use (Cimons, 2004)—this despite the strong associations between alcohol use and trauma and the effectiveness of screening and brief interventions in reducing substance use (D'Onofrio and Degutis, 2002; Gentilello et al., 2005; Moyer et al., 2002).

Insurance discrimination is not limited to private-sector insurance programs. The traditional Medicare indemnity program (the fee-for-service program in which the great majority of Medicare beneficiaries are enrolled) covers mental health and substance-use care. However the outpatient benefit requires relatively high cost sharing (50 percent), except for medication management (20 percent copayment).

Other Discriminatory Public Policies

Restrictions on access to student loans for some drug offenses Because federal student loan programs can help pay for higher education, they can play an important part in helping individuals realize their plans for recovery from substance-use illnesses. However, the 1998 Amendments to the Higher Education Act of 1965 added a provision[9] that makes an individual convicted (in the criminal as opposed to juvenile justice system) of the possession or sale of a controlled substance ineligible to receive any federal grant, loan, or work assistance funding for higher education. The period of

---

[8]Joan M. Pearson, Principal, Towers Perrin. Personal communication July 8, 2005.

[9]20 USC Chapter 28, Higher Education Resources and Student Assistance, Subchapter IV, Part F, Section 1091(r). Regulations at 34 CFR Chapter VI, Subpart D, section 668.40.

ineligibility varies from 1 year to an "indefinite" length of time according to whether the conviction is for possession or sale and whether it is for a first, second, or subsequent offense. These restrictions are placed on an individual in addition to the sentence imposed by the criminal justice system. Eligibility can be reinstated subsequent to satisfactory completion of an approved drug rehabilitation program (which is defined liberally but must include at least two unannounced drug tests). This law does not include alcohol-related convictions, such as multiple drunk-driving convictions or manslaughter as a result of drunk driving. Nor does it prohibit student loans for individuals convicted of non–drug-related violent crimes, such as assault, rape, or murder.

Potential lifetime ban on receipt of food stamps or welfare for felony drug conviction Under section 115 of the Personal Responsibility and Work Opportunity Reconciliation Act of 1996 (often referred to as the "Welfare Reform Act"), individuals convicted of a state or federal felony offense of possession, use, or sale of drugs (i.e., controlled substances, not alcohol) are subject to a ban on receiving federal cash assistance (Temporary Assistance for Needy Families [TANF] or "welfare") and food stamps, even if they serve the full term of their sentence, unless the state in which they reside has passed legislation opting out of or mitigating this restriction.[10,11]

Moreover, although a convicted individual cannot be included in the calculation of household size for TANF benefits or food stamps, his or her income and resources are included in calculating eligibility for food stamps.[12] Including the ineligible person's income in determining food stamp benefits penalizes the entire household, which is thereby eligible for less assistance each month. This and the TANF provisions diminish the resources available to convicted individuals living in poverty to change their life circumstances in ways that are important to achieving recovery. For example, they are less capable of paying for child care, securing transportation, and paying for education—all of which may be necessary in securing and retaining employment. These resources may also be critical to removing these individuals from contact with people, places, and situations associated with their former drug use. Such contact creates a biological response

---

[10]21 US Code Chapter 13, Subchapter I, Part D, Section 862a. Accessed at http://uscode.house.gov on February 2, 2005.

[11]As of 1997, 21 states had done so by opting out entirely (10 states), allowing individuals convicted of felonies who are in substance abuse treatment programs to receive benefits (6 states), or implementing a shorter disqualification period or reduced benefits (4 states) (Gabor and Botsko, 1998).

[12] Implementing regulations for the Food Stamp Program are at 7 CFR Chapter II Part 273 sections 273.11 (c) and (m).

in an individual with a drug dependence that induces cravings for the addictive substance (Hyman and Malenka, 2001).

EVIDENCE COUNTERS STEREOTYPES OF IMPAIRED DECISION MAKING AND DANGEROUSNESS

Two Harmful Stereotypes: Incompetent Decision Making and Dangerousness

The 1996 General Social Survey of the attitudes, beliefs, and behaviors of Americans documented the extent to which Americans believe individuals with M/SU illnesses are incompetent to make decisions and are a danger to themselves or others (Pescosolido et al., 1999):

- More than a third (36 percent) of Americans believed that individuals with major depression are "not very able" or "not able at all" to make decisions about their treatment; 74 percent believed this to be true for individuals with schizophrenia. A minority (6.8 percent) further believed that an individual with a mental health "problem" not severe enough to be considered a mental illness also is not very able or not able at all to make treatment decisions.
- The public perceived those with drug problems as least competent in decision making. About half (51 percent) believed individuals with alcohol dependence are not very able or not able at all to make decisions about their treatment; 72.1 percent believed this of individuals with cocaine dependence.
- The belief that individuals with major depression are "very likely" to do something violent to others was held by 9.2 percent; 12.8 percent believed this of individuals with schizophrenia. The percentages were higher for individuals with dependence on alcohol (17.5 percent) and cocaine (42 percent).
- As the public's perception of the seriousness of an individual's condition increased, so, too, did the belief in that individual's dangerousness, while belief in the person's competence to make decisions decreased.
- Significantly, the proportion of Americans who associated mental illness with "violent or dangerous behavior" in 1996 was nearly double that found in the 1950 General Social Survey (Pescosolido et al., undated).

Such beliefs are inconsistent with the evidence (discussed below) that a clear majority of individuals with mental illnesses (including those with severe illnesses such as schizophrenia) and substance-use illnesses are able to make treatment and other life decisions, and do not represent a danger to themselves or others. Stereotypes of incompetent decision making and dangerousness are refuted by strong evidence showing great diversity in the decision-making abilities of individuals with M/SU illnesses—just as there is in the population without these illnesses. Variable proportions of "normal" research subjects have been found to have deficits in decision making. Many situations (e.g., stress, serious illness, pain, or, more commonly, poor judgment) can undermine mentally healthy people's decision-making capacity. Moreover, individuals with M/SU illnesses are a minor source of the acts of violence committed in society; most acts of violence are committed by individuals who traditionally would not be considered mentally ill.

Evidence on Decision-Making Capacity[13]

Conceptual Framework

The process of determining the decision-making capacity of any individual (whether with or without an M/SU illness) can be conceptualized as involving three interrelated sets of factors: (1) the individual's innate abilities at a point in time to understand, appreciate, reason, and communicate preferences; (2) the risks and benefits inherent in the specific decision to be made; and (3) the knowledge and biases of the person making the judgment about the capacity of the individual in question. The influence of each of these factors on decision-making capability is discussed below.

Ability to understand, appreciate, reason, and communicate preferences
Analyses and reviews of the legal and ethics literature over many years have identified several abilities as integral to the concept of "competence" (Appelbaum and Grisso, 1988; Brody, 1998; Culver and Gert, 1990; Faden and Beauchamp, 1986; Roth et al., 1977). The abilities to understand, appreciate, reason, and communicate one's preferences are those most often accepted as salient in the clinical setting, cited in major policy recommendations, and used in clinical reports on competence (American Psychiatric Association, 1998; Appelbaum and Grisso, 1995; Berg et al., 1996; National Bioethics Advisory Commission, 1998). The model based on these four abilities was developed, operationalized, and tested over the past two decades

---

[13]Much of the evidence and discussion in this section is from three papers commissioned by the committee: "Impact of Mental Illness and Substance-Related Disorders on Decision-Making Capacity and Its Implications for Patient-Centered Mental Health Care Delivery" by Scott Kim, MD, PhD, Department of Psychiatry and the Program for Improving Health Care Decisions, University of Michigan Medical School; "Capacity to Consent to or Refuse Treatment and/or Research: Theoretical Considerations" by Elyn R. Saks, JD, Orrin B. Evans, Professor of Law, Psychology, and Psychiatry and the Behavioral Sciences, University of Southern California Law School, and Dilip V. Jeste, MD, Professor of Psychiatry and Neurosciences, University of California, San Diego; and "Decisional Capacity in Mental Illness and Substance Use Disorders: Empirical Database and Policy Implications," also by Drs. Jeste and Saks.

(Appelbaum and Grisso, 1988, 1995; Appelbaum et al., 1999; Berg, 1996; Grisso and Appelbaum, 1995; Grisso et al., 1997). This model is the basis for three generations of instruments (Appelbaum et al., 1999; Grisso et al., 1995, 1997) employed in studies of decision making involving persons with general medical illness (heart disease) (Grisso and Appelbaum, 1995; Grisso et al., 1995), schizophrenia (Carpenter et al., 2000; Grisso and Appelbaum, 1995; Grisso et al., 1997), major depression (Appelbaum et al., 1999; Grisso and Appelbaum, 1995), HIV (Moser et al., 2002), and Alzheimer's disease (Kim et al., 2001) disease.[14] In this model:

- *Understanding* refers to an individual's ability to comprehend relevant facts. The individual need not be able to apply, believe, or acknowledge that the facts pertain to him or herself. For instance, one might be able to explain that doctors are recommending a specific course of treatment and clearly articulate their rationale, and yet refuse to believe that this rationale applies to one's own case (Appelbaum et al., 1982). The concept of understanding thus has a fairly narrow meaning.
- *Appreciation* is the ability to apply the facts of a situation to oneself.
- *Reasoning* refers to the formal aspects of decision making, such as the ability to compare, make judgments about probability, and think about the consequences of potential actions (Grisso and Appelbaum, 1998). It does not refer to the reasonableness of the content of a belief; rather, the focus is on the process of arriving at a decision.
- *Evidencing a choice* is a minimal, necessary requirement.

When these functional abilities are fully intact, the person's decision-making capability is not in question (Meisel, 1998). When these functional abilities are obviously absent (for example, when a patient is in a catatonic state and unable even to express a preference), the determination of incapacity also is straightforward. The determination is more difficult when decision-making abilities fall somewhere in between. For example, as discussed below, multiple studies using various methodologies have shown that persons with schizophrenia have impairments in the abilities needed for informed consent (Grisso and Appelbaum, 1995; Grisso et al., 1997; Grossman and Summers, 1980). Given such impairment, how do we decide whether individuals are competent to decide for themselves? Two other sets of factors have been identified as influencing the competency determination

---

[14]Although this is the most widely cited model, it is not without its critics (Charland, 1998; Kapp and Mossman, 1996; Saks, 1999; Slobogin, 1996) since what is being attempted is measurement of a fairly abstract and (at least in part) socially constructed concept. Also, while this terminology is that used most frequently, there is some variability in the way these terms are interpreted (Saks and Jeste, 2004).

process: the risk context, and the knowledge and characteristics of those making the judgment about decision-making capacity.

Contextual risk–benefit factors It is widely accepted that decision-making capacity should be measured separately for different types of decisions, rather than inferring a uniform ability or inability to make all decisions on the basis of a specific diagnosis or a generic cognitive screening test (Grisso and Appelbaum, 1998). Thus there are many types of decision-making competencies, such as competence to give informed consent to research, to give informed consent to medical treatment, to make a will, and to manage finances.

It also is widely held that the threshold for finding an individual capable of making a decision (Grisso and Appelbaum, 1998) and/or the criteria used to make such a finding (Appelbaum et al., 1998; Cournos et al., 1993) should vary depending upon the risks and benefits involved (i.e., when the stakes are higher, a higher level of ability is necessary). Although there is some philosophical debate about this risk-related model of competence (Brock, 1991; Cale, 1999; Wicclair, 1991), it is reflected in major policy statements (American Psychiatric Association, 1998; Keyserlingk, 1995; National Bioethics Advisory Commission, 1998; New York Department of Health Advisory Work Group on Human Subject Research Involving the Protected Classes, 1999; Office of the Maryland Attorney General, 1998). Moreover, many clinicians report adhering to this model in practice (Masand et al., 1998; Umapathy et al., 1999). The application of this model has implications for designing and implementing an overall evaluation process, especially when standards for competence are being set. For example, whether a person is capable of participating in a self-directed mental health services program may depend not only on that person's abilities, but also on the extent to which decision-making assistance is provided and safety net practices are in place so that any adverse events are anticipated and procedures exist for their prevention and management.

Characteristics of the competency evaluator Ideally, individuals making judgments about others' decision-making capability would use only objective evidence on the relevant abilities of the subject and information on the risks and benefits of the situation to make such a judgment. However, an evaluator who places greater value on protecting an individual from potential harm may, for any given risk–benefit scenario, require a higher threshold of ability than another evaluator who tends to err on the side of allowing the person to determine his or her own course (Faden and Beauchamp, 1986). Thus, determinations of competency status inevitably involve value judgments (National Bioethics Advisory Commission, 1998; Roth et al., 1977).

Most studies of decision-making capability conducted to date have focused on the abilities of the individual; however, application of the data from these research studies will inevitably involve the contextual and evaluator elements as well. Currently, there is no "gold standard" or algorithm that can be used by competency evaluators to make a final decision about an individual's decision-making capability (Grisso and Appelbaum, 1998).

Decision-Making Abilities of Individuals with and without M/SU Illnesses

Mental illnesses Most research on decision-making capability in mental health has involved persons who might be expected to have the greatest impairments in this capability—those with chronic psychoses such as schizophrenia and schizoaffective disorder. Individuals with less severe illnesses, such as depression, have less often been the subjects of such research; however, findings to date suggest that this lack of research attention may be appropriate. Mild to moderate depression, for example, appears to have little effect on decision-making capability; even inpatients with depression tend to perform quite well on decision-making capacity interviews (Appelbaum et al., 1999; Grisso and Appelbaum, 1995; Stiles et al., 2001; Vollmann et al., 2003). Severe depression without dementia or psychosis also is not associated with severe impairments in decision-making capability (Bean et al., 1994; Lapid et al., 2003).

The findings of research on decision-making capability involving individuals with psychotic symptoms also are encouraging:

• Although as a group, persons with psychotic symptoms exhibit impaired decision-making capability to a greater extent than non–mentally ill individuals, there is considerable heterogeneity within the group.
• Psychotic symptoms have less influence on decision-making capability than do cognitive abilities (i.e., the ability to remember, learn, understand, and reason). In this respect, individuals with severe mental illnesses, such as schizophrenia, that can affect cognition (Goldman-Rakic, 1994) may have much in common with those having other chronic general medical conditions, such as Parkinson's disease, multiple sclerosis, or brain injury, that can impair brain functioning, memory, and cognition, as well as individuals who are otherwise considered healthy but make poor decisions.
• There is substantial evidence that understanding of factual information (even among persons with psychotic symptoms) can be improved through interventions.

Difference in decision-making ability Despite methodological heterogeneity and idiosyncrasies, studies over time consistently have found impaired understanding in persons with schizophrenia as a group (Benson et al., 1988; Grossman and Summers, 1980; Irwin et al., 1985; Munetz and Roth, 1985; Roth et al., 1982; Schacter et al., 1994). The most significant study to date, the MacArthur Treatment Competence Study (Grisso and Appelbaum, 1995), found that persons with schizophrenia performed worse than their normal counterparts on every measure of decision-making ability. Using a psychometrically derived threshold score defined as the bottom 5 percent of the normal controls, about 25 percent of those with schizophrenia failed on any given measure of decision-making ability. Further, 52 percent of those with schizophrenia failed on at least one such measure. Subsequent studies have yielded similar findings (Carpenter et al., 2000; Grisso et al., 1997; Moser et al., 2002; Vollmann et al., 2003). Even when the capacity construct is operationalized very differently, the pattern of group impairment is found (Saks et al., 2002).

Despite this unequivocal evidence for impaired decision-making capability in persons with chronic psychoses as a group, there is tremendous within-group heterogeneity (Palmer et al., 2004). For example, in the MacArthur study of acutely ill psychotic patients with symptoms severe enough for psychiatric inpatient admission, nearly half performed adequately on all the subscales relevant to decision-making capability. This heterogeneity is so great that any policy that ignores it will be either too restrictive or too permissive for large proportions of this population. For example, while it may appear from an intuitive standpoint that patients with obvious and severe psychotic symptoms (e.g., actively hallucinating or delusional) may be readily identified as lacking decision-making capability, this is apparently not the case.

Poor decision-making abilities better predicted by cognitive than by psychotic symptoms Some contemporary models of decision-making capacity suggest that certain cognitive abilities (e.g., memory, information processing, and executive functions) underlie specific tasks involved in decisional capacity (Dymek et al., 2001; Marson and Harrell, 1999; Marson et al., 1996, 1997). Among older persons with schizophrenia, diabetes, or Alzheimer's disease, cognitive impairment has been shown to be a significant predictor of decisional capacity (Palmer et al., 2004); this is the case even within diagnostic groups. Consistent with these findings, research has shown that although patients' decision-making performance is correlated modestly with psychotic symptoms, it is correlated more strongly with cognitive dysfunction (Moser et al., 2002; Palmer et al., 2004; Saks et al., 2002). In total, these findings suggest that decisional incapacity is best conceptualized as a reflection of brain dysfunction resulting in cognitive impairment, rather than as a direct by-product of positive symptoms of psychosis, such as hallucinations and delusions. The lay perception of schizophrenia, defined largely by positive symptoms, thus poorly predicts decision-making incapacity. Decisional capacity is a multidimensional construct reflecting the interaction of a wide range of patient characteristics and contextual/environmental factors.

Ability of interventions to improve decision-making capability The ability to understand the factual elements of informed consent has been shown to be highly responsive to interventions aimed at improving performance (Moser et al., 2002; Stiles et al., 2001; Wirshing et al., 1998; Wong et al., 2000). For example, a comparison of routine informed consent and consent enhanced by an educational session for older, chronically psychotic individuals and normal controls found that although the patient group performed worse than the controls on a comprehension test, the patient group that received education to enhance consent showed comprehension similar to that of the normal group (Dunn et al., 2002). In another study, even those who performed very poorly on an understanding scale tended to improve considerably with a remediation session, to the point where their performance as a group became comparable to that of the normal control group (Carpenter et al., 2000). However, few data exist on the effects of such interventions on other decision-making abilities, such as appreciation and reasoning.

Summary The evidence detailed above shows that it is inappropriate to draw conclusions about individuals' capacity for decision making solely on the basis of whether they are mentally ill, or even whether they have a particular mental illness, such as schizophrenia. Many people with mental illnesses—indeed, many with severe mental illnesses—are not incompetent on most measures of competency. Even among patients hospitalized with schizophrenia, the MacArthur researchers found only 25 percent incompetent on any given measure, and only 50 percent if the measures were aggregated (Grisso and Appelbaum, 1998). Other studies have found a higher proportion of individuals with schizophrenia to be competent in decision making (Saks et al., 2002). The evidence shows that poor decision making has a stronger relationship to cognitive problems (e.g., problems with memory, attention, learning, and thought) and deficiencies in higher-level executive functions than to the symptoms of mental illness, such as psychosis. The minority who experience a decline in such cognitive abilities because of their mental illness may not be very different from individuals who have general medical conditions such as cerebrovascular disease, are under the effects of serious emotional stress or in pain, or generally have lower abilities to understand and analyze information. Simple screening instruments are needed to allow evaluators to determine when a more thorough investigation is warranted, and it may be that such screening is just as appropriate when patients are seriously physically ill as when they are seriously mentally ill.

Effects of substance use on decision making and compulsive behavior Individuals with substance-use problems and illnesses can experience varying degrees of impaired decision making, as well as compulsive behaviors, depending upon a variety of factors, including the substance in use, whether use extends to dependence, and whether the individual is in a state of intoxication or withdrawal. For example, although manifestations of intoxication vary greatly—according to the individual, the substance, the dose, the duration of exposure to the drug, the period of time since the last dose, and other factors—individuals intoxicated from use of any substance are likely to have impaired cognition and judgment, including disturbances of perception, attention, and thinking; mood lability; belligerence; and impaired social functioning. These symptoms may be short-lived or persist for hours or days beyond the time when the substance is detectable in bodily fluids (American Psychiatric Association, 2000).

Apart from these known cognitive and behavioral characteristics of intoxication, decision-making capacity has not been examined as closely in substance-use illnesses as in mental illnesses. This is in part because with substance-related problems and illnesses, there are fewer concerns about decision-making capability in a nonintoxicated state than about the ability to maintain a desired pattern of behavior over time (Hazelton et al., 2003; Rosen and Rosenheck, 1999). For example, although nonintoxicated individuals with substance-use problems or illnesses may perform quite well on a typical interview assessing decision-making capability (unless there are other issues, such as dementia due to substance use), they may still relapse in the face of drug-related cravings and cues in their environment. According to the usual criteria, such persons would be considered to have intact decision-making capability. Indeed, this is the way researchers treat decision-making capability for the purposes of enrolling patients in studies of substance-use problems and illnesses (Gorelick et al., 1999).

However, substance dependence is characterized by compulsive alcohol- and other drug-taking behaviors, even in the face of serious adverse consequences (Hyman and Malenka, 2001). Research designed to shed light on these behaviors has produced findings similar to those for individuals with mental illnesses: although nonintoxicated individuals with substance dependence as a group exhibit problems in decision making, there are great within-group differences in decision-making abilities (Grant et al., 2000). Studies of decision making by individuals dependent upon alcohol, cocaine, or methamphetamines, for example, revealed three different decision-making subgroups. The first did not differ from normal comparison subjects in decision-making abilities. The second performed similarly to people with certain types of brain lesions; they made choices that were insensitive to future consequences and favored short-term rewards, even though this strategy resulted in long-term losses. The third subgroup made choices that offered the promise of high rewards, regardless of short- or long-term consequences, and the presence or prospect of obtaining those rewards dominated their behavior (Bechara and Damasio, 2002; Bechara et al., 2002).

Impaired decision making by individuals not mentally ill or using substances As mentioned above, the absence of an M/SU illness does not necessarily mean that one is unimpaired in decision-making ability. There are many situations that stress mentally healthy people's decision-making capacity. They may be under the sway of a strong emotion, desperate because of bad medical news, physically frail in a way that affects their thinking, under severe stress, or in great pain. Any of those factors, and many others, can affect a mentally healthy person's ability to process medical information and make a competent decision.

In addition, even when not under such stress, mentally healthy people regularly process information in ways that are not completely rational. They overvalue vivid memories, misunderstand probabilities, depart from the laws of logic, and let irrational ideas affect their judgment (Kahneman et al. 1982). Indeed, there is a separate branch of cognitive psychology that identifies such reasoning frailties in much of the population (Garnham and Oakhill, 1994; Connolly et al., 2000). Not surprisingly, variable proportions of "normal" research subjects have been found to have deficits in decision-making capability (Davis et al., 1998; Roth et al., 1982).

In short, *not all*, but also *not only*, individuals with M/SU illnesses are sometimes less than competent in their decision making.

Risk of Dangerousness

As noted above, fear of individuals with severe mental illnesses because of their perceived greater dangerousness is a significant factor in the development of stigma and discrimination (Corrigan et al., 2002; Martin et al., 2000). However, findings of population-based epidemiological and cohort studies show that the vast majority of individuals with a mental illness and no concurrent substance use pose no greater risk of violent behavior than those without M/SU illnesses.[15]

The empirical literature on violence and mental illnesses is copious. Samples and methods differ greatly across studies, making comparisons

---

[15]We focus here on studies of violence in the community because public fears of persons with mental illness typically are based on concerns about the likelihood of their perpetrating violence in the places where most people live and work. A separate literature, not reviewed here, addresses violent behavior by persons with mental illnesses in institutions, which can be a major problem for front-line staff and directly contributes to difficulties in recruitment and retention and to quality-of-care issues in these settings.

difficult and rendering each study susceptible to challenge on one basis or another. The following summary of the data is illustrative of the major studies, rather than exhaustive, and does not attempt a detailed methodological critique.

The first large-scale epidemiological data on the prevalence and incidence of violence (assaultive behavior) among individuals with M/SU illnesses were produced in the early 1980s as a part of the Epidemiological Catchment Area (ECA) study, which was designed primarily to determine the prevalence of untreated psychiatric illnesses in community populations across the United States.[16] A secondary analysis of these data (Swanson, 1994) found that the vast majority of individuals with mental illness who had not qualified for a substance-use or -dependence diagnosis in the past year were not violent. Even among individuals with major mental illnesses (such as schizophrenia) having no co-occurring substance-use diagnosis, the proportion committing an act of violence was only somewhat higher than that in the population without mental illness. Only about 7 percent of those with a major mental illness (but without a substance-use or dependence diagnosis) had engaged in any assaultive behavior in the preceding year, compared with slightly more than 2 percent of individuals without any major psychiatric diagnosis. Individuals with less-severe mental illness were at no greater risk of committing an act of violence than those with no mental illness. Because major mental illness is a relatively rare occurrence, individuals with mental illnesses (but without a substance-use or -dependence diagnosis) account for a very small proportion (about 3–5 percent) of the risk of violence in a community.

Substance-use illnesses by themselves and in combination with major mental illnesses were found to be related more strongly to violence. The ECA study found a 1-year violence prevalence rate of 19.7 percent among respondents with a substance-use or -dependence diagnosis without the presence of a major mental illness, and rate of 22 percent among those with dual mental and substance-use or -dependence diagnoses. Individuals with substance-use or -dependence diagnoses alone represented 26–27 percent of the risk of violence in the community, while those with both diagnoses contributed a much smaller share of the risk (5–6 percent) because of their smaller numbers.[17]

The ECA study also found that the presence of severe M/SU illnesses is only one factor helping explain (and statistically predict) violence. Other

---

[16]The study conducted a series of parallel surveys in New Haven, Baltimore, Saint Louis, Durham, and Los Angeles.

[17]The contribution of any group to overall rates of violence is a function of three factors: the number of individuals in the group, the prevalence of violence within the group, and the size of the group relative to the total population (Swanson, 1994).

factors, such as age, gender, and socioeconomic status, also are associated with violent behavior.

A number of subsequent studies have examined cohorts selected from the general population and followed them at one or more points in time to determine their rates of violence and mental illness. These studies have tended to be performed in countries other than the United States—Denmark (Brennan et al., 2000), Sweden (Hodgins and Janson, 2002), New Zealand (Arsenault et al., 2000), and Finland (Tiihonen et al., 1997)—where comprehensive databases are available. Many of these studies focused on individuals with psychotic illnesses and major depression. All found a link between individuals with these illnesses and violence: persons with these severe illnesses had 2–27 times higher rates of violence, depending on diagnosis and gender, compared with persons without such illnesses. Many of the studies controlled for substance-use diagnoses, socioeconomic status, and other variables likely to inflate rates of violence (Monahan, 1981). However, studies from countries with lower overall rates of violence than the United States, such as the Scandinavian countries where many of these studies were conducted, are likely to show a greater effect of mental illnesses, and hence the results cannot be extrapolated directly to this country (Simpson et al., 2003). In the United States, however, an epidemiological sample in an economically impoverished, largely immigrant neighborhood in New York City (Link et al., 1992) found that a group of current psychiatric outpatients and former psychiatric inpatients had significantly elevated rates of reported violence compared with the never-treated members of the study sample.

In contrast to the above epidemiological and cohort studies, the MacArthur Violence Risk Assessment Study, the largest prospective study to date of a clinical sample (i.e., newly discharged psychiatric inpatients) found that persons with severe mental illnesses were at no greater risk for community violence than nonhospitalized persons in their neighborhoods, as long as they did not have concurrent symptoms of a substance-use diagnosis. However rates of substance-use problems and illnesses were significantly elevated in the patient sample compared with the community comparison group (31.5 percent at the first 10-week follow-up versus 17.5 percent) (Steadman et al., 1998). Other studies that attempted to control for a co-occurring substance-use diagnosis, however, including the ECA analysis, found that its presence did not fully account for the effect of mental illnesses on violence. Further emphasizing the discrepancies in the data, the MacArthur study found that persons with schizophrenia had the lowest violence risk of the major diagnostic categories, whereas several other studies have found schizophrenia to have the strongest relationship with violence (Arsenault et al., 2000; Wessely, 1997). Two studies that followed patients after their first episode of schizophrenia found an increased risk of violence compared with other psychiatric patients (in England [Wessely, 1997]) and compared with a matched sample from the general population (in Australia [Wallace et al., 2004]).

In summary, although findings of many studies suggest a link between mental illnesses and violence, the contribution of people with mental illnesses to overall rates of violence is small. Based on the ECA data, Swanson (1994) and colleagues estimated that roughly 3–5 percent of violence in the United States could be attributed to persons with mental illnesses. Moreover, results of studies from England and New Zealand indicate that in those countries, the percentage of homicides accounted for by persons with major mental illnesses has fallen in recent decades despite policies of deinstitutionalization that have placed more people with severe mental illnesses in the community (Monahan, 1981; Shaw et al., 2004; Taylor and Gunn, 1999). Data also suggest that most violence committed by persons with mental illnesses is directed at family members and friends rather than at strangers (Simpson et al., 2003; Steadman et al., 1998) and tends to occur in the perpetrator's or the victim's residence rather than in public places (Steadman et al, 1998). Indeed, persons without mental illnesses are more likely to attack strangers and to be violent in public (Shaw et al., 2004; Steadman et al., 1998). Thus while there may be a causal relationship between mental illnesses and violence, the magnitude of the relationship is greatly exaggerated in the minds of the general population.

COERCED TREATMENT[18]

Individuals with substance-use illnesses, and to a lesser extent those with mental illnesses, are more likely to be forced or coerced into treatment than are individuals with general medical illnesses.[19] Coerced treatment sometimes occurs as the result of a legal order; sometimes as the result of pressure from other formal organizations, such as employers or social agencies; and at other times through informal pressures exerted by family members or friends. Forms of coercion exist along a continuum, ranging from friendly persuasion, to interpersonal pressure, to control of resources, to force. How individuals perceive this coercion is variable and is influenced by the nature of the coercive process, that is, the extent to

---

[18]In this report, the term "coercion" is not used in its narrow legal sense, but refers to the full range of pressures applied to individuals to secure their participation in treatment, encompassing workplace mandates; criminal justice diversion programs (including drug and mental health courts); and other sources of leverage, such as social programs that require treatment adherence to receive housing, disability, or welfare benefits.

[19]Individuals are also coerced into treatment for general medical conditions, such as tuberculosis, but this occurs less frequently.

which they view those who are coercive as acting out of concern for them, treating them fairly, with respect, and without deception; providing them a chance to tell "their side of the story"; and considering what they have to say about treatment decisions (Dennis and Monahan, 1996). Within the legal system, specialty drug or mental health courts offer individuals with M/SU problems or illnesses the option of treatment as an alternative to criminal processing or sentencing. This and other types of coercion are intended to compensate for poor decision making, compulsive behavior, or a risk of danger to oneself or others. These practices generate great controversy and raise the question of how patient-centered care with the patient as the source of control can and should be provided in their presence.

Coercion and Mental Illnesses

Until relatively recently in the history of the treatment of mental illnesses, coercive interventions were the norm. In the United States, the first statute authorizing voluntary hospitalization of persons with mental illness was not enacted until 1882, and even through the 1960s, the vast majority of psychiatric hospitalizations took place on an involuntary basis. (Voluntary hospitalizations accounted for only 10 percent of admissions in 1949 and 24 percent in 1961 [Brakel, 1985].) Once hospitalized, even voluntarily, patients were assumed to have no right to decide whether to accept the treatment chosen for them. And under provisions for conditional or probationary discharge, many patients in the public system of care could be called back to the hospital at their psychiatrist's discretion (Lindman and McIntyre, 1961).

There are several reasons for this reliance on involuntary hospitalization and treatment, and they relate to the themes discussed earlier. Violence committed by some individuals with mental illnesses led to a general misperception of all such persons as dangerous and thereby in need of confinement. This attitude was compounded by the belief that mental illnesses usually rendered persons incompetent to make decisions for themselves; asking them whether they desired hospitalization or treatment was therefore regarded as pointless. The convenience for caregivers and treaters of making decisions *for* rather than *with* persons with mental illnesses may also have contributed to the use of coercive approaches.

In the 1960s and 1970s, as the rights of underrepresented groups in general received attention, involuntary commitment statutes were narrowed in every state to limit nonconsensual hospitalization to persons who manifested clear dangerousness to themselves or others. Procedures were revamped simultaneously to afford protections, such as judicial hearings and assistance of an attorney, characteristic of the criminal process. By the

1980s, many states—often prompted by judicial decisions—had instituted substantial rights for even involuntarily hospitalized patients to refuse unwanted treatment. A large number of these states required a formal finding of decisional incapacity before a patient's decisions could be overridden (Appelbaum, 1994).

Compared with the situation in 1960, today's mental health system is substantially less coercive. But coercive approaches remain significant features of the system, and as the majority of treatment episodes have shifted to the community, new mechanisms for pressuring or compelling persons with mental illnesses to undergo treatment have evolved (Monahan et al., 2001b). These developments have been motivated by the concerns about impaired decisional capacity and dangerousness described above, as well as by more recent concerns about reducing the burden on the criminal justice system for treating mental illnesses and addressing the needs of untreated persons with severe mental illnesses.

Outpatient commitment is probably the most discussed of the community-based mechanisms for compelling persons with mental illnesses to receive care (Swartz and Monahan, 2001).[20] A majority of states now have statutes permitting commitment to outpatient treatment (Judge David L. Bazelon Center for Mental Health Law, 2000a). Criteria in the newer statutes are typically broader than those for inpatient commitment, often being predicated on the likelihood that without treatment, the person will deteriorate to the point that standards for inpatient commitment will be met. In most statutes, this prediction must be based on a pattern of previous deterioration after release from the hospital. For persons who are found eligible for outpatient commitment, courts can require compliance with a treatment plan, including outpatient visits and medication. Although findings of a number of uncontrolled studies suggest positive effects from outpatient commitment (e.g., reduced rates of hospitalization), the only two controlled studies had methodological problems that rendered their results ambiguous (Appelbaum, 2001).

While outpatient commitment has garnered the most attention, with critics claiming both that it unfairly extends the state's coercive powers and that it would be unnecessary if enough high-quality outpatient services existed (Brown, 2003; Judge David L. Bazelon Center for Mental Health Law, 2000b), less visible approaches can be more coercive and may be more common as well. This is because outpatient commitment statutes are generally without effective enforcement mechanisms. Statutes may allow noncompliant persons to be picked up by the police and brought for evalu-

---

[20]Seclusion and restraint are more intense forms of coercion used in inpatient settings and are addressed in Chapter 4 in a discussion of threats to safe care.

ation to a mental health center, but they generally do not permit involuntary administration of medication or hospitalization unless the usual criteria required for those interventions are met.

The criminal justice system also exercises coercion in several ways. Persons who have been arrested and convicted of an offense can be required by the terms of their probation or parole to participate in treatment of their mental illness, at the risk of being incarcerated if they fail to comply. The extent and effectiveness of this process are essentially unstudied (Skeem et al., 2003). In addition, the last decade has seen the growth of mental health courts in many jurisdictions, modeled on specialty drug courts that are common nationwide (Steadman et al., 2001). Defendants identified as having a mental illness may be given the option of referral to a mental health court prior to or following trial; ongoing compliance with treatment may be required to avoid incarceration. As yet, there is no unitary model for mental health courts, and as with interventions by the probation and parole systems, their effectiveness is unknown (Redlich et al., 2005; Wolff, 2004).

More-informal means of leveraging persons with mental illnesses into treatment also exist but are less visible (Monahan et al., 2001b). These include control of their money by family members or formally appointed representative payees. The latter can be designated by the Social Security Administration to receive payments on behalf of recipients who are believed to be too impaired to manage their money; the Veterans Administration has a similar mechanism. Recent data suggest that formal and informal money managers are common for persons with severe mental illnesses, and that control over a person's finances is often used in an attempt to promote compliance with treatment (Luchins et al., 2003; Monahan et al., 2005; Redlich et al., 2005). Access to housing may similarly be conditioned on treatment involvement, even where laws would appear to preclude such conditions (Monahan et al., 2001b, 2005).

Overall, the degree of coerciveness in the current mental health system may be underestimated and the source of the majority of coercive pressures misidentified. A recent cross-sectional study of the extent to which four types of coercion were experienced by chronically mentally ill individuals receiving mental health services in public-sector settings in five states during 2002–2003 found that across all sites, 44 to 59 percent of individuals experienced at least one of four types of coercion into treatment. Making housing contingent upon compliance was the most frequently used form of leverage (experienced by 23–40 percent of individuals). Other types of leverage and the frequency with which they were encountered across sites were use of criminal sanctions (15–30 percent), outpatient commitment (12–20 percent), and withholding access to money (7–19 percent) (Monahan et al., 2005). Questions remain about both the extent to which such practices are used more broadly and their impact—both positive and negative—on persons subjected to them.

Coercion and Substance-Use Illnesses

The majority of individuals entering treatment for substance-use illnesses do so as a result of coercion (Weisner and Schmidt, 2001). As is the case with mental health care, this coercion takes many forms and can be thought of as ranging along a continuum. Thus coercion ranges from subtle forms, as when an individual acts to please family, friends, or significant others, to more overt forms, such as coercion by an employer through a stated risk of loss of employment, or a situation in which an individual is threatened with the loss of custody of a child or liberty and the establishment of a criminal record, as is the case in the criminal justice system. In the private sector, for example, many clients enter treatment with some degree of coercion from the workplace, either by employers, employee assistance programs, or unions (Polcin and Weisner, 1999; Roman and Blum, 2002; Weisner et al., 2002). These referrals are due to positive drug tests on the job or to alcohol or drugs interfering with job performance. Public benefit programs also exercise coercion. For example, local welfare agencies sometimes exert pressure on individuals with alcohol or drug problems to receive treatment for their substance use in order to maintain their benefits and become ready to work (Capitani et al., 2001).

In addition, most states have mechanisms in place for involuntary civil commitment of individuals with substance-use illnesses and involuntary treatment mechanisms in the criminal justice system (e.g., through drug courts) (Hall and Appelbaum, 2002). Drug courts are increasing in number throughout the country. They focus on criminal behavior related to illicit drugs (rather than alcohol) and are designed to reduce the number of nonviolent substance-using offenders who are incarcerated, as well as potentially to provide better outcomes (Longshore et al., 2005; Marlowe, 2003, Marlow et al., 2004). Drug courts rely upon the identification of substance-use offenders during the pretrial or presentencing period and in return for a guilty plea offer these individuals the option of receiving community-based treatment for their substance use in lieu of incarceration (Belenko, 1999, 2002; Longshore et al., 2005; Marlowe et al., 2004). Successful treatment (completion of a year or more) results in dismissal of the original charges, while failure to complete treatment results in immediate incarceration, since the individual has already pled guilty. In some states, such as California, specific legislation exists to offer treatment for individuals arrested for nonviolent felony offenses related to alcohol or drug use.

Research on the effects of coerced treatment (through the legal system, the workplace, welfare, and informal pressure) for substance-use illnesses has yielded mixed results but on the whole has found higher retention and similar outcomes relative to voluntary clients (Farabee et al., 1998; Lawental et al., 1996). A review of 18 longitudinal studies of the effectiveness of compulsory substance-use treatment published between 1988 and 2001 found that compulsory treatment (legal, formal, informal, and mixed) generally achieved better treatment retention, but no reduction of substance use or criminal behavior (Wild et al., 2002). This same review identified the need for stronger research and analytic models to illuminate the utility of compulsory treatment. Further, agreement needs to be reached on appropriate measures of the outcomes of coerced treatment; these can range from increased attendance at treatment appointments for outpatients; to the absence of illicit drugs in urine/blood; to improved functioning in family, work, and educational roles. Finally, when patients are mandated to treatment, it is not always clear that they are getting the most appropriate treatment, or that they are aware of the consequences of not doing well in treatment. Thus, issues relating to patient-centered care and decision making in health care for both mental and substance-use conditions are important here. When patients make choices between treatment and criminal justice sanctions, it is essential that they be informed about the treatment they will receive, have as much choice in the decision as feasible, and be informed about the "usual" outcomes of that treatment so they can make an informed decision.

Summary

The phenomenon of coercion, like the consequences of stigma and discrimination, has implications for the implementation of the *Quality Chasm* rule of patients being able to "exercise the degree of control they choose over health care decisions that affect them." Despite these difficulties, however, the committee finds that the aim of patient-centered care applies equally to individuals with and without M/SU illnesses. To compensate for the obstacles presented by coercion, as well as those posed by stigma and discrimination, the committee finds that health care clinicians, organizations, insurance plans, accrediting bodies, and federal and state governments will need to undertake specific actions to actively support all M/SU patients' decision-making abilities and preferences, including those of individuals who are coerced into treatment.

ACTIONS TO SUPPORT PATIENT-CENTERED CARE

Our knowledge of how stigma develops, how it affects stigmatized individuals, and how it can be eradicated is incomplete but growing (Corrigan, 2004; Farina, 1998). Many advocacy, governmental, and public service organizations in the United States and elsewhere have used this knowledge to establish campaigns to combat the stigma of M/SU illnesses, usually through the use of one or more of the following strategies: (1) educating the public about M/SU illnesses; (2) creating opportunities for the public to have contact with individuals with these illnesses; (3) protesting against erroneous, stereotyped portrayal of these individuals by the media[21]; and (4) pursuing legal action to guarantee rights to health care, housing, employment, and other justice-related concerns (Corrigan and Penn, 1999; Smith, 2002). These initiatives include those of SAMHSA's Resource Center to Address Discrimination and Stigma (SAMHSA, 2000); SAMHSA's National Addiction Technology Transfer Centers Network initiative to develop and disseminate a training module on stigma for treatment providers, and to collect and distribute research-based information on fighting the stigma of drug and alcohol dependence (Woll, 2001); Faces & Voices of Recovery, a national recovery advocacy campaign and organization that promotes public policies and actions to end discrimination against individuals with substance-use illnesses[22]; the National Alliance for the Mentally Ill's (NAMI) "In Our Own Voices" and "StigmaBusters" initiatives; the National Institute of Mental Health's (NIMH) Outreach Partnership Program (NIMH, 2005); and the efforts of many other consumer and advocacy organizations, such as the National Mental Health Association and the National Council on Alcoholism and Drug Dependence, that fight stigma by using a combination of the above strategies. Some consumers report that becoming involved in these initiatives helps them cope with the adverse effects of stigma and develop feelings of self-empowerment and self-enhancement (Wahl, 1999).

The committee applauds and supports the continuation of these campaigns. However, national, state, and local initiatives to eliminate stigma and discrimination often are targeted at changing the attitudes of society at large. Research has shown that public attitudes are not the sole determinant of behaviors; behaviors are also influenced by a number of personal and situational features present in the interactions of stigmatized individuals with others. Thus, to combat the effects of stigma on patient-centered care, additional actions are required of (1) health care organizations and clinicians providing treatment services; (2) insurance plans that shape patient–provider relationships; and (3) public policy makers and quality oversight organizations, who are able to address other situational conditions that

---

[21]There is less empirical evidence in support of protest as an effective mechanism for reducing stigma than is the case for the other three strategies (Corrigan and Penn, 1999; Corrigan et al., 2001).

[22]Pat Taylor, Faces & Voices of Recovery, e-mail communication, October 11, 2004.

foster and permit stigmatizing attitudes and behaviors at the locus of care delivery.

Combating Stigma and Supporting Decision Making at the Locus of Care Delivery

Health care clinicians, organizations, insurance plans, accrediting organizations, and government bodies can counter the adverse effects of stigma on patient-centered M/SU health care by taking several concrete actions. These include (1) endorsing and supporting decision making by M/SU health care consumers as the default policy in their organizational polices and practices; (2) involving M/SU health care consumers in service design, administration, and delivery; (3) providing decision-making support to all M/SU health care consumers, including those under coercion and making decisions about diversion programs; and (4) supporting illness self-management *practices* for all consumers and formal self-management *programs* for individuals with chronic illnesses.

Endorsing and Supporting Consumer Decision Making in Organizational Polices and Practices

All organizations have cultures, defined as the dominant and commonly held beliefs, attitudes, values, and behaviors that shape organizational goals, policies, and procedures (Schein, 1992). In health care, the effect of an organization's beliefs, attitudes, values, and behaviors on the practices of its individual members is so widely accepted that substantial analysis and tool development have taken place to help organizations create, for example, "cultures of safety" (Bagian and Gosbee, 2000; Wong et al., 2002). Desired cultures can be consciously built and objectively assessed. Recently, for example, the Agency for Healthcare Research and Quality (AHRQ) developed a survey instrument for use by hospitals in assessing the extent to which they have been effective in creating an internal culture of safety (AHRQ, 2005). Organizations similarly can create cultures that endorse and support consumer decision making through their leadership and formal policies, and through employee education in the adverse effects of stigma and the capabilities of M/SU consumers to engage in decision making.

Leadership and policy practices Effective leadership within an organization is essential to achieving cultural change (Davenport et al., 1998; Heifetz and Laurie, 2001). If patient-centered care is to be provided and decision making by consumers of M/SU services is to be ensured, leaders within treatment organizations must see that their organizational culture actively supports these practices. Organizational leaders can take many different actions to create such a culture. First, organizational managers and leaders can demonstrate behaviors that recognize and support consumer decision making in their interactions with other organizational employees. As noted above, each patient's right to make treatment decisions and receive support in doing so should be clinicians' and organizations' default policy unless there is evidence of a danger to the patient or others, or the patient has been determined to be incompetent to make decisions. Organizations' formal, written policy documents, such as mission statements and policies and procedures manuals, can explicitly endorse and specify this default policy and other organizational actions to support consumer decision making. If the organization has a consumer bill of rights, it can include content on consumer decision making. The orientation of new providers and ongoing training of existing providers also should include content on the adverse effects of stigma on patients' self-efficacy and recovery, and reaffirm organizational polices and practices that support patient decision making.

Continuing education of clinicians and other service personnel Because it is not reasonable to expect that all clinicians (especially those newly licensed) will come to their practice settings possessing all of the necessary knowledge and skills, organizations need to provide for their clinicians' ongoing training (IOM, 2004b) and education (see Chapter 7). Education has been shown to decrease stigma and improve clinicians' attitudes regarding persons with mental illnesses (Corrigan and Penn, 1999; Farina, 1998). Empirical evidence also indicates that having credible and competent leaders deliver this education is important if some of these messages (e.g., those related to stigma) are to be taken up by learners (Corrigan et al., 2001). The education and training provided should include, for example, content on patient-centered care and decision making, erroneous beliefs about dangerousness, and the clinician's and the organization's need to tolerate "bad" choices and achieve the right balance between "beneficence" and autonomy (Murdach, 1996).

Tolerance for "bad" decisions[23] The *Quality Chasm* report (IOM, 2001) notes that among all consumers, there can at times be a tension between the aim of providing patient-centered care and that of providing effective (evidence–based) care. For example, a patient may have received information on and desire to receive a particular type of treatment, but the provider

---

[23]The discussion in this section incorporates content from the paper "Patient-Centered Care/Self-Directed Care: Legal, Policy and Programmatic Considerations," prepared for the committee by Susan Stefan of the Center for Public Representation.

may know that evidence of the treatment's effectiveness is lacking or incon-
clusive, or has shown the treatment to be ineffective. The provider may have
evidence that an alternative treatment may be more or equally effective at
lower cost. The *Quality Chasm* report notes that in such instances, health
care institutions, clinicians, and patients need to work together to reconcile
competing and conflicting aims through *shared* decision making.

A more difficult situation exists when patients, particularly individuals
with severe mental illnesses, propose a course of action that their mental
health professional believes to be misguided. Without guidance in such
situations, clinicians may react in ways that may reflect their own values
more than the patient's, and thereby undermine patient-centered care. For
example, some clinicians may believe that the apparent irrationality of a
patient's treatment decision raises questions about the individual's competence to make such decisions, and use this to justify excluding the patient
from decision making about his or her care. Others may formally respect
their patient's autonomy and decision making but do so in a way that
distances them from the patient and his or her decisions. For example,
when a patient disagrees with a mental health professional about the course
of treatment, the professional may "respect" the patient's decision but
formally or informally withdraw from the treatment partnership. Patient
decision making is preserved, but the treatment relationship is weakened,
and the patient has in effect been punished for disagreeing with the mental
health professional (Stefan, 2004).

In contrast, in her autobiographical book *An Unquiet Mind*, Kay Red-
field Jamison paints a vivid portrait of patient-centered care as she describes
her relationship with her psychiatrist, who remained steadfast through her
many disagreements with his recommendations that she take lithium for
her bipolar illness. While Jamison does not represent a "typical" patient,
her concerns, her reluctance to pursue a recommended course of treatment,
and the concomitant risks are not unusual. Moreover, the manner in which
she was involved in decision making is a strong example of patient-centered
care.

Jamison explains that over a 1-year period, she started and stopped
taking lithium multiple times:

> . . . I still somehow thought that I ought to be able to carry on without
> drugs, that I ought to be able to continue to do things my own way. My
> psychiatrist, who took all of these complaints very seriously—existential
> qualms, side effects, matters of value from upbringing—never wavered in
> his conviction that I needed to take lithium. . . . (Jamison, 1995:102)

Her psychiatrist stayed with her, recording her decisions and their
consequences and continuing his attempts to help her. He never took steps

to commit her involuntarily[24] or medicate her against her will, although her "depressions were getting worse and far more suicidal" (p. 103). Jamison eventually decided that she needed to take lithium and, because she had made the decision herself after struggling with it, has continued to do so despite experiencing adverse effects. Her psychiatrist discussed and persuaded but did not coerce. Instead, he listened to, respected, and responded to her concerns, exemplifying being "respectful of and responsive to individual patient preferences, needs, and values and ensuring that patient values guide all clinical decisions" (IOM, 2001:40).

Jamison's experience can be contrasted with that of a patient involved in the research of the MacArthur Research Network on Mental Health and the Law on coercion. That experience illustrates the opposite of Jamison's—the absence of patient-centeredness:

> I talked to him [the therapist who had arranged for his commitment] this morning. I said, "You . . . didn't even listen to me. You . . . call yourself a counselor. . . . Why did you decide to do this instead of . . . try to listen to me and understand . . . what I was going through." And he said, "Well, it doesn't matter, you know, you're going anyway." He didn't listen to what I had to say. . . . He didn't listen to the situation. . . . He had decided before he ever got to the house . . . that I was coming up here. Either I come freely or the officers would have to subdue me and bring me in. (Bennett et al., 1993:298)

It is important to be clear about what patient-centered care does and does not mean. Patient-centered care does not mean that professionals must agree with all of the patient's decisions. Nor does it mean that a provider should abandon a patient if the patient's decisions disagree with the provider's own. A Michigan policy on self-directed care explicitly provides that "self-determination shall not serve as a method for a [community mental health support program] to reduce its obligations to the consumer, or to avoid the provision of needed specialty mental health services or supports" (Michigan Department of Community Health, 2003). Patient-centered care does involve supporting the patient through disagreements about treatment decisions, asking about the patient's goals for recovery, and factoring these into shared decision making for the recovery process.

Taking these and other actions to endorse and support the primacy of consumer decision making in treatment polices and practices lays the groundwork for implementing three additional practices that can support

---

[24]This may have been influenced in part by his stated belief that she could not be involuntarily committed under the state's laws (Jamison, 1995).

consumer decision making more directly: (1) involving M/SU health care consumers in service design, administration, and delivery; (2) providing decision-making support to all M/SU health care consumers; and (3) supporting illness self-management *practices* for all consumers and formal self-management *programs* for individuals with chronic illnesses.

Involving Consumers in Service Design, Administration, and Delivery

Contact with individuals with mental illnesses improves health care workers' attitudes toward them and decreases negative stereotyping (Corrigan et al., 2001; Kolodziej and Johnson, 1996), including erroneous perceptions of dangerousness (Corrigan et al., 2002; Farina, 1998). The same is true for the public at large (Rasinski, 2003). Contact is most effective in countering erroneous beliefs and stigma when participants have equal status, interact in a highly collaborative manner, have personal rather than formal interactions, and have support from the institution in which the contact occurs (Corrigan and Penn, 1999; Kolodziej and Johnson, 1996). Equal status is facilitated when individuals work together on specified activities giving those in a stigmatized group the opportunity to apply and demonstrate their own knowledge and skills. Such contact can be achieved by involving individuals with M/SU illnesses in administrative, clinical care delivery, and policy-making roles.

Consumer participation in service design and administration Consumers have served in key administrative and service design roles in a number of M/SU health care organizations. For example, they have served on key policy-making bodies that plan, design, and oversee internal performance measurement and quality improvement (Hibbard, 2003; Sabin and Daniels, 1999, 2001), and that design and implement mechanisms for soliciting consumer feedback on the quality of delivered services (Sabin and Daniels, 1999). Serving on bodies that develop and oversee utilization management policies (when the care-providing organization is also a health plan) is another way for consumers to participate in service design and administration (Sabin et al., 2001). These mechanisms for direct involvement in service design and administration are more effective in reducing stigma than simply having consumers serve on separate advisory councils because they provide opportunities for consumers to work side by side with care providers in a collaborative manner.

Consumers as service providers People with M/SU illnesses have for many years served as providers of treatment and recovery support services by leading and participating in self-help or mutual help groups such as Alcoholics Anonymous (Humphreys et al., 2004); serving as case managers, counselors, crisis workers, job coaches, and residential managers; and providing care in a variety of other positions supporting psychiatric rehabilitation and recovery (Kaskutas and Ammon, 2003–2004; Mowbray et al., 1997; Solomon and Draine, 2001). These positions range from those that are unpaid, to those that are paid but created or set aside exclusively for consumers (available only to people with mental illnesses), to those that are paid and competitive (available to consumers and nonconsumers) (Cook, 2004).

Consumers also serve as providers in peer support programs that help individuals with severe M/SU illnesses achieve recovery. Georgia's Peer Support program, for example, employs individuals who (1) are current or former recipients of mental health services for a major mental illness, (2) openly identify themselves as consumers, (3) have had advocacy or advisory experience, (4) have made a demonstrated effort at self-directed mental health recovery, and (5) have successfully passed a written and oral examination after completing a 2-week training program. The Georgia Division of Mental Health, Developmental Disabilities, and Addictive Diseases trains and certifies these peer specialists to model competence and recovery by providing (under the direct supervision of a mental health professional) structured, scheduled activities that promote socialization, recovery, self-advocacy, development of natural supports, and maintenance of community living skills to individuals with "serious and persistent" mental illnesses. Their primary responsibility is to assist consumers in regaining control over their recovery process and developing the attitudes and skills that facilitate recovery. They do this through a variety of activities ranging from helping consumers create a wellness recovery action plan, to supporting consumers in their vocational choices, to informing them about community and other supports and how to utilize them in the recovery process (Sabin and Daniels, 2003).

SAMHSA's Recovery Community Services Program similarly uses peer support to help consumers of substance-use treatment services prevent relapse, promote timely reentry into treatment when relapse occurs, and aid in achieving sustained recovery and an enhanced quality of life. Grants made through this program support peer-to-peer recovery assistance, including help in securing housing, education, and employment; building constructive family and other personal relationships; managing stress; participating in alcohol- and other drug-free social and recreational activities; and obtaining services from multiple systems, such as the primary and mental health care, child welfare, and criminal justice systems (SAMHSA, 2004a).

Peer support programs are discussed further below as an important mechanism for increasing consumers' self-efficacy beliefs and decision-making capabilities.

Providing Decision-Making Support to All M/SU Health Care Consumers

Supporting consumer decision making means providing consumers with (1) a choice of treatments and providers; (2) information about the benefits and risks of different treatment options; (3) assistance in making choices; and (4) for those individuals with significantly impaired cognition or diminished self-efficacy beliefs, compensatory mechanisms such as peer support programs and advance directives.

Providing consumers with real choices Decision making is less relevant if the only choice presented is that between one treatment and no treatment. As evidence presented in Chapter 5 shows, there may be multiple different therapeutic approaches for a given M/SU illness—different medications, medication alone without psychotherapy, psychotherapy alone without medication, and medication combined with psychotherapy (frequently shown to be most effective). Some of these approaches have more proven effectiveness than others; others may have less evidence to support their effectiveness but offer the promise of fewer side effects. Because of this and other factors, patient preferences are likely to differ. The *Quality Chasm* report notes, for example, that among all patients, some people are "risk averse," while others may choose a riskier intervention despite a lesser likelihood of benefit.[25] Moreover, patients with more chronic medical conditions often have been shown to be more willing to take risks in the hopes of achieving better health. Their preferences also have been shown to be motivated in part by a concern for social health (defined as the ability to develop, maintain, and nurture major social relations), not solely by a desire for physical or mental health (Sherbourne et al., 1999).

When consumers are coerced into treatment or have no choice of provider, offering them a choice of treatment is especially important. In general, few inpatients—whether voluntarily or involuntarily admitted—choose the psychiatrist, therapist, or nurse who is assigned to their care. A similar situation occurs for the many individuals who receive care in a clinic setting. In these inpatient and outpatient settings, individuals receive care from the providers scheduled to provide care on that day. For patients receiving care from a specialized team (e.g., an assertive community treatment [ACT] team), there is typically only one team available. With respect to choice of treatments, rules for involuntary treatment of committed patients vary across states, with some states (but not all) precluding involuntary treatment with medications unless patients are first declared incompetent to make decisions about their care. Whatever rule is in effect, and regardless

---

[25]The report further notes that patient preferences are likely to change over time and as a consequence of the issues at hand.

of whether patients are able to choose their providers, individuals can still exercise choice by selecting among different treatment approaches, medications, and strategies for treating and recovering from their illness. Patients should be supported in expressing their treatment preferences and having them incorporated into treatment decision making. Supporting decision making and treatment preferences requires that patients have information on the various treatment options available.

Providing information about the benefits and risks of different treatment options Information needs to be available to consumers to support their decision making and to promote their exercise of choice. Clinicians and their sponsoring health care organizations should provide patients with information (in a user-friendly format) about the comparative effectiveness of different treatment approaches (regardless of whether those approaches are offered by the clinician or health care organization) and any risks/contraindications/side effects that may be present given the patient's clinical profile. When information on the comparative effectiveness of different treatment approaches is not available (see the discussion of the limited evidence base in Chapter 4), this lack of information should be made known to the consumer. Patients should also be given information on whether a specific therapeutic approach is available from their clinician, organization, or health plan.

Providing decision support to all patients It is widely acknowledged that all clinicians need support in their clinical decision making to stay abreast of recent developments in therapeutics. If patient are truly to share in clinical decision making, it is likely that they, too, will need information to support that decision making. However, decision-support tools are just beginning to be used in general health care to help consumers select among different treatment options for a limited number of medical conditions, for example, problems with vision or specific diseases such as benign prostatic hypertrophy (Stanton, 2002). Consumers of M/SU health care services also need such decision-support tools, although their availability is currently very limited.

In the interim, clinicians and health care organizations can support all M/SU consumers in their decision making by (1) providing them with the information described above (in a user-friendly format); (2) avoiding undermining their decision-making abilities (verbal support is effective in increasing individuals' belief in their ability to make treatment decisions, or their self-efficacy; see the discussion earlier in this chapter [Bandura, 1997b]); and (3) appreciating the changing nature of consumers' decision-making preferences. The *Quality Chasm* report, for example, underscores that shared decision making is a dynamic process that changes as patients' circumstances and preferences change. As evidence presented in the preceding section indicates, decision-making capacity appears to be less a fixed, unchangeable trait and more a state dependent on a variety of factors. The capacity for decision making should therefore be viewed not as an all-or-nothing state, but as the result of the interplay of multiple functional abilities that can vary according to the context and over time. For example, a person may understand a consent form one day but not the next when he or she is distracted, confused, under duress, in pain, or delirious. Similarly, a person may be impaired in the acute phases of a severe mental illness, such as schizophrenia or bipolar illness, but may return to normal when in remission. The *Quality Chasm* report also acknowledges that patients vary in their preferences and views about how active they want to be in decision making: some patients desire a very active role, while others may prefer to delegate decision making to their providers or a proxy.

Providing stronger decision support mechanisms for individuals with significantly impaired cognition or diminished self-efficacy beliefs Peer support services and advance directives can be used to assist individuals with significantly impaired cognition or diminished self-efficacy beliefs.

Peer support programs As noted earlier in this chapter, evidence shows that individuals' belief in their self-efficacy can be increased through four mechanisms: (1) their own success in mastering a task or activity, (2) observation of others' success in the same area, (3) verbal persuasion and social influences, and (4) individuals' own physiological and affective states. Vicarious experience is particularly powerful when the observer can identify with some of the characteristics of the person performing the activity. Observing the successes of a model with whom one identifies enhances one's belief in one's own capabilities. Empowerment and belief in one's self-efficacy are also influenced by the verbal encouragement of others (Bandura, 1997b).

The positive effects of seeing or visualizing people similar to oneself successfully perform specific activities are proportionate to the degree of similarity between the person performing the activities and the observer. Modeling that conveys effective coping strategies by individuals who begin timorously, but who gradually overcome their difficulties through persistent efforts can be more helpful than "masterful" models, that is, individuals who perform calmly and faultlessly. Observers are persuaded that if others can do it, they can too (conversely, observing the failures of others similar to themselves decreases the self-efficacy beliefs of observers) (Bandura, 1997b).

Peer support programs involve individuals who serve as models of self-efficacy. These programs provide verbal persuasion and social influences, as well as the opportunity to observe others' success in facing the same challenges. Peer leadership has been found to be a key component of successful self-management programs (Lorig et al., 2001). Peer support programs also are identified in the Chronic Care Model of illness management (described in Chapter 5) as a useful mechanism for supporting patients in their illness self-management (Bodenheimer et al., 2002b). Studies of illness self-management programs have shown that when peers are well trained and given a detailed protocol, they teach as well as and possibly better than health professionals (Lorig and Holman, 2003).

Peer support programs are a strong component of mental health care, as described above. Peer-based support services in recovery from substance-use problems and illnesses have an even longer history, extending from the eighteenth century to the present and encompassing Native American "recovery circles"; fraternal temperance societies; and social support provided within inebriate homes and asylums, half-way houses, and self-managed recovery homes (White, 2002, 2004). Twelve-step mutual support groups such as Alcoholics Anonymous (AA), Narcotics Anonymous (NA), and Cocaine Anonymous (CA) are used as a routine adjunct to treatment and are relied on as a form of long-term aftercare for many alcohol and drug treatment programs today (McElrath, 1997; Troyer et al., 1995). The efficacy or effectiveness of the largest addiction-oriented mutual aid/self-help group, AA, has been the focus of increased research and several reviews in recent years (e.g., Emrick et al., 1993; Kaskutas et al., 2003; Kelly et al., 2002; Tonigan and Toscova, 1996). This work has documented correlational evidence of a relationship between AA attendance and, more strongly, AA "involvement" (e.g., having a sponsor, being a sponsor, working the steps) and positive drinking-related outcomes. In addition, participation in self-help groups has been associated with lower subsequent health care costs (Humphreys and Moos, 1996, 2001).

Advance directives[26,27] Psychiatric advance directives, like advance directives used in general health care, are intended to preserve consumers' ability to engage in self-direction during times when their decision-making capacity or ability to communicate their preferences might be impaired. Psychiatric *instructional* directives typically address such issues as preferred medications, treatments, service providers and locations, and who is to be notified about hospitalizations and allowed to visit. Psychiatric *proxy* di-

---

[26]Advance directives for mental health care are legally executed documents stating an individual's preferences regarding various aspects of psychiatric treatment in times of crisis, inpatient care, or otherwise impaired decision making.

[27]Information in this section incorporates content from the commissioned paper "'Patient-Centered' and 'Consumer-Directed' Mental Health Services" by Judith A. Cook, PhD, Professor and Director, Center on Mental Health Services Research and Policy, University of Illinois at Chicago.

rectives (sometimes combined with instructional directives) allow people to designate someone to make treatment decisions on their behalf (Srebnik and La Fond, 1999). Allowing individuals to state their treatment preferences ahead of time increases the likelihood that care during times of psychiatric crisis and/or lack of decision-making competency will reflect their values and preferences. A number of approaches to preparing mental health advance directives have been developed, including completion of paper-and-pencil checklists, use of templates available on the Internet, and use of an interactive CD-ROM on a computer. Duke University's Program on Advance Psychiatric Directives provides tool kits and user-friendly instructions for consumers, clinicians, and family members to use in completing psychiatric advance directives (Cook, 2004).

Although there is much interest in advance directives for mental health care, few people with mental illnesses create such directives or find them honored in times of crisis. The reasons for failing to honor an advance directive include lack of provider awareness of the directive; concerns about an individual's competency at the time the directive was prepared; written directives that are unclear; poor communication with proxies about treatment preferences; limited availability of desired services in many communities; revocation issues, such as who can revoke a directive and under what circumstances; and legal and ethical issues involved in implementing directives that physicians disagree with or perceive as harmful to the individual (Cook, 2004). Moreover, although this option appears sensible and potentially applicable within the substance-use treatment field, there are as yet no published studies of its use in this field, and very few treatment programs have employed this approach with alcohol- or drug-dependent patients.

Several evaluation studies have found psychiatric advance directives to be feasible for use (with support) by individuals with severe and chronic mental illnesses (Peto et al., 2004; Sherman, 1998; Srebnik et al., 2004). Use of such directives is also perceived positively by consumers and associated with decreased feelings of coercion and increased perception of having a choice in their treatment decisions (Srebnik et al., 2004; Sutherby et al., 1999). Psychiatric advance directives, like advance directives for general medical conditions, can help ensure patient-centered care in times of diminished medical decision-making capacity (Backlar et al., 2001; Swanson et al., 2000).

Supporting Illness Self-Management Practices and Programs

The evidence reviewed earlier in this chapter shows the value of patients' self-management of their illnesses. However, it is important to underscore that successful self-management programs go far beyond traditional patient education programs by requiring teaching, supporting, and working closely with patients. Also, as cited earlier in this chapter, expert designers and researchers on these programs caution that many programs calling themselves self-management programs do not teach all the core skills involved and fail to address the necessary scope of issues (Lorig and Holman, 2003). Self-management support is defined as the "systematic provision of education *and supportive interventions* to increase patients' skills and confidence in managing their health problems, including regular assessment of progress and problems, goal setting, and problem-solving support" (IOM, 2003:52 [emphasis added]). Whereas traditional patient education offers technical information and skills training (typically in areas defined by the clinician), self-management education supports patients in identifying their problems and provides techniques to help them make decisions, take appropriate actions, and modify these plans as circumstances or the course of their illness changes. Patient self-management thus requires that a clinician utilize a collaborative model of practice in which the patient and clinician are equal partners, with equal expertise (Bodenheimer et al., 2002a). Whereas the clinician brings expertise in the illness and therapeutics, patients are experts in their own lives and in what concerns them and motivates and enables them to make changes in their lives. This model is the basis for a collaborative process between the health care provider and patient in which attainable, short-term goals are identified by the patient, discussed jointly, and agreed upon.

Several approaches have been developed in recent years to support individuals' self-management. One example, the Wellness Recovery Action Plan (WRAP), is a structured approach designed to help individuals with mental illnesses identify internal and external resources for facilitating recovery, and then use these tools to create a plan for successful living (Copeland, 2002). Creating a WRAP plan generally begins with development of a personal Wellness Toolbox, consisting of simple, safe, and (usually) free self-management strategies such as a healthy diet, exercise, good sleep patterns, and pursuit of adult life roles. The person then uses this toolbox to create an individualized plan for using each strategy to attain and/or maintain recovery. The plan also includes identification of early warning signs of symptom exacerbations or crisis, and ways in which the toolbox can help people manage and feel better. In addition, WRAP encourages development of a crisis plan, which states how the person would like to be treated in times of crisis (similar to an advance directive), as well as a postcrisis plan for getting back on the road to recovery.

Patient self-management of chronic illness also has become one of the pillars of the Chronic Care Model, reflecting recognition of the fact that for chronic illnesses, patients themselves are their principal caregivers—

assuming such responsibilities as regulation of diet and exercise, self-measurement of laboratory values (e.g., blood glucose levels), and medication use. The Chronic Care Model helps patients and their families develop the skills and confidence to manage their chronic illness, providing self-management tools (e.g., symptom-monitoring flow charts, diets) and routinely assessing the patient's and family's problems and accomplishments in illness management (Bodenheimer et al., 2002b). Components of the Chronic Care Model have been applied successfully to the treatment of depression (Badamgarev et al., 2003; Gilbody et al., 2003; Pincus et al., 2003), and the model has been identified as having potential applicability to the care of persons with chronic substance-use illnesses as well (Watkins et al., 2003).

Eliminating Discriminatory Legal and Administrative Policies

In addition to the practices recommended above to be undertaken at the locus of care, public policy needs to be aligned to support patient-centered care. One very important policy change needed is ending insurance discrimination. Restrictions on access to student loans and the potential lifetime ban on receipt of food stamps or welfare (discussed earlier in this chapter) also need to be reexamined to determine whether their success in deterring drug use or achieving other purposes outweighs the obstacles they pose to the recovery of individuals with substance-use illnesses.

Attention needs to be paid as well to how coerced treatment is used for individuals with M/SU illnesses. Although the use of coercion is somewhat different for mental and substance-use illnesses, it is likely to continue for the foreseeable future for many individuals with substance-use illnesses, as well as for a minority of individuals with mental illnesses. For this reason, it is important that policies governing the use of coercion (1) reduce the risk of its use in situations in which it is not needed by making transparent the policies and practices used to assess decision-making capacity and dangerousness; (2) preserve as much patient decision making as possible whenever coercion is used, in part by providing comparative information on treatment and providers; and (3) minimize the risks associated with coerced treatment. Research also is needed to better understand the need for, appropriate use of, and outcomes of coercive practices for treatment of M/SU illnesses. Moreover, coercion can sometimes be avoided altogether. In a study of inpatient psychiatric admissions in two states, many individuals who experienced involuntary legal commitment reported that they were not offered the opportunity to enter the hospital voluntarily, and more than half indicated that they would have entered voluntarily had the offer been made (Hoge et al., 1997).

Transparent Policies and Practices for Assessing Decision-Making Capacity and Dangerousness

As previously discussed, the source of coercion into treatment for M/SU illnesses can be either informal (e.g., family and friends) or formal or governmental (e.g., mandatory outpatient treatment for individuals with mental illnesses because of a perceived danger to themselves or others, or criminal justice diversion programs such as drug courts for individuals with substance-use illnesses). Moreover, pressure for treatment can be expressed in both positive (persuasion or inducements) or negative (threats or force) forms. Evidence shows that threats and force lead to high levels of perceived coercion relative to persuasion and inducement. For this reason, positive pressure, such as persuasion, should be the strategy of choice to get people to accept treatment. Negative approaches should be used in emergencies or when all other options have failed (Dennis and Monahan, 1996).

With respect to involuntary commitment or treatment for mental illness or other governmentally imposed treatment for substance use, carefully crafted criteria for applying governmentally imposed coercion and due process protections would help minimize the risk that involuntary treatment mechanisms will be used to serve other than therapeutic ends (Hall and Appelbaum, 2002). However, application of even the best-crafted criteria is hampered by the lack of standardization in the approaches used by evaluators and the courts to determine both decision-making capacity and the risk of violence for individuals with mental illnesses. Variation is due both to infrequent (though growing) reliance on standardized assessment measures and to a lack of consensus on the relevant normative questions. These normative questions include (1) how much impairment of decision making is tolerable, or at what level of impaired decision making it is appropriate to override a patient's preference to avoid treatment; and (2) how much risk of violence should be tolerated before a person is confined for treatment or other coercive interventions are undertaken. These questions cannot be answered solely by empirical research because they involve identifying and reaching agreement on matters of values. As noted in the previous discussion of decision making, for example, decisions about a person's competency status inevitably involve the value judgments of the individual performing the evaluation (National Bioethics Advisory Commission, 1998; Roth et al., 1977). For this reason, some recommend that these judgments be made by a group of individuals from diverse backgrounds (Saks and Jeste, 2004).

Until more standardized instruments with better normative data and consensus on standards and processes for making such a determination are available, following the *Quality Chasm's* rule of transparency could help minimize the risk that coerced treatment will be used for other than thera-peutic purposes or for protection of the public, as well as help establish a normative database to guide decision making in this area. The rule of transparency states:

> The health care system should make information available to patients and their families that allows them to make informed decisions when selecting a health plan, hospital, or clinical practice, or choosing among alternative treatments. This should include information describing the system's per-formance on safety, evidence-based practice, and patient satisfaction. (IOM, 2001:8)

In M/SU health care, the health care "system" encompasses other soci-etal systems that are not as strongly involved in the delivery of general health care—the criminal and juvenile justice, education, and child welfare systems. The health care delivered under the auspices of these systems and the policies that influence the delivery of that care also must be transparent to clients, their families, and the public at large so that individuals in need of care, their families, and society can make informed decisions about when and how coerced treatment is to be used. Policies and practices not only for initiating coercive treatment, but also for terminating it should be transpar-ent, providing information on what one has to do to be discharged from involuntary inpatient or outpatient treatment or to have one's status changed to voluntary. Moreover, documenting the tools and approaches used in the judicial system to arrive at decisions to invoke mandatory outpatient treatment would be of help in developing the normative data-base needed to provide better guidance to individuals charged with making these decisions.

Preserving Patient-Centered Care and Patient Decision Making in Coerced Treatment

As previously discussed, the ways in which individuals perceive coer-cion vary and are influenced by the nature of the coercive process—the extent to which patients perceive those who are coercive as acting out of concern for them; treating them fairly, with respect, and without deception; giving them a chance to tell "their side of the story"; and considering what they have to say about treatment decisions (Dennis and Monahan, 1996). In all circumstances then, but especially when negative pressures are being used, patients need to be afforded "as much process as possible." Further, individuals who are coerced into treatment should still be involved in deci-sion making about the types of treatment to be used for their illness and in the choice of provider.

Minimizing Risks in Involuntary Treatment

As evidence in Chapter 4 shows, treatment itself is not without risks. These risks can result from errors in care as well as from the delivery of ineffective care. As discussed earlier, while unsafe and ineffective care permeates all of health care, individuals with M/SU illnesses may be especially at risk for errors and vulnerable to their effects. This is the case because the symptoms of some severe M/SU illnesses, such as major depression or schizophrenia, when not alleviated by therapy, may decrease patients' ability to be involved in the management of their care and therefore to detect and report errors in their care. Moreover, the stigma attached to individuals with M/SU illnesses may render them less likely to be believed when reporting information about errors and adverse events. These risks may be multiplied for an individual who has been committed involuntarily to inpatient or outpatient mental health treatment or coerced into treatment for substance use. When the patient's autonomy and treatment preferences are superseded, it is critically important that those responsible for making treatment decisions use comparative information on provider and treatment safety and effectiveness and continue to involve the patient in selecting and evaluating treatment alternatives.

Ensuring safe and effective care and preserving patient decision making can be accomplished by providing patients and their family members or other proxy decision makers with information about the illness to be treated; the range of available, evidence-based treatments for the illness and evidence on their relative effectiveness; and comparative information on the performance of individual providers and organizations in treating the illness (see Chapter 4).

Needed Research

More research is needed on how best to minimize the use of coercion and how to use it most effectively when it is unavoidable. In mental health care:

> Little hard information exists on the pervasiveness of the various forms of mandated treatment for people with mental disorders, how leverage is imposed, or what the measurable outcomes of using leverage actually are. The many vexing legal and ethical questions surrounding mandated treatment have not been thoroughly aired. . . . If policy makers and practitioners in mental health care are to embrace—or repudiate—some or all forms of mandated community treatment, an evidence-based approach must soon replace polemics. (Monahan et al., 2003:37)

With respect to the use of coercion in treatment for substance use, research is needed to determine the effects, both positive and negative, of outpatient commitment, drug courts, the use of treatment conditions in probation and parole, and less formal mechanisms of pressure on persons with substance-use problems and illnesses. Empirical data will not resolve the debate about the legitimacy of these approaches, but to the extent that their consequences are known, such data can inform treatment interventions and policy making. Data can also help identify how involuntary interventions can be avoided.

Recommendations

The committee finds that actions in all of the areas addressed in this chapter can help to counteract the effects of stigma and discrimination on patient-centered care. To this end, the committee makes two recommendations.

Recommendation 3-1. To promote patient-centered care, all parties involved in health care for mental or substance-use conditions should support the decision-making abilities and preferences for treatment and recovery of persons with M/SU problems and illnesses.

- Clinicians and organizations providing M/SU treatment services should:
  - Incorporate informed, patient-centered decision making throughout their practices, including active patient participation in the design and revision of patient treatment and recovery plans, the use of psychiatric advance directives, and (for children) informed family decision making. To ensure informed decision making, information on the availability and effectiveness of M/SU treatment options should be provided.
  - Adopt recovery-oriented and illness self-management practices that support patient preferences for treatment (including medications), peer support, and other elements of the wellness recovery plan.
  - Maintain effective, formal linkages with community resources to support patient illness self-management and recovery.
- Organizations providing M/SU treatment should also:
  - Have in place policies that implement informed, patient-centered participation and decision making in treatment, illness self-management, and recovery plans.
  - Involve patients and their families in the design, administration, and delivery of treatment and recovery services.
- Accrediting bodies should adopt accreditation standards that require the implementation of these practices.

- Health plans and direct payers of M/SU treatment services should:
  - For persons with chronic mental illnesses or substance-use dependence, pay for peer support and illness self-management programs that meet evidence-based standards.
  - Provide consumers with comparative information on the quality of care provided by practitioners and organizations, and use this information themselves when making their purchasing decisions.
  - Remove barriers to and restrictions on effective and appropriate treatment that may be created by copayments, service exclusions, benefit limits, and other coverage policies.

The committee wishes to underscore that, with respect to the recommendation that health plans and direct payers of M/SU treatment services pay for peer support and illness self-management programs for individuals with chronic mental and substance-use illnesses, we are not calling for payment for all programs that involve peer support (including self- and mutual-help 12-step programs) or all programs that aim to teach illness self-management. Rather, the committee recommends funding of peer support and illness self-management programs that provide a standardized intervention encompassing all components found necessary through empirical testing and modeling, that have themselves been empirically tested, and that have been shown to improve health outcomes. The Georgia Peer Support program and the Stanford University School of Medicine's standardized approach for illness self-management are two examples of such programs.

Recommendation 3-2. Coercion should be avoided whenever possible. When coercion is legally authorized, patient-centered care is still applicable and should be undertaken by:

- Making the policies and practices used for determining dangerousness and decision-making capacity transparent to patients and their caregivers.
- Obtaining the best available comparative information on safety, effectiveness, and availability of care and providers, and using that information to guide treatment decisions.
- Maximizing patient decision making and involvement in the selection of treatments and providers.

The committee notes that the above recommendations will be ineffective if the receipt of care by those who need it is not timely, if the care received is of poor quality, and if the necessary linkages with supportive human services are not in place. Improving the quality of M/SU therapies is addressed in the next chapter, while coordinating M/SU health care with other needed services is addressed in Chapter 5. Implementation of the above recommendations, as well as those made in succeeding chapters, is necessary to ensure the provision of patient-centered care.

REFERENCES

AHRQ (Agency for Healthcare Research and Quality). 2005. *Hospital Survey on Patient Safety Culture.* [Online]. Available: http:www.ahrq.gov/qual/hospculture [accessed July 7, 2005]. Rockville, MD: AHRQ.

AMA (American Medical Association). 2001. *International Classification of Diseases,* 9th Revision Clinical Modification 2002, Volumes 1 and 2. Chicago, IL: AMA Press.

American Psychiatric Association. 1998. Guidelines for assessing the decision-making capacities of potential research subjects with cognitive impairment. *American Journal of Psychiatry* 155(11):1649–1650.

American Psychiatric Association. 2000. *Diagnostic and Statistical Manual of Mental Disorders.* Fourth Edition, Text Revision, DSM-IV-TR ed. Washington, DC: American Psychiatric Association.

Appelbaum PS. 1994. *Almost a Revolution: Mental Health Law and the Limits of Change.* New York: Oxford University Press.

Appelbaum P. 2001. Thinking carefully about outpatient commitment. *Psychiatric Services* 52(3):347–350.

Appelbaum PS, Grisso T. 1988. Assessing patients' capacities to consent to treatment. *New England Journal of Medicine* (319):1635–1638.

Appelbaum PS, Grisso T. 1995. The MacArthur Treatment Competence Study. I: Mental illness and competence to consent to treatment. *Law and Human Behavior* 19(2):105–126.

Appelbaum PS, Roth LH, Lidz C. 1982. The therapeutic misconception: Informed consent in psychiatric research. *International Journal of Law and Psychiatry* 5(3–4):319–329.

Appelbaum BC, Appelbaum PS, Grisso T. 1998. Competence to consent to voluntary psychiatric hospitalization: A test of a standard by APA. *Psychiatric Services* 49(9):1193–1196.

Appelbaum PS, Grisso T, Frank E, O'Donnell S, Kupfer D. 1999. Competence of depressed patients for consent to research. *American Journal of Psychiatry* 156(9):1380–1384.

Arsenault L, Moffitt T, Caspi A, Taylor P, Silva P. 2000. Mental disorders and violence in a total birth cohort: Results form the Dunedin study. *Archives of General Psychiatry* 57(10):979–986.

Backlar P, McFarland BH, Swanson JW, Mahler J. 2001. Consumer, provider, and informal caregiver opinions on psychiatric advance directives. *Administration and Policy in Mental Health* 28(6):427–441.

Badamgarev E, Weingarten S, Henning J, Knight K, Hasselblad V, Gano A Jr, Ofman J. 2003. Effectiveness of disease management programs in depression: A systematic review. *American Journal of Psychiatry* 160(12):2080–2090.

Bagian JP, Gosbee JW. 2000. Developing a culture of patient safety at the VA. *Ambulatory Outreach,* Spring:25–29.

Bandura A. 1997a. Clinical functioning. In: Bandura A, ed. *Self-Efficacy: The Exercise of Control.* New York, NY: W.H. Freeman and Company. Pp. 319–368.

Bandura A. 1997b. *Self-Efficacy: The Exercise of Control.* New York: W.H. Freeman.

Barry CL, Gabel JR, Frank RG, Hawkins S, Whitmore HH, Pickreign JD. 2003. Design of mental health benefits: Still unequal after all these years. *Health Affairs* 22(5):127–137.

Bean G, Nishisato S, Rector NA, Glancy G. 1994. The psychometric properties of the Competency Interview Schedule. *Canadian Journal of Psychiatry—Revue Canadienne De Psychiatrie* 39(8):368–376.

Bechara A, Damasio H. 2002. Decision-making and addiction (Part I): Impaired activation of somatic states in substance dependent individuals when pondering decisions with negative future consequences. *Neuropsychologia* 40(10):1675–1689.

Bechara A, Dolan S, Hindes A. 2002. Decision-making and addiction (part II): Myopia for the future or hypersensitivity to reward? *Neuropsychologia* 40(10):1690–1705.

Belenko S. 1999. Research on drug courts: A critical review. *National Drug Court Institute Review* 2(2):1–58.

Belenko S. 2002. Drug courts. In: Leukefeld C, Tims F, Farabee D, eds. *Treatment of Drug Offenders: Policies and Issues.* New York: Springer. Pp. 301–318.

Bennett NS, Lidz CW, Monahan J, Mulvey EP, Hoge SK, Roth LH, Gardner W. 1993. Inclusion, motivation, and good faith: The morality of coercion in mental hospital admission. *Behavioral Sciences and the Law* 11(3):295–306.

Benson P, Roth LH, Appelbaum PS, Lidz C, Winslade W. 1988. Information disclosure, subject understanding, and informed consent in psychiatric research. *Law and Human Behavior* 12(4):455–475.

Berg JW. 1996. Legal and ethical complexities of consent with cognitively impaired research subjects: Proposed guidelines. *Journal of Law, Medicine & Ethics* 24(1):18–35.

Berg JW, Appelbaum PS, Grisso T. 1996. Constructing competence: Formulating standards of legal competence to make medical decisions. *Rutgers Law Review* 48:345–396.

Bergeson S. 2004. Testimony before the Institute of Medicine Committee on Crossing the Quality Chasm: Adaptation to Mental Health and Addictive Disorders. Washington, DC, July 14. Available from the Institute of Medicine.

Bodenheimer T, Lorig K, Holman H, Grumbach K. 2002a. Patient self-management of chronic disease in primary care. *Journal of the American Medical Association* 288(19):2469–2475.

Bodenheimer T, Wagner EH, Grumbach K. 2002b. Improving primary care for patients with chronic illness. *Journal of the American Medical Association* 288(14):1775–1779.

Brakel S. 1985. Voluntary admission. In: Brakel S, Parry J, Wesiner B, eds. *The Mentally Disabled and the Law.* 3rd ed. Chicago, IL: American Bar Foundation.

Brennan PA, Mednick. SA, Hodgins S. 2000. Major mental disorders and criminal violence in a Danish birth cohort. *Archives of General Psychiatry* 57(5):494–500.

Brock DW. 1991. Decision-making competence and risk. *Bioethics* 5(2):105–112.

Brody BA. 1998. *The Ethics of Biomedical Research.* New York: Oxford University Press.

Brown JD. 2003. Is involuntary outpatient commitment a remedy for community mental health service failure? *Ethical Human Sciences and Services* 5(1):7–20.

Bureau of Labor Statistics. 2003. *National Compensation Survey: Employee Benefits in Private Industry in the United States, 2000.* Bulletin 2555. Washington, DC: U.S. Department of Labor. [Online]. Available: http://stats.bls.gov/ncs/ebs/sp/ebbl0019.pdf [accessed February 25, 2004].

Cale GS. 1999. Risk-related standards of competence: Continuing the debate over risk-related standards of competence. *Bioethics* 13(2):131–148.

Capitani J, Hercik J, Kakuska C, Schwacter N, Welfare Peer Technical Assistance Network. 2001. *Pathways to Self-Sufficiency: Findings of the National Needs Assessment.* Prerelease draft. [Online]. Available: http://peerta.acf.hhs.gov/pdf/needsassessment.pdf [accessed May 26, 2005].

Carpenter WT Jr, Gold J, Lahti A, Queen C, Conley R, Bartko J, Kovnick J, Appelbaum PS. 2000. Decisional capacity for informed consent in schizophrenia research. *Archives of General Psychiatry* 57(6):533–538.

Charland L. 1998. Appreciation and emotion: Theoretical reflections on the MacArthur Treatment Competence Study. *Kennedy Institute of Ethics Journal* 8(4):359–376.

Cimons M. 2004. *Challenging a Hidden Obstacle to Alcohol Treatment: Little Known Insurance Laws Thwart Screening in Emergency Rooms.* Washington, DC: The George Washington University Medical Center.

Claxton G, Holve E, Finder B, Gabel J, Pickreign J, Whitmore H, Hawkins S, Dhont K. 2003. *Employer Health Benefits: 2003 Annual Survey.* Menlo Park, CA and Chicago, IL: Henry J. Kaiser Foundation and Health Research and Educational Trust.

Connoly T, Arkes HR, Hammond KR, eds. 2000. *Judgment and Decision Making: An Interdisciplinary Reader.* 2nd ed. Cambridge, MA: Cambridge University Press.

Cook JA. 2004. *"Patient-Centered" and "Consumer-Directed" Mental Health Services.* Paper commissioned by the Institute of Medicine Committee on Crossing the Quality Chasm: Adaptation to Mental Health and Addictive Disorders. Available from the Institute of Medicine.

Copeland ME. 2002. *Wellness Recovery Action Plan.* West Dummerston, VT: Peach Press.

Corrigan PW. 2004. Don't call me nuts: An international perspective on the stigma of mental illness. *Acta Psychiatrica Scandinavica* 109(6):403–404.

Corrigan PW, Penn DL. 1999. Lessons from social psychology on discrediting psychiatric stigma. *American Psychologist* 54(9):765–776.

Corrigan PW, Watson AC. 2003. Factors that explain how policy makers distribute resources to mental health services. *Psychiatric Services* 54(4):501–507.

Corrigan PW, River LP, Lundin RK, Penn DL, Uphoff-Wasowski K, Campion J, Mathisen J, Gagnon C, Bargman M, Goldstein H, Kubiak MA. 2001. Three strategies for changing attributions about severe mental illness. *Schizophrenia Bulletin* 27(2):187–195.

Corrigan PW, Rowan D, Green A, Lunding R, River P, Uphoff-Wasowski K, White K, Kubiak MA. 2002. Challenging two mental illness stigmas: Personal responsibility and dangerousness. *Schizophrenia Bulletin* 28(2):293–309.

Cournos F, Faulkner LR, Fitzgerald L, Griffith E, Munetz MR, Winick B. 1993. Report of the Task Force on Consent to Voluntary Hospitalization. *Bulletin of the American Academy of Psychiatry and the Law* 21(3):293–307.

Cronkite RC, Moos RH, Twohey J, Cohen C, Swindle R Jr. 1998. Life circumstances and personal resources as predictors of the ten-year course of depression. *American Journal of Community Psychology* 26(2):255–279.

Culver CM, Gert B. 1990. The inadequacy of incompetence. *Milbank Quarterly* 68(4): 619–643.

Davenport T, DeLong D, Beers M. 1998. Successful knowledge management projects. *Sloan Management Review* 39(2):43–57.

Davis TC, Holcombe RF, Berkel HJ, Pramanik S, Divers SG. 1998. Informed consent for clinical trials: A comparative study of standard versus simplified forms. *Journal of the National Cancer Institute* 90(9):668–674.

Dennis DL, Monahan J, eds. 1996. *Coercion and Aggressive Community Treatment: A New Frontier in Mental Health Law.* New York: Plenum Press.

D'Onofrio G, Degutis LC. 2002. Preventive care in the emergency department: Screening and brief intervention for alcohol problems in the emergency department—A systematic review. *Academic Emergency Medicine* 9(6):627–637.

Dunn L, Lindamer L, Palmer BW, Golshan S, Schneider L, Jeste DV. 2002. Improving understanding of research consent in middle-aged and elderly patients with psychotic disorders. *American Journal of Geriatric Psychiatry* 10(2):142–150.

Dymek MP, Atchinson P, Harrell L, Marson DC. 2001. Competency to consent to medical treatment in cognitively impaired patients with Parkinson's disease. *Neurology* 56(1):17–24.

Emrick CD, Tonigan JS, Montgomery H, Little L. Alcoholics Anonymous: What is currently known? 1993. In: McCrady BS, Miller WR, eds. *Research on Alcoholics Anonymous: Opportunities and Alternatives.* New Brunswick, NJ: Rutgers Center of Alcohol Studies. Pp. 41–78.

Faden R, Beauchamp T. 1986. *A History and Theory of Informed Consent.* New York: Oxford University Press.

Farabee D, Prendergast ML, Anglin MD. 1998. The effectiveness of coerced treatment for drug-abusing offenders. *Federal Probation* 62(1):3–10.

Farina A. 1998. Stigma. In: Mueser KT, Tarrier N, eds. *Handbook of Social Functioning in Schizophrenia.* Needham Heights, MA: Allyn & Bacon. Pp. 247–279.

Gabor V, Botsko C. 1998. *State Food Stamp Policy Choices under Welfare Reform: Findings of 1997 50-State Survey.* [Online]. Available: http:www.fns.usda.gov/oane/MENU/Published/FSP/FILES/ProgramDesign/finsum.pdf [accessed January 12, 2005].

GAO (U.S. Government Accountability Office). 2000. *Mental Health Parity Act: Despite New Federal Standards, Mental Health Benefits Remain Limited.* GAO/HEHS-00-95. Washington, DC: GAO.

GAO. 2003. *Child Welfare and Juvenile Justice: Federal Agencies Could Play a Stronger Role in Helping States Reduce the Number of Children Placed Solely to Obtain Mental Health Services.* GAO-03-397. Washington, DC: GAO. [Online]. Available: http://www.gao.gov/new.items/d03397.pdf [accessed October 25, 2004].

Garnham A, Oakhill J. 1994. *Thinking and Reasoning.* Cambridge, MA: Blackwell.

Gentilello LM, Ebel BE, Wickizer TM, Salkever DS, Rivara FP. 2005. Alcohol interventions for trauma patients treated in emergency departments and hospitals: A cost benefit analysis. *Annals of Surgery* 241(4):541–550

Gilbody S, Whitty P, Grimshaw J, Thomas R. 2003. Educational and organizational interventions to improve the management of depression in primary care: A systematic review. *Journal of the American Medical Association* 289(23):3145–3151.

Giliberti M, Schulzinger R. 2000. *Relinquishing Custody: The Tragic Result of Failure to Meet Children's Mental Health Needs.* Washington, DC: Bazelon Center for Mental Health Law.

Goldman-Rakic P. 1994. Working memory dysfunction in schizophrenia. *Journal of Neuropsychiatry and Clinical Neurosciences* 6(4):348–357.

Gorelick D, Pickens R, Bonkovsky F. 1999. Clinical research in substance abuse: Human subjects issues. In: Pincus H, Lieberman J, Ferris S, eds. *Ethics in Psychiatric Research: A Resource Manual for Human Subjects Protection.* Washington, DC: American Psychiatric Association. Pp. 177–218.

Grant S, Contoreggi C, London E. 2000. Drug abusers show impaired performance in a laboratory test of decision making. *Neuropsychologia* 38(8):1180–1187.

Grisso T, Appelbaum PS. 1995. The MacArthur treatment competence study. III: Abilities of patients to consent to psychiatric and medical treatments. *Law and Human Behavior* 19(2):149–174.

Grisso T, Appelbaum PS. 1998. *Assessing Competence to Consent to Treatment: A Guide for Physicians and Other Health Professionals.* New York: Oxford University Press.

Grisso T, Appelbaum PS, Mulvey EP, Fletcher K. 1995. The MacArthur Treatment Competence Study. II: Measures of abilities related to competence to consent to treatment. *Law and Human Behavior* 19(2):127–148.

Grisso T, Appelbaum PS, Hill-Fotouhi C. 1997. The MacCAT-T: A clinical tool to assess patients' capacities to make treatment decisions. *Psychiatric Services* 48(11):1415–1419.

Grossman L, Summers F. 1980. A study of the capacity of schizophrenia patients to give informed consent. *Hospital and Community Psychiatry* 31(3):205–206.

Hall KT, Appelbaum PS. 2002. The origins of commitment for substance abuse in the United States. *Journal of the American Academy of Psychiatry and the Law.* 30(1):33–45; discussion 46-48.

Hall LL, Graf AC, Fitzpatrick MJ, Lane T, Birkel RC. 2003. *Shattered Lives: Results of a National Survey of NAMI Members Living with Mental Illnesses and Their Families.* Arlington, VA: National Alliance for the Mentally Ill.

Hazelton LD, Sterns GL, Chisolm T. 2003. Decision-making capacity and alcohol abuse: Clinical and ethical considerations in personal care choices. *General Hospital Psychiatry* 25(2):130–135.

Health Policy Tracking Service. 2004. Parity and Other Insurance Mandates for the Treatment of Mental Illness and Substance Abuse. *Issue Brief*, December 31.

Heifetz R, Laurie D. 2001. The work of leadership. *Harvard Business Review* 79(11):131–140.

Hibbard JH. 2003. Engaging health care consumers to improve the quality of care. *Medical Care* 41(Supplement 1):I-61–I-70.

Hodgins S, Janson CG. 2002. *Criminality and Violence among the Mentally Disordered: The Stockholm Metropolitan Project.* Cambridge, UK: Cambridge University Press.

Hoge MA, Jacobs S, Belitsky R, Migdole S. 2002. Graduate education and training for contemporary behavioral health practice. *Administration and Policy in Mental Health* 29(4/5):335–357.

Hoge SK, Lidz CW, Eisenberg M, Gardner W, Monahan J, Mulvey E, Roth L, Bennett N. 1997. Perceptions of coercion in the admission of voluntary and involuntary psychiatric patients. *International Journal of Law and Psychiatry* 20(2):167–181.

Humphreys K, Moos R. 1996. Reduced substance abuse-related health care costs among voluntary participants in Alcoholics Anonymous. *Psychiatric Services* 47(7):709–713.

Humphreys K, Moos RH. 2001. Can encouraging substance abuse inpatients to participate in self-help groups reduce the demand for out-patient care? A quasi-experimental study. *Alcoholism: Clinical and Experimental Research* 25(5):711–716.

Humphreys K, Wing S, McCarty D, Chappel J, Gallant L, Haberle B, Horvath AT, Kaskutas LA, Kirk T, Kivlahan D, Laudet A, McCrady BS, McLellan AT, Morgenstern J, Townsend M, Weiss R. 2004. Self-help organizations for alcohol and drug problems: Towards evidence-based practice and policy. *Journal of Substance Abuse Treatment* 26(3):151–158.

Hyman SE, Malenka RC. 2001. Addiction and the brain: The neurobiology of compulsion and its persistence. *Nature Reviews Neuroscience* 2(10):695–703.

IOM (Institute of Medicine). 2001. *Crossing the Quality Chasm: A New Health System for the 21st Century.* Washington, DC: National Academy Press.

IOM. 2003. In: Adams K, Corrigan JM, eds. *Priority Areas for National Attention: Transforming Health Care Quality.* Washington, DC: The National Academies Press.

IOM. 2004a. *Health Literacy: A Prescription to End Confusion.* Washington, DC: The National Academies Press.

IOM. 2004b. In: Page A, ed. *Keeping Patients Safe: Transforming the Work Environment of Nurses.* Washington, DC: The National Academies Press.

Irwin M, Lovitz A, Marder SR, Mintz J, Winslade W, Van Putten T, Mills M. 1985. Psychotic patients understanding of informed consent. *American Journal of Psychiatry* 142(11):1351–1354.

Jamison KR. 1995. *An Unquiet Mind.* New York, NY: Alfred A. Knopf, Inc.

Jenkins CL. 2004, November 29. Mental illness sends many to foster care. *The Washington Post.* Metro Section. Pp. B1 and B4, Column 1.

Join Together. 2003. *Ending Discrimination against People with Alcohol and Drug Problems: Recommendations from a National Policy Panel.* Boston, MA: Join Together, Boston University School of Public Health. [Online]. Available: http://www.jointogether.org/sa/files/pdf/discrimination.pdf [accessed October 3, 2004].

Judge David L. Bazelon Center for Mental Health Law. 2000a. *Involuntary Outpatient Commitment: Summary of State Statutes.* Washington DC: Judge David L. Bazelon Center for Mental Health Law. [Online]. Available: http://www.bazelon.org/issues/commitment/ioc/iocchart.pdf [accessed January 25, 2005].

Judge David L. Bazelon Center for Mental Health Law. 2000b. *Position Statement on Involuntary Commitment.* Washington DC: Judge David L. Bazelon Center for Mental Health Law. [Online]. Available: http://www.bazelon.org/issues/commitment/bazelonposition.htm on [accessed January 25, 2005].

Kahneman D, Slovic P, Tversky A, eds. 1982. *Judgment under Uncertainty: Heuristics and Biases.* Cambridge, UK: Cambridge University Press.

Kapp MB, Mossman D. 1996. Measuring decisional capacity: Cautions on the construction of a "capacimeter." *Psychology, Public Policy, and Law* 2(1):73–95.

Kaskutas LA, Ammon L. 2003–2004. A naturalistic comparison of outcomes at social and clinical model substance abuse treatment programs. *International Journal of Self-Help and Self-Care* 2(2):111–133.

Kaskutas LA, Turk N, Bond J, Weisner C. 2003. The role of religion, spirituality and Alcoholics Anonymous in sustained sobriety. *Alcoholism Treatment Quarterly* 21(1):1–16.

Kelly JF, Myers MG, Brown SA. 2002. Do adolescents affiliate with 12-step groups? A multivariate process model of effects. *Journal of Studies on Alcohol* 63(3):293–304.

Keyserlingk EW. 1995. Proposed guidelines for the participation of persons with dementia as research subjects. *Perspectives in Biology and Medicine* 38(2):319–362.

Kim SYH, Caine ED, Currier GW, Leibovici A, Ryan JM. 2001. Assessing the competence of persons with Alzheimer's disease in providing informed consent for participation in research. *American Journal of Psychiatry* 158(5):712–717.

Kolodziej ME, Johnson BT. 1996. Interpersonal contact and acceptance of persons with psychiatric disorders: A research synthesis. *Journal of Consulting and Clinical Psychology* 64(6):1387–1396.

Lapid M, Rummans T, Poole K, Pankratz S, Maurer M, Rasmussen K, Philbrick K, Appelbaum P. 2003. Decisional capacity of severely depressed patients requiring electroconvulsive therapy. *Journal of ECT* 19(2):67–72.

Lawental E, McLellan AT, Grissom GR, Brill P, O'Brien C. 1996. Coerced treatment for substance abuse problems detected through workplace urine surveillance: Is it effective? *Journal of Substance Abuse* 8(1):115–128.

Leibfried T. 2004. Testimony before the Institute of Medicine Committee on Crossing the Quality Chasm: Adaptation to Mental Health and Addictive Disorders. Washington, DC, July 14. Available from the Institute of Medicine.

Lindman F, McIntyre D. 1961. *The Mentally Disabled and the Law.* Chicago, IL: University of Chicago Press.

Link BG, Phelan JC. 2001. Conceptualizing stigma. *Annual Review of Sociology* 27(1): 363–385.

Link B, Andrews A, Cullen F. 1992. The violent and illegal behavior of mental patients reconsidered. *American Sociological Review* 57(3):275–292.

Link BG, Phelan JC, Bresnahan M, Stueve A, Pescosolido BA. 1999. Public conceptions of mental illness: Labels, causes, dangerousness, and social distance. *American Journal of Public Health* 89(9):1328–1333.

Link B, Struening E, Neese-Todd S, Asmussen S, Phelan JC. 2001. Stigma as a barrier to recovery: The consequences of stigma for the self-esteem of people with mental illnesses. *Psychiatric Services* 52(12):1621–1626.

Longshore D, Urada D, Evans E, Hser YH, Prendergast M, Hawken A. 2005. *Evaluation of the Substance Abuse and Crime Prevention Act: 2004 Report.* Los Angeles, CA: UCLA Integrated Substance Abuse Programs. [Online]. Available: http://www.uclaisap.org/Prop36/documents/sacpa080405.pdf [accessed October 10, 2005].

Lorig KR, Holman HR. 2003. Self-management education: History, definition, outcomes, and mechanisms. *Annals of Behavioral Medicine* 26(1):1–7.

Lorig KR, Ritter P, Stewart AA, Sobel D, Brown BW, Bandura A, Gonzalez VM, Laurent DD, Holman HR. 2001. Chronic disease self-management program: 2-year health status and health care utilization outcomes. *Medical Care* 39(11):1217–1223.

Luchins D, Roberts D, Hanrahan P. 2003. Representative payeeship and mental illness: A review. *Administration and Policy in Mental Health* 30(4):341–353.

Mann CE, Himelein MJ. 2004. Factors associated with stigmatization of persons with mental illness. *Psychiatric Services* 55(2):185–187.

Markowitz FE. 1998. The effects of stigma on the psychological well-being and life satisfaction of persons with mental illness. *Journal of Health and Social Behavior* 39(4):335–347.

Marlowe DB. 2003. Integrating substance abuse treatment and criminal justice supervision. *NIDA Science & Practice Perspectives* 2(1):4–14.

Marlowe DB, Festinger DS, Lee PA. 2004. The judge is a key component of drug court. *Drug Court Review* IV(2):1–34.

Marson D, Harrell L. 1999. Executive dysfunction and loss of capacity to consent to medical treatment in patients with Alzheimer's disease. *Seminars in Clinical Neuropsychiatry* 4:41–49.

Marson DC, Chatterjee A, Ingram KK, Harrell LE. 1996. Toward a neurological model of competency: Cognitive predictors of capacity to consent in Alzheimer's disease using three different legal standards. *Neurology* 46(3):666–672.

Marson DC, Hawkins L, McInturff B, Harrell LE. 1997. Cognitive models that predict physician judgements of capacity to consent in mild Alzheimer's disease. *Journal of the American Geriatrics Society* 45(4):458–464.

Martin JK, Pescosolido BA, Tuch SA. 2000. Of fear and loathing: The role of "disturbing behavior," labels, and causal attributions in shaping public attitudes toward people with mental illness. *Journal of Health and Social Behavior* 41(2):208–223.

Masand PS, Bouckoms AJ, Fischel SV, Calabrese LV, Stern TA. 1998. A prospective multi-center study of competency evaluations by psychiatric consultation services. *Psychosomatics* 39(1):55–60.

McElrath, D. 1997. The Minnesota model. *Journal of Psychoactive Drugs* 29(2):141–144.

McGlynn EA, Asch SM, Adams J, Keesey J, Hicks J, DeCristofaro A, Kerr EA. 2003. The quality of health care delivered to adults in the United States. *New England Journal of Medicine* 348(26):2635–2645.

Meisel A. 1998. Legal aspects of end-of-life decision making. In: Steinberg M, Youngner S, eds. *End of Life Decisions: A Psychosocial Perspective*. Washington, DC: American Psychiatric Press, Inc. Pp. 235–258.

Michigan Department of Community Health. 2003. *Self-Determination Policy and Practice Guideline*. [Online]. Available: http://www.michigan.gov/documents/SelfDetermination Policy_70262_7.pdf [accessed May 26, 2005].

Monahan J. 1981. *The Clinical Prediction of Violent Behavior*. National Institute of Mental Health. Washington, DC: U.S Government Printing Office. Reprinted as *Predicting Violent Behavior: An Assessment of Clinical Techniques* (Sage Publications, 1981).

Monahan J, Steadman H, Silver E, Appelbaum PS, Robbins PC, Mulvey EP, Roth LH, Grisso T, Banks S. 2001a. *Rethinking Risk Assessment: The MacArthur Study of Mental Disorder and Violence*. New York: Oxford University Press.

Monahan J, Bonnie RJ, Appelbaum PS, Hyde P, Steadman H, Swartz M. 2001b. Mandated community treatment: Beyond outpatient commitment. *Psychiatric Services* 52(9):1198–1205.

Monahan J, Swartz M, Bonnie RJ. 2003. Mandated treatment in the community for people with mental disorders. *Health Affairs* 22(5):28–38.

Monahan J, Redlich AD, Swanson J, Robbins PC, Appelbaum PS, Petrilla J, Steadman HJ, Swartz M, Angell B, McNiel DE. 2005. Use of leverage to improve adherence to psychiatric treatment in the community. *Psychiatric Services* 56(1):37–44.

Moser DJ, Schultz SK, Arndt S, Benjamin ML, Fleming FW, Brems CS, Paulsen JS, Appelbaum PS, Andreasen NC. 2002. Capacity to provide informed consent for participation in schizophrenia and HIV research. *American Journal of Psychiatry* 159(7):1201–1207.

Mowbray CT, Moxley DP, Jasper CA, Howell LL, eds. 1997. *Consumers as Providers in Psychiatric Rehabilitation.* Columbia, MD: International Association of Psychosocial Rehabilitation Services.

Moyer A, Finney J, Swearingen C, Vergun P. 2002. Brief interventions for alcohol problems: A meta-analytic review of controlled investigations in treatment-seeking and non-treatment-seeking populations. *Addiction* 97(3):279–292.

Mueser KT, Corrigan PW, Hilton DW, Tanzman B, Schaub A, Gingerich S, Essock SM, Tarrier N, Morey B, Vogel-Scibilia S, Herz MI. 2002. Illness management and recovery: A review of the research. *Psychiatric Services* 53(10):1272–1284.

Munetz M, Roth LH. 1985. Informing patients about tardive dyskinesia. *Archives of General Psychiatry* 42(9):866–871.

Murdach AD. 1996. Beneficence re-examined: Protective intervention in mental health. *Social Work* 41(1):26–32.

National Bioethics Advisory Commission. 1998. *Research Involving Persons with Mental Disorders That May Affect Decision-making Capacity.* Volume 1. Rockville, MD: National Bioethics Advisory Commission.

New York State Department of Health Advisory Work Group on Human Subject Research Involving the Protected Classes. 1999. *Recommendations on the Oversight of Human Subject Research Involving the Protected Classes.* [Online]. Available: http://nysl.nysed.gov/ Archimages/14195.PDF [accessed October 7, 2005].

NIMH (National Institute of Mental Health). 2005. *NIMH Outreach Partnership Program.* [Online]. Available: http://www.nimh.nih.gov/outreach/partners/index.cfm [accessed July 30, 2005].

Office of the Maryland Attorney General. 1998. *Final Report of the Attorney General's Research Working Group.* Baltimore, MD: Office of the Maryland Attorney General.

Pajares F. 2002. *Overview of Social Cognitive Theory and of Self-Efficacy.* Emory University. [Online]. Available: http://www.emory.edu/EDUCATION/mfp/eff.html [accessed October 8, 2004].

Palmer BW, Dunn LB, Appelbaum PS, Jeste DV. 2004. Correlates of treatment-related decision-making capacity among middle-aged and older patients with schizophrenia. *Archives of General Psychiatry* 61(3):230–236.

Peck MC, Scheffler RM. 2002. An analysis of the definitions of mental illness used in state parity laws. *Psychiatric Services* 53(9):1089–1095.

Peele PB, Lave JR, Xu Y. 1999. Benefit limits in managed behavioral health care: Do they matter? *The Journal of Behavioral Health Services & Research* 26(4):430–441.

Peele PB, Lave JR, Kelleher KJ. 2002. Exclusions and limitations in children's behavioral health care coverage. *Psychiatric Services* 53(5):591–594.

Perlick DA, Rosenheck RA, Clarkin JF, Sirey JA, Salahi J, Struening LE, Link BG. 2001. Adverse effects of perceived stigma on social adaptation of persons diagnosed with bipolar affective disorder. *Psychiatric Services* 52(12):1627–1632.

Pescosolido BA, Martin JK, Link BG, Kikuzawa S, Burgos G, Swindle R, Phelan J. Undated. *Americans' Views of Mental Health and Illness at Century's End: Continuity and Change.* Public Report on the MacArthur Mental Health Module, 1996 General Social Survey. Bloomington, IN: The Indiana Consortium of Mental Health Services Research, Indiana University and The Joseph P. Mailman School of Public Health, Columbia University. [Online]. Available: http://www.indiana.edu/~icmhsr/amerview1.pdf [accessed August 18, 2004].

Pescosolido BA, Monahan J, Link BG, Stueve A, Kikuzawa S. 1999. The public's view of the competence, dangerousness, and need for legal coercion of persons with mental health problems. *American Journal of Public Health* 89(9):1339–1345.

Peto T, Srebnik D, Zick E, Russo J. 2004. Support needed to create psychiatric advance directives. *Administration and Policy in Mental Health* 31(5):409–419.

Pincus HA, Hough L, Houtsinger JK, Rollman BL, Frank R. 2003. Emerging models of depression care: Multi-level ("6P") strategies. *International Journal of Methods in Psychiatric Research* 12(1):54–63.

Polcin D, Weisner C. 1999. Factors associated with coercion in entering treatment for alcohol problems. *Drug and Alcohol Dependence* 54(1):63–68.

Project MATCH Research Group. 1998. Matching alcoholism treatments to client heterogeneity: Project MATCH three-year drinking outcomes. *Alcoholism: Clinical and Experimental Research* 22(6):1300–1311.

Rasinski KA. 2003. *Stigma Associated With Drug Addiction: Report of a Language Audit Based on the Results of a National Survey of Drug Policy.* Chicago, IL: University of Chicago, National Opinion Research Center.

Redlich AD, Steadman HJ, Monahan J, Petrila J, Griffin P. 2005. The second generation of mental health courts. *Psychology, Public Policy, and Law* 11(4):527–538.

Rivara FP, Tollefson S, Tesh E, Gentilello L. 2000. Screening trauma patients for alcohol problems: Are insurance companies barriers? *Journal of Trauma: Injury, Infection, and Critical Care* 48(1):115–118.

Roman PM, Blum TC. 2002. The workplace and alcohol problem prevention. *Alcohol Research and Health* 26(1):49–57.

Rosen M, Rosenheck R. 1999. Substance use and assignment of representative payees. *Psychiatric Services* 50(1):95–98.

Roth LH, Meisel A, Lidz CW. 1977. Tests of competency to consent to treatment. *American Journal of Psychiatry* (134):279–284.

Roth LH, Lidz CW, Meisel A, Soloff PH, Kaufman K, Spiker DG, Foster FG. 1982. Competency to decide about treatment or research: An overview of some empirical data. *International Journal of Law and Psychiatry* 5(1):29–50.

Ryan R, Deci E. 2000. Self-determination theory and the facilitation of intrinsic motivation, social development, and well-being. *American Psychologist* 55(1):68–78.

Sabin JE, Daniels N. 1999. Public-sector managed behavioral health care: III. Meaningful consumer and family participation. *Psychiatric Services* 50(7):883–885.

Sabin JF, Daniels N. 2001. Managed care: Strengthening the consumer voice in managed care: I. Can the private sector meet the public sector standard? *Psychiatric Services* 52(4):461–464.

Sabin JE, Daniels N. 2003. Strengthening the consumers voice in managed care: VII. The Georgia Peer Specialist Program. *Psychiatric Services* 54(4):497–498.

Sabin JE, O'Brien MF, Daniels N. 2001. Managed care: Strengthening the consumer voice in managed care: II. Moving NCQA standards from rights to empowerment. *Psychiatric Services* 52(10):1303–1305.

Saks ER. 1999. Competency to decide on treatment and research: The MacArthur capacity instruments. In: National Bioethics Advisory Commission, ed. *Research Involving Persons with Mental Disorders That May Affect Decision-Making Capacity: Volume II, Commissioned Papers.* Rockville, MD: National Bioethics Advisory Commission. Pp 59–78.

Saks ER, Jeste DV. 2004. *Capacity to Consent to or Refuse Treatment and/or Research: Theoretical Considerations.* Paper commissioned by the Institute of Medicine Committee on Crossing the Quality Chasm: Adaptation to Mental Health and Addictive Disorders. Available from Institute of Medicine.

Saks ER, Dunn LB, Maershall BJ, Nayak GV, Golsan S, Jeste DV. 2002. The California Scale of Appreciation: A new instrument to measure the appreciation component of capacity to consent to research. *American Journal of Geriatric Psychiatry* 10(2): 166–174.

Samet JH, Rollnick S, Barnes H. 1996. Beyond CAGE: A brief clinical approach after detection of substance abuse. *Archives of Internal Medicine* 156(20):2287–2293.

SAMHSA (Substance Abuse and Mental Health Services Administration). 2000. *Changing the Conversation: Improving Substance Abuse Treatment: The National Treatment Plan Initiative*. DHHS Publication No. (SMA) 00-3479. Rockville, MD: U.S. Department of Health and Human Services.

SAMHSA. 2004a. *Recovery Community Services Program*. [Online]. Available: http://rcsp. samhsa.gov/about/history.htm [accessed May 26, 2005].

SAMHSA. 2004b. *Results From the 2003 National Survey on Drug Use and Health: National Findings*. DHHS Publication Number SMA 04-3964. NSDUH Series H-25. Rockville, MD: U.S. Department of Health and Human Services.

Schacter D, Kleinman I, Prendergast P, Remington G, Schertzer S. 1994. The effect of psychopathology on the ability of schizophrenic patients to give informed consent. *Journal of Nervous and Mental Disorders* 182(6):360–362.

Schein EH. 1992. *Organizational Culture and Leadership*. 2nd ed. San Francisco, CA: Jossey-Bass.

Shaw J, Amos T, Hunt IM, Flynn S, Turnbull P, Kapur N, Appleby L. 2004. Mental illness in people who kill strangers: Longitudinal study and national clinical survey. *British Medical Journal* 328(7442):734–737.

Sherbourne C, Hays RD, Wells KB. 1995. Personal and psychological risk factors for physical and mental health outcomes and course of depression and depressed patients. *Journal of Consulting and Clinical Psychology* 63(3):345–355.

Sherbourne CD, Sturm R, Wells KB. 1999. What outcomes matter to patients? *Journal of General Internal Medicine* 14(6):357–363.

Sherman P. 1998. Computer-assisted creation of psychiatric advance directives. *Community Mental Health Journal* 34(4):351–362.

Shoor S, Lorig K. 2002. Self-care and the doctor-patient relationship. *Medical Care* 40(4):II-40–II-44.

Simpson A, McKenna B, Moskowitz A, Skipworth J, Barry-Walsh J. 2003. *Myth and Reality: The Relationship between Mental Illness and Homicide in New Zealand*. Auckland, NZ: Health Research Council of New Zealand.

Sirey JA, Bruce ML, Alexopoulos GS, Perlick DA, Friedman SJ, Meyers BS. 2001. Perceived stigma and patient-rated severity of illness as predictors of antidepressant drug adherence. *Psychiatric Services* 52(12):1615–1620.

Skeem JL, Encandela J, Louden JE. 2003. Perspectives on probation and mandated mental health treatment in specialized and traditional probation departments. *Behavioral Sciences and the Law* 21(4):429–458.

Slobogin C. 1996. "Appreciation" as a measure of competence: Some thoughts about the MacArthur Group's approach. *Psychology, Public Policy, and Law* 2:18–30.

Smith M. 2002. Stigma. *Advances in Psychiatric Treatment* 8(5):317–323.

Solomon P, Draine J. 2001. The state of knowledge of the effectiveness of consumer provided services. *Psychiatric Rehabilitation Journal* 25(1):20–27.

Srebnik DS, La Fond JQ. 1999. Advance directives for mental health treatment. *Psychiatric Services* 50(7):919–925.

Srebnik D, Appelbaum PS, Russo J. 2004. Assessing competence to complete psychiatric advance directives with the competence assessment tool for psychiatric advance directives. *Comprehensive Psychiatry* 45(4):239–245.

Stanford University School of Medicine. 2005. *Chronic Disease Self-Management Program.* [Online]. Available: http://patienteducation.stanford.edu/programs/cdsmp.html [accessed January 27, 2005].

Stanton M. 2002. *Expanding Patient-Centered Care to Empower Patients and Assist Providers.* AHRQ Publication Number: 02-0024. Rockville, MD: AHRQ and DHHS. [Online]. Available: http://www.ahrq.gov/qual/ptcareria.pdf [accessed February 8, 2005].

Steadman HJ, Mulvey EP, Monahan J, Robbins PC, Appelbaum PS, Grisso T, Roth LH, Silver E. 1998. Violence by people discharged from acute psychiatric inpatient facilities and by others in the same neighborhoods. *Archives of General Psychiatry* 55(5):393–401.

Steadman H, Davidson S, Brown C. 2001. Mental health courts: Their promise and unanswered questions. *Psychiatric Services* 52(4):457–458.

Stefan S. 2004. *Patient Centered Care/Self Directed Care: Legal, Policy and Programmatic Considerations.* Paper commissioned by the Institute of Medicine Committee on Crossing the Quality Chasm: Adaptation to Mental Health and Addictive Disorders.

Stiles PG, Poythress NG, Hall A, Falkenbach D, Williams R. 2001. Improving understanding of research consent disclosures among persons with mental illness. *Psychiatric Services* 52(6):780–785.

Stuart G, Tondora J, Hoge M. 2004. Evidence-based teaching practice: Implications for behavioral health. *Administration and Policy in Mental Health* 32(2):107–130.

Sutherby K, Szmukler GI, Halpern A, Alexander M, Thornicroft G, Johnson C, Wright S. 1999. A study of "crisis cards" in a community psychiatric service. *Acta Psychiatrica Scandinavica* 100(1):56–61.

Swanson J. 1994. Mental disorder, substance abuse, and community violence: An epidemiologic approach. In: Monahan J, Steadman HJ, eds. *Violence and Mental Disorder.* Chicago, IL: University of Chicago Press. Pp. 101–136.

Swanson JW, Tepper MC, Backlar P, Swartz MS. 2000. Psychiatric advance directives: An alternative to coercive treatment? *Psychiatry* 63(2):160–172.

Swartz M, Monahan J. 2001. Special section on involuntary outpatient commitment: Introduction. *Psychiatric Services* 52(3):323–324.

Taylor PJ, Gunn J. 1999. Homicides by people with mental illness: Myth and reality. *British Journal of Psychiatry* 174(1):9–14.

Tiihonen J, Isohanni M, Raesaenen P, Koiranen M, Moring J. 1997. Specific major mental disorders and criminality: A 26-year prospective study of the 1996 northern Finland birth cohort. *American Journal of Psychiatry* 154(6):840–845.

Tonigan JS, Toscova R. 1996. Meta-analysis of the literature on Alcoholics Anonymous: Sample and study characteristics moderate findings. *Journal of Studies on Alcohol* 57(1):65–72.

Troyer TN, Acampora AP, O'Connor LE, Berry JW. 1995. The changing relationship between therapeutic communities and 12-step programs: a survey. *Journal of Psychoactive Drugs* 27(2):177–180.

Umapathy C, Ramchandani D, Lamdan R, Kishel L, Schindler B. 1999. Competency evaluations on the consultation-liaison service: Some overt and covert aspects. *Psychosomatics* 40(1):28–32.

Vollmann J, Bauer A, Danker-Hopfe H, Helmchen H. 2003. Competence of mentally ill patients: A comparative empirical study. *Psychological Medicine* 33(8):1463–1471.

Von Korff M, Gruman J, Schaefer J, Curry SJ, Wagner EH. 1997. Collaborative management of chronic illness. *Annals of Internal Medicine* 127(12):1097–1102.

Wahl OF. 1999. Mental health consumers' experience of stigma. *Schizophrenia Bulletin* 25(3):467–478.

Wallace C, Mullen PE, Burgess P. 2004. Criminal offending in schizophrenia over a 25-year period marked by deinstitutionalization and increasing prevalence of comorbid substance use. *American Journal of Psychiatry* 161(4):716–727.

Warsi A, Wang PS, LaValley MP, Avorn J, Solomon DH. 2004. Self-management education programs in chronic disease. *Archives of Internal Medicine* 164(15):1641–1649.

Watkins K, Pincus HA, Tanielian TL, Lloyd J. 2003. Using the chronic care model to improve treatment of alcohol use disorders in primary care settings. *Journal of Studies on Alcohol* 64(2):209–218.

Weisner C, Schmidt L. 2001. Rethinking access to alcohol treatment. In: Galanter M, ed. *Services Research in the Era of Managed Care*. New York: Kluwer Academic/Plenum Press. Pp. 107–136.

Weisner C, Matzger H, Tam T, Schmidt L. 2002. Who goes to alcohol and drug treatment? Understanding utilization within the context of insurance. *Journal of Studies on Alcohol* 63(6):673–682.

Wessely S. 1997. The epidemiology of crime, violence and schizophrenia. *British Journal of Psychiatry* 170 (Supplement 32):8–11.

White WL. 2002. Addiction treatment in the United States: Early pioneers and institutions. *Addiction* 97(9):1087–1092.

White WL. 2004. Addiction recovery mutual aid groups: An enduring international phenomenon. *Addiction* 99(5):532–538.

White WL. undated. *The Rhetoric of Recovery Advocacy: An Essay on the Power of Language*. [Online]. Available: http://facesandvoicesofrecovery.org/pdf/rhetoric_of_advocacy.pdf [accessed September 13, 2005].

Wicclair MR. 1991. Patient decision-making capacity and risk. *Bioethics* 5(2):91–104.

Wild TC, Roberts AB, Cooper EL. 2002. Compulsory substance abuse treatment: An overview of recent findings and issues. *European Addiction Research* 8(2):84–93.

Wirshing DA, Wirshing WC, Marder SR, Liberman RP, Mintz J. 1998. Informed consent: Assessment of comprehension. *American Journal of Psychiatry* 155(11):1508–1511.

Wolff NP. 2004. *Law and Disorder: The Case against Diminished Responsibility*. Paper commissioned by the Institute of Medicine Committee on Crossing the Quality Chasm: Adaptation to Mental Health and Addictive Disorders. Available from the Institute of Medicine.

Woll P. 2001. *Healing the Stigma of Addiction: A Guide for Treatment Professionals*. Chicago, IL: Great Lakes Addiction Technology Transfer Center.

Wong J, Clare I, Holland A, Watson P, Gunn M. 2000. The capacity of people with a "mental disability" to make a healthcare decision. *Psychological Medicine* 30(2):295–306.

Wong P, Helsinger D, Petry J. 2002. Providing the right infrastructure to lead the culture change for patient safety. *Joint Commission Journal on Quality Improvement*. 28(7):363–372.

Wright ER, Gronfein WP, Owens TJ. 2000. Deinstitutionalization, social rejection, and the self-esteem of former mental patients. *Journal of Health and Social Behavior* 41(1):68–90.

4

Strengthening the
Evidence Base and
Quality Improvement Infrastructure

Summary

Despite substantial evidence documenting the efficacy of numerous treatments for mental and substance-use problems and illnesses, mental and/or substance-use (M/SU) health care (like all health care) often is not consistent with this evidence base. Further, in the absence of evidence on how best to treat some M/SU conditions, treatment for the same condition often varies inappropriately from provider to provider. Moreover, medication errors and the use of restraints and seclusion threaten patient safety, while many individuals with serious symptoms of M/SU illnesses receive no treatment despite having health insurance and geographic access to health care. Finally, although we know about risk factors for the development of some M/SU illnesses, the health care system fails to apply this knowledge in prevention initiatives. As a result, large numbers of people who are at risk of developing M/SU illnesses go on to do so, even as those with existing illnesses cannot always count on receiving safe and effective care.

Remedies for these problems are the same as those for general health care: identifying and disseminating effective practices, providing decision support for clinicians at the point of care delivery, measuring the extent to which effective practices are applied, and incorporating measurement results into ongoing quality improvement activities. For multiple reasons, however, the infrastructure to support these activities is less well developed for M/SU than for general health care. Clinical assessment and treatment practices (especially psychosocial interventions) have not been standardized and classified for inclusion in the administrative datasets widely used to analyze variations in care and other quality-related issues in general health care. Initiatives to disseminate advances in evidence-based care often fail to use effective strategies and available resources. The development of performance measures for M/SU health care has not received sufficient attention in the private sector, and efforts in the public sector have not yet achieved widespread consensus. Finally, the understanding and use of modern quality improvement methods have not yet permeated the day-to-day operations of organizations and individual clinicians delivering M/SU services— both those in the general health care sector and those providing specialty M/SU health care.

The committee recommends a five-part strategy to build this infrastructure and improve the safety and effectiveness of M/SU health care: (1) a more coordinated strategy for filling the gaps in the evidence base; (2) a stronger, more coordinated, and evidence-based approach to disseminating evidence to clinicians; (3) improved diagnostic and assessment strategies; (4) a stronger infrastructure for measuring and reporting the quality of M/SU health care; and (5) support for quality improvement practices at the locus of health care.

PROBLEMS IN THE QUALITY OF CARE

As in general health care, there is ample evidence of problems in the quality of care for mental and/or substance-use (M/SU) problems and illnesses. These problems include (1) failure to provide care consistent with existing scientific evidence, (2) variations in care that occur when clear evidence on effective care is lacking, (3) failure to provide *any* treatment for an M/SU illness or to address the risk factors associated with the development of these illnesses, and (4) unsafe care.

Failure to Provide Care Consistent with Scientific Evidence

Numerous studies document the discrepancy between M/SU care that is known to be effective and the care that is actually delivered. An extensive review of all peer-reviewed studies published from 1992 through 2000 in Medline, the Cochrane Collaborative, and related sources that assessed rates of adherence to specific clinical practice guidelines for treating diverse M/SU clinical conditions (including alcohol withdrawal, bipolar disorder, depression, panic disorder, psychosis, schizophrenia, and substance abuse) found that of the 21 cross-sectional studies showing unequivocal results, only 24 percent documented adequate adherence to the aspect(s) of the practice guidelines under study. Of 5 pre/post studies, only 2 showed adequate adherence rates. When these two groups of naturalistic studies were combined, only 27 percent demonstrated adequate rates of adherence. Better adherence was observed in 6 of the 9 controlled trials reviewed[1] (Bauer, 2002). Subsequent studies have continued to document clinicians' departures from evidence-based practice guidelines for conditions as varied as attention deficit hyperactivity disorder (ADHD) (Rushton et al., 2004), anxiety disorders (Stein et al., 2004), conduct disorders in children (Zima et al., 2005), comorbid mental and substance-use illnesses (Watkins et al., 2001), depression in adults (Simon et al., 2001) and children (Richardson et al., 2004), opioid dependence (D'Aunno and Pollack, 2002), use of illicit drugs (Friedmann et al., 2001), and schizophrenia (Buchanan et al., 2002).

As in general health care, M/SU care received by members of racial and ethnic minorities is even less consistent with standards for effective care than that received by nonminority members. Two nationally representative studies found that members of ethnic minorities were less likely to receive appropriate care for depression or anxiety than were white Americans (Wang et al., 2000; Young et al., 2001). Likewise, facilities dispensing methadone for the treatment of opioid dependence that have a greater percentage of African American patients have been shown to be more likely to dispense low and ineffective doses (D'Aunno and Pollack, 2002).

A 1999 comparison of the performance of 67.7 percent of the nation's health maintenance organizations (HMOs) on five measures of the quality of mental health care[2] and nine measures[3] of the quality of general health care found that the HMOs delivered mental health care in accordance with standards of care on average 48 percent of the time, compared with an average of 69 percent for the nine general health care measures (Druss et al., 2002). In a landmark study of the quality of a wide variety of health care received by U.S. citizens, individuals with many different types of illnesses received guideline-concordant care about 50 percent of the time, whereas those with alcohol dependence received care consistent with scientific knowledge only about 10.5 percent of the time (McGlynn et al., 2003).

---

[1]This was attributed to the multifaceted and intensive strategies employed to facilitate and maintain the uptake of these practice guidelines.

[2]Timely ambulatory care after inpatient hospitalization (two measures), medication management of depression (two measures), and outpatient care for depression (one measure).

[3]Adolescent immunizations, use of specific drugs after a heart attack, breast cancer screening, child immunizations, delivery of prenatal care in the first trimester, postpartum checkups, cervical cancer screening, cholesterol screening, and eye examinations for diabetics.

This failure to provide care consistent with evidence also is manifest in the failure to offer ongoing care for substance dependence consistent with the condition's chronic nature. Historically, drug dependence has been conceptualized as a disease, a bad habit, or a sin (Musto, 1973). Despite significant differences among these perspectives, all are based on a view that often persists today: that some limited (often very limited) amount, duration, and/or intensity of therapies, medications, and services should be adequate to cause patients with a drug dependence illness to "learn their lesson," "achieve insight," and especially "change their ways." The expectation is that once patients have achieved that insight or learned that lesson, they will be ready for discharge from treatment and will continue as recovered for a substantial period of time. This view has led to the universally applied convention of evaluating the outcomes of treatment through measurement of patient performance 6–12 (or more) months following discharge from treatment (see Finney et al., 1996; Gerstein and Harwood, 1990; Gossop et al., 2001; Hubbard et al., 1989; McLellan et al., 1993a,b; Project MATCH Research Group, 1997; Simpson et al., 1997, 1999).

In fact, however, most alcohol- and drug-dependent patients relapse following cessation of treatment (IOM, 1998; McLellan, 2002). In general, about 50–60 percent of patients begin reusing within 6 months of treatment cessation, regardless of the type of discharge, patient characteristics, or the particular substance(s) used (IOM, 1998; McKay et al., 1999, 2004; McLellan, 2002). It is increasingly apparent that patients with more chronic forms of substance-use illnesses require and do well with appropriately tailored continuing care and monitoring (McKay, 2005; McLellan et al., 2000). Indeed, accumulating evidence suggests that many cases of substance-use illness are best treated with the same type and level of ongoing clinical support as other chronic illnesses, such as cardiovascular disease and diabetes (McLellan et al., 2000).

Variations in Care Due to a Lack of Evidence

Variations in health care are driven by a variety of factors—some appropriate and therapeutic, others not. Appropriate variations in care result when clinicians tailor therapeutic regimens to patients' unique clinical conditions, in consultation with patients about their expressed preferences and values. Undesirable variations reflect departures from widely accepted evidence-based standards of care (as described above) due to provider preferences, traditions, ignorance of evidence-based standards, or administrative or financial constraints. Variations also result from inconsistencies in diagnosis (described later in this chapter) and from the absence of widely accepted standards of care. Variations in the absence of clinical practice guidelines have been documented, for example, in the use of seclusion and restraint (Busch and Shore, 2000), patterns of prescribing psychotropic medications for preschoolers and older children (Rawal et al., 2004; Zito et al., 2000), the use of combinations of antipsychotics (Miller and Craig, 2002), and inpatient care lengths of stay (Harman et al., 2003). A 1999–2000 cross-sectional study of the care of children and adolescents at residential treatment centers in four states, for instance, found that 42.9 percent of youths receiving antipsychotic medications had no history of or current psychosis and were thus receiving those medications for "off-label" purposes. Significant regional differences in the prescription of antipsychotic drugs were found across the four states and were associated with the presence of attention deficit/impulsivity, substance use, the duration of symptoms, danger to others, sexually abusive behavior, elopement, and crime/delinquency. The use of antipsychotic medications to treat aggression and conduct disorders has been reported in the clinical literature and identified as an off-label use. Yet positive outcomes for their use in children to treat attention deficit/impulsivity disorders is not well documented and raises concerns, as does the widespread use of antipsychotics for off-label purposes generally and the regional variations in this practice (Rawal et al., 2004).

There is historical evidence that race and ethnicity account for some of these variations. African Americans have been more likely to receive antipsychotics across the diagnostic spectrum, even without indications for their use (Strickland et al., 1991), and more likely than whites to receive these medications "PRN" (as needed) and in higher doses (Chung et al., 1995; Strakowski et al., 1993).

Failure to Treat and Prevent

Failure to Treat

More than a decade ago, the 1990–1992 National Comorbidity Study documented the high proportion of individuals with symptoms of serious mental illness who failed to receive any treatment for their condition (Wang et al., 2002). Since that time, progress has been made. Recent studies have shown improvements in access to and receipt of care for those with the most severe mental illnesses (Kessler et al., 2005; Mechanic and Bilder, 2004). And although the prevalence of M/SU illnesses has remained the same over the past decade, a greater proportion of all non-aged adults with M/SU problems and illnesses have received treatment. Between 1990 and 1992, 20.3 percent of individuals with a mental "disorder" received treatment; between 2001 and 2003 this proportion was 32.9 percent (Kessler et al., 2005). Improvements also have been noted in the access to care for children with these illnesses (Glied and Cuellar, 2003).

Despite this progress, however, the same reports showing improved access to care for some reveal that many others who need treatment still do not receive it (Mechanic and Bilder, 2004); this is true especially for ethnic minorities (Kessler et al., 2005). Between 2001 and 2003, fewer than half (40.5 percent) of individuals with symptoms of a serious mental illness received treatment (Kessler et al., 2005), and there is evidence of a decline in access for those with less severe mental illnesses (Kessler et al., 2005; Mechanic and Bilder, 2004). Findings of recent studies similarly reaffirm the continuing failure to treat substance-use problems and illnesses (Watkins et al., 2001).

These failures to treat persist, even when individuals are receiving some type of health care and have financial and geographic access to care. For example, data for 1998–2001 from a seven-site longitudinal study of 1,088 youths in residential, outpatient, and inpatient treatment for drug use show that 43 percent of the youths reported receiving no mental health services in the 3 months after being admitted, despite having severe mental health problems at the time of admission. At three sites where mental health services were provided at no additional charge, rates of service receipt for those with severe mental illnesses were 6 percent, 28 percent, and 79 percent, respectively. In contrast, rates of receipt of care for comorbid general health problems among these youths ranged from 64 to 71 percent (Jaycox et al., 2003). Results of the 2003 National Survey on Drug Use and Health document a similar failure to treat adults. Data from another national survey conducted in 1997–1998 reveal that among persons with probable comorbid mental and substance-use disorders who received treatment for one of these conditions, fewer than a third (28.6 percent) received treatment for the other (Watkins et al., 2001).

Reasons for the failure to treat M/SU illnesses have not been fully determined, but the finding of low treatment rates in the presence of access to services and no additional cost to the patient indicates that access and ability to pay are not always the only contributing factors. This point is confirmed by responses of civilian, noninstitutionalized adults aged 18 and older to the 2003 National Survey on Drug Use and Health, which captured separately information on mental and substance-use problems and illnesses. These respondents reported the following reasons for not receiving mental health treatment that they believe they needed: cost/insurance issues (45.1 percent), did not feel the need for treatment at the time/could handle the problem without treatment (40.6 percent), did not know where to go for services (22.9 percent), stigma (22.8 percent), did not have time (18.1 percent), believed treatment would not help (10.3 percent), fear of being committed/having to take medication (7.2 percent), and other access barriers (3.7 percent). Reasons given by respondents who felt they needed treatment for a substance-use problem but did not receive it were somewhat different: not ready to stop using (41.2 percent), cost or insurance barriers (33.2 percent), stigma (19.6 percent), did not feel the need for treatment (at the time) or could handle the problem without treatment (17.2 percent), access barriers other than cost (12.3 percent), did not know where to go for treatment (8.7 percent), believed treatment would not help (6.3 percent), and did not have time (5.3 percent) (SAMHSA, 2004a).

Other studies of factors that influence consumers' entry into alcohol and drug treatment have found that individuals with alcohol or drug problems who do not experience recovery on their own typically do not go into treatment until their problems become severe or until social circumstances, such as workplace problems or criminal offenses, send them there. In a 2001 nationally representative survey of individuals in recovery from alcohol or drug illnesses and their families, 60 percent reported that denial of addiction or refusal to admit the severity of the problem was the greatest barrier to their recovery. Embarrassment or shame was the second most frequently cited obstacle (Peter D. Hart Research Associates, Inc., 2001). Factors that drive these individuals to seek help vary over the course of their alcohol or drug use. Early on, these factors include adverse social consequences in the workplace, criminal convictions, or serious disturbances in interpersonal relationships. As substance use progresses over time, health problems related to use are associated with seeking treatment (Satre et al., 2004; Weisner and Matzger, 2002).

Individuals who are members of ethnic minorities face additional obstacles to receiving needed mental health services (DHHS, 2001). Despite roughly similar levels of need, ethnic minorities are less likely to receive mental health care than are white Americans. Blacks, for example, are only 50 percent as likely to receive psychiatric treatment as whites when both receive a diagnosis of the same severity (Kessler et al., 2005). Latino children also have higher rates of unmet need relative to other children (Kataoka et al., 2002). Access to mental health services may be restricted for ethnic minorities for multiple reasons—for example, because they are more apt to be uninsured (Brown et al., 2000), because ethnic minority providers and/or providers with appropriate language capabilities are often unavailable, and because they may have less trust in the health care system (LaVeist et al., 2000).

Failure to Prevent

Sometimes failure to provide care occurs at the level of the health system, rather than at the patient–provider level. The United States, like other developed countries, has structures and mechanisms in place to address threats to the public's health that arise from both external environmental conditions and an individual's personal health practices. An earlier

Institute of Medicine report on reducing risks for mental disorders (IOM, 1994) notes that prevention activities for many general health conditions take place even when the etiology of an illness and how to prevent it are not fully understood. Examples are primary prevention of cancer and heart disease, for which the public health system has targeted known risk factors (e.g., diet, exercise, lipid levels, smoking) despite the lack of such knowledge. This risk reduction model of prevention targets the risk factors known to be associated with an illness or injury. By contrast, despite scientific evidence on risk factors associated with some mental illnesses (predominantly in children and adolescents) and effective interventions to mitigate these factors (see, e.g., Beardslee et al., 2003; Hollon et al., 2002; Mojtabai et al., 2003), this evidence has not yet been widely applied in practice (Davis, 2002), and the prevalence[4] of M/SU problems and illnesses does not appear to have declined over the past decade (Kessler et al., 2005).

Although there is not yet clear evidence to support preventive interventions for specific diagnoses (e.g., ADHD, anxiety, or depression), risk factors have been identified that have been helpful for developing broad, school-based preventive programs that generally target "behavior problems." This prevention literature for children is focused largely in two areas: (1) risk factors for conduct problems, serious disruptive behaviors, and violence, and testing of interventions aimed at preventing the onset of those problems (Kazdin, 2003; Patterson et al., 1989, 1993; Webster-Stratton and Hammond, 1997, 1999); and (2) prevention of depression among adolescents (Clarke et al., 1995; Lewinsohn, 1987) or children (Beardslee et al., 1996, 1997; Podorefsky et al., 2001). The U.S. Surgeon General's report on youth violence also clearly sets forth the evidence for prevention of violent behavior (Office of the Surgeon General, 2001).

Unsafe Care

As with the quality of M/SU health care overall, less is known about errors in or injuries due to M/SU treatment services than is the case for general health care (Bates et al., 2003; Moos, 2005). This is especially true for errors that occur in outpatient settings, where the greatest proportion of treatment for individuals with M/SU problems and illnesses is provided. Some mental health "interventions" have been found to be harmful subsequent to their use; examples are organized visits to jails and prisons by children or adolescents to deter their future delinquency (sometimes known as "scared straight" programs) (Petrosino et al., 2005) and rebirthing therapy (Lilienfeld et al., 2003). Others, such as critical incidence stress

---

[4]Data on incidence are not available.

debriefing, have been found to be potentially harmful (Rose et al., 2005). Most data on threats to safety have been collected on medication errors and the use of seclusion and restraints in mental health care. Errors or injuries from treatment for substance-use problems and illnesses have not yet received substantial attention. Although an estimated 7–15 percent of patients who receive psychosocial treatment for substance use may be worse off after treatment, a conceptual model to help distinguish the iatrogenic effects of the intervention from other factors that can cause worsening of substance-use problems (e.g., social isolation) has only recently been proposed (Moos, 2005).

Medication Errors

A Medline search for articles published between 1996 and 2003 on medication errors (one of the most common types of health care errors) in psychiatric treatment revealed relatively few data available, and only a handful of studies of adverse drug events in inpatient psychiatric settings. Although studies of adverse drug events in general hospitals have yielded data on errors involving psychotropic drugs, less is known about medication errors in psychiatric hospitals and psychiatric units of general hospitals. Moreover, as recently as 2002, terms such as "adverse drug events," "medication errors," and "adverse drug reactions" were not even listed as key search words in several widely read psychiatric journals (Grasso et al., 2003b). Errors committed in substance-use treatment also have received little attention.

What is known from the few published studies gives cause for concern. A retrospective, multidisciplinary review of the charts of 31 randomly selected patients in a state psychiatric hospital discharged during a 4 1/2-month study period detected 2,194 medication errors during these patients' entire 1,448 inpatient days.[5] Of the 2,194 errors, 19 percent were rated as having the potential to cause minor harm, 23 percent moderate harm, and 58 percent severe harm (Grasso et al., 2003a). Another 12-month study of all long-term residents of 18 community-based nursing homes in Massachusetts found that psychoactive medications (antipsychotics, antidepressants, and sedatives/hypnotics) were among the most common medications

---

[5]These medication error rates are consistent with rates reported in studies occurring in general medical hospitals, but the distribution of the types of errors is markedly different. A much higher proportion of errors (66 percent) occurred during the administration of the medication as opposed to its prescribing, transcription, or dispensing. The authors note that at the time the study was conducted, medication administration was performed by medical technicians as opposed to licensed nurses—a practice that was discontinued subsequent to the study (Grasso et al., 2003a).

associated with preventable adverse drug events, and neuropsychiatric events were the most common type of preventable adverse drug events (Gurwitz et al., 2000).

With respect to ambulatory care, additional safety concerns have been raised about the practice of long-term treatment with combinations of antipsychotic medications (except in instances of failures of monotherapy using different drugs). The use of combinations of antipsychotic medications continues despite (1) the absence of evidence to support the practice, (2) the lack of evidence to inform clinicians about how to adjust dosages in the face of increased symptoms or side effects, and (3) increased risks to the patient from problematic side effects and failure to adhere to treatment (Miller and Craig, 2002). Similarly, experts in children's mental health care express concern about the growing use of atypical antipsychotics to treat aggression in children and adolescents in the face of limited basic and clinical research supporting the rationale, efficacy, and safety of using these agents for this purpose (Patel et al., 2005).

Seclusion and Restraint

Use of seclusion and restraint, while necessary in some emergency situations to prevent harm to a patient or others, also is associated with substantial psychological and physical harm to patients (GAO, 1999). The federal government estimates that each year approximately 150 individuals in the United States die as the direct result of these practices (SAMHSA, 2004b). In 1998, the death of an 11-year-old boy who died while secluded and restrained in a psychiatric hospital focused national attention on the risks to patients when these approaches are used. A follow-up report of the U.S. General Accounting Office (now the Government Accountability Office) (GAO) confirmed the danger of improper use of seclusion and restraint and called attention to inadequate monitoring and reporting of their use, inconsistent and insufficient standards for their use and reporting by licensing and accreditation bodies, and widespread failure to employ strategies that can prevent their use and reduce the risk of related injuries. Children experience higher rates of seclusion and restraint relative to adults and are at greater risk of injury from their use (GAO, 1999).

Consumers and their advocates, professional associations, provider organizations, and the federal government recommend substantial reductions in the use of seclusion and restraint (American Association of Community Psychiatrists, 2003; NAMI, 2003; NASMHPD, 1999, 2005; SAMHSA, 2004b). GAO found that these practices can be greatly reduced through strong management commitment and leadership, defined principles and policies regarding when and how they may be used, a requirement to report their use, staff training in their safe use and alternative approaches, and oversight and monitoring (GAO, 1999).[6] Several initiatives incorporating these practices have greatly reduced the use of seclusion and restraint (American Psychiatric Association et al., 2003; Hennessy, 2002), some achieving near elimination of the practices. Pennsylvania's state psychiatric hospital system, for example, which called attention to the use of seclusion and restraints as an indicator of "treatment failure," sharply decreased their use from 107.9 hours per 1,000 patient days in 1993 to 2.72 hours per 1,000 patient days in 2000 through quality improvement initiatives in all state psychiatric hospitals (Smith et al., 2005).

Use of seclusion and restraint continues, however, despite a Cochrane Collaboration finding that "few other forms of treatment which are applied to patients with various psychiatric diagnoses are so lacking in basic information about their proper use and efficacy (Sailas and Fenton, 2005:4). As a result, seclusion and restraints are frequently applied without clear indications for their use (Finke, 2001) and can lead to death (Denogean, 2003; Schnaars, 2003), physical harm (Mohr et al., 2003), or severe psychological trauma (Pflueger, 2002).[7] Individuals admitted to inpatient psychiatric care often have a history of sexual or other physical abuse (Goodman et al., 1997; Mueser et al., 2002). Being physically overpowered, restrained, or placed in a locked room may have many features in common with the abuse experienced earlier by these individuals.

Heightened Safety Concerns and Need for Multiple Actions

The limited information on the safety of M/SU health care is of particular concern because some of the unique features of M/SU illnesses and their treatments could make patients less able to detect and avoid errors and more vulnerable to errors and adverse events when they occur. For example, the stigma experienced by individuals with M/SU illnesses may make them less willing to report errors and adverse events and less likely to be believed when they do so. The symptoms of some severe illnesses, such as major depression or schizophrenia, when not alleviated by therapy, also could interfere with a patient's ability to detect and report medication errors.

The departures from scientific knowledge, variations in care, failures to treat and prevent, and unsafe practices discussed above have multiple causes. These include (1) gaps in the evidence base, (2) problems in disseminating existing evidence to clinicians and ensuring its uptake, (3) greater subjectiv-

---

[6]These initiatives are intended to complement other essential elements, such as adequate numbers of well-trained staff and the use of proven psychological and medication treatments.

[7]Because reporting of the use of seclusion and restraints is not required, however, data on prevalence rates for their use and rates of adverse consequences are not available.

ity in diagnosing mental problems and illnesses relative to general health conditions, (4) a less-well-developed infrastructure for measuring and reporting the quality of M/SU health care, and (5) inadequate adoption of quality improvement practices at the locus of M/SU care delivery. The following sections of this chapter present evidence on these issues and describe actions that can be taken to address them, specifically by:

- Improving the production of evidence.
- Improving diagnosis and assessment.
- Using evidence-based practices and untapped resources to better disseminate the evidence.
- Strengthening the quality measurement and reporting infrastructure.
- Applying quality improvement methods at the locus of care.

Related issues of improved care coordination, use of information technology, implications of a more diverse workforce, and creation of incentives in the marketplace to support this five-part strategy are addressed in succeeding chapters.

IMPROVING THE PRODUCTION OF EVIDENCE

Gaps in the Evidence Base

Efficacious Treatments

Over the past two decades, there has been an impressive increase in the number and quality of studies on M/SU problems, illnesses, and therapies for both children (Burns and Hoagwood, 2004, 2005; Pappadopulos et al., 2004; Weisz, 2004) and adults (IOM, 1997; Johnson et al., 2000). Nonetheless, gaps remain in our knowledge of how to treat some M/SU conditions, how to care simultaneously for multiple comorbidities, how to care for some population subgroups, and which evidence-based therapies are better than others or best of all (see Box 4-1).

Such gaps in knowledge mean that evidence-based clinical practice guidelines are unavailable for many M/SU problems and illnesses.

The Efficacy–Effectiveness Gap

In addition to the above gaps in knowledge of efficacious therapies, there has been more research on the *efficacy* of specific treatments than on the *effectiveness* of these treatments when delivered in usual settings of care; in the presence of comorbid conditions, social stressors, and varying degrees of social support; and when administered by service providers with-

---

**BOX 4-1   Some of the Knowledge Gaps
in Treatment for M/SU Conditions**

Therapies for children and older adults. Knowledge about how to best care for
individuals at both ends of the age continuum is limited, including how to incorporate effective treatment for the most prevalent disorders of childhood (i.e., anxiety,
ADHD, depression, conduct disorders) into routine care (Hoagwood et al., 2001;
Stein, 2002), the effect of multiple medications on children's outcomes, and the
comparative efficacy of different therapies for severe conditions (e.g., bipolar disorder, childhood depression) (Kane et al., 2003). Evidence is also needed on how
to better care for older adults with comorbid conditions and the frail elderly in usual
settings of care (Borson et al., 2001).

Treatment of multiple conditions. In spite of the high frequency of comorbid
mental, substance-use, and general illnesses (see Chapters 1 and 5), there is a
substantial lack of knowledge about effective treatment for individuals with complex comorbidity (Kessler, 2004).

Posttraumatic Stress Disorder/Acute Stress Disorder. Better evidence is
needed about effective treatment for posttraumatic stress disorder (PTSD) and
acute stress disorder (ASD), e.g., how best to combine pharmacotherapy and psychotherapy, and how to relieve some specific symptoms, such as insomnia or
nightmares, and in the presence of other medications. Moreover, although cognitive and behavioral therapies have demonstrated efficacy in treating victims of
sexual assault, interpersonal violence, and industrial or vehicular accidents, their
effectiveness in treating PTSD or ASD in combat veterans or victims of mass violence requires further study (Work Group on ASD and PTSD, 2004).

---

out specialized education in their use (DHHS, 1999; Essock et al., 2003;
Kazdin, 2004). For example, while numerous clinical efficacy studies have
documented that psychostimulant medications reduce the core symptoms
of ADHD, accumulating evidence suggests that this drug treatment is much
less effective as currently delivered in routine community settings (Lefever
et al., 2003). For people with severe mental illnesses and many substance-
use problems and illnesses, how well the clinical aspects of treatment work
is often closely related to such factors as housing, income support, and
employment-related activities. This complicates considerations regarding
effectiveness and has resulted in calls for improved research efforts (discussed below) that can provide information on both the effectiveness and
efficacy of interventions (Carroll and Rounsaville, 2003; Tunis et al., 2003;
Wolff, 2000).

Although the knowledge gaps discussed above also exist for general
health care, some of the tools and strategies used to build the evidence base

Psychotic illnesses. Questions remain about which antipsychotic medication should be the first line of therapy, what constitutes a sufficient period of time for a trial of a new medication to see if it is effective, and how to handle poor response to the initial prescribed medication (Kane et al., 2003). Moreover, the use of multiple antipsychotic medications takes place despite a lack of evidence about their combined efficacy and how to manage their dosing when increased symptoms or side effects occur (Miller and Craig, 2002).

Amphetamine or marijuana dependence. No medications have yet been found effective in treating these dependencies.

Cocaine dependence. No medications are currently approved by the U.S. Food and Drug Administration to treat this dependency.

Relative effectiveness of different treatments. Multiple therapies are used to treat the same illness. For example, more than 550 psychotherapies are currently in use for children and adolescents, with little helpful information for clinicians or consumers about their comparative effectiveness (Kazdin, 2000, 2004). As in other areas of health care, the federal government's drug approval rules give little incentive for head-to-head clinical trials (Pincus, 2003), and there is a lack of substantial capital investment in developing and testing psychosocial interventions.

Therapies for other population subgroups. Ethnic and cultural minorities are largely missing from efficacy studies for many treatments (DHHS, 2001) in spite of growing evidence that drug dosages may vary by ethnic status (Lin et al., 1997). Few of these studies had the power necessary to examine the impact of care on specific minorities.

in general health care are less frequently utilized in M/SU health care. Research on M/SU health care needs to make greater use of these approaches to generating evidence on effective therapies.

Filling the Gaps in the Evidence Base

As is the case for general health care, federal agencies, philanthropic organizations, and other private-sector entities undertake many efforts to identify priority areas in M/SU health care in need of evidence, fund and conduct research, and support systematic reviews of research findings to identify evidence-based therapies. A strategy for coordinating these various efforts is articulated in Chapter 9. However, the large number of gaps in the evidence base for M/SU health care also requires that all sources of valid and reliable information be used to produce as much evidence as quickly, comprehensively, and accurately as possible. Three sources of information have been under-utilized: (1) studies other than randomized controlled trials, (2) administrative datasets that often exist electronically, and (3) patients and their ability to report changes in their symptoms and well-being (outcomes of care). Steps can be taken to make better use of each of these sources.

Studies Other Than Randomized Controlled Trials

While well-designed randomized controlled trials are recognized as the gold standard for generating sound clinical evidence, experts note that the sheer number of possible pharmacological and nonpharmacological treatments for many M/SU illnesses makes relying solely on such studies to identify evidence-based care infeasible (Essock et al., 2003). Others add that some features of mental health care make use of randomized controlled trials methodologically problematic as well. For example, in studies of the effectiveness of psychotherapy, the therapist and the patient cannot be blinded to the intervention, delivery of a placebo psychotherapeutic intervention is difficult to conceptualize, and standardization of the intervention is problematic because therapists must respond to what happens in a psychotherapy session as it unfolds (Tanenbaum, 2003). For such reasons, the behavioral and social sciences have often used quasi-experimental as well as qualitative research designs (National Academy of Sciences, undated), practices that are sometimes a source of contention.

Some assert that quasi-experimental studies often are more useful than randomized controlled trials in generating practical information on how to provide effective mental health interventions in some clinical areas (Essock et al., 2003). Consistent with this assertion, the U.S. Preventive Services Task Force notes that a well-designed cohort study may be more compelling than a poorly designed or weakly powered randomized controlled trial (Harris et al., 2001). Observational studies also have been identified as a valid source of evidence that is useful in determining aspects of better quality of care (West et al., 2002). However, others note the comparative weakness of these study designs in controlling for bias and other sources of error and exclude them from systematic reviews of evidence for the determination of evidence-based practices.

A discussion of variations in study design and their implications for systematic reviews of evidence is beyond the scope of this report; many researchers and methodologists are considering strategies for addressing these difficult issues (Wolff, 2000). As this study was under way, the National Research Council had established a planning committee to oversee the development of a broad, multiyear effort—the Standards of Evidence–Strategic Planning Initiative—to identify critical issues affecting the quality and utility of research in the behavioral and social sciences and education (National Academy of Sciences, undated). The committee believes such discussions are critical to strengthening the appropriate use of all of the above types of research in building the evidence base on effective treatments for M/SU illnesses.

Better Capture of Mental and Substance-Use Health Care Data in Administrative Datasets

In general health care, routinely collected administrative data (e.g., claims or encounter data) that are generally produced each time a patient is admitted to a hospital or makes a visit to an ambulatory heath care provider are widely used for health services research, epidemiologic studies, and quality assessment and improvement initiatives (Iezzoni, 1997; Zhan and Miller, 2003). While these datasets have limitations with respect to their completeness, accuracy, and level of detail (AHRQ, 2004a; Iezzoni, 1997), administrative data remain a preferred and routinely used source of information for multiple quality-related purposes because they are readily available, inexpensive, and computer readable (AHRQ, 2004b; Zhan and Miller, 2003). For example, analysis of administrative data revealed the now well-known and sizable variations that exist in clinical care within the United States, an analysis that continues today (Mullan, 2004; Wennberg, 1999). Consequently, administrative data produce a variety of clinical quality indicators for hospital care (AHRQ, 2004b), underpin many of the quality measures found in the National Committee for Quality Assurance's (NCQA) Healthplan Employer Data and Information Set (HEDIS) performance measures (NCQA, 2004a), and are the data source for the Agency for Healthcare Research and Quality's (AHRQ) new patient safety indicators (Zhan and Miller, 2003). Because of their utility, administrative data are viewed as a mainstay of health services research on quality of care (Iezzoni, 1997) and are likely to become even more so as the National Health Information Infrastructure is developed (see Chapter 6).

These inpatient and outpatient datasets typically contain standardized information on each individual's diagnosis (using International Classification of Diseases [ICD] codes) and on the specific therapies and procedures performed for that diagnosis (using the American Medical Association's [AMA] Current Procedural Terminology [CPT] codes, the Centers for Medicare and Medicaid Services' (CMS) Healthcare Common Procedure Coding System [HCPCS] for outpatient care, and ICD, ninth revision, Clinical Modification (ICD-9-CM) procedure codes for inpatient care). However, these codes are less useful at present for the study of M/SU care than for the study of general health care for several reasons. Psychotherapy codes are few and imprecise and differ across inpatient and outpatient settings. Codes for other psychosocial services generally are absent, as are codes for the use of restraints. And the new CPT II codes for use in performance measurement, a significant development, do not yet include codes for measuring the quality of M/SU health care.

CPT codes CPT psychotherapy codes generally do not indicate what specific type of psychotherapy was provided, only that psychotherapy in general was provided and how long the session lasted. The 2005 CPT codes (AMA, 2004a) include only two main codes for psychotherapy:

> *"Insight Oriented, Behavior Modifying and/or Supportive Psychotherapy"* in an office or other outpatient facility, approximately 20 to 30, or 45 to 50, or 75 to 80 minutes face-to-face with the patient (codes 90804, 90806, and 90808 respectively) without or with (codes 90805, 90807, or 90809) accompanying medical evaluation and management services.

> *"Interactive Psychotherapy"* which consists of individual psychotherapy, interactive, using play equipment, physical devices, language interpreter, or other mechanism of non-verbal communication, in an office or outpatient facility for approximately 20 to 30, or 45 to 50, or 75 to 80 minutes face-to-face with the patient (codes 90810, 90812, and 90814, respectively). These codes are typically used for children or others who have not yet developed or who have lost language communication skills.

A similar number of codes exist for these same services when provided in an inpatient hospital, partial hospital, or residential care facility. Six other codes for psychoanalysis and group, family, and interactive psychotherapy exist, as well as 10 codes for "Other Psychiatric Services or Procedures," such as electroconvulsive treatments, hypnotherapy, and biofeedback. With the exception of a code for psychoanalysis, none of these codes identify the specific type of psychotherapy administered (e.g., cognitive therapy, behavior modification, cognitive behavioral therapy, interpersonal therapy, dialectical behavioral therapy, prolonged exposure therapy for individuals suffering from posttraumatic stress disorder, Gestalt therapy, movement/dance/art therapy, humanistic therapy, existential therapy, eye movement desensitization therapy, primal therapy, person-centered therapy, multisystemic therapy, and the many variants of these. Nor are there procedure codes for the use of diagnostic or behavioral assessment instruments. Other evidence-based psychotherapies, as well as psychosocial interventions such as family psychoeducation, multisystemic therapy, illness self-management programs, and assertive community treatment also do not have designated CPT codes. Moreover, a recent initiative of the AMA and the CPT Editorial Panel to develop codes for performance measurement (CPT II codes) and emerging technologies, services, and procedures (CPT III codes) has not yet adequately addressed M/SU health care.

The new CPT II codes are optional codes to support nationally established performance measures by allowing the electronic capture of information that otherwise would have to be obtained through medical record abstraction or chart review. The growing use of administrative data for research purposes also instigated their development. The CPT II codes currently address specific types of patient management (e.g., prenatal care); patient history-taking activities (e.g., assessment of tobacco use, anginal symptoms and level of activity); physical examination processes (e.g., measurement of blood pressure); and therapeutic, preventive, or other interventions (e.g., counseling or intervention for cessation of tobacco use and prescription of certain medications).[8] CPT III codes for new and emerging technologies include a new code for online medical evaluation service using the Internet or similar electronic communications network (AMA, 2004a). NCQA is proposing to use the new CPT II codes for the first time in HEDIS 2006 to capture data on blood pressure ($\leq$140/90 mm Hg or > 140/90), prenatal and postpartum care, beta-blocker treatment after heart attacks, diabetes care, and cholesterol management after a cardiovascular event (NCQA, 2005).

Category II codes are reviewed by a Performance Measures Advisory Group (PMAG) made up of performance measurement experts representing AHRQ, CMS, the Joint Commission on Accreditation of Healthcare Organizations (JCAHO), NCQA, and the AMA's Physician Consortium for Performance Improvement (the Consortium). The PMAG may seek additional expertise and/or input as necessary from other national health care organizations, including national medical specialty societies, other national health care professional associations, accrediting bodies, and federal regulatory agencies, and will consider code proposals submitted by national regulatory agencies, accrediting bodies, national professional and medical specialty societies, and other organizations (AMA, 2004a).

ICD-9 procedure codes ICD-9 procedure codes for inpatient care are somewhat more detailed than the CPT codes with respect to psychotherapy. For example, they include a separate code for behavior therapies such as "aversion therapy, behavior modification, desensitization therapy, extinction therapy, relaxation therapy, and token economy." They do not, however, include a code for use of restraints in psychiatric care, although there are two codes for use of "isolation." Similarly, ICD-9-E codes, used to classify external events or circumstances that can cause injury or other adverse events, do not include a specific code for injuries obtained during the appli-

---

[8]Codes for diagnostic/screening processes or results, follow-up or other outcomes, and patient safety are planned but not yet included in the 2005 version.

cation or use of restraints, in contrast with the codes provided for a variety of other "misadventures to patients during surgical and medical care," ranging from errors caused by a surgical operation (Code E870.0) to errors caused by administration of an enema (Code E870.7) (AMA, 2004b).

As a result, when psychotherapy is delivered to a patient and paid for by insurers, it is essentially a "black box." In child and adolescent therapy alone, for example, it is conservatively estimated that, even if one omits various combinations of treatments and variants of treatments that are not substantially different, there are more than 550 psychotherapies in use (Kazdin, 2000). Because of their lack of specificity, however, administrative data currently cannot document the extent of variation in therapeutic practice and trends over time as they have done for general health care. More-detailed therapy codes, type-of-provider codes,[9] and codes that use consistent terminology across inpatient and outpatient settings could help in measuring the use and variation in use of the many hundreds of types of psychotherapy. Moreover, if the type of psychotherapy were routinely captured in administrative data and combined with data on patients' reports regarding the results of their care (as are currently obtained in some consumer surveys now in use), such information could assist in evaluating the *effectiveness* of different therapies in the field, in contrast to evaluation of their *efficacy* in experimentally controlled settings (see above and the discussion of outcome data below). The absence of detailed administrative data linked to patient outcomes makes it difficult to discern the relative effectiveness of different therapies or whether, as some assert, the effectiveness of the therapist's relationship with the client may be equally or more important than the type of therapy provided (Levant, 2004; Norcross, 2002). Moreover, performance measurement and improvement would be facilitated by this type of administrative data. Performance measures based on administrative data, such as claims data, are more likely to be used than measures based on more costly or labor-intensive sources of data, such as medical records or patient surveys (Hermann et al., 2000).

Following the issuance of regulations implementing the administrative simplification provisions of the Health Insurance Portability and Accountability Act (HIPAA), the Substance Abuse and Mental Health Services Administration (SAMHSA), the National Association of State Mental Health Directors, Inc. (NASMHPD), and the National Association of State Alcohol and Drug Abuse Directors, Inc. (NASADAD) took steps to identify some additional procedure codes to capture the range of treat-

---

[9]If codes existed for each type of provider (e.g., marriage and family therapist, clinical psychologist, psychiatrist), variations in care by provider type would be visible and aid efforts to reduce variation.

ment services provided (see http://hipaa.samhsa.gov). Similar, expanded efforts in coordination with public- and private-sector experts in coding, evidence-based practices, and use of administrative datasets could help substantially in building the evidence base on the effectiveness of different M/SU treatments.

Collection of Outcome Data from Patients

Patients are increasingly recognized as valid judges of the quality of their health care (Iezzoni, 1997); this applies equally to general and M/SU health care. In addition to reporting on their experiences with care delivery processes—such as the extent to which they were able to participate in decisions about their own care and gain skill in the self-management of their illness—consumers can provide information on the effectiveness of treatment in reducing symptoms and improving functioning (Hibbard, 2003). Moreover, "the shift toward patient-centered care has meant that a broader range of *outcomes from the patient's perspective* needs to be measured in order to understand the true benefits and risks of healthcare interventions." (emphasis added) (Stanton, 2002:2) Patient questionnaires that ask about the extent to which patients' symptoms have been reduced as a result of treatment are already being used to measure outcomes for treatment of general medical conditions such as benign prostatic hypertrophy and cataracts. These questionnaires have been found to yield accurate and reliable information on the extent of improvement in symptoms, providing detailed and sensitive measures of treatment effectiveness from the patient's perspective. For example, the VF-14, a 14-item questionnaire on eyesight, asks patients about the amount of difficulty they experience in pursuing usual daily activities, such as driving and reading fine print. Many insurers (including Medicare) require that the results of the VF-14 be reported as part of claims payment. The questionnaire also is required by the National Eye Institute to test the benefits of new technologies and procedures for cataract patients (Stanton, 2002).

Such consumer surveys may be an even more appropriate and valuable source of data on the outcomes of M/SU health care than on those of general health care. Laboratory tests or other physical measures, such as blood glucose levels, blood pressure, and forced expiratory lung volume, can measure outcomes of general health care accurately and easily. In contrast, fewer laboratory or other physical examination findings can measure whether mental illness or drug dependence is remitting. Thus patients are likely to be the best source of information on the extent to which their symptoms are abating and functioning is improved.

Patient reports of symptoms and functioning (outcomes of care) can readily be gathered using several clinically feasible, valid, and reliable questionnaires, such as the Behavior and Symptom Identification Scale (BASIS-32) (Eisen et al., 1999, 2004) and the Patient Health Questionnaire (PHQ-9) (Lowe et al., 2004). Alternatively, clinicians can assess response to treatment systematically and reliably by obtaining information from the patient, combined with other data, and following up over time by using such instruments as the Global Assessment of Functioning (GAF), the Brief Psychiatric Rating Scale (BPRS), and the Health of the Nation Outcome Scales (HoNOS) (VA Technology Assessment Program, 2002). In the alcohol and drug field, instruments such as the Addiction Severity Index (ASI), the Global Appraisal of Individual Needs (GAIN), and the Project MATCH Form 90 are widely used to measure function. In addition, patient surveys used for quality measurement purposes, such as the Experience of Care and Health Outcomes (ECHO) Survey (Anonymous, 2001) and the Mental Health Statistical Improvement Project (MHSIP) surveys, include questions on patients' perceptions of their improvements in functioning.

If the more detailed administrative data on treatment described above were linked to patient reports of improvement in clinical symptoms and other outcomes, additional evidence could be generated on what treatments and treatment approaches are more effective than others in usual settings of care. For example, the annual Medicare Current Beneficiary Survey asks aged and disabled Medicare beneficiaries living in the community and in institutions to answer questions about many aspects of their health and health care, including their health status and ability to function. These patient self-report data are often combined with Medicare claims and expenditure data to answer a variety of questions about Medicare-covered services (CMS, 2004), such as whether particular services improve beneficiaries' functional status (Hadley et al., 2000) and what effects variations in Medicare spending have on the delivery of care and patient outcomes (Fisher et al., 2003). In addition, the analysis of administrative data and patient outcomes can be used to facilitate experimental research by identifying target population groups that are using therapies or medications of interest and have experienced either treatment failures, partial symptom abatement, or more complete recovery (Miller and Craig, 2002). In the Veterans Health Administration (VHA), linking outcome data on patients treated for posttraumatic stress disorder with administrative data showed that long-term, intensive inpatient treatment was not more effective than short-term treatment and cost $18,000 more per patient per year (Fontana and Rosenheck, 1997; Rosenheck and Fontana, 2001). In 1999, the VHA mandated that all mental health inpatients be rated at discharge using the GAF instrument, and that all outpatients be similarly rated at least once every 90 days during active treatment. The agency now includes GAF outcome measures in its National Mental Health Program Performance Monitoring System (Greenberg and Rosenheck, 2005) (see the discussion in Appendix C).

How Mechanisms for Analyzing the Evidence
Can Be Strengthened and Coordinated

As evidence is generated, systematic analysis is essential to translate it into clinically useful practice guidelines and other clinician decision-support tools. Many organizations and initiatives in the United States are performing such analyses for M/SU health care. However, there is often little coordination of those efforts. Moreover, although the practice of evidence-based care is widely endorsed, there is not yet a shared understanding in M/SU health care (as is also the case in general health care [Steinberg and Luce, 2005]) of what constitutes a finding that a given practice is evidence-based. Views differ about the acceptability of various forms of evidence, what level of evidence is necessary for a practice to be recommended or endorsed as evidence-based (Tanenbaum, 2003), and whether knowledge of evidence-based care for a population can be adapted to meet each individual's unique needs (Tanenbaum, 2005).

This lack of consensus prompted a call from Congress in 1999 for AHRQ to identify and describe sound methods for rating the strength of scientific evidence. AHRQ found several acceptable systems that address the essential considerations of (1) the aggregate quality ratings for individual studies; (2) the quantity of studies (number of studies, magnitude of observed effects, and sample size or power); and (3) consistency, or the extent to which similar and different study designs yield similar findings (West et al., 2002). However, AHRQ's findings while helpful, do not resolve debates about whether a given intervention is evidence-based. Most evidence reviewers acknowledge that many interventions have varying degrees of evidence in their favor, ultimately necessitating a judgment as to whether the evidence supports recommending their use.

This judgment can often differ according to the entity conducting the evidence review but may be more susceptible to variation in M/SU than in general health care for several reasons. First, a greater number of organizations are involved in making determinations with regard to evidence-based practices in M/SU health care. As Chapter 7 attests, a greater number of professions (e.g., physicians, psychologists, counselors, marriage and family therapists) with their diverse traditions and training are involved in independently diagnosing and treating M/SU conditions than is the case for general health care. Their professional organizations are increasingly conducting evidence reviews and promulgating their own practice guidelines. Moreover, because M/SU problems and illnesses are addressed not only by the health care system, but also by the welfare, justice, and education systems, organizations and disciplines involved in these latter systems also are dedicating resources to evaluating the evidence and identifying evidence-based M/SU health care practices (see the Department of Justice's What Works initiative in Table

4-1). Second, the biological and social sciences often have employed different types of research designs, with resulting differences in the types of empirical evidence produced. Because M/SU health care involves both medical and psychosocial issues and professions that have their historical origins in either the biological or social sciences, reviews are conducted by entities with different origins and research traditions and sometimes produce different types of empirical evidence and judgments about their meaning. Table 4-1 lists some of the leading organizations or initiatives that conduct evidence reviews of M/SU health care services and make determinations with regard to effective practices.

The commitment of these and other organizations to promoting the delivery of evidence-based care is to be applauded. "Reinvention" has been identified as a key ingredient in ensuring acceptance of new concepts and necessary change (Greenhalgh et al., 2004). At the same time, however, variations in review and rating methodologies can result in different practice guidelines for treating the same condition and a lack of consensus on what guidelines are best (Manderscheid et al., 2001). The lack of coordination and consensus across the multiple existing review efforts also contributes to significant confusion about what constitutes "evidence-based" health care for mental and substance-use conditions (Ganju, 2004). These variations and sometimes duplication in the topics reviewed create challenges to the promotion of evidence-based care. Moreover, the lack of coordination among these initiatives means there are fewer resources available for other quality improvement activities.

There is also a contrast between the evidence review infrastructure for psychotherapies and that for drug safety and efficacy, as well for how new treatments and therapies are deployed. The U.S. Food and Drug Administration (FDA) oversees the development, delivery, and dissemination of safe and effective medication therapies by subjecting new medications to a safety review before they are released into the marketplace for use by consumers. FDA review mechanisms also assess the strength of the evidence for the effectiveness of certain drugs prior to their release. Medications cannot be distributed or advertised to the public unless they have been approved by the FDA. However, no such safety and efficacy reviews are required for psychotherapies. As a consequence, those seeking psychotherapy cannot always be confident that the treatment they are receiving has met any standards for safe and effective care. In one extreme example, this situation resulted in the death of a 10-year-old child who was subjected to "rebirthing therapy" (Associated Press, 2005), a practice subsequently discredited (Lilienfeld et al., 2003). Moreover, while many new therapies in general health care, such as surgical procedures not involving a new medical device, can be used without an FDA-type review, individual patients for whom such therapies are used generally receive information about the evidence for

TABLE 4-1   Organizations and Initiatives Conducting Systematic
Evidence Reviews in M/SU Health Care

The Cochrane Collaboration	The standard setter for evidence-based reviews, its Database of Systematic Reviews and other products are the output of over 50 international Collaborative Review Groups (CRGs), which follow detailed procedures contained in a 234-page handbook. CRGs review primarily randomized controlled trials (Alderson et al., 2004). The Cochrane Collaboration maintains four CRGs related to M/SU illnesses: the Depression, Anxiety and Neurosis Group; the Developmental, Psychosocial, and Learning Problems Group; the Drug and Alcohol Group; and the Schizophrenia Group, which together have produced over 100 evidence reports for these areas (The Cochrane Collaboration, 2004).
The U.S. Preventive Services Task Force	Congressionally mandated, it is the "gold standard" for reviewing preventive services in the United States (AHRQ, 2002–2003). Its standardized methodology has been adopted by others, including the Veterans Health Administration and Department of Defense. Because of its focus on prevention, its evidence reviews are limited to screening practices, counseling interventions, and other preventive interventions delivered in primary care settings (Harrison et al., 2001). To date, the task force's recommendations pertaining to M/SU illnesses have addressed screening and/or counseling in primary care settings for alcohol misuse by adults, depression in adults, and suicide risk in the general population (Harris et al., 2001).
National Registry of Evidence-based Programs and Practices (NREPP)	The Substance Abuse and Mental Health Services Administration's (SAMHSA) rating and classification system for M/SU prevention and treatment interventions designates evidence-based programs and practices as "model," "effective" or "promising." As of June 2005, NREPP listed more than 50 model, 30 effective, and 50 promising programs. In contrast to the evaluation of generic practice interventions (e.g., screening, cognitive behavioral therapy), as is the focus of the Cochrane Collaboration and the U.S. Preventive Services Task Force, the majority of NREPP's reviews to date have evaluated specific "brand-name" programs for prevention (e.g., the Keep A Clear Mind drug education program), but it also reviews generic practices such as multisystemic therapy and cognitive behavioral treatments. NREPP

(continued on next page)

TABLE 4-1   continued

	also differs in that its reviews evaluate evidence accompanying an entity's application for review whereas Cochrane, AHRQ EPCs, and Campbell reviews (described below) consist of an independent search for all evidence on a particular generic intervention. Originally developed to evaluate substance-use prevention interventions, the scope of NREPP's reviews has been expanded to include both prevention and treatment of all mental and addictive disorders (SAMHSA, 2005). In a Federal Register notice in August 2005, SAMHSA solicited formal public comment on NREPP's review processes and criteria (SAMHSA, 2005).
Agency for Healthcare Research and Quality's (AHRQ) Evidence-based Practice Centers (EPCs)	Through AHRQ, the United States funds 13 EPCs that address topics particularly relevant to the Medicare and Medicaid programs. One EPC specializes in technology assessments for the Center for Medicare and Medicaid Services; another supports the work of the U.S. Preventive Services Task Force. EPC reviews are developed from comprehensive syntheses and analyses of the scientific literature, and can include meta-analyses and cost analyses. EPCs also provide technical assistance to stakeholders to help translate the reports into quality improvement tools, curriculums, and policy. EPCs are located predominantly in academic research centers. Of the 123 EPC evidence reports listed on AHRQ's website as of November 2004, 4 addressed M/SU health care: the diagnosis of ADHD, the treatment of ADHD, pharmacotherapy for alcohol dependence, and new drug therapies for depression—all published in 1999 (AHRQ, undated).
Veterans Health Administration (VHA)	VHA performs systematic reviews of health care technologies through its national Technology Assessment Program (VATAP) and development of clinical practice guidelines. VATAP's reviews of devices, drugs, procedures, and organizational and supportive systems used in health care have focused on outcome measurement in mental health services (Department of Veterans Affairs, 2004). Practice guidelines have addressed major depression, psychoses, posttraumatic stress disorder, and substance use.
Department of Justice's (DOJ) Federal Collaboration on What Works	Like the efforts of NREPP, DOJ's What Works initiative aims to develop and apply consistent federal standards to determine what constitutes evidence-based programs. In conjunction with the U.S. Department of Education, SAMHSA, the National Institute on Drug Abuse, and the National Institute on Alcohol

TABLE 4-1 continued

	Abuse and Alcoholism, as well as selected private organizations, DOJ in 2004 convened the Federal Collaboration on What Works, which spawned a working group whose early efforts focused on the development of a framework for assessing the evidence for program effectiveness. This Hierarchical Classification Framework for Program Effectiveness is intended to be applied initially to programs relevant to the mission of the Office of Justice Programs (i.e., primarily prevention, intervention, supervision, and treatment of drug abuse, juvenile delinquency, and adult crime), but the working group has identified it as potentially contributing to the development of a common standard of program effectiveness for use throughout the federal government (Department of Justice, 2005).
The Campbell Collaboration	Created in 2000 as a sibling of the Cochrane Collaboration, the Campbell Collaboration conducts systematic reviews of evidence in the fields of education, criminal justice, and social welfare. Its systematic reviews are carried out in accordance with explicit review protocols published in the Campbell Database of Systematic Reviews and are subject to comment and criticisms from users of that database. As of March 1, 2005, seven completed systemic reviews were listed on its website, along with an additional 35 registered titles or protocols for forthcoming reviews. Because the education, criminal justice, and social welfare systems play key roles in the funding and delivery of M/SU treatment services, there is some expected overlap between Cochrane and Campbell reviews, and seven completed Campbell reviews are also registered as Cochrane reviews. To address this overlap, the Cochrane and Campbell Collaborations are pursuing coordination of their activities, including joint registration of methods groups, as well as links with other conveners and members of Cochrane and Campbell methods groups and with the steering group representatives of both organizations* (The Campbell Collaboration, undated).
State Governments	Some states conduct or sponsor their own evidence reviews. For example, in 1999 Hawaii created a panel to review the efficacy and effectiveness of treatments for a range of child and adolescent mental health conditions (Chorpita et al., 2002). Using methods and rating criteria adapted from those of the American

(continued on next page)

TABLE 4-1 continued

	Psychological Association, its Evidence-based Services Committee's 10 subcommittees review evidence on treatment for anxious or avoidant behavior, depression or withdrawn behavior problems, disruptive behavior and willful misconduct problems, substance use, attention and hyperactivity behavior problems, bipolar disorder, schizophrenia, and autism; school-based programs; and service interventions (Hawaii Department of Health, 2004). The reviews are used to specify services that will and will not be provided to the state's mental health clients. State mental health commissioners as a group have identified the need for a central location where they can obtain the latest research related to evidence-based practices. As a result, the National Association of State Mental Health Program Directors' National Research Institute created a Center for Mental Health Quality and Accountability to collate research on such practices, foster the development of new evidence-based practices, and facilitate the dissemination of this knowledge to state mental health programs (Ganju, 2003).
Professional Associations	Professional associations for many disciplines (e.g., the American Psychiatric Association, American Society of Addiction Medicine, American Psychological Association, and American Academy of Pediatrics) conduct reviews of the evidence as a prelude to promulgating clinical practice guidelines. The American Psychological Association's criteria for determining effective practices (American Psychological Association, undated) also have been adopted by other organizations for use in reviews of the evidence. The Interdisciplinary Committee on Evidence-Based Youth Mental Health (a consortium of the American Academy of Pediatrics, the American Academy of Child and Adolescent Psychiatry, and the American Psychological Association's divisions of clinical child psychology and school psychology) also has identified a goal of developing and periodically updating an archive of data from clinical trials in order to provide a synthesis of the research on child and adolescent mental health (Hoagwood et al., 2001).

*Personal communication, Sally Hopewell, coeditor *Cochrane Methods Groups Newsletter*, via e-mail on March 4, 2005.

their potential advantages and risks through the informed consent process. If a new treatment in general health care is considered experimental, review by an institutional review board is required. Psychotherapies are unique in this regard in that a given therapist may offer a new therapeutic approach without its undergoing a safety or effectiveness review and without having to inform the patient about the extent to which its safety and effectiveness have been established.

The committee concludes that a more comprehensive, systematic, and coordinated approach is needed to describe, assess, and classify M/SU treatments and practices according to the level of evidence that supports their use. Better coordination of current national and international review activities, as well as coordination of those efforts with the evidence review activities that underlie the guideline development process of many organizations, could prevent redundancy and waste, produce more evidence reviews on a timelier basis, and avoid conflicting interpretations of the data for clinicians and consumers. The organizations engaged in these activities are natural partners for building a more comprehensive, coordinated, and systematic review network. Many of these same organizations are also involved with the dissemination of their review findings in the form of practice guidelines and other clinical decision-support tools.

IMPROVING DIAGNOSIS AND ASSESSMENT

The production of evidence will be less fruitful if it is not accompanied by accurate diagnosis and comprehensive longitudinal assessment. Because having a mental illness or alcohol- or other substance-use diagnosis is a leading risk factor for suicide (Maris, 2002), failure to diagnose these conditions can be lethal. An inaccurate diagnosis also can lead to ineffective treatment and even harmful outcomes. Yet individuals with the same symptoms presenting to different mental health clinicians can receive different diagnoses. For example, variations have been documented in the extent to which depression is diagnosed in individuals with similar symptoms by both psychiatrists (Kramer et al., 2000) and primary care providers (Mojtabai, 2002) and in the extent to which ADHD is diagnosed within different communities (Lefever et al., 2003). Recently, the diagnosis of bipolar illness in children, especially preschoolers, has been the subject of considerable controversy among psychiatrists (McClellan, 2005). For many conditions, significant discrepancies have been observed among diagnoses generated from structured interviews for research purposes and those resulting from clinician judgments (Lewczyk et al., 2003) and diagnostic tools developed for clinical purposes (Eaton et al., 2000).

In children, diagnoses may have an even greater range of variability because diagnostic manifestations change over the course of development.

Moreover, clinicians are greatly dependant upon parents' perceptions of the nature of the presenting problems. Parents may differ, for example, in the extent to which they perceive very active behavior as problematic versus being "all boy," or view a quiet and introspective child as being "shy" versus having a "social disorder." Subjectivity in diagnosis also is manifest in the variable diagnoses received by white patients and individuals who are members of ethnic minorities. African American patients with manic-depressive illness, for example, have been found to be at higher risk for being misdiagnosed as having schizophrenia than are whites (Bell and Mehta, 1980, 1981; Mukherjee et al., 1983). Such racial differences have tended to disappear when structured interviews rather than clinical diagnoses are used (Adebimpe, 1994; Simon and Fleiss, 1973), suggesting the existence of differences in clinician assessment by patient ethnicity.

A number of factors account for variations in diagnosis of M/SU illnesses. Foremost, in contrast with general health conditions, relatively few laboratory, imaging, or other physical measures can detect the presence of a mental illness or substance dependence.[10] Accurate diagnosis relies instead upon descriptive methods whereby patients or their caregivers inform clinicians about symptoms, and clinicians apply their expert judgment to determine whether diagnostic criteria for a condition are met. Moreover, individual clinicians vary in the breadth, depth, and theoretical basis of their training (see Chapter 7). Because diagnosis requires a subjective interpretation of reported symptoms, these variations result in inconsistency and unreliability in how individuals are diagnosed. Administrative rules and financial incentives can also influence diagnostic practices.

Criteria for diagnosing M/SU problems and illnesses reliably are found in the American Psychiatric Association's *Diagnostic and Statistical Manual of Mental Disorders* (DSM), which has been a highly significant milestone in the diagnosis and treatment of mental and substance-use problems and illnesses and is now in its revised fourth edition (DSM-IV-R). However, adherence to these guidelines is not uniform. Fully 56 percent of primary care physicians in Michigan surveyed in 2002 reported that they did not use DSM criteria to diagnose ADHD (Rushton et al., 2004). This may be because DSM-IV is not easy to use in primary care settings, in part because of its focus on specialty care, its length, and its complexity (Pincus, 2003).

Several different approaches have been undertaken to improve the accuracy of diagnosis of M/SU illnesses. System-level interventions, such as routine screening, have been shown to help (Gilbody et al., 2001; Rollman et al., 2001). Structured diagnostic interview instruments have also been developed to reduce variability in information gathering and biases that can inadvertently influence individual clinicians' decision making. While these

---

[10]Substance use, but not dependence, can be detected by laboratory tests.

instruments have demonstrated reasonable reliability, their clinical feasibility and accuracy in routine practice are not well established (Lewczyk et al., 2003). Other initiatives have provided clinicians with education and guidelines to improve their recognition and treatment of mental illnesses (Lin et al., 2001; Thompson et al., 2000).

The committee concludes that multiple strategies are needed to improve diagnostic accuracy in M/SU health care. First, existing evidence-based diagnostic tools and assessment practices should be identified and applied in practice, just as must be done for evidence-based treatment. More age-appropriate diagnostic instruments also should be developed that are reliable and practicable for routine use, and information about these tools should be included in initiatives to better disseminate evidence-based practices. Further, clinicians should be encouraged to employ standardized clinical assessment instruments to measure target symptoms consistently and systematically, and document results over the course of treatment (American Psychiatric Association Task Force for the Handbook of Psychiatric Measures, 2000).

As discussed earlier in this chapter, however, even when evidence-based practices are known, their adoption by all relevant practitioners—in both general and M/SU health care—is too slow. Accordingly, many public and private organizations are actively engaged in efforts to strengthen the dissemination and uptake of effective clinical practices. Yet these activities themselves are not always consistent with the evidence on effective dissemination and uptake of new knowledge. Improving the effectiveness of dissemination activities is thus the next essential step in improving the effectiveness of M/SU health care.

BETTER DISSEMINATION OF THE EVIDENCE

Research has been under way for many years, in health care as well as other fields of study, to identify the multiple contributors to successful dissemination and adoption of new practices and innovations by their targeted users. An extensive and systematic review of empirical evidence and related theoretical literature from multiple disciplines (Greenhalgh et al., 2004) identified the following key factors in successful dissemination and adoption of innovations: (1) the characteristics of the innovation itself, (2) the characteristics of the individuals targeted to adopt it, (3) sources of communication and influence regarding the innovation, (4) structural and cultural characteristics of organizations targeted to adopt it, (5) external influences on targeted individuals or organizations, (6) organizations' uptake processes, and (7) the linkages among these six factors (see Box 4-2).

Although some of the factors affecting the adoption of new practices (e.g., characteristics of individual adopters) may not be very amenable to

BOX 4-2 Key Factors Associated with Successful Dissemination and Adoption of Innovations

Characteristics of the Innovation
Innovation more likely to be adopted if it:
- Offers unambiguous advantages in effectiveness or cost-effectiveness.
- Is compatible with adopters' values, norms, needs.
- Is simple to implement.
- Can be experimented with on a trial basis.
- Has benefits that are easily observed.
- Can be adapted, refined, modified for adopter's needs.
- Is low risk.
- Is relevant to adopter's current work.
- Is accompanied by easily available or provided knowledge required for its use.

Sources of Communication and Influence
Uptake of innovation influenced by:
- Structure and quality of social and communication networks.
- Similarity of sources of information to targeted adopters; e.g., in terms of socioeconomic, educational, professional, and cultural backgrounds.
- Use of opinion leaders, champions, and change agents.

External Influences
Uptake of innovation influenced by:
- Nature of an organization's relationships with other organizations.
- Nature of an organization's participation in formal dissemination and uptake initiatives.
- Policy mandates.

Linkages Among the Components
Innovation more likely to be adopted if there are:
- Formal linkages between developers and users early in development.
- Effective relationships between any designated "change agents" and targeted adopters.

Characteristics of Individual Adopters
Uptake of innovation influenced by individual's:
- General cognitive and psychological traits conducive to trying innovations (e.g., tolerance of ambiguity, intellectual ability, learning style).
- Context-specific psychological characteristics; e.g., motivation and ability to use the intervention in the given context.
- Finding the intervention personally relevant.

Structural and Cultural Characteristics of Potential Organizational Adopters
Innovation more likely to be adopted if organization:
- Is large, mature, functionally differentiated, and specialized; has slack in resources; and has decentralized decision making.
- Can identify, capture, interpret, share, and integrate new knowledge.
- Is receptive to change through strong leadership, clear strategic vision, good management and key staff, and climate conducive to experimentation and risk taking.
- Has effective data systems.
- Is "ready" for change because of difficulties in current situation, fit between organization and innovation, anticipated benefits, internal support and advocacy, available time and resources for change, and capacity to evaluate innovation's implementation.

The Uptake Process
Innovation more likely to be adopted with:
- Flexible organizational structure that supports decentralized decision making.
- Leadership and management support.
- Personnel motivation, capacity, and competence.
- Funding.
- Internal communication and networks.
- Feedback.
- Adaptation and reinvention.

SOURCE: Greenhalgh et al., 2004.

external change, others are. For example, the sources of communication and influence used in dissemination of information can be chosen. While many initiatives are now under way to disseminate evidence-based M/SU practices, these initiatives are generally being undertaken by specialty M/SU organizations, as opposed to those associated with general health care. Evidence indicates that integrating the dissemination of evidence-based M/SU health care practices into the scope and initiatives of mainstream general health care dissemination activities is essential to reaching the vast numbers of general health care clinicians who now treat M/SU problems and illnesses and have an essential role in ensuring the early detection, appropriate treatment, and referral of these conditions.

Key Dissemination Efforts

Substance Abuse and Mental Health Services Administration

As part of its Science to Service Initiative, SAMHSA has multiple activities under way to disseminate information on evidence-based practices, promote the incorporation of such practices into general and M/SU health care, and facilitate feedback from the field to guide research. For example, SAMHSA's Center for Mental Health Services is developing six "tool kits" addressing Illness Management and Recovery, Medication Management, Assertive Community Treatment, Family Psychoeducation, Supported Employment, and Integrated Dual Diagnosis Treatment for Co-Occurring Disorders. The kits include information sheets for all stakeholder groups, introductory videos, practice demonstration videos, and workbooks or manuals for practitioners. The tool kits will be finalized through a national demonstration project to be completed at the end of 2005 (SAMHSA, undated-a). SAMHSA also funds the Center for Mental Health Quality and Accountability of the National Association of State Mental Health Program Directors (NASMHPD) Research Institute (NRI) to provide an overview of evidence-based practices to the association's constituents and other stakeholders (NASMHPD Research Institute, undated).

SAMHSA's dissemination mechanisms for substance-use prevention and treatment include Treatment Improvement Protocols, the National Addiction Technology Transfer Centers (ATTC) Network (1 national and 13 regional centers), the Network for the Improvement of Addiction Treatment, and the Centers for the Application of Prevention Technology. Further, SAMHSA's State Systems Development Program—an enhanced technical assistance program involving conferences and workshops, development of training materials and knowledge transfer manuals, and on-site consultation—assists states with the administration and implementation of Substance Abuse Prevention and Treatment Block Grant activities. The program's Treatment Improvement Exchange, the hub for the full range of its technical assistance services, also facilitates and promotes information exchange between SAMHSA's Center for Substance Abuse Treatment (CSAT) and state and local alcohol and substance abuse agencies. These activities include information development and dissemination; state, regional, and national conferences; and on-site expert consultation (SAMHSA, undated-c). In addition, SAMHSA is partnering with the National Institute of Mental Health (NIMH) and the National Institute on Drug Abuse (NIDA) to jointly fund planning activities and research on the adoption of evidence-based practices by state M/SU agencies.

National Institutes of Health

NIMH is partnering with SAMHSA to promote and support the dissemination of evidence-based mental health treatment practices and their adoption by state mental health systems through Bridging Science and Service grants to states (NIMH, 2004). NIDA and CSAT have a similar joint initiative—the NIDA/SAMHSA-ATTC Blending Initiative—which encourages the use of evidence-based treatments by professionals in the drug abuse field. NIDA has identified specific research practices (e.g., motivational interviewing) as ready for use by the field at large. Blending teams comprising staff from CSAT's ATTC network and NIDA researchers then develop strategic dissemination plans for the adoption and implementation of these practices (NIDA, 2005).

In addition, NIMH, NIDA, and the National Institute on Alcohol Abuse and Alcoholism (NIAAA) have multiple publication, interpersonal, electronic media, and other initiatives to help disseminate information on evidence-based practices. For example, NIDA's Office of Science Policy and Communications, responsible for research dissemination activities, produces a number of periodical publication (e.g., *NIDA Notes, Perspectives*), as well as topic-specific publications. NIDA's *Principles of Drug Addiction Treatment: A Research-based Guide*, for example, is a synthesis of the treatment research organized into 13 key principles, questions and answers, and a listing of some programs for which a strong evidence base exists.[11]

Veterans Health Administration

VHA's clinical practice guidelines initiative (described in Table 4-1) also identifies, disseminates, and promotes the adoption of evidence-based practices. Practice guidelines resulting from evidence reviews are frequently

---

[11]E-mail communication, Jack B. Stein PhD, Deputy Director of Division of Epidemiology, Services, and Prevention Research, National Institute on Drug Abuse on December 15, 2004.

displayed in clinical flowcharts that offer decision support to VHA clinicians (VHA, 2005). VHA's Quality Enhancement Research Initiative facilitates the translation of research findings into routine care by (1) conducting research to fill gaps in knowledge about what constitutes best treatment practices, (2) undertaking demonstration projects that implement already known best practices, (3) identifying enhancements to VHA's information systems, and (4) conducting research and demonstration projects to accelerate the uptake of evidence-based practices (Fischer et al., 2000). The initiative includes projects in mental health (schizophrenia and depression) and substance-use illnesses (improving the quality of methadone maintenance therapy).

Professional Associations

As discussed above, many professional bodies are actively engaged in dissemination activities. These activities are often connected with their development and distribution of practice guidelines.

Underused Sources of Communication and Influence

The dissemination activities described above are conducted by organizations that generally are perceived as specialty M/SU organizations and thus may be most likely to communicate and have influence with specialty M/SU health care providers. As described in Chapter 7, however, primary care providers deliver a substantial portion of mental health services and are a critical source for the detection of M/SU conditions, referral, and subsequent treatment. Other non–M/SU specialty providers also have key roles to play in detection, treatment, and referral. However, data show that these general health care providers need to adopt evidence-based practices to better detect, treat, and appropriately refer individuals in need of M/SU health care. Thus it is important that dissemination of the evidence on effective M/SU health care reach all providers, not just those specializing in M/SU care.

However, the key current dissemination efforts described above may be less likely to influence primary care providers and other non–M/SU specialty clinicians. Research on the effective dissemination of innovations described above (Box 4-2) shows that individuals' and organizations' adoption of new practices is greatly influenced by their social networks. Successful dissemination occurs most easily among individuals with similar educational, professional, and cultural backgrounds. Opinion leaders within a field also strongly influence the dissemination and uptake of innovations. Formal dissemination programs will be more successful if they are aware of and address potential adopters' needs and perspectives, and tailor their dissemination strategies to the demographic, structural, and cultural characteristics of different subgroups (Greenhalgh et al., 2004). To this end, resources routinely tapped by general and other non–M/SU specialty health care practitioners and policy makers should be used to help disseminate evidence on effective detection and treatment of M/SU illnesses. In short, M/SU health care needs to be better addressed in evidence dissemination efforts that are routinely employed to address providers of general health promotion and disease and disability prevention and treatment. The U.S. Centers for Disease Control and Prevention (CDC) and AHRQ's Division of User Liaison and Research Translation (formerly called the User Liaison Program) are two highly regarded organizations with expertise in knowledge dissemination that can be utilized more fully for this purpose.

Centers for Disease Control and Prevention

CDC's mission is "to promote health and quality of life by preventing and controlling disease, injury, and disability" (CDC, 2005a:1). It does so by serving as "the principal agency in the United States government for protecting the health and safety of all Americans and for providing essential human services, especially for those people who are least able to help themselves" (CDC, 2005b:1). Despite this mandate, CDC's substantial and highly regarded expertise in these areas, and the large contribution of M/SU illnesses to morbidity, disability, and injury (see Chapter 1), M/SU illnesses could be better represented in CDC's organizational structures, programs, and initiatives.

CDC encompasses multiple centers, institutes, and offices (CDC, 2005c) (see Box 4-3). Of these, the National Center for Chronic Disease Prevention and Health Promotion might reasonably be expected to address M/SU problems and illnesses, given their substantial contribution to chronic disease and general health problems. Yet the listing of chronic disease programs on the center's website includes arthritis, cancer, diabetes, epilepsy, global health, healthy aging, healthy youth, heart disease and stroke, nutrition and physical activity, oral health, a block grant program to implement national objectives contained in the Healthy People report, prevention research programs, elimination of racial disparities, pregnancy-related illnesses, tobacco use, and an initiative for uninsured women (addressing high blood pressure and cholesterol, nutrition and weight management, physical inactivity, and tobacco use)—but not M/SU illnesses. Another key initiative of the center—Steps to a HealthierUS—is designed to advance the goal of helping Americans live longer, better, and healthier lives through 5-year cooperative agreements with states, cities, and tribal entities to implement chronic disease prevention efforts focused on reducing the burden of diabetes, overweight, obesity, and asthma and three related risk factors—

BOX 4-3 Centers, Offices, and Institute of the Centers for Disease Control and Prevention

- **Coordinating Center for Environmental Health and Injury Prevention**
  - **National Center for Environmental Health/Agency for Toxic Substances and Disease Registry** provides national leadership in preventing and controlling disease and death resulting from the interactions between people and their environment.
  - **National Center for Injury Prevention and Control** prevents death and disability from nonoccupational injuries, including those that are unintentional and those that result from violence.
- **Coordinating Center for Health Information and Services**
  - **National Center for Health Statistics** provides statistical information intended to guide actions and policies to improve the health of the American people.
  - **National Center for Public Health Informatics** provides national leadership in the application of information technology in the pursuit of public health.
  - **National Center for Health Marketing** provides national leadership in health marketing science and in its application to impact public health.
- **Coordinating Center for Health Promotion**
  - **National Center on Birth Defects and Developmental Disabilities** provides national leadership for preventing birth defects and developmental disabilities and for improving the health and wellness of people with disabilities.
  - **National Center for Chronic Disease Prevention and Health Promotion** prevents premature death and disability from chronic diseases and promotes healthy personal behaviors.
  - **Office of Genomics and Disease Prevention** provides national leadership in fostering understanding of human genomic discoveries and how they can be used to improve health and prevent disease.
- **Coordinating Center for Infectious Diseases**
  - **National Center for Infectious Diseases** prevents illness, disability, and death caused by infectious diseases in the United States and around the world.
  - **National Immunization Program** prevents disease, disability, and death from vaccine-preventable diseases in children and adults.
  - **National Center for HIV, STD, and TB Prevention** provides national leadership in preventing and controlling human immunodeficiency virus infection, sexually transmitted diseases, and tuberculosis.
- **Coordinating Office for Global Health** provides national leadership, coordination, and support for CDC's global health activities in collaboration with CDC's global health partners.
- **Coordinating Office for Terrorism Preparedness and Emergency Response** provides strategic direction for the agency to support terrorism preparedness and emergency response efforts.
- **National Institute for Occupational Safety and Health** ensures safety and health for all people in the workplace through research and prevention.

physical inactivity, poor nutrition, and tobacco use (CDC, 2005d). The prevention and treatment of M/SU illnesses are not mentioned in these and similar CDC initiatives

Moreover, the CDC website providing an overview of chronic illness (http://www.cdc.gov/nccdphp/overview.htm)[12] fails to list any M/SU problems or illnesses among the Leading Causes of Disability among Persons Aged 15 Years or Older, United States (although the source for the data cited is dated 1991–1992). This omission is in spite of the evidence presented in Chapter 1 and acknowledged in the President's New Freedom Commission report that mental illnesses rank first among conditions that cause disability in the United States (New Freedom Commission on Mental Health, 2003).

Instead of being included explicitly in these and other structures or formal initiatives, mental health is addressed in CDC through a Mental Health Work Group that is not part of any of the agency's formal centers, programs, or offices and has no formal budget allocation, personnel positions, or other dedicated administrative support. "Staff members participating in this work group do so voluntarily as an add-on to their other CDC responsibilities because of their commitment to advancing the field of mental health within the context of the overall mission of CDC" (CDC, 2005e:1). Although CDC has undertaken important work on alcohol use (see, for example, http://www.cdc.gov/alcohol/about.htm) and alcohol and drug use among youth (see http://www.cdc.gov/HealthyYouth/alcoholdrug/index.htm), M/SU health care could benefit greatly from a larger commitment of CDC resources and expertise.

Agency for Healthcare Research and Quality's User Liaison Program

For more than 22 years, AHRQ's User Liaison Program (ULP) has focused on bringing information on science-based health care services to policy makers at the state and local levels, including the staff of governors' offices, state legislators and their staffs, and executive branch agency heads such as Medicaid and public health directors, to help them develop more effective policies and programs. The ULP historically has relied on workshops, seminars, and conferences to provide this information, but in the past few years has also been conducting audio and web conferencing. The ULP has addressed a wide variety of topics identified through regular formal and informal mechanisms, including biennial needs assessment meetings across the country, conference calls with stakeholders, and portions of workshops devoted to audience feedback regarding topics to be addressed

---

[12]As of October 10, 2005.

each year. As of 2004, the ULP's mission had been expanded to encompass a wider range of knowledge transfer activities (e.g., technical assistance, distance learning, electronic and face-to-face networking, web and teleconferencing). Its target audience has also been expanded to include providers and purchasers in addition to policy makers. To better carry out these new mandates, AHRQ has revised the ULP to focus on long-term knowledge transfer strategies for a few critical health care issues. As of December 2004, these issues were (1) developing high-reliability organizations, (2) care management, (3) purchaser–provider synergies for improving health care quality, and (4) decreasing disparities. This change in direction means that the ULP will likely not offer specific disease-focused programs in the future. Rather, multiple clinical areas of concern can be addressed within the four targeted issues identified above.[13] M/SU health care policy makers, administrators, and clinicians ought to be targeted as part of ULP activities.

Conclusions and Recommendation

The committee concludes that dissemination strategies for effective M/SU treatment innovations should use the sources of communication and influence that are highly regarded in general health care in addition to those so regarded in M/SU health care. Moreover, organizations that are especially influential with private-sector providers and other policy makers and purchasers because of their past relationships should be included in a coordinated strategy. For example, with its new focus on policy makers and purchasers, as well as clinicians, AHRQ's ULP could be an instrument for bringing M/SU health care to the attention of these key leaders.

> **Recommendation 4-1. To better build and disseminate the evidence base, the Department of Health and Human Services (DHHS) should strengthen, coordinate, and consolidate the synthesis and dissemination of evidence on effective M/SU treatments and services by the Substance Abuse and Mental Health Services Administration; the National Institute of Mental Health; the National Institute on Drug Abuse; the National Institute on Alcohol Abuse and Alcoholism; the National Institute of Child Health and Human Development; the Agency for Healthcare Research and Quality; the Department of Justice; the Department of Veterans Affairs; the Department of Defense; the Department of Education; the Centers for Disease Control and Prevention; the Centers for Medicare and Medicaid Services; the Administration for**

---

[13]Personal communication with Steve Seitz, User Liaison Program, Agency for Healthcare Research and Quality on December 9, 2004.

Children, Youth, and Families; states; professional associations; and other private-sector entities.

To implement this recommendation, DHHS should charge or create one or more entities to:

- Describe and categorize available M/SU preventive, diagnostic, and therapeutic interventions (including screening, diagnostic, and symptom-monitoring tools), and develop individual procedure codes and definitions for these interventions and tools for their use in administrative datasets approved under the Health Insurance Portability and Accountability Act.
- Assemble the scientific evidence on the efficacy and effectiveness of these interventions, including their use in varied age and ethnic groups; use a well-established approach to rate the strength of this evidence, and categorize the interventions accordingly; and recommend or endorse guidelines for the use of the evidence-based interventions for specific M/SU problems and illnesses.
- Substantially expand efforts to attain widespread adoption of evidence-based practices through the use of evidence-based approaches to knowledge dissemination and uptake. Dissemination strategies should always include entities that are commonly viewed as knowledge experts by general health care providers and makers of public policy, including the Centers for Disease Control and Prevention, the Agency for Healthcare Research and Quality, the Centers for Medicare and Medicaid Services, the Office of Minority Health, and professional associations and health care organizations.

The committee calls attention to three important considerations involved in implementing this recommendation. First, implementing this recommendation will require a long-term commitment on the part of DHHS. An ongoing process accommodating changes in the science base over time will be necessary to synthesize the evidence base; assess interventions based on the strength of their scientific evidence; and develop and continually update a reliable categorization and coding scheme for individual M/SU prevention, screening, assessment, psychotherapy, psychosocial, and other treatment interventions. Given fiscal constraints, and in an effort to mainstream M/SU health care, the committee recommends that DHHS make use of public- and private-sector structures and processes already in place that synthesize evidence, develop procedure codes such as the HCPCS codes and CPT codes for administrative datasets, develop performance measures and measurement approaches for the public and private sectors, and carry out related activities. To marshal the substantial expertise and resources of these entities and assist them in dedicating additional resources to M/SU health care, DHHS will need to provide them with formal support and financial and nonfinancial resources to enable and sustain these activities until they are firmly in place.

In addition, the committee notes that a wide variety of M/SU health care interventions are important to the effective treatment of M/SU conditions and need to be included in the recommended evidence review, coding, and performance measurement initiatives. In addition to traditional psychotherapy, these initiatives should encompass screening and diagnostic questionnaires and assessment tools with practical utility in routine primary and specialty care settings (as opposed to tools used for research purposes); other clinically practicable tools used to monitor symptoms and patient outcomes; and the range of psychosocial services with proven effectiveness, such as family psychoeducation, illness self-management, and assertive community treatment. In addition to procedure codes, codes should be developed that indicate the type of clinician providing care (e.g., psychiatrist, psychologist, marriage and family therapist, or counselor).

Finally, the committee reaffirms its view that the development of more precise procedure and provider codes is a critical pathway to improvements in quality. The development of an analytic database comparable to that which exists for general health is critical to informing our understanding of factors that influence utilization of care, variations in care, and the relationship between health outcomes and various types of treatments. Such information also will provide transparency as to what health care purchasers are paying for and what consumers are actually receiving. As these codes are developed, the federal government should require their use in all federally mandated and supported administrative data collection activities.

In addition, as discussed above, the committee believes that the collection of outcome data can both inform clinical care at the point of care delivery and contribute to the development of evidence on effective treatments. It therefore makes the following recommendation:

Recommendation 4-2. Clinicians and organizations providing M/SU services should:

- Increase their use of valid and reliable patient questionnaires or other patient-assessment instruments that are feasible for routine use to assess the progress and outcomes of treatment systematically and reliably.
- Use measures of the processes and outcomes of care to continuously improve the quality of the care provided.

The committee points out that this recommendation refers to general health care providers who offer M/SU health care, as well as to specialty M/SU health care providers.

STRENGTHENING THE QUALITY MEASUREMENT[14] AND REPORTING INFRASTRUCTURE

A frequently stated maxim across many industries is, "You can't improve what you can't measure." This holds true in health care. Measuring the quality of care provided by individuals, organizations, and health plans and reporting back the results is linked both conceptually and empirically to reductions in variations in care and increases in the delivery of effective care (Berwick et al., 2003; Jha et al., 2003). However, this successful strategy has not yet seen widespread application in M/SU health care. Less measurement of the safety, effectiveness, and timeliness of M/SU health care has taken place than is the case for general health care (AHRQ, 2003; Garnick et al., 2002). In 1998, the President's Advisory Commission on Consumer Protection and Quality in the Health Care Industry identified mental health care as an aspect of health care not well addressed by existing quality measures and measure sets (The President's Advisory Commission on Consumer Protection and Quality in the Health Care Industry, 1998). Five years later, the first National Healthcare Quality Report published by DHHS continued to identify mental illness as a clinical area lacking "broadly accepted" and "widely used" measures of quality. Of 107 measures of the effectiveness of health care, only 7 addressed mental health: 3 the treatment of depression in adults, 1 suicide, and 3 management of delirium and confusion in nursing homes and home health. None addressed the quality of care for substance-use problems and illnesses. The only measure that pertained to children was that for suicide (AHRQ, 2003). No additional measures of the quality of mental health care were included in the second annual report published in 2004, and measures of the quality of substance-use care remained absent (AHRQ, 2004a).

This lack of measurement is not caused by a lack of organizations and initiatives developing measures of M/SU health care quality. A National Inventory of Mental Health Quality Measures, funded by AHRQ, NIMH, SAMHSA, and The Evaluation Center@HSRI (The Human Services Re-

---

[14]The terms "performance measurement" and "quality measurement," like "performance measures" and "quality measures," are often used interchangeably because quality measures are a type of performance measures (financial performance, for example, is another type). In this report, we follow that practice, using "performance measures/measurement" and "quality measures/measurement" interchangeably to refer to all aspects of quality health care—the structures, processes, and outcomes of care.

search Institute) identified more than 100 measures of the processes of M/SU health care developed by government agencies, researchers, clinician/ professional organizations, accreditors, health systems/facilities, employer purchasers, consumer coalitions, and commercial organizations (Hermann et al., 2004). A significant number of outcome measurement instruments also have been identified by VHA (VA Technology Assessment Program, 2002). The failure of mainstream health care quality measurement and improvement efforts to incorporate a greater number of M/SU quality measures is due in part to the separation of M/SU and general health care, as discussed in Chapters 2 and 5. Because of this separation, many M/SU health care advocates, professional associations, and other organizations have undertaken efforts to develop and apply measures of the quality of M/SU health care. However, a major factor inhibiting both mainstream and specialty efforts is the lack of a quality measurement and reporting infrastructure addressing M/SU health care.

Necessary Components of a Quality Measurement and Reporting Infrastructure

Effectively measuring quality and reporting results to providers, consumers, and oversight organizations requires structures, resources, and expertise to perform several related functions:

- Conceptualizing the aspects of care to be measured.
- Translating the quality-of-care measurement concepts into performance measure specifications.
- Pilot testing the performance measure specifications to determine their validity, reliability, feasibility, and cost.
- Ensuring calculation of the performance measures and their submission to a performance measure repository.
- Auditing to ensure that the performance measures have been calculated accurately and in accordance with specifications.
- Analyzing and displaying the performance measures in a format or formats suitable for understanding by the multiple intended audience(s), such as consumers, health care delivery entities, purchasers, and quality oversight organizations.
- Maintaining the effectiveness of individual performance measures and performance measure sets and policies over time.

These seven functions are currently performed to varying degrees for M/SU health care by multiple organizations—again often separately from general health care, but in this case the separation also exists across the public and private health care sectors. The result is the rudiments of a quality measurement and reporting infrastructure, but with some redundancy and gaps in the measures, measurement functions, and entities whose performance is being measured, and without a coordinated approach that maximizes the efficiency and effectives of the various efforts. What is needed is one or more infrastructures that perform these seven functions for the four different levels of health care delivery: (1) individual clinicians or groups of clinicians; (2) health care organizations, such as inpatient facilities; (3) health plans; and (4) public health systems (national, state, and local). Below we discuss for each of the seven functions special issues related to the delivery of M/SU health care that should influence the implementation of that function and the development of a quality measurement and reporting infrastructure for M/SU health care.

Conceptualizing the Aspects of Care to Be Measured

Because of the large number of existing process and outcome quality indicators and measures, the multiple populations of interest (e.g., children; older adults; individuals with less-frequent but severe and chronic mental illnesses, such as schizophrenia; and inpatients), the different units of analysis (clinicians; inpatient and outpatient organizations; health plans; and local, state, and national systems), and the importance of not overburdening the clinicians and organizations that will produce the measures, a framework is needed for identifying a finite number (often termed a "core" set) of valid, reliable, effective, and efficient measures that can best serve the multiple interested parties and purposes. The best-documented example of such a framework is that of the Strategic Framework Board, which designed a National Quality Measurement and Reporting System (NQMRS) for U.S. health care overall to guide such efforts as those of the National Quality Forum (McGlynn, 2003).

Within M/SU health care, multiple organizations and initiatives also have put forth frameworks or core measure sets, using different approaches to identify aspects of care delivery to be measured and select measures of the structures, processes, and outcomes of M/SU care. These initiatives include the Forum on Performance Measures in Behavioral Health and Related Service Systems (Teague et al., 2004), the Mental Health Statistics Improvement Program Quality Report (Ganju et al., 2004), the Center for Quality Assessment and Improvement in Mental Health (Hermann and Palmer, 2002; Hermann et al., 2004), the Behavioral Healthcare Performance Measurement System for inpatient care of the NRI, the Outcomes Roundtable for Children and Families (Doucette, 2003), and the Washington Circle Group (McCorry et al., 2000) (all of which are convened and/or funded by SAMHSA), as well as the previous efforts of the American College of Mental Health Administrators Accreditation Workgroup (ACMHA,

2001) and the American Managed Behavioral Health Association. The federal government also has adopted a framework through its State Outcomes Measurement and Management System (described below) (SAMHSA, undated-b). These efforts are in addition to performance measure sets that address health care overall and include some M/SU performance measures, such as NCQA's HEDIS and measures used by VHA (see Appendix C).

All of these efforts have tackled two enduring and related problems that are encountered in all performance measurement efforts: (1) the tension between having measures of high validity, reliability, and ease of calculation and having a broader set of measures that is more representative of the populations and conditions of interest; and (2) the difficulty of achieving consensus on the measure set across all stakeholders (Hermann and Palmer, 2002). In addition to these problems, conceptualizing a framework for M/SU health care is more complex than doing so for general health care for the reasons discussed below.

More-diverse stakeholders The larger number of disciplines licensed to diagnose and treat M/SU problems and illnesses relative to those licensed to diagnose and treat general health conditions potentially requires the involvement of a greater number of stakeholder groups in a consensus process. Moreover, as discussed earlier, M/SU health care involves both specialty and general medical providers. In addition, the involvement of the education, juvenile and criminal justice, and child welfare systems as payers and providers of M/SU services means performance measures selected for M/SU health care must be determined with input from these stakeholders, who are not typically involved in general health care. Consumer advocates also have been very active in shaping the delivery of M/SU health care, again with implications for the numbers and diversity of stakeholders in a consensus process.

Difference between the public and private sectors Although general health care is delivered in both the public and private sectors, in M/SU health care the public sector serves a population with a clinical profile much different from that of the population served by the private sector—most often those with severe and chronic illnesses. Thus, measures that may be meaningful to private-sector stakeholders may be less useful to those in the public sector. In NCQA's HEDIS measures for general health care, for example, some measures[15] are designated for calculation for Medicaid populations but not for privately insured populations (NCQA, 2004b). This practice may need to be employed more widely for M/SU health care. Even measures appropriate for multiple populations may need to be reported separately.

---

[15]Frequency of ongoing prenatal care and annual dental visit.

Different types of evidence As discussed earlier, M/SU health care has often relied on evidence generated by quasi-experimental studies rather than randomized controlled trials. Some performance measures that are deemed valid by M/SU stakeholders may therefore be less credible to performance measurement stakeholders in the general health care sector.

Unclear locus of accountability The separation of the delivery of M/SU and general health care discussed earlier impairs performance measurement in two ways. First, it can create confusion as to whether a given performance measure can be used because it is unclear to whom the measure should apply. There is confusion about the entity accountable for care quality when care can be delivered through multiple delivery arrangements (e.g., primary or specialty care, general or carve-out health plans, school-based programs). For example, the HEDIS performance measures addressing M/SU health care apply to general health plans seeking accreditation, but not to managed behavioral health care organizations.[16]

Another problem caused by the separation of M/SU and general health care, as well as by the separation of mental and substance-use care, relates to access to data. To produce many performance measures, data on the patient's entire illness—from detection through ongoing treatment—are needed. When patients are served by entities separate from their general health care plan or from each other, such as carved-out managed behavioral health plans, employee assistance programs, school-based health care services, and child welfare agencies, the ability to link necessary data is impaired, making many performance measures infeasible (Bethell, 2004; Garnick et al., 2002). Moreover, the voluntary support sector is not typically viewed as formal treatment despite the fact that self-help groups such as Alcoholics Anonymous and other types of peer counseling play an important role in recovery for many individuals with M/SU illnesses. Indeed, the voluntary support sector has been characterized by a lack of data and, in some cases, a commitment to anonymity (Horgan and Garnick, 2005).

As articulated in a paper on performance measurement for child and adolescent M/SU health care that was commissioned by the committee (Bethell, 2004:30):

> Perhaps one of the most significant findings . . . is the lack of coordination in the field among the many actors engaged in measurement development in the area of mental and behavioral health care for children and adolescents. It seems new activities evolve daily with no coordinating center to ensure activities address priority needs and strategic goals as

---

[16]Personal communication Phil Renner, Vice President, NCQA on March 22, 2005.

reflected in the *Crossing the Quality Chasm* reform model. The lack of coordination is especially evident between efforts occurring primarily from the vantage point of the medical arena (e.g., Medicaid, health plan and pediatric practice-based measurement) and those taking place in the more community-based, public health mental health arena (state mental health agencies, community-based clinics, etc.). Ironically, this lack of coordination on the measurement front exactly mirrors the very frustrating lack of coordination between the medical and psychiatric-based mental health services also experienced by families with children with mental and behavioral health care problems.

Translating Quality-of-Care Measurement Concepts into Performance Measure Specifications

Some quality measures address structural and qualitative characteristics of care providers and require a "yes/no" answer. The Leapfrog Group's measure of whether inpatient facilities use computerized physician order entry exemplifies such a structural measure. Most quality measures in use today, however, measure processes of care and require a numerical calculation of the rate at which an appropriate activity is performed for a defined population. These calculations require detailed instructions for calculating the numerators and denominators of the rates to guarantee the accuracy and reliability of the measures. The instructions specify, for example, data sources to be used to calculate a measure, rules for including and excluding some individuals from the rate, time frames for data capture, and sampling strategy if sampling is used. Translating measurement concepts into quality measures also requires detailed knowledge of multiple data sources, including health plan enrollment and encounter data, inpatient and outpatient claims data, pharmacy and laboratory databases, administrative data coding sets, and patient surveys, as well as knowledge of the capabilities of organizations' information systems and of the appropriateness of and techniques for case-mix adjustment.

Appreciation of and knowledge in all these areas is not universal. As a result, many entities that put forth intended quality *measures* are actually putting forth quality measure *concepts*, as opposed to well-developed measures with accompanying specifications for their calculation. A comprehensive 1999–2000 search for and review of mental health performance measures developed in the United States that met a minimum threshold of development (i.e., had a specific numerator and denominator, a designated data source, and an ostensible relationship to quality) found that half of the first 86 measures reviewed were insufficiently developed for implementation, and few measures had been tested for reliability or validity (Hermann et al., 2000). A quality measurement infrastructure for M/SU health care will need to have ongoing formal structures and processes to translate quality measurement concepts into measures that are ready for deployment. NCQA, for example, conducts this translation activity using both internal staff and a formal structure of measurement advisory panels that provide clinical and technical expert knowledge, ad hoc expert panels, and a technical advisory group (NCQA, 2004b).

Pilot Testing the Performance Measure Specifications

Frequently, measures that appear to be theoretically sound are operationally complex, very costly to produce, or unreliable and invalid for reasons not apparent during their design. For example, with respect to M/SU quality measures, the fact that a population is covered by both a general health plan and a separate employee assistance program or carved-out behavioral health plan means that the clinical data required to calculate a measure may be in the possession of multiple separate organizations and difficult to access and link. Stigma and discriminatory benefit designs (discussed in Chapter 3) also mean that many individuals choose to or must pay for M/SU services out of pocket; in such cases, no claim record is produced, so that a major data source for the calculation of quality measures is lacking. For the same reasons, providers sometimes deliver an M/SU service but code it as a general medical problem. Because of these impediments to accurate and reliable measurement of the quality of M/SU health care, new quality measures almost always require some type of pilot testing before being implemented and used for decision making (Garnick et al., 2002). For example, prior to NCQA's incorporation of quality measures addressing health plans' treatment of alcohol and other drug problems into the HEDIS measurement process, these measures were pilot tested by six health care organizations that delivered services to approximately 5 million people so as to evaluate the measures' feasibility and quality improvement potential (Hon, 2003).

Ensuring Calculation and Submission of the Performance Measures

Successful quality measurement initiatives in general health care have taken place under one of two conditions: (1) a critical mass of influential supporters is committed to either requiring or carrying out the calculation and submission of measures (e.g., HEDIS), or (2) there is an ongoing commitment of sufficient resources to enable the analysis of quality measures, making them so useful that those calculating and submitting them do so voluntarily (e.g., NRI's Behavioral Healthcare Performance Measurement System and AHRQ's Healthcare Cost and Utilization Project [H-CUP] Quality Indicators).

For example, the success of the HEDIS performance measures dataset can be traced to its initiation by a small but committed and influential group of employers and health plans. These employers, who purchased health care for their employees, were seeking meaningful data to require of their contracting health plans. The health plans wished to reduce costly variations in the data they were required to submit to multiple purchasers. This critical mass of employer-purchasers and health plans ensured the calculation and submission of the HEDIS measures while they were still in a preliminary state, which subsequently attracted other influential supporters. CMS, for example, now requires health plans participating in the Medicare program to submit data on HEDIS measures. Many state Medicaid agencies also require the submission of HEDIS or HEDIS-like measures. In contrast, submission of the Behavioral Healthcare Performance Measurement System inpatient hospital measures to NASMHPD or NRI is not required, but facilities that choose to do so may use those measures to fulfill accreditation reporting requirements.

Auditing to Ensure That Performance Measures Have Been Calculated Accurately and According with Specifications

Reported measures may not accurately represent an individual's or organization's performance. Information systems and internal data recording conventions used by individual clinicians and health care organizations vary greatly. Data also may not be collected or stored in ways that facilitate collection of a measure as requested. When measures further require data to be linked across organizations, there may be incompatible data formats. All these factors can introduce error, as can less-than-scrupulous adherence to a measure's specifications. Because the reporting of quality measures to external bodies for public disclosure to consumers, for use in financial reimbursement strategies to reward best performance, or in response to other quality oversight requirements can have significant consequences for the entity being measured, it is important for the accuracy of the reported measures to be verified. This is typically accomplished through systematic audits of the measures' calculation. NCQA, for example, has developed standardized auditing procedures for use in verifying the integrity of the calculation of HEDIS measures (NCQA, undated).

Analyzing and Displaying the Performance Measures in Suitable Formats

Ensuring that quality measures are useful for multiple audiences requires analytic and communication capabilities that can respond to the sometimes differing needs of consumers, health care providers (both individual clinicians and organizations), purchasers, and quality oversight organizations. For example, while clinicians and health care organizations may want numerous, detailed data on their performance on individual procedures and a variety of individual treatments, strong evidence shows that consumers can attend to a limited number of variables when making decisions such as which clinician or health plan to select (Office of Technology Assessment, 1988). Thus, in addition to providing detailed performance measures, there is a need to aggregate such measures into a smaller set. Data also need to show real differences in performance to help consumers select among care providers. In addition, health care delivery entities require benchmarking data so they can compare their performance with that of others in their field. Purchasers and quality oversight organizations also need comparative information for incentivizing and rewarding best performance. Risk adjustment of performance measures may sometimes be necessary, especially when reporting measures of patient outcomes as opposed to measures of the processes of care delivery.

Maintaining the Effectiveness of Performance Measures and Measure Sets and Policies

Individual performance measures and their deployment require ongoing maintenance. Performance measures' specifications often change over time; for example, administrative coding systems may change, health care entities calculating the measures may discover issues not anticipated in the original specifications, and health care delivery systems themselves change. Also, some measures need to be retired as priorities shift over time and as new, needed measures are developed. For example, a comprehensive review of mental health performance measures found several gaps in the available set of M/SU measures. First, only a handful of adequately developed process-of-care measures exist for children, older adults, individuals with prevalent but not severe mental illnesses (e.g., anxiety disorders, dysthymia, or personality disorders), and individuals with dual mental health and substance-use disorders. The review further documented a lack of measures assessing the content of psychotherapy; instead measures focused on whether psychotherapy was provided and how frequently.[17] And there were fewer process-of-care measures for substance-use problems and illnesses compared with those for mental illnesses (Hermann et al., 2000).

There is also a need for performance measure deployment policies and practices that guard against the unintended consequences of measuring only a small portion of the care that is delivered. Because it is not possible to measure everything, and because how an entity performs on one measure does not indicate how it will perform on another or in an area not measured

---

[17]This is likely due in part to the poor specificity of administrative codes discussed earlier in this chapter.

(Brook et al., 1996), focusing on only a small set of performance measures may have the unintended consequence of drawing quality improvement resources away from care delivery practices that are not in the measurement set. Periodic rotation of the measures to be calculated may therefore be needed, especially as new performance measures are developed.

Need for Public–Private Leadership and Partnership to Create a Quality Measurement and Reporting Infrastructure

Ensuring the existence of a quality measurement and reporting infrastructure that is responsive to the issues outlined above requires leadership. The committee also notes that, as with successful efforts in performance measurement in general health care, leadership is required from a critical mass of influential stakeholders; no one entity has sufficient influence or control over the vast array of M/SU providers and delivery systems or command over the many diverse technical and other resources needed to develop, test, ensure reporting of, audit, analyze, display, and continuously improve a set of M/SU health care performance measures for the nation. Moreover, although much M/SU health care is delivered in the public sector, many individuals also receive care in the private sector, often from general as opposed to specialty M/SU providers. And the many clinicians providing M/SU health care receive both public and private reimbursement. To ensure that these providers (both general and M/SU) are not required to report different quality measures to different purchasers or to report measures that are purportedly the same but calculated in different ways to multiple purchasers, public- and private-sector purchasers must reach agreement on a common set of quality measures and specifications for their reporting.

The committee acknowledges the primary leadership role played by the public sector to date in developing M/SU performance measures. While the private sector has exhibited strong leadership in the development of performance measures and measurement initiatives for general health care, leadership in M/SU performance measurement has come primarily from the public sector, most notably from SAMHSA and the Department of Veterans Affairs (DVA). For example, the successful efforts of the Washington Circle Group to identify a set of performance measures for substance-use health care and the subsequent inclusion of these measures in HEDIS came about as a result of SAMHSA's convening and nurturing these efforts. All of the efforts to conceptualize and define a comprehensive set of performance measures in mental health described above also have occurred under the auspices of SAMHSA.

Given its role in stimulating and supporting the existing M/SU health care performance measurement initiatives, together with the fact that government funding (much of it federal) is the source of 76 percent of funding for substance-use health care and 63 percent of funding for mental health services (Mark et al., 2005) (see Chapter 8), the federal government can be a prime mover in creating consensus across the public and private sectors on standard sets of measures of the quality of M/SU health care. It can do so by (1) partnering more strongly in initiatives located in the private sector, (2) requiring the submission of jointly agreed-upon public- and private-sector measures in state grants and directly administered programs, and (3) continuing its historical efforts to develop and test new performance measures. However, the public sector alone cannot achieve a performance measurement and reporting system for M/SU health care. Private-sector initiatives to build the components of the performance measurement and reporting infrastructure for health care overall need to reach out to M/SU communities to ensure their strong participation in these initiatives.

Considering currently available resources, influence, and expertise, the committee believes a partnership of public and private leaders is needed to build a quality measurement and reporting infrastructure for M/SU health care. The committee further believes that this infrastructure should build on existing structures. It should also aim to achieve maximal consistency and integration of public and private performance measurement and reporting efforts, as well as the efforts of M/SU and general health care.

Establishing Collaborative Public- and Private-Sector Efforts

There is ample precedent for collaborative public–private quality measurement efforts, as is seen in the agreement reached by public-sector (i.e., Medicaid) and private-sector (private insurance) purchasers and other stakeholders on the reporting of standardized measures of child health care in HEDIS, in the endorsement of a wide variety of performance measures by both the public and private sectors through the National Quality Forum, and in the agreement reached by the public and private sectors on a common set of performance measures for inpatient psychiatric care through a partnership among NASMHPD, NRI, the National Association of Psychiatric Health Systems (NAPHS), the American Psychiatric Association, and JCAHO. The core measures developed by NASMHPD, NRI, and NAPHS have been accepted by JCAHO as meeting its ORYX© reporting requirements for accredited inpatient psychiatric facilities (Ghinassi, 2004).

DHHS could further its collaboration with the private sector by participating more strongly in general health care and private-sector performance measurement initiatives. For example, while VHA and DHHS's CMS and AHRQ have liaison positions on NCQA's policy-making Committee on Performance Measurement, SAMHSA has no such position. Similarly, the National Quality Forum, a private, not-for-profit, open-membership organization that endorses consensus-based national standards for measurement and public reporting of health care performance data, involves more than 250 public- and private-sector consumer, purchaser, provider, health plan, research, and quality improvement members in its consensus process for endorsing performance measures for multiple types of inpatient and outpatient health care. The forum has begun to address the quality of M/SU health care by convening a workshop to identify evidence-based practices for substance-use treatment and a workshop on behavioral health funded in part by DVA (Kizer, 2005; National Quality Forum, 2004).[18] Continued involvement and support of SAMHSA and DVA in this and other national performance measurement and reporting initiatives for general health care, as well as their encouraging other M/SU organizations to participate, would help bring the resources of the private sector to bear on M/SU performance measurement and achieve consistency across the public and private sectors—both of which would facilitate the creation of a performance measurement and reporting infrastructure for M/SU health care.

An additional benefit is that M/SU health care would be able to participate on the ground floor in quality measurement initiatives, such as the development of new CPT II codes to capture outcome and otherwise non-reimbursed process-of-care measures in administrative datasets. As described earlier in this chapter, this advance has taken place through a Performance Measures Advisory Group comprising representatives of AHRQ, CMS, JCAHO, NCQA, and the AMA's Physician Consortium for Performance Improvement (AMA, 2004a). Had representatives of M/SU health care been a part of this effort and the precursor efforts of the constituent agencies, improvements in M/SU performance measurement might have occurred alongside the development of CPT II codes for general health care. While the federal government can take action to become more involved in such private-sector initiatives, these private initiatives must also take action to ensure strong representation of M/SU health care providers and delivery systems (both public and private).

Requiring Submission of Jointly Agreed-Upon Public- and Private-Sector Measures in Public and Publicly Funded Programs

The federal government also can do much to promote the collection and reporting of M/SU quality measures in both the private and public sectors. This is illustrated by the inclusion of measures developed for the Medicare and Medicaid programs in HEDIS and their subsequent application to privately enrolled populations. Both SAMHSA and DVA have ini-

---

[18]Elaine J. Power, Vice President, The National Quality Forum, personal communication on March 23, 2005.

tiatives under way to measure the performance of their M/SU programs that can contribute to the development and use of M/SU performance measures in the private sector.

SAMHSA is beginning to require performance measurement and reporting in all its grant programs for substance-use prevention and treatment and mental health as part of its National Outcome Measures initiative. This initiative aims to measure 10 outcomes of care: (1) abstinence from substance use and decreased mental illness symptomotology, (2) increased/retained employment or return to/stay in school, (3) decreased criminal justice involvement, (4) increased stability in housing, (5) increased access to services, (6) increased retention in treatment for substance abuse and reduced utilization of inpatient psychiatric care, (7) increased social supports/social connectedness, (8) clients' perception of care, (9) cost-effectiveness, and (10) use of evidence-based practices. While several of the actual measures (e.g., for evidence-based substance-use practices) are still being developed, SAHMSA achieved a major milestone in this initiative when, in 2004, it reached agreement with a representative body of states on the measures to be reported in 2005, on measures that required developmental work, and on a plan for preparing all states to report fully on the measures by the end of fiscal year 2007. SAMHSA's State Outcomes Measurement and Management System will support the expansion of state data collection efforts to meet the requirements of the agreed-upon National Outcome Measures (SAMHSA, undated-b).

DVA similarly has a National Mental Health Program Performance Monitoring System, which uses internal VHA performance measures to evaluate the work of the VA's 21 Veterans Integrated Services Networks (VISNs) and the medical centers within each of these networks. Many of these measures address the quality of M/SU health care, including the new outcome measures of each patient's functional status (Greenberg and Rosenheck, 2005).

While these performance measurement initiatives are noteworthy, their benefits could be even greater if the information obtained by the federal government were shared with the private sector as part of formal public and private collaboration.

Continuing Public-Sector Efforts to Develop, Test, and Implement New Performance Measures

While DHHS and DVA are reaching out to become an integral part of private-sector performance measurement and reporting initiatives, they should not discontinue their internal efforts to develop, test, and implement performance measures, for several reasons. First, SAMHSA and DVA are the primary payers for much of the M/SU health care provided in the United

States. They have an obligation to move forward to ensure that the quality of the care they secure and provide to their beneficiaries is as good as it can be. Second, there is not yet an agreed-upon National Quality Measurement and Reporting System in place. Until such a system begins to take shape, SAMHSA and DVA need to develop as much expertise as possible in quality measurement and reporting so they can be strong partners in the system's development and implementation. Finally, SAMHSA and DVA will be more attractive partners if they bring to the table both experience and influence in shaping the quality measurement activities of a large portion of the marketplace, as has the Medicare program.

APPLYING QUALITY IMPROVEMENT METHODS AT THE LOCUS OF CARE

Measuring and reporting on quality by themselves will not achieve improvements in care (Berwick et al., 2003). Since quality improvement is, at its heart, a change initiative, successful quality improvement requires that quality measurement be linked with activities at the locus of care to effect change and that understanding and use of these change (quality improvement) techniques be woven into the day-to-day operations of health care organizations and provider practices.

Although a systematic review and analysis of quality improvement strategies reveals remarkably little information about the most effective ways to secure the consistent incorporation of research findings into routine clinical practice (Shojania et al., 2004), many published reports of successful quality improvement initiatives clearly show that it is possible for organizations to change the quality of their health care for the better (Shojania and Grimshaw, 2005), just as it is possible to increase the quality of other industries' products (Deming, 1986). While the susceptibility to successful change is a function of some intrinsic characteristics of individuals (Berwick, 2003), the types of activities that organizations and clinicians need to undertake to achieve and sustain quality improvement can be surmised from research on and studies of organizational change (Shojania and Grimshaw, 2005). A large body of research and other published work on organizational change, for example, consistently calls attention to five predominantly human resource management practices[19] (and one other organizational practice) that are key to successful change implementation: (1) ongoing communication about the desired change with those who are to effect it; (2) training in the new practice; (3) worker involvement in designing the change process; (4) sustained attention to progress in making the

---

[19]The human resource side of change tends to be undermanaged as compared with management of the implementation of technological changes (Kimberly and Quinn, 1984).

change; (5) use of mechanisms for measurement, feedback, and redesign; and (6) functioning as a learning organization. All of these practices require the exercise of effective leadership (IOM, 2004).

These practices are illustrated in some of the leading quality improvement initiatives in health care, including those of VHA (Jha et al., 2003) and the Institute for Healthcare Improvement (http://www.ihi.org/ihi/programs). Most recently, they have been employed by some of the smallest and least resource-rich health care providers—providers of substance-use treatment services—through the Network for the Improvement of Addiction Treatment (NIATx) (see Box 4-4).

More-widespread application of quality improvement techniques would be facilitated by similar initiatives in mental health care, additional substance-use treatment sites, and provider sites offering combined M/SU treatment that could undertake research, demonstration, and dissemination of quality improvement strategies across more diverse clinicians, organizations, and systems delivering M/SU health care.

**BOX 4-4   The Network for the Improvement
of Addiction Treatment (NIATx)**

NIATx is a partnership between The Robert Wood Johnson Foundation's "Paths to Recovery" program and the Center for Substance Abuse Treatment's "Strengthening Treatment Access and Retention" program. The mission of NIATx is to help providers learn approaches that make more efficient use of their treatment capacity and produce improvements in care delivery that affect access to and retention in addiction treatment.

Of the millions of Americans who need substance-use treatment, only a small minority receive it. Fifty percent of those who do leave treatment before its benefits can be realized. While finances and psychological readiness explain some of this deficit, the issue that often keeps clients from treatment is the way services are delivered. Systems engineering, process improvement, and innovative uses of technology have been shown in other industries to dramatically improve the quality and efficiency of service delivery processes. NIATx brings these resources to substance-use treatment. The National Program Office at the University of Wisconsin's Industrial and Systems Engineering Department provides coaching, phone, and face-to-face educational sessions; a process improvement website and other communications to the field; and administrative support.

NIATx aims to reduce waiting time, reduce the percentage of no shows for treatment, reduce the percentage of clients that leave treatment early, and increase the number of clients admitted to treatment through three initiatives.

The Treatment Provider Initiative. The 39 treatment agencies (including 9 mental health agencies with addiction services) in 25 states that participate in NIATx are demonstrating the potential of process improvement to help treatment providers improve nine work processes that influence treatment access and retention: (1) the first contact a client has with the treatment agency, (2) the intake and

A PUBLIC–PRIVATE STRATEGY FOR QUALITY MEASUREMENT AND IMPROVEMENT

To address the need for strengthened quality measurement and improvement and the application of quality improvement at the locus of care, the committee recommends a public–private collaborative strategy.

Recommendation 4-3. To measure quality better, DHHS, in partnership with the private sector, should charge and financially support an entity similar to the National Quality Forum to convene government regulators, accrediting organizations, consumer representatives, providers, and purchasers exercising leadership in quality-based purchasing for the purpose of reaching consensus on and implementing a common, continuously improving set of M/SU health care quality measures for providers, organizations, and systems of care. Participants in this consortium should commit to:

---

assessment process, (3) the process by which clients are transferred between levels of care, (4) paperwork burden, (5) client and employee scheduling, (6) support systems (e.g., day care) that can help clients stay in treatment, (7) processes for reaching out to clients and referral agencies, (8) techniques for engaging clients, and (9) strategies to improve the agency's financial condition.

The Single State Agency Initiative. While the Provider Initiative demonstrates the potential to substantially improve access and retention, the state initiative tests the potential of Single State Agencies to improve their own work processes and to widely disseminate improvements (such as those identified in the Provider Initiative) across all treatment agencies in each of five states.

The Innovation Initiative. The innovation initiative examines ways to take full advantage of the technologies (e.g., consumer health informatics, virtual reality simulation, sensors, computer-mediated communication) currently or soon to be available to enhance the efficiency and effectiveness of addiction prevention and treatment.

NIATx members have demonstrated that work processes can be improved, which in turn improves the quality of care clients receive, as well as the fiscal health of treatment agencies. Within the first 18 months of the initiative, members reported improvements in each of the four project aims. Thirty-seven change projects resulted in an average reduction of 51 percent in waiting times between first contact and first treatment session. Twenty-eight change projects produced an average reduction in no-show rates of 41 percent. Twenty-three change projects produced an average increase of 56 percent in admissions, while 39 change projects produced improvements in continuation averaging 39 percent. The extent to which those improvements can be sustained and diffused to other parts of the organization is now being examined, and early results are encouraging.

- Requiring the reporting and submission of the quality measures to a performance measure repository or repositories.
- Requiring validation of the measures for accuracy and adherence to specifications.
- Ensuring the analysis and display of measurement results in formats understandable by multiple audiences, including consumers, those reporting the measures, purchasers, and quality oversight organizations.
- Establishing models for the use of the measures for benchmarking and quality improvement purposes at sites of care delivery.
- Performing continuing review of the measures' effectiveness in improving care.

Recommendation 4-4. To increase quality improvement capacity, DHHS, in collaboration with other government agencies, states, philanthropic organizations, and professional associations, should create or charge one or more entities as national or regional resources to test, disseminate knowledge about, and provide technical assistance and leadership on quality improvement practices for M/SU health care in public- and private-sector settings.

Recommendation 4-5. Public and private sponsors of research on M/SU and general health care should include the following in their research funding priorities:

- Development of reliable screening, diagnostic, and monitoring instruments that can validly assess response to treatment and that are practicable for routine use. These instruments should include a set of M/SU "vital signs": a brief set of indicators—measurable at the patient level and suitable for screening and early identification of problems and illnesses and for repeated administration during and following treatment—to monitor symptoms and functional status. The indicators should be accompanied by a specified standardized approach for routine collection and reporting as part of regular health care. Instruments should be age- and culturally appropriate.
- Refinement and improvement of these instruments, procedures for categorizing M/SU interventions, and methods for providing public information on the effectiveness of those interventions.
- Development of strategies to reduce the administrative burden of quality monitoring systems and to increase their effectiveness in improving quality.

REFERENCES

ACMHA (American College of Mental Health Administration). 2001. *A Proposed Consensus Set of Indicators for Behavioral Health*. Pittsburg, PA: ACMHA. [Online]. Available: http://www.acmha.org/publications/acmha_20.pdf [accessed March 18, 2005].

Adebimpe VR. 1994. Race, racism, and epidemiological surveys. *Hospital and Community Psychiatry* 45(1):27–31.

AHRQ (Agency for Healthcare Research and Quality). 2002–2003. *U.S. Preventive Services Task Force Ratings: Strength of Recommendations and Quality of Evidence. Guide to Clinical Preventive Services*. Rockville, MD: AHRQ. [Online]. Available: http:www.ahrq.gov/clinic/3rduspstf/ratings.htm [accessed February 28, 2005].

AHRQ. 2003. *National Healthcare Quality Report*. Rockville, MD: U.S. Department of Health and Human Services.

AHRQ. 2004a. *2004 National Healthcare Quality Report*. AHRQ Publication Number: 05-0013. Rockville, MD: U.S. Department of Health and Human Services. [Online]. Available: http://www.Quality Tools.Ahrq.Gov/Qualityreport/Documents/Nhrq2004.Pdf [accessed July 22, 2005].

AHRQ. 2004b. *AHRQ Quality Indicators—Guide to Inpatient Quality Indicators: Quality of Care in Hospitals—Volume, Mortality, and Utilization*. AHRQ Publication Number: 02-RO204 (June 2002), Revision 4 (December 22, 2004). Rockville, MD: AHRQ. [Online]. Available: http:www.qualityindicators.ahrq.gov/downloads/iqi/iqi_guide_rev4.pdf [accessed February 25, 2005].

AHRQ. undated. *EPC Evidence Reports*. [Online]. Available: http://www.ahrq.gov/clinic/epcindex.htm [accessed November 26, 2004].

Alderson P, Green S, Higgins J, eds. 2004. *Cochrane Reviewers' Handbook 4.2.2 [Updated March 2004]*. Chichester, UK: John Wiley & Sons. The Cochrane Library.

AMA (American Medical Association). 2004a. *Current Procedural Terminology: CPT 2005* 2nd ed. Chicago, IL: AMA Press.

AMA. 2004b. *Hospital ICD-9-CM 2005, Volumes 1, 2, & 3 Compact*. Chicago, IL: AMA Press.

American Association of Community Psychiatrists. 2003. *AACP Guidelines for Recovery Oriented Services*. [Online]. Available: http://www.comm.psych.pitt.edu/finds/ROSMenu.html [accessed February 18, 2005].

American Psychiatric Association Task Force for the Handbook of Psychiatric Measures. 2000. *Handbook of Psychiatric Measures*. Washington, DC: American Psychiatric Association.

American Psychiatric Association, American Psychiatric Nurses Association, National Association of Psychiatric Health Systems. 2003. *Learning from Each Other: Success Stories and Ideas for Reducing Restraint/Seclusion in Behavioral Health*. [Online]. Available: http://www.psych.org/psych_pract/treatg/pg/LearningfromEachOther.pdf [accessed February 20, 2005].

American Psychological Association. undated. *A Guide to Beneficial Psychotherapy: Empirically Supported Treatments*. [Online]. Available: http://www.apa.org/divisions/div12/rev_est/index.html [accessed March 7, 2005].

Anonymous. 2001. *ECHO Experience of Care and Health Outcomes Survey*. [Online]. Available: http://www.hcp.med.harvard.edu/echo/home.html [accessed March 18, 2005].

Associated Press. 2005, February 14. Colorado Supreme Court refuses to hear therapist's appeal in "rebirthing" death. State and Regional. Denver, CO: *Summit Daily News*.

Bates DW, Shore MF, Gibson R, Bosk C. 2003. Examining the evidence. *Psychiatric Services* 54(12):1–5.

Bauer MS. 2002. A review of quantitative studies of adherence to mental health clinical practice guidelines. *Harvard Review of Psychiatry* 10(3):138–153.

Beardslee WR, Wright EJ, Rothberg PC, Salt P, Versage E. 1996. Response of families to two preventive intervention strategies: Long-term differences in behavior and attitude change. *Journal of the American Academy of Child and Adolescent Psychiatry* 35(6):774–782.

Beardslee WR, Wright EJ, Salt P, Drezner K, Gladstone TR, Versage EM, Rothberg PC. 1997. Examination of children's responses to two preventive intervention strategies over time. *Journal of the American Academy of Child and Adolescent Psychiatry* 36(2):196–204.

Beardslee WR, Gladstone TR, Wright EJ, Cooper AB. 2003. A family-based approach to the prevention of depressive symptoms in children at risk: Evidence of parental and child change. *Pediatrics* 112(2):119–131.

Bell CC, Mehta H. 1980. The misdiagnosis of black patients with manic depressive illness. *Journal of the National Medical Association* 73(2):141–145.

Bell CC, Mehta H. 1981. Misdiagnosis of black patients with manic depressive illness: Second in a series. *Journal of the National Medical Association* 73(2):101–107.

Berwick DM. 2003. Dissemination innovations in health care. *Journal of the American Medical Association* 289(15):1969–1975.

Berwick DM, James B, Coye MJ. 2003. Connections between quality measurement and improvement. *Medical Care* 41(1):Supplement I-30–I-38.

Bethell C. 2004. *Taking the Next Step to Improve the Quality of Child and Adolescent Mental and Behavioral Health Care Services.* Paper commissioned by the Institute of Medicine Committee on Crossing the Quality Chasm: Adaptation to Mental Health and Addictive Disorders.

Borson S, Bartels SJ, Colenda CC, Gottlieb G. 2001. Geriatric mental health services research: Strategic plan for an aging population. *American Journal of Geriatric Psychiatry* 9(3): 191–204.

Brook RH, McGlynn EA, Cleary PD. 1996. Quality of health care. Part 2: Measuring quality of care. *New England Journal of Medicine* 335(13):966–969.

Brown ER, Ojeda VD, Wyn R, Levan R. 2000. *Racial and Ethnic Disparities in Access to Health Insurance and Health Care.* Los Angeles, CA: UCLA Center for Health Policy Research and The Henry J. Kaiser Family Foundation. [Online]. Available: http:www.kff.org/uninsured/loader.cfm?url=/commonspot/security/getfile.cfm&PageID=13443 [accessed July 10, 2005].

Buchanan RW, Kreyenbuhl J, Zito JM, Lehman A. 2002. The schizophrenia PORT pharmacological treatment recommendations: Conformance and implications for symptoms and functional outcome. *Schizophrenia Bulletin* 28(1):63–73.

Burns BJ, Hoagwood K, eds. 2004. Evidence-based practices Part I: A research update. *Child and Adolescent Psychiatric Clinics of North America* 13(4).

Burns BJ, Hoagwood K, eds. 2005. Evidence-based practices Part II: Effecting change. *Child and Adolescent Psychiatric Clinics of North America* 14(2).

Busch AB, Shore MF. 2000. Seclusion and restraint: A review of recent literature. *Harvard Review of Psychiatry* 8(5):261–270.

Carroll KM, Rounsaville BJ. 2003. Bridging the gap: A hybrid model to link efficacy and effectiveness research in substance abuse treatment. *Psychiatric Services* 54(3):333–339.

CDC (Centers for Disease Control and Prevention). 2005a. *United States Department of Health and Human Services Centers for Disease Control and Prevention.* [Online]. Available: http://www.cdc.gov/about/mission.htm [accessed October 10, 2005].

CDC. 2005b. *United States Department of Health and Human Services Centers for Disease Control and Prevention.* [Online]. Available: http://www.cdc.gov/about/default.htm [accessed October 10, 2005].

CDC. 2005c. *United States Department of Health and Human Services Centers for Disease Control and Prevention.* [Online]. Available: http://www.cdc.gov/about/cio.htm [accessed October 10, 2005].

CDC. 2005d. *Chronic Disease Prevention: United States Department of Health and Human Services, Centers for Disease Control and Prevention, National Center for Chronic Disease Prevention and Health Promotion.* [Online]. Available: http://www.cdc.gov/nccdphp [accessed October 10, 2005].

CDC. 2005e. *About the Mental Health Work Group.* [Online]. Available: http://www.cdc.gov/mentalhealth/about.htm [accessed September 20, 2005].

Chorpita BF, Yim LM, Dankervoet JC, Arensdorf A, Amundsen MJ, McGee C, Serrano A, Yates A, Burns JA, Morelli P. 2002. Toward large-scale implementation of empirically supported treatments for children: A review and observations by the Hawaii Empirical Basis to Services Task Force. *Clinical Psychology: Science and Practice* 9(2):165–190.

Chung H, Mahler JC, Kakuma T. 1995. Racial differences in treatment of psychiatric inpatients. *Psychiatric Services* 46(6):586–591.

Clarke GN, Hawkins W, Murphy M, Sheeber LB, Lewisohn PM, Seeley JR. 1995. Targeted prevention of unipolar depressive disorder in an at-risk sample of high school adolescents: A randomized trial of a group cognitive intervention. *Journal of the American Academy of Child and Adolescent Psychiatry* 34(3):312–321.

CMS (Centers for Medicare and Medicaid Services). 2004. *Medicare Current Beneficiary Survey: Survey Overview.* [Online]. Available: http://www.cms.hhs.gov/MCBS/Overview.asp [accessed February 23, 2005].

D'Aunno T, Pollack HA. 2002. Changes in methadone treatment practices: Results from a national panel study, 1988–2000. *Journal of the American Medical Association* 288(7):850–856.

Davis NJ. 2002. The promotion of mental health and the prevention of mental and behavioral disorders: Surely the time is right. *International Journal of Emergency Mental Health* 4(1):3–29.

Deming WE. 1986. *Out of the Crisis.* Cambridge, MA: Massachusetts Institute of Technology, Center for Advanced Engineering Study.

Denogean AT. 2003, October 18. No charges in death of woman at Kino. *Tucson Citizen.* p. 1A. [Arizona].

Department of Justice. 2005. *The What Works Repository—Working Group of the Federal Collaboration on What Works.* Washington, DC: Community Capacity Development Office, Office of Justice Programs, U.S. Department of Justice.

Department of Veterans Affairs. 2004. *VA Technology Assessment Program (VATAP).* [Online]. Available: http://www.va.gov/vatap/publications.htm [accessed March 7, 2005].

DHHS (U.S. Department of Health and Human Services). 1999. *Mental Health: A Report of the Surgeon General.* Rockville, MD: DHHS. Substance Abuse and Mental Health Services Administration, Center for Mental Health Services, and National Institutes of Health, National Institute of Mental Health.

DHHS. 2001. *Mental Health: Culture, Race, and Ethnicity—A Supplement to Mental Health: A Report of the Surgeon General.* Rockville, MD: DHHS.

Doucette A. 2003. *Outcomes Roundtable for Children and Families Performance Measurement Survey: Summary of Findings.* Paper presented at a conference, Advancing Mental and Behavioral Health Care Quality Measurement and Improvement for Children and Adolescents. Baltimore, MD, March 30, 2004.

Druss BG, Miller CL, Rosenheck RA, Shih SC, Bost JE. 2002. Mental health care quality under managed care in the United States: A view from the Health Employer Data and Information Set (HEDIS). *American Journal of Psychiatry* 159(5):860–862.

Eaton WW, Neufeld K, Chen L, Cai G. 2000. A comparison of self-report and clinical diagnostic interviews for depression: Diagnostic interview schedule and schedules for clinical assessment in neuropsychiatry in the Baltimore Epidemiologic Catchment Area Follow-up. *Archives of General Psychiatry* 57(3):217–222.

Eisen SV, Normand SL, Belanger, AJ, Spiro A, Esch D. 2004. The Revised Behavior and Symptom Identification Scale (BASIS-R): Reliability and validity. *Medical Care* 42(12):1230–1241.

Eisen SV, Wilcox M, Leff HS, Schaefer E, Culhane MA. 1999. Assessing behavioral health outcomes in outpatient programs: Reliability and validity of the BASIS-32. *Journal of Behavioral Health Services and Research* 26(1):5–17.

Essock SM, Drake RE, Frank RG, McGuire TG. 2003. Randomized controlled trials in evidence-based mental health care: Getting the right answer to the right question. *Schizophrenia Bulletin* 29(1):115–123.

Finke L. 2001. The use of seclusion is not evidence-based practice. *Journal of Child and Adolescent Psychiatric Nursing* 14(4):186–189.

Finney JW, Hahn AC, Moos RH. (1996). The effectiveness of inpatient and outpatient treatment for alcohol abuse: The need to focus on mediators and moderators of setting effects. *Addiction* 91(12):1773–1796.

Fischer EP, Marder SR, Smith GR, Owen RR, Rubenstein L, Hedrick SC, Curran GM. 2000. Quality Enhancement Research Initiative in Mental Health. *Medical Care* 38(6 Supplement 1):I70–I81.

Fisher ES, Wennberg DE, Stukel TA, Gottlieb DJ, Lucas FL, Pinder E. 2003. The implications of regional variations in Medicare spending. Part 2: Health outcomes and satisfaction with care. *Annals of Internal Medicine* 138(4):288–298.

Fontana A, Rosenheck RA. 1997. Effectiveness and cost of the inpatient treatment of post-traumatic stress disorder: Comparison of three models of treatment. *American Journal of Psychiatry* 154(6):758–765.

Friedmann PD, McCullough D, Saitz R. 2001. Screening and intervention for illicit drug abuse: A national survey of primary care physicians and psychiatrists. *Archives of Internal Medicine* 161(2):248–251.

Ganju V. 2003. Implementation of evidence-based practices in state mental health systems: Implications for research and effectiveness studies. *Schizophrenia Bulletin* 29(1):125–131.

Ganju V. 2004. *Quality and Accountability: An Agenda for Public Mental Health Systems.* A paper developed for the Institute of Medicine Meeting on Crossing the Quality Chasm—An Adaptation to Mental Health and Addictive Disorders. Washington, DC. Available from the Institute of Medicine.

Ganju V, Smith ME, Adams N, Allen J Jr, Bible J, Danforth M, Davis S, Dumont J, Gibson G, Gonzalez O, Greenberg P, Hall LL, Hopkins C, Koch RJ, Kupfer D, Lutterman T, Manderscheid R, Onken S, Osher T, Stange JL, Wieman D. 2004. *The MHSIP Quality Report: The Next Generation of Mental Health Performance Measures.* Rockville, MD: SAMHSA.

GAO (Government Accounting Office). 1999. *Mental Health: Improper Restraint or Seclusion Use Places People at Risk.* GAO/HEHS-99-176. Washington, DC: GAO. [Online]. Available: http://www/gao.gov/archive/1999/he99176.pdf [accessed on October 10, 2005].

Garnick DW, Lee MT, Chalk M, Gastfriend D, Horgan CM, McCorry F, McLellan AT, Merrick EL. 2002. Establishing the feasibility of performance measures for alcohol and other drugs. *Journal of Substance Abuse Treatment* 23(4):375–385.

Gerstein D, Harwood H, eds. 1990. *Treating Drug Problems.* Volume 1. Washington, DC: National Academy Press.

Ghinassi FA. 2004. Testimony before the Institute of Medicine Committee on Crossing the Quality Chasm: Adaptation to Mental Health and Addictive Disorders. Washington, DC. July 14, 2004. Available from the Institute of Medicine.

Gilbody S, House A, Sheldon T. 2001. Routinely administered questionnaires for depression and anxiety: Systematic review. *British Medical Journal* 322(7283):406–409.

Glied S, Cuellar AE. 2003. Trends and issues in child and adolescent mental health. *Health Affairs* 22(5):39–50.

Goodman LA, Rosenberg SD, Mueser KT, Drake RE. 1997. Physical and sexual assault history in women with serious mental illness: Prevalence, correlates, treatment, and future research directions. *Schizophrenia Bulletin* 23(4):685–696.

Gossop M, Marsden J, Stewart D, Treacy S. 2001. Outcomes after methadone maintenance and methadone reduction treatments: Two year follow-up results from the National Treatment Outcome Research Study. *Drug and Alcohol Dependence* 62(3):255–264.

Grasso BC, Genest R, Jordan CW, Bates DW. 2003a. Use of chart and record reviews to detect medication errors in a state psychiatric hospital. *Psychiatric Services* 54(5): 677–681.

Grasso BC, Rothschild JM, Genest R, Bates DW. 2003b. What do we know about medication errors in inpatient psychiatry? *Joint Commission Journal on Quality and Safety* 29(8): 391–400.

Greenberg G, Rosenheck R. 2005. *Department of Veterans Affairs National Mental Health Program Performance Monitoring System: Fiscal Year 2004 Report*. West Haven, CT: Northeast Program Evaluation Center (182), VA Connecticut Healthcare System. [Online]. Available: http://nepec.org/NMHPPMS/default.htm [accessed May 30, 2005].

Greenhalgh T, Robert G, MacFarlane F, Bate P, Kyriakidou O. 2004. Diffusion of innovations in service organizations: Systematic review and recommendations. *The Milbank Quarterly* 82(4):581–629.

Gurwitz JH, Field TS, Avorn J, McCormick D, Jain S, Eckler M, Benser M, Edmondson AC, Bates DW. 2000. Incidence and preventability of adverse drug events in nursing homes. *American Journal of Medicine* 109(2):87–94.

Hadley J, Rabin D, Epstein A, Stein S, Rimes C. 2000. Post hospitalization home health care use and changes in functional status in a Medicare population. *Medical Care* 38(5): 494–507.

Harman JS, Manning WG, Lurie N, Christianson JB. 2003. Association between interruptions in Medicaid coverage and use of inpatient psychiatric services. *Psychiatric Services* 54(7):999–1005.

Harris RP, Helfand M, Woolf SH, Lohr KN, Mulrow CD, Teutsch SM, Atkins D. 2001. Current methods of the U.S. Preventive Services Task Force: A review of the process. *American Journal of Preventive Medicine* 20(3S):21–35.

Harrison PA, Beebe TJ, Park E. 2001. The Adolescent Health Review: A brief, multidimensional screening instrument. *Journal of Adolescent Health* 29(2):131–139.

Hawaii Department of Health. 2004. *Evidence Based Services Committee 2004 Biennial Report—Summary of Effective Interventions for Youth With Behavioral and Emotional Needs*. [Online]. Available: http://www.state.hi.us/health/mental-health/camhd/library/pdf/ebs/ebso11.pdf [accessed March 8, 2005].

Hennessy R. 2002. Focus on the states: Hospitals in Florida, Georgia and Utah drastically reduce seclusion and restraint. *Networks* (1–2)10–11. [Online]. Available: http://www.nasmhpd.org/general_files/publications/ntac_pubs/networks/SummerFall2002.pdf [accessed February 20, 2005].

Hermann RC, Palmer RH. 2002. Common ground: A framework for selecting core quality measures for mental health and substance abuse care. *Psychiatric Services* 53(3): 281–287.

Hermann RC, Leff HS, Palmer RH, Yang D, Teller T, Provost S, Jakubiak C, Chan J. 2000. Quality measures for mental health care: Results from a national inventory. *Medical Care Research and Review* 57(Supplement 2):136–154.

Hermann RC, Palmer H, Leff S, Schwartz M, Provost S, Chan J, Chiu WT, Lagodmos G. 2004. Achieving consensus across diverse stakeholders on quality measures for mental healthcare. *Medical Care* 42(12):1246–1253.

Hibbard JH. 2003. Engaging health care consumers to improve the quality of care. *Medical Care* 41(Supplement 1):I-61–I-70.

Hoagwood K, Burns BJ, Kiser L, Ringeisen H, Schoenwald SK. 2001. Evidence-based practice in child and adolescent mental health services. *Psychiatric Services* 52(9):1179–1189.

Hollon SD, Munoz RF, Barlow DH, Beardslee WR, Bell CC, Bernal G, Clarke GN, Franciosi LP, Kazdin AE, Kohn L, Linehan MM, Markowitz JC, Miklowitz DJ, Persons JB, Niederehe G, Sommers D. 2002. Psychosocial intervention development for the prevention and treatment of depression: Promoting innovation and increasing access. *Biological Psychiatry* 52(6):610–630.

Hon J. 2003. *Using Performance Measurement to Improve the Quality of Alcohol Treatment.* Washington, DC: The George Washington University Medical Center.

Horgan C, Garnick D. 2005. *The Quality of Care for Adults with Mental and Addictive Disorders: Issues in Performance Measurement.* Paper commissioned by the Institute of Medicine Committee on Crossing the Quality Chasm: Adaptation to Mental Health and Addictive Disorders. Available from the Institute of Medicine.

Hubbard RL, Marsden ME, Rachal JV, Harwood HJ, Cavanaugh ER, Ginzburg HM. 1989. *Drug Abuse Treatment: A National Study of Effectiveness.* Chapel Hill, NC: University of North Carolina Press.

Iezzoni LI. 1997. Data sources and implications: Administrative databases. In: Iezzoni LI, ed. *Risk Adjustment for Measuring Healthcare Outcomes* 2nd ed. Chicago, IL: Health Administration Press. Pp. 169–242.

IOM (Institute of Medicine). 1994. Mrazek PJ, Haggerty RJ, eds. *Reducing Risks for Mental Disorders: Frontiers for Prevention Intervention Research.* Washington, DC: National Academy Press.

IOM. 1997. *Dispelling the Myths about Addiction: Strategies to Increase Understanding and Strengthen Research.* Washington, DC: National Academy Press.

IOM. 1998. *Bridging the Gap Between Practice and Research: Forging Partnerships with Community-based Drug and Alcohol Treatment.* Washington, DC: National Academy Press.

IOM. 2004. Page A, ed. *Keeping Patients Safe: Transforming the Work Environment of Nurses.* Washington, DC: The National Academies Press.

Jaycox LH, Morral AR, Juvonen J. 2003. Mental health and medical problems and service use among adolescent substance users. *Journal of the American Academy of Child and Adolescent Psychiatry* 42(6):701–709.

Jha AK, Perlin JB, Kizer KW, Dudley RA. 2003. Effect of the transformation of the Veterans Affairs Health Care System on the Quality of Care. *New England Journal of Medicine* 348(22):2218–2227.

Johnson R, Chatuape M, Strain E, Walsh S, Stitzer M, Bigelow G. 2000. A comparison of levomethadyl acetate, buprenorphine, and methadone for opioid dependence. *New England Journal of Medicine* 343(18):1290–1297.

Kane JM, Leucht S, Carpenter D, Docherty JP. 2003. Optimizing pharmacologic treatment of psychotic disorders. *Journal of Clinical Psychiatry* 64 Supplement 12(1–100): 5–19.

Kataoka SH, Zhang L, Wells KB. 2002. Unmet need for mental health care among U.S. children: Variation by ethnicity and insurance status. *American Journal of Psychiatry* 159(9):1548–1555.

Kazdin A. 2000. *Psychotherapy for Children and Adolescents: Directions for Research and Practice.* New York: Oxford University Press.

Kazdin AE. 2003. *Evidence-Based Psychotherapies for Children and Adolescents*. New York: Guilford Press.

Kazdin AE. 2004. Evidence-based treatments: Challenges and priorities for practice and research. *Child and Adolescent Psychiatric Clinics of North America* 13(4):923–940.

Kessler RC. 2004. Impact of substance abuse on the diagnosis, course, and treatment of mood disorders: The epidemiology of dual diagnosis. *Biological Psychiatry* 56:730–737.

Kessler RC, Demler O, Frank RG, Olfson M, Pincus HA, Walters EE, Wang P, Wells KB, Zaslavsky AM. 2005. Prevalence and treatment of mental disorders, 1990 to 2003. *New England Journal of Medicine* 352(24):2515–2523.

Kimberly J, Quinn R. 1984. *Managing Organizational Transitions*. Homewood, IL: Dow Jones—Irwin.

Kizer K. 2005. Conducting a dissonant symphony. *Modern Healthcare* 34(14):20.

Kramer TL, Daniels AS, Zieman GL, Willimas C, Dewan N. 2000. Psychiatric practice variations in the diagnosis and treatment of major depression. *Psychiatric Services* 51(3):336–340.

LaVeist TA., Diala C, Jarrett NC. 2000. Social status and perceived discrimination: Who experiences discrimination in the health care system, how and why? In: Hogue C, Hargraves M, Scott-Collins K, eds. *Minority Health in America—Findings and Policy Implications from the Commonwealth Fund Minority Health Survey*. Baltimore, MD: Johns Hopkins University Press. Pp 194–208.

Lefever G, Arcona A, Antonuccio D. 2003. ADHD among American schoolchildren: Evidence of overdiagnosis and overuse of medication. *The Scientific Review of Mental Health Practice* 21(1). [Online]. Available: http://www.srmph.org/0201-adhd.html [accessed November 2, 2004].

Levant RF. 2004. The empirically validated treatments movement: A practitioner/educator perspective. *Clinical Psychology: Science and Practice* 11(2):219–224.

Lewczyk CM, Garland AF, Hurlburt MS, Gearity J, Hough RL. 2003. Comparing DISC-IV and clinician diagnoses among youths receiving public mental health services. *Journal of the American Academy of Child and Adolescent Psychiatry* 42(3):349–356.

Lewinsohn PM. 1987. The coping-with-depression course. In: Munoz RF, ed. *Depression Prevention: Research Directions*. Washington, DC: Hemisphere Publishing Corporation. Pp. 159–170.

Lilienfeld SO, Lynn SJ, Lohr JM, eds. 2003. *Science and Pseudoscience in Clinical Psychology*. New York: Guilford Press.

Lin EH, Simon GE, Katzelnick DJ, Pearson SD. 2001. Does physician education on depression management improve treatment in primary care? *Journal of General Internal Medicine* 16(9):614–619.

Lin KM, Anderson D, Poland RE. 1997. Ethnic and cultural considerations in psychopharmacology. In: Dunner D, ed. *Current Psychiatric Therapy II*. Philadelphia, PA: W.B. Saunders. Pp. 75–81.

Lowe B, Unutzer J, Callahan CM, Perkins A, Kroenke K. 2004. Monitoring depression treatment outcomes with the Patient Health Questionnaire-9. *Medical Care* 42(12):1194–1201.

Manderscheid RW, Henderson MJ, Brown DY. 2001. Status of national accountability efforts at the millenium. In: Manderscheid RW, Henderson MJ, eds. *Mental Health, United States, 2000*. DHHS Publication Number: (SMA) 01-3537. Washington DC: U.S. Government Printing Office. Pp. 43–52.

Maris RW. 2002. Suicide. *The Lancet* 360(9329):319–326.

Mark TL, Coffey RM, Vandivort-Warren R, Harwood HJ, King EC, the MHSA Spending Estimates Team. 2005. U.S. spending for mental health and substance abuse treatment, 1991–2001. *Health Affairs Web Exclusive* W5-133–W5-142.

McClellan J. 2005. Commentary: Treatment guidelines for child and adolescent bipolar disorder. *Journal of the American Academy of Child and Adolescent Psychiatry* 44(3): 236–239.

McCorry F, Garnick DW, Bartlett J, Cotter F, Chalk M. 2000. Developing performance measures for alcohol and other drug services in managed care plans. *Joint Commission Journal on Quality Improvement* 26(11):633–643.

McGlynn EA. 2003. Introduction and overview of the conceptual framework for a national quality measurement and reporting system. *Medical Care* 41(Supplement 1):I-1–I-7.

McGlynn EA, Asch SM, Adams J, Keesey J, Hicks J, DeCristofaro A, Kerr EA. 2003. The quality of health care delivered to adults in the United States. *New England Journal of Medicine* 348(26):2635–2645.

McKay J. 2005. Is there a case for extended interventions for alcohol and drug use disorders? *Addiction* 100(11):1594–1610.

McKay JR, Alterman AI, Cacciola JS, Rutherford MR, O'Brien CP, Koppenhaver J, Shepard D. 1999. Continuing care for cocaine dependence: Comprehensive 2-year outcomes. *Journal of Consulting and Clinical Psychology* 67(3):420–427.

McKay JR, Lynch KG, Shepard DS, Ratichek S, Morrison R, Koppenhaver J, Pettinati HM. 2004. The effectiveness of telephone-based continuing care in the clinical management of alcohol and cocaine use disorders: 12 month outcomes. *Journal of Consulting and Clinical Psychology* 72(6):967–979.

McLellan AT. 2002. Contemporary drug abuse treatment: A review of the evidence base. In: *Investing in Drug Abuse Treatment: A Discussion Paper for Policy Makers*. New York: United Nations Press.

McLellan AT, Grissom G, Brill P, Durell J, Metzger DS, O'Brien CP. 1993a. Private substance abuse treatments: Are some programs more effective than others? *Journal of Substance Abuse Treatment* 10(3):243–254.

McLellan AT, Arndt IO, Woody GE, Metzger D. 1993b. Psychosocial services in substance abuse treatment: A dose-ranging study of psychosocial services. *Journal of the American Medical Association* 269(15):1953–1959.

McLellan AT, Lewis DL, O'Brien CP, Kleber HD. 2000. Drug dependence, a chronic medical illness: Implications for treatment, insurance and outcomes evaluation. *Journal of the American Medical Association* 284(13):1689–1695.

Mechanic D, Bilder S. 2004. Treatment of people with mental illness: A decade-long perspective. *Health Affairs* 23(4):84–95.

Miller AL, Craig CS. 2002. Combination antipsychotics: Pros, cons, and questions. *Schizophrenia Bulletin* 28(1):105–109.

Mohr WK, Petti TA, Mohr B. 2003. Adverse effects associated with physical restraint. *Canadian Journal of Psychiatry* 48(5):330–337.

Mojtabai R. 2002. Diagnosing depression and prescribing antidepressants by primary care physicians: The impact of practice style variations. *Mental Health Services Research* 4(2):109–118.

Mojtabai R, Malaspina D, Susser E. 2003. The concept of population prevention: Application to schizophrenia. *Schizophrenia Bulletin* 29(4):791–801.

Moos RH. 2005. Iatrogenic effects of psychosocial interventions for substance use disorders: Prevalence, predictors, prevention. *Addiction* 100(5):595–604.

Mueser KT, Rosenberg SD, Goodman LA, Trumbetta SL. 2002. Trauma, PTSD, and the course of severe mental illness: An interactive model. *Schizophrenia Research* 53 (1–2):123–143.

Mukherjee S, Shukla S, Woodle J, Rosen AM, Olarte S. 1983. Misdiagnosis of schizophrenia in bipolar patients: A multiethnic comparison. *American Journal of Psychiatry* 140(12): 1571–1574.

Mullan F. 2004. Wrestling with variation: An interview with Jack Wennberg. *Health Affairs.* [Online]. Available: http://content.healthaffairs.org/cgi/content/full/healthaff.var.73/DC2 [accessed February 25, 2005].

Musto DF. 1973. *The American Disease: The Origins of Narcotic Control.* New Haven, CT: Yale University Press.

NAMI (National Alliance for the Mentally Ill). 2003. *Seclusion and Restraint: Task Force Report.* Arlington, VA: NAMI. [Online]. Available: http://ww.nami.org/content/ NavigationMenu/Inform_Yourself/About_Public_Policy/Policy_Research_Institute/ seclusion_and_restraints.pdf [accessed February 20, 2005].

NASMHPD (National Association of State Mental Health Directors, Inc.). 1999. *Position Statement on Seclusion and Restraint.* [Online]. Available: http://www.nasmhpd.org/ general_files/position_statement/posses1.html [accessed February 20, 2005].

NASMHPD. 2005. *NASMHPD Position Statement on Services and Supports to Trauma Survivors.* [Online]. Available: http://www.nasmhpd.org/general_files/position_statement/ NASMHPD%20TRAUMA%20Position%20statementFinal.pdf [accessed February 20, 2005].

NASMHPD Research Institute. undated. *NRI Center for Mental Health Quality and Accountability: Evidence-Based Practices.* [Online]. Available: http://ebp.networkofcare.net/ index.cfm?pageName=index [accessed March 7, 2005].

National Academy of Sciences. undated. *Standards of Evidence: Strategic Planning Initiative.* [Online]. Available: http://www7.nationalacademies.org/dbasse/Standards%20of%20 Evidence%20Description.html [accessed March 2, 2005].

National Quality Forum. 2004. *National Quality Forum Home.* [Online]. Available: http:// www.qualityforum.org [accessed March 21, 2005].

NCQA (National Committee for Quality Assurance). 2004a. *HEDIS 2005 Technical Specifications.* Washington, DC: NCQA.

NCQA. 2004b. *HEDIS 2005 Technical Specifications Volume 2.* Washington, DC: NCQA.

NCQA. 2005. *Draft Document for HEDIS 2006 Public Comment.* [Online]. Available: http:// www.ncqa.org/Programs/HEDIS/Public%20Comments/overview/pdf with notation [accessed March 18, 2005].

NCQA. undated. *NCQA HEDIS Compliance Audit Program.* [Online]. Available: http:// ww.ncqa.org/programs/hedis/audit/auditex.htm [accessed June 8, 2005].

New Freedom Commission on Mental Health. 2003. *Achieving the Promise: Transforming Mental Health Care in America. Final Report.* DHHS Publication Number SMA-03-3832. Rockville, MD: U.S. Department of Health and Human Services.

NIDA (National Institute of Drug Abuse). 2005. *NIDA/SAMHSA-ATTC Blending Initiative.* [Online]. Available: http://www.drugabuse.gov/CTN/whatisblending.html [accessed June 6, 2005].

NIMH (National Institute of Mental Health). 2004. *State Implementation of Evidence-Based Practices II: Bridging Science and Service RFA MH-05-004.* [Online]. Available: http:// grants.nih.gov/grants/guide/rfa-files/RFA-MH-05-004.html [accessed June 7, 2005].

Norcross JC, ed. 2002. *Psychotherapy Relationships That Work: Therapist Contributions and Responsiveness to Patients.* New York: Oxford University Press.

Office of Technology Assessment. 1988. *The Quality of Medical Care: Information for Consumers.* OTA-H-386. Washington, DC: U.S. Government Printing Office.

Office of the Surgeon General. 2001. *Youth Violence: A Report of the Surgeon General.* Washington, DC: U.S. Department of Health and Human Services.

Pappadopulos EA, Guelzow BT, Wong C, Ortega M, Jensen PS. 2004. A review of the growing evidence base for pediatric psychopharmacology. In: Burns BJ, Hoagwood KE, eds. Evidence-Based Practice Part I: Research Update. *Child and Adolescent Psychiatric Clinics of North America* Vol. 13, No. 4. Pp. 817–856.

Patel NC, Crismon ML, Hoagwood K, Jensen PS. 2005. Unanswered questions regarding atypical antipsychotic use in aggressive children and adolescents. *Journal of Child and Adolescent Psychopharmacology* 15(2):270–284.

Patterson GR, DeBaryshe BD, Ramsey E. 1989. A developmental perspective on antisocial behavior. *American Psychologist* 44(2):329–335.

Patterson GR, Dishion TJ, Chamberlain P. 1993. Outcomes and methodological issues relating to treatment of antisocial children. In: Giles TR, ed. *Handbook of Effective Psychotherapy*. New York: Plenum Press. Pp. 43–88.

Peter D. Hart Research Associates, Inc. 2001. *The Face of Recovery*. Washington, DC: Peter D. Hart Research Associates, Inc.

Petrosino A, Turpin-Petrosino C, Buehler J. 2005. "Scared Straight" and other juvenile awareness programs for preventing juvenile delinquency. Cochrane Developmental, Psychosocial and Learning Problems Group *The Cochrane Database of Systematic Reviews* 4.

Pflueger W. 2002. Consumer view: Restraint is not therapeutic. *Networks* (1–2):7. [Online]. Available: http://www.nasmhpd.org/general_files/publications/ntac_pubs/networks/SummerFall2002.pdf [accessed February 20, 2005].

Pincus HA. 2003. The future of behavioral health and primary care: Drowning in the mainstream or left on the bank? *Psychosomatics* 44(1):1–11.

Podorefsky DL, McDonald-Dowdell M, Beardslee WR. 2001. Adaptation of preventive interventions for a low-income, culturally diverse community. *Journal of the American Academy of Child & Adolescent Psychiatry* 40(8):879–886.

Project MATCH Research Group. 1997. Matching alcoholism treatments to client heterogeneity: Project MATCH post treatment drinking outcomes. *Journal of Studies on Alcohol* 58(1):7–29.

Rawal PH, Lyons JS, MacIntyre II JC, Hunter JC. 2004. Regional variation and clinical indicators of antipsychotic use in residential treatment: A four state comparison. *The Journal of Behavioral Health Services & Research* 31(2):178–188.

Richardson LP, Di Giuseppe D, Christakis DA, McCauley E, Katon W. 2004. Quality of care for Medicaid-covered youth treated with antidepressant therapy. *Archives of General Psychiatry* 61(5):475–480.

Rollman BL, Hanusa BH, Gilbert T, Lowe HJ, Kapoor WN, Schulberg HC. 2001. The electronic medical record. A randomized trial of its impact on primary care physicians' initial management of major depression. *Archives of Internal Medicine* 161(2):189–197.

Rose S, Bison J, Churchill R, Wessely S. 2005. Psychological debriefing for preventing post traumatic stress disorder. *The Cochrane Database of Systematic Reviews* 2.

Rosenheck RA, Fontana A. 2001. Impact of efforts to reduce inpatient costs on clinical effectiveness: Treatment of Post Traumatic Stress Disorder in the Department of Veterans Affairs. *Medical Care* 39(2):168–180.

Rushton JL, Fant K, Clark SJ. 2004. Use of practice guidelines in the primary care of children with Attention-Deficit Hyperactivity Disorder. *Pediatrics* 114(1):e23–e28. [Online]. Available: http://www.pediatrics.aappublications.org/cgi/reprint/114/1/e23 [accessed on September 1, 2005].

Sailas E, Fenton M. 2005. Seclusion and restraint for people with serious mental illness. *The Cochrane Database of Systematic Reviews* 1.

SAMHSA (Substance Abuse and Mental Health Services Administration). 2004a. *Results from the 2003 National Survey on Drug Use and Health: National Findings*. DHHS Publication Number SMA 04-3964. Rockville, MD: SAMHSA.

SAMHSA. 2004b. *SAMHSA Action Plan: Seclusion and Restraint—Fiscal Years 2004 and 2005*. [Online]. Available: http://www.samhsa.gov/Matrix/SAP_seclusion.aspx [accessed February 20, 2005].

SAMHSA. 2005. *SAMHSA's National Registry of Evidence-Based Programs and Practices (NREPP).* [Online]. Available: http://www.modelprograms.samhsa.gov/template.cfm?page=nreppover [accessed June 6, 2005].

SAMHSA. undated-a. *About Evidence-Based Practices: Shaping Mental Health Services toward Recovery.* [Online]. Available: http://mentalhealth.samhsa.gov/cmhs/community support/toolkits/about.asp [accessed March 6, 2005].

SAMHSA. undated-b. *Fiscal Year 2006 Justification of Estimates for Appropriations Committees.* [Online]. Available: http://www.samhsa.gov/budget/FY2006/FY2006Budget.doc [accessed March 26, 2005].

SAMHSA. undated-c. *Report to Congress on the Prevention and Treatment of Co-Occurring Substance Abuse Disorders and Mental Disorders.* [Online]. Available: http://www.samhsa.gov/reports/congress2002/CoOccurringRpt.pdf [accessed April 25, 2004].

Satre DD, Knight BG, Dickson-Fuhrmann E, Jarvik LF. 2004. Substance abuse treatment initiation among older adults in the GET SMART program: Effects of depression and cognitive status. *Aging & Mental Health* 8(4):346–354.

Schnaars C. 2003, April 13. Tape called strong evidence in boy's death. *Daily Press.* Local News. p. C1. Newport News, Virginia.

Shojania KG, Grimshaw JM. 2005. Evidence-based quality improvement: The state of the science. *Health Affairs* 24(1):138–150.

Shojania KG, McDonald KM, Wachter RM, Owens DK. 2004. *Closing the Quality Gap: A Critical Analysis of Quality Improvement Strategies, Volume 1—Series Overview and Methodology.* AHRQ Publication Number: 04-0051-1. Rockville, MD: Agency for Healthcare Research and Quality.

Simon GE, Von Korff M, Rutter CM, Peterson DA. 2001. Treatment processes and outcomes for managed care patients receiving new antidepressant prescriptions from psychiatrists and primary care physicians. *Archives of General Psychiatry* 58(4):395–401.

Simon R, Fleiss J, Gurland B, Stiller P, Sharpe L. 1973. Depression and schizophrenia in hospitalized black and white mental patients. *Archives of General Psychiatry* 28(4): 509–512.

Simpson DD, Joe GW, Brown BS. 1997. Treatment retention and follow-up outcomes in the Drug Abuse Treatment Outcome Study (DATOS). *Psychology of Addictive Behaviors* 11(4):294–301.

Simpson DD, Joe GW, Fletcher BW, Hubbard RL, Anglin MD. 1999. A national evaluation of treatment outcomes for cocaine dependence. *Archives of General Psychiatry* 56(6):507–514.

Smith G, Davis R, Bixler E, Lin H, Altenor A, Altenor R, Hardenstein B, Kopchik G. 2005. Special section on seclusion and restraint: Pennsylvania state hospital system's seclusion and restraint reduction program: Timeline of change. *Psychiatric Services* 56:1115–1122.

Stanton M. 2002. *Expanding Patient-Centered Care to Empower Patients and Assist Providers.* AHRQ Publication Number: 02-0024. Rockville, MD: Agency for Healthcare Research and Quality. [Online]. Available: http://www.ahrq.gov/qual/ptcareria.pdf [accessed February 8, 2005].

Stein M. 2002. The role of attention-deficit/hyperactivity disorder diagnostic and treatment guidelines in changing physician practices. *Pediatric Annals* 31(8):496–504.

Stein MB, Sherbourne CD, Craske MG, Means-Christensen A, Bystritsky A, Katon W, Sullivan G, Roy-Byrne PP. 2004. Quality of care for primary care patients with anxiety disorders. *American Journal of Psychiatry* 161(12):2230–2237.

Steinberg EP, Luce BR. 2005. Evidence based? Caveat emptor! *Health Affairs* 24(1):80–92.

Strakowski SM, Shelton RC, Kolbrener ML. 1993. The effects of race and comorbidity on clinical diagnosis in patients with psychosis. *Journal of Clinical Psychiatry* 54(3): 96–102.

Strickland TL, Ranganath V, Lin K, Poland RE, Mendoza R, Smith MW. 1991. Psychopharmacologic considerations in the treatment of Black American populations. *Psychopharmacology Bulletin* 27(4):441–448.

Tanenbaum S. 2003. Evidence-based practice in mental health: Practical weaknesses meet political strengths. *Journal of Evaluation in Clinical Practice* 9(2):287–301.

Tanenbaum SJ. 2005. Evidence-based practice as mental health policy: Three controversies and a caveat. *Health Affairs* 24(1):163–173.

Teague GB, Trabin T, Ray C. 2004. Toward common performance indicators and measures for accountability in behavioral health care. In: Roberts AR, Yeager K, eds. *Evidence-Based Practice Manual: Research and Outcome Measures in Health and Human Services.* New York: Oxford University Press. Pp. 46–61.

The Campbell Collaboration. undated. *The Campbell Collaboration.* [Online]. Available: http://www.campbellcollaboration.org/index.html [accessed December 3, 2004].

The Cochrane Collaboration. 2004. *What Is The Cochrane Collaboration?* [Online]. Available: http://www.cochrane.org/docs/descrip.htm [accessed December 3, 2004].

The President's Advisory Commission on Consumer Protection and Quality in the Health Care Industry. 1998. *Quality First: Better Health Care for All Americans.* Washington, DC: U.S. Government Printing Office.

Thompson C, Kinmonth A, Stevens L, Peveler R, Stevens A, Ostler K, Pickering R, Baker N, Hensen A, Preece J, Cooper D, Campbell M. 2000. Effects of a clinical-practice guideline and practice-based education on detection and outcome of depression in primary care: Hampshire Depression Project randomized controlled trial. *Lancet* 355(9199): 185–191.

Tunis SR, Stryer DB, Clancy CM. 2003. Practical clinical trials: Increasing the value of clinical research for decision-making in clinical and health policy. *Journal of the American Medical Association* 290(12):1624–1632.

VA Technology Assessment Program. 2002. *Outcome Measurement—Mental Health Overview: Final Report.* [Online]. Available: http://www.va.gov/vatap [accessed February 28, 2005].

VHA (Veterans Health Administration). 2005. *Clinical Practice Guidelines.* [Online]. Available: http://www.oqp.med.va.gov/cpg/cpg.htm [accessed February 28, 2005].

Wang PS, Berglund P, Kessler RC. 2000. Recent care of common mental disorders in the United States: Prevalence and conformance with evidence-based recommendations. *Journal of General Internal Medicine* 15(5):284–292.

Wang P, Demler M, Kessler RC. 2002. Adequacy of treatment for serious mental illness in the United States. *American Journal of Public Health* 92(1):92–98.

Watkins KE, Burnam A, Kung F-Y, Paddock S. 2001. A national survey of care for persons with co-occurring mental and substance use disorders. *Psychiatric Services* 52(8):1062– 1068.

Webster-Stratton C, Hammond M. 1997. Treating children with early-onset conduct problems: A comparison of child and parent training interventions. *Journal of Consulting and Clinical Psychology* 65(1):93–109.

Webster-Stratton C, Hammond M. 1999. Marital conflict management skills, parenting style, and early-onset conduct problems: Processes and pathways. *Journal of Child Psychology and Psychiatry, and Allied Disciplines* 40(6):917–927.

Weisner C, Matzger H. 2002. A prospective study of the factors influencing entry to alcohol and drug treatment. *Journal of Behavioral Health Services & Research* 29(2):126–137.

Weisz JR. 2004. *Psychotherapy for Children and Adolescents: Evidence-Based Treatments and Case Examples.* Cambridge, MA: Cambridge University Press.

Wennberg JE, ed. 1999. *The Dartmouth Atlas of Health Care in the United States.* [Online]. Available: http://www.dartmouthatlas.org/pdffiles/99atlas.pdf [accessed November 24, 2004].

West S, King V, Carey TS, Lohr K, McKoy N, Sutton S, Lux L. 2002. *Systems to Rate the Strength of Scientific Evidence.* AHRQ Publication No. 02-E016. Rockville, MD: Agency for Healthcare Research and Quality.

Wolff N. 2000. Using randomized controlled trials to evaluate socially complex services: Problems, challenges, and recommendations. *Journal of Mental Health Policy and Economics* 3(2):97–109.

Work Group on ASD and PTSD. 2004. *Practice Guideline for the Treatment of Patients with Acute Stress Disorder and Posttraumatic Stress Disorder.* [Online]. Available: http://www.psych.org/psych_prac/treatg/pg/PTSD-PG-PartsA-B-CNew.pdf [accessed June 6, 2005].

Young AS, Klap R, Sherbourne C, Wells KB. 2001. The quality of care for depressive and anxiety disorders in the United States. *Archives of General Psychiatry* 58(1):55–61.

Zhan C, Miller MR. 2003. Administrative data based patient safety research: A critical review. *Quality & Safety in Health Care* 12(Supplement II):ii58–ii63.

Zima BT, Hurlburt MS, Knapp P, Ladd H, Tang L, Duan N, Wallace P, Rosenblatt A, Landsverk J, Wells KB. 2005. Quality of publicly-funded outpatient specialty mental health care for common childhood psychiatric disorders in California. *Journal of the American Academy of Child & Adolescent Psychiatry* 44(2):130–144.

Zito JM, Safer DJ, dosReis S, Gardner JF, Boles M, Lynch F. 2000. Trends in the prescribing of psychotropic medications to preschoolers. *Journal of the American Medical Association* 283(8):1025–1030.

5

Coordinating Care for Better Mental, Substance-Use, and General Health

Summary

Mental and substance-use problems and illnesses seldom occur in isolation. They frequently accompany each other, as well as a substantial number of general medical illnesses such as heart disease, cancers, diabetes, and neurological illnesses. Sometimes they masquerade as separate somatic problems. Consequently, mental, substance-use, and general health problems and illnesses are frequently intertwined, and coordination of all these types of health care is essential to improved health outcomes, especially for chronic illnesses. Moreover, mental and/or substance-use (M/SU) problems and illnesses frequently affect and are addressed by education, child welfare, and other human service systems. Improving the quality of M/SU health care— and general health care—depends upon the effective collaboration of all mental, substance-use, general health care, and other human service providers in coordinating the care of their patients.

However, these diverse providers often fail to detect and treat (or refer to other providers to treat) these co-occurring problems and also fail to collaborate in the care of these multiple health conditions—placing their patients' health and recovery in jeopardy. Collaboration by mental, substance-use, and general health care clinicians is especially difficult because of the multiple separations that characterize mental and substance-use health care: (1) the greater separation of mental and substance-use health care from general health care; (2) the separation of mental and substance-

210

use health care from each other; (3) society's reliance on the education, child welfare, and other non–health care sectors to secure M/SU services for many children and adults; and (4) the location of services needed by individuals with more-severe M/SU illnesses in public-sector programs apart from private-sector health care.

This mass of disconnected care delivery arrangements requires numerous patient interactions with different providers, organizations, and government agencies. It also requires multiple provider "handoffs" of patients for different services and transmittal of information to and joint planning by all these providers, organizations, and agencies if coordination is to occur. Overcoming these separations also is made difficult because of legal and organizational prohibitions on clinicians' sharing information about mental and substance-use diagnoses, medications, and other features of clinical care, as well as a failure to implement effective structures and processes for linking the multiple clinicians and organizations caring for patients. To overcome these obstacles, the committee recommends that individual treatment providers create clinically effective linkages among mental, substance-use, and general health care and other human service agencies caring for these patients. Complementary actions are also needed from government agencies, purchasers, and accrediting bodies to promote the creation of these linkages.

To enable these actions, changes are needed as well to address the less-evolved infrastructure for using information technology, some unique features of the M/SU treatment workforce that also have implication for effective care coordination, and marketplace practices. Because these issues are of such consequence, they are addressed separately in Chapters 6, 7, and 8, respectively.

CARE COORDINATION AND RELATED PRACTICES DEFINED

Crossing the Quality Chasm notes that the multiple clinicians and health care organizations serving patients in the American health care system typically fail to coordinate their care. That report further states that the resulting gaps in care, miscommunication, and redundancy are sources of significant patient suffering (IOM, 2001).[1] The *Quality Chasm's* health care quality framework addresses the need for better care coordination in

---

[1]In a subsequent report, produced at the request of the U.S. Department of Health and Human Services, the Institute of Medicine identified "care coordination" as one of 20 priority health care areas deserving of immediate attention by all participants in American health care (IOM, 2003a).

one of its ten rules and in another rule calls attention to the need for provider communication and collaboration to achieve this goal:

> *Cooperation among clinicians.* Clinicians and institutions should actively collaborate and communicate to ensure an appropriate exchange of information and coordination of care.

> *Shared knowledge and the free flow of information.* Patients should have unfettered access to their own medical information and to clinical knowledge. Clinicians and patients should communicate effectively and share information. (IOM, 2001:62)

These two rules highlight two prerequisites to coordination of care: communication and collaboration across providers and within and across institutions. *Communication* exists when each clinician or treatment provider caring for a patient shares needed treatment information with other clinicians and providers caring for the patient. Information can be shared verbally; manually in writing; or through information technology, such as a shared electronic health record. *Collaboration* is multidimensional and requires the aggregation of several behaviors, including the following:

- **A shared understanding of goals and roles**—Collaboration is enhanced by a shared understanding of an agreed-upon collective goal (Gittell et al., 2000) and clarity regarding each clinician's role. Role confusion and role conflict are frequent barriers to interdisciplinary collaboration (Rice, 2000).
- **Effective communication**—Multiple studies have identified effective communication as a key feature of collaboration (Baggs and Schmitt, 1988; Knaus et al., 1986; Schmitt, 2001; Shortell et al., 1994). "Effective" is defined variously as frequent, timely, understandable, accurate, and satisfying (Gittell et al., 2000; Shortell et al., 1994).
- **Shared decision making**—In shared decision making, problems and strategies are openly discussed (Baggs and Schmitt, 1997; Baggs et al., 1999; Rice, 2000; Schmitt, 2001), and consensus is often used to arrive at a decision. Disagreements over treatment approaches and philosophies, roles and responsibilities, and ethical questions are common in health care settings. Positive ways of addressing these inevitable differences are identified as a key component of effective caregiver collaboration (Shortell et al., 1994).

It is important to note that, according to health services researchers, collaboration is not a dichotomous variable, simply present or absent. Rather, it is present to varying degrees (Schmitt, 2001).

Collaboration also is typically characterized by necessary precursors. Clinicians are more likely to collaborate when they perceive each other as having the knowledge necessary for good clinical care (Baggs and Schmitt, 1997). Mutual respect and trust are necessary precursors to collaboration as well (Baggs and Schmitt, 1988; Rice, 2000); personal respect and trust are intertwined with respect for and trust in clinical competence.

Care coordination is the outcome of effective collaboration. Coordinated care prevents drug–drug interactions and redundant care processes. It does not waste the patient's time or the resources of the health care system. Moreover, it promotes accurate diagnosis and treatment because all providers receive relevant diagnostic and treatment information from all other providers caring for a patient.

Care integration is related to care coordination. As defined by experts in health care organization and management (Shortell et al., 2000), integration of care and services can be of three types:

- *"Clinical integration* is the extent to which patient care services are *coordinated* across people, functions, activities, and sites over time so as to maximize the value of services delivered to patients" (p. 129).
- *Physician (or clinician) integration* is the extent to which clinicians are economically linked to an organized delivery system, use its facilities and services, and actively participate in its planning, management and governance.
- *Functional integration* is "the extent to which key support functions and activities (such as financial management, strategic planning, human resources management, and information management) are coordinated across operating units so as to add the greatest overall value to the system" (p. 31). The most important of these functions and activities are human resources deployment strategies, information technologies, and continuous improvement processes.

Shortell et al.'s *clinical* integration corresponds to care coordination as addressed in the *Quality Chasm* report.

In the context of co-occurring mental and substance-use problems and illnesses, the Substance Abuse and Mental Health Services Administration (SAMHSA) similarly identifies three levels of integration (SAMHSA, undated):

- *Integrated treatment* refers to interactions *between clinicians* to address the individual needs of the client/patient, and consists of "any mechanism by which treatment interventions for co-occurring disorders are combined within the context of a primary treatment relationship or service setting" (p. 61).

- *Integrated program* refers to an organizational structure that ensures the provision of staff or linkages with other programs to address all of a client's needs.

- *Integrated systems* refers to an organizational structure that supports an array of programs for individuals with different needs through funding, credentialing/licensing, data collection/reporting, needs assessment, planning, and other system planning and operation functions.

SAMHSA's *integrated treatment* corresponds to Shortell et al.'s *clinical integration;* both appear to equate to *coordination of care* as used in the *Quality Chasm* report. In this report, we use the *Quality Chasm* terminology of *care coordination* and address the coordination of care at the level of the patient. We do not address issues surrounding the other levels of coordination or integration represented by Shortell et al.'s *clinician* and *functional integration* or SAMHSA's *integrated programs* and *systems.*

FAILED COORDINATION OF CARE FOR CO-OCCURRING CONDITIONS

Co-Occurring Mental, Substance-Use, and General Health Problems and Illnesses

Mental or substance-use problems and illnesses seldom occur in isolation. Approximately 15–43 percent of the time they occur together (Kessler et al., 1996; Kessler, 2004; Grant et al., 2004a,b; SAMHSA, 2004). They also accompany a wide variety of general medical conditions (Katon, 2003; Mertens et al., 2003), sometimes masquerade as separate somatic problems (Katon, 2003; Kroenke, 2003), and often go undetected (Kroenke et al., 2000; Saitz et al., 1997). As a result, individuals with M/SU problems and illnesses have a heightened need for coordinated care.

Co-Occurring Mental and Substance-Use Problems and Illnesses

The 1990–1992 National Comorbidity Survey well documented the high rates of co-occurring mental and substance use conditions, finding an estimated 42.7 percent of adults aged 15–54 with an alcohol or drug "disorder" also having a mental disorder, and 14.7 percent of those with a mental disorder also having an alcohol or drug disorder (Kessler et al., 1996; Kessler 2004). These findings are reaffirmed by more recent studies. According to the National Institute on Alcohol Abuse and Alcoholism (NIAAA) 2001–2002 National Epidemiologic Survey on Alcohol and Related Conditions, 19.7 percent of the general adult (18 and older) U.S. population with any substance-use disorder is estimated to have at least one co-occurring independent (non–substance-induced) mood disorder, and 17.7 percent to have at least one co-occurring independent anxiety disorder. Among respondents with a mood disorder, 20 percent had at least one substance-use disorder, as did 15 percent of those with an anxiety disorder. Rates of co-occurrence are higher among individuals who seek treatment for substance-use disorders; 40.7 percent, 33.4 percent, and 33.1 percent of those who sought treatment for an alcohol-use disorder had at least one independent mood disorder, anxiety disorder, or other drug use disorder, respectively. Among those seeking treatment for a drug-use disorder, 60.3 percent had at least one independent mood disorder, 42.6 percent at least one independent anxiety disorder, and 55.2 percent a comorbid alcohol-use disorder (Grant et al., 2004a).

Similar or higher rates of co-occurrence are found for other types of mental problems and illnesses (Grant et al., 2004b), as well as for serious mental illnesses generally. The 2003 National Survey on Drug Use and Health documented that among adults aged 18 and older not living in an institution or inpatient facility, an estimated 18 percent of those who had used illicit drugs in the past year also had a serious mental illness.[2] Over 21 percent of adults with substance "abuse" or dependence were estimated to have a serious mental illness, and 21.3 percent of adults with such an illness had been dependent on or "abused" alcohol or illicit drugs in the past year (SAMHSA, 2004).

One longitudinal study of patients in both mental health and drug treatment settings found that mental illnesses were as prevalent and serious among individuals treated in substance-use treatment facilities as among patients in mental health treatment facilities. Similarly, individuals served in mental health treatment facilities had substance-use illnesses at rates and severity comparable to those among individuals served in substance-use treatment facilities (Havassy et al., 2004).

Co-occurrence with General Health Conditions

M/SU problems and illnesses frequently accompany a substantial number of chronic general medical illnesses, such as diabetes, heart disease, neurologic illnesses, and cancers, sometimes masquerading as separate somatic problems (Katon, 2003). Approximately one in five patients hospitalized for a heart attack, for example, suffers from major depression, and evidence from multiple studies is "strikingly consistent" that post–heart attack depres-

---

[2]A serious mental illness was defined for this study as a diagnosable mental, behavioral, or emotional disorder that met criteria in the *Diagnostic and Statistical Manual*, fourth edition (DSM-IV) and resulted in functional impairment that substantially interfered with or limited one or more major life activities.

sion significantly increases one's risk for death: patients with depression are about three times more likely to die from a future attack or other heart problem (Bush et al., 2005:5). Depression and anxiety also are strongly associated with somatic symptoms such as headache, fatigue, dizziness, and pain, which are the leading cause of outpatient medical visits and often medically unexplained (Kroenke, 2003). They also are more often present in individuals with a number of medical conditions as yet not well understood, including chronic fatigue syndrome, fibromyalgia, irritable bowel syndrome, and nonulcer dyspepsia (Henningsen et al., 2003).

The converse also is true. Individuals with M/SU conditions often have increased prevalence of general medical conditions such as cardiovascular disease, high blood pressure, diabetes, arthritis, digestive disorders, and asthma (De Alba et al., 2004; Mertens et al., 2003; Miller et al., 2003; Sokol et al., 2004; Upshur, 2005). Persons with severe mental illnesses have much higher rates of HIV and hepatitis C than those found in the general population (Brunette et al., 2003; Rosenberg et al., 2001; Sullivan et al., 1999). Moreover, specific mental or substance-use diagnoses place individuals at higher risk for certain general medical conditions. For example, those in treatment for schizophrenia, depression, and bipolar illness are more likely than the general population to have asthma, chronic bronchitis, and emphysema (Sokol et al., 2004). Persons with anxiety disorders have higher rates of cardiac problems, hypertension, gastrointestinal problems, genitourinary disorders, and migraine (Harter et al., 2003). Individuals with schizophrenia are at increased risk for obesity, heart disease, diabetes, hyperlipidemia, hepatitis, and osteoporosis (American Diabetes Association et al., 2004; Goff et al., 2005; Green et al., 2003). And chronic heavy alcohol use is associated with liver disease, immune system disorders, cardiovascular diseases, and diabetes (Carlsson et al., 2000; Corrao et al., 2000; NIAAA, 2000).

Substance use, particularly injection drug use, carries a high risk of other serious illnesses. In a large cohort study of middle-class substance-using patients, the prevalence of hepatitis C was 27 percent in all substance users and 76 percent in injection drug users (Abraham et al., 1999). Injection drug use accounts for about 60 percent of new cases of hepatitis C (Alter, 1999) and remains the second most common risk behavior for acquisition of HIV in the United States (CDC, 2001). Evidence of past infection with hepatitis B also is common in injection drug users (Garfein, et al., 1996). Hepatitis C and coinfection with HIV and active hepatitis B are associated with more-severe liver disease (Zarski et al., 1998). Alcohol use is prevalent among HIV-infected patients (Conigliaro et al., 2003), and accelerates cognitive impairment in HIV-associated dementia complex (Fein et al., 1998; Tyor and Middaugh, 1999).

Given that patients with HIV infection are now living longer, the impact of comorbid conditions in these patients, including alcohol and drug-use problems, has become increasingly important. Hepatitis C–related liver injury progresses more rapidly in both HIV coinfected persons and alcohol users. Laboratory and preliminary clinical evidence indicates that both alcohol use and hepatitis C can negatively affect immunologic and clinical HIV outcomes. Furthermore, both alcohol and drug use may adversely affect the prescription and efficacy of and adherence to HIV medications (Moore et al., 2004; Palepu et al., 2003; Samet et al., 2004).

The co-occurrence of mental, substance-use, and general health problems and illnesses has important implications for the recovery of individuals with these illnesses. All of these conditions need to be to be detected and treated; however, this often does not happen, and even when it does, providers dealing with one condition often fail to detect and treat the co-occurring illness and to collaborate in the coordinated care of these patients.

Failure to Detect, Treat, and Collaborate in the Care of Co-Occurring Illnesses

Although detection of some common mental illnesses, such as depression, has increased over the past decade, general medical providers still too often fail to detect alcohol, drug, or mental problems and illnesses (Friedmann et al., 2000b; Miller et al., 2003; Saitz et al., 1997, 2002). In a nationally representative survey of general internal medicine physicians, family medicine physicians, obstetrician/gynecologists, and psychiatrists, for example, 12 percent reported that they did not usually ask their new patients whether they drank alcohol, and fewer than 20 percent used any formal screening tool to detect problems among those who did drink (Friedmann et al., 2000b). Moreover, evidence indicates that general medical providers often assume that the health complaints of patients with a prior psychiatric diagnosis are psychologically rather than medically based (Graber et al., 2000).

Similarly, mental health and substance-use treatment providers frequently do not screen, assess, or address co-occurring mental or substance-use conditions (Friedmann et al., 2000b) or co-occurring general medical health problems. In a survey of patients of one community mental health center, 45 percent of respondents reported that their mental health provider did not ask about general medical issues (Miller et al., 2003).

Evidence presented in Chapter 4 documents some of the failures of providers to treat co-occurring conditions. Other studies have added to the evidence that even when co-occurring M/SU conditions are known, they are not treated (Edlund et al., 2004; Friedmann et al., 2000b, 2001). The above-cited longitudinal study of patients with comorbid conditions at four public residential treatment facilities for seriously mentally ill patients and three residential treatment facilities for individuals with substance-use illnesses found no listings of co-occurring problems or illnesses in patient charts despite the existence of significant comorbidity. "Patient charts in the public mental health system generally include a primary psychiatric disorder; co-occurring psychiatric or substance use disorders are not systematically included. Substance abuse treatment sites only documented substance use disorders" (Havassy et al., 2004:140). In the national survey of primary care providers and psychiatrists described above, 18 percent of physicians reported that they typically offered no intervention (including a referral) to their problem-drinking patients, in part because of misplaced concern about patients' sensitivity on these issues (Friedmann et al., 2000b). Nearly the same proportion (15 percent) reported that they did not intervene when use of illicit drugs was detected (Friedmann et al., 2001). A 1997–1998 national survey found that among persons with probable co-occurring mental and substance-use disorders who received treatment for either condition, fewer than a third (28.6 percent) received treatment for the other (Watkins et al., 2001).

Additional evidence of the failure to coordinate care is found in the complaints of consumers of M/SU services. The President's New Freedom Commission reported that consumers often feel overwhelmed and bewildered when they must access and integrate mental health care and related services across multiple, disconnected providers in the public and private sectors (New Freedom Commission on Mental Health, 2003).

These failures to detect and treat co-occurring conditions take place in a health care system that has historically and currently separates care for mental and substance-use problems and illnesses from each other and from general health care, to a greater extent than is the case for other specialty health care. Absent or poor linkages characterize these separate care delivery arrangements. Numerous demonstration projects and strategies have been developed to better link health care for general, mental, and substance-use health conditions and related services. These include The Robert Wood Johnson Foundation's Depression in Primary Care: Linking Clinical and Systems Strategies Project (Upshur, 2005) and the MacArthur Foundation's RESPECT—Depression Project (Dietrich et al., 2004).

NUMEROUS, DISCONNECTED CARE DELIVERY ARRANGEMENTS

"Every system is perfectly designed to achieve exactly the results it gets."
(Berwick, 1998)

Organizations and providers offering treatment and services for mental, substance-use, and general health care conditions typically do so through separate care delivery arrangements:

• Arrangements for the delivery of health care for mental and substance-use conditions are typically separate from general health care (financially and organizationally more so than other specialty health care services).

• In spite of the frequent co-occurrence of M/SU problems and illnesses, the delivery of health care for these conditions also typically occurs through separate treatment providers and organizations.

• Some health care for mental and substance-use conditions and related services are delivered through governmental programs that are separate from private insurance—requiring coordination across public and private sectors of care.

• Non–health care sectors—education, child welfare, and juvenile and criminal justice systems—also separately arrange for M/SU services.

Traversing these separations is made difficult by a failure to put in place effective strategies for linking general, mental, and substance-use health care and the other human services systems that also deliver much-needed services for M/SU problems and illnesses; by a lack of agreement about which entity or entities should be held accountable for coordinating care; and by state and federal laws (and the policies and practices of some health care organizations) that limit information sharing across providers.[3]

Separation of M/SU Health Care from General Health Care

Although the proportion has been declining in recent years, two-thirds of Americans (64 percent in 2002) under the age of 65 receive health care through private insurance offered by their or their family member's employer (Fronstin, 2003). Over the past two decades, employers and other group purchasers of health care (e.g., state Medicaid agencies) have increasingly provided mental and substance-use health care benefits through health insurance plans that are separate administratively and financially from the plans through which individuals receive their general health care. These separate M/SU health plans are informally referred to as "carved out." In *payer* carve-outs, an employer or other payer offers prospective enrollees one or more health plans encompassing all of their covered health care except that for mental and substance-use conditions. Covered individuals are then enrolled in another health plan that includes a network of M/SU

---

[3]In addition, the less-evolved infrastructure for deploying information technology among mental health and substance-use treatment providers inhibits ease of coordination (see Chapter 6). Some of the unique features of the M/SU treatment workforce (e.g., the greater number of provider types, variation in their training and focus, and their greater location in solo or small group practices) that also contribute to this problem are addressed in Chapter 7.

providers chosen separately by the employer/payer. In *health plan* carve-outs, employees enroll in just one comprehensive health plan, and the administrators of that plan arrange internally to have M/SU health care provided and managed through a separate vendor. Estimates of the proportion of employees receiving M/SU health services through carve-out arrangements with managed behavioral health organizations (MBHOs) vary from 36 to 66 percent, reflecting differences in targeted survey respondents (e.g., employers, MBHOs, or employees) and what is being measured (e.g., carved-out services can include utilization review or case management only, or the provision of a full array of M/SU services) (Barry et al., 2003).

The MBHOs that provide these carve-out M/SU services arose in part in response to financial concerns. In the 1980s, employers' costs for behavioral health services were increasing at twice the rate of medical care overall and four times the rate of inflation. Evidence is clear that MBHOs have been successful in reducing these costs and also in achieving greater use of community-based care as opposed to institutionalization. They also have been credited with playing a role in keeping costs down in the face of broadened benefits, which has assisted in securing support for greater parity of mental health benefit coverage. Moreover, MBHOs have helped move clinicians from solo into group practices (Feldman, 2003), which, as discussed in Chapter 7, can facilitate quality improvement. Carve-out arrangements can nurture recognition and support for specialized knowledge of M/SU problems and illnesses and treatment expertise. They also can attenuate problems involving the adverse selection of individuals with M/SU illnesses in insurance plans (see Chapter 8).

In contrast to the clear evidence for the benefits described above, evidence for the effects of carve-out arrangements on quality of care is limited and mixed (Donohue and Frank, 2000; Grazier and Eselius, 1999; Hutchinson and Foster, 2003). However, models of safety and errors in health care suggest that whenever individuals are cared for by separate organizations, functional units, or providers, discontinuities in care can result unless the unavoidable gaps in care are anticipated, and strategies to bridge those gaps are implemented (Cook et al., 2000). A previous Institute of Medicine (IOM) report found that carved-out M/SU services "do not necessarily lead to poor coordination of care. . . . However the separation of primary care and behavioral health care systems brings risks to coordination and integration. . ." (IOM, 1997:116). The President's New Freedom Commission on Mental Health care deemed the separation between systems for mental and general health care so large as to constitute a "chasm" (New Freedom Commission on Mental Health, 2003).

Several factors could help account for problems with coordinating care in the presence of M/SU carve-outs. First, under carve-out arrangements, primary care physicians generally are not expected to treat (and may not always be able to be reimbursed for treating) M/SU problems and illnesses (Feldman et al., 2005; Upshur, 2005). The employer or other purchaser of health insurance benefits for the individual has, by contract, specified that general health care is to be provided by one network of providers though a health plan covering that care, and M/SU care through a different health plan's network of specialty M/SU providers. This is different from the situation with other medical problems and illnesses. For example, when a patient seeks care for diabetes, asthma, allergies, heart problems, or other general medical conditions, the patient's primary care provider is allowed to treat these illnesses and can be reimbursed for those services. When the primary care provider and/or the patient decides that the problem requires the attention of a specialist, the provider makes a referral or the patient self-refers to a specialist. Use of a specialist comes about based generally on the primary care provider's and/or patient's judgment. In contrast, under M/SU carve-out arrangements, M/SU health care often is predetermined by the employer or other group purchaser to require the attention of a specialist and must therefore be provided by a second provider. As a result, one method of care coordination—care by the same provider—is not available to the patient. While not all primary care providers have the expertise and/or desire to treat M/SU illnesses (see Chapters 4 and 7), some do, and evidence indicates that many patients typically turn initially to their primary care provider for help with M/SU problems and illnesses (Mickus et al., 2000).

A second obstacle to care coordination is that information about the patient's health problem or illness, medications, and other treatments must now be shared across and meet the often differing privacy, confidentiality, and additional administrative requirements imposed by the different health plans. Consumers also are required to navigate the administrative requirements of both health plans.

Finally, as described in Chapter 4, the use of carve-outs poses difficulties for quality measurement and improvement—including measurement and improvement of coordination—in two ways. First, because primary care providers cannot always be reimbursed for M/SU health care, they sometimes provide the care but code the visit according to the patient's somatic complaint (for which the treatment they provide can be reimbursed) (Rost et al., 1994). This situation masks the true prevalence of M/SU illnesses in primary care and impedes quality measurement and improvement efforts. Moreover, the existence of two parallel health plans serving the patient creates some confusion about accountability for quality and coordination. For example, the National Committee for Quality Assurance's mental and substance-use quality measures (i.e., those contained in its Health Plan Employer Data and Information Set [HEDIS] measurement set) are required to be reported by comprehensive managed care plans seeking accreditation, but not by MBHOs seeking accreditation.[4] Also, as discussed later in this chapter, accreditation standards do not always make clear the responsibilities for care coordination when an individual is served by two health plans, such as a managed care plan providing general health care and an MBHO.

Separation of Health Services for Mental and Substance-Use Conditions from Each Other

The mental health and substance-use treatment systems evolved separately in the United States as a result of the different historical understandings of and responses to these illnesses described in Chapter 2. This separation became increasingly institutionalized with the evolution of three separate institutes of the National Institutes of Health (NIH) (the National Institute of Mental Health [NIMH] in 1949 and National Institute on Alcohol Abuse and Alcoholism [NIAAA] and the National Institute on Drug Abuse [NIDA] in 1974) and separate programming and funding divisions within SAMHSA. This separation at the federal policy level is frequently mirrored at the state level, where separate state mental health and substance-use agencies exist (although they are combined in some states).

The separation of service delivery that mirrors this separation of policy making and funding does not optimally serve individuals with co-occurring mental and substance-use illnesses. A congressionally mandated study of the prevention and treatment of co-occurring substance-use and mental conditions (SAMHSA, undated) found that the difficulties faced by individuals with these co-occurring conditions in receiving successful treatment and achieving recovery are due in part to the existence of these two separate service systems. The study notes: "Too often, when individuals with co-occurring disorders do enter specialty care, they are likely to bounce back and forth between the mental health and substance abuse services systems, receiving treatment for the co-occurring disorder serially, at best" (SAMHSA, undated:*i*). The study further states that this separation of public-sector substance-use and mental health service systems is accompanied by marked differences in "staffing resources, philosophy of treatment, funding sources, community political factors, regulations, prior training of staff, credentials of staff, treatment approaches, medical staff resources, assertive community outreach capabilities, and routine types of evaluations and testing procedures performed" (SAMHSA, undated:*v*). Of greatest concern, the study found that individuals with these co-occurring conditions also may be

---

[4]Personal communication, Philip Renner, MBA, Assistant Vice President for Quality Measurement, NCQA on March 22, 2005.

excluded from mental health programs because of their substance-use condition and from substance-use treatment programs because of their mental condition (SAMHSA, undated).

Frequent Need for Individuals with Severe Mental Illnesses to Receive Care Through a Separate Public-Sector Delivery System

Treatment for M/SU conditions also is unique in that state and local governments manage public-sector health care systems that are separate from the private-sector health care system for individuals with M/SU illnesses. Indeed, "behavioral disorders remain essentially the only set of health problems for which state and local governments finance and manage a specialty treatment system. [Although] public funds pay for a large portion of the costs of care for certain other disorders (such as Medicare financing of dialysis), and public services exist for a few rare disorders such as leprosy, . . . the public mental health system is the only substantial disorder-specific treatment system in existence today" (Hogan, 1999:106).

Because (as discussed in Chapter 3) individuals with M/SU illnesses face greater limitations in their insurance coverage than is the case with coverage for other illnesses, some individuals with M/SU illnesses who start receiving their care through private insurance must switch to public insurance (Medicaid or the State Children's Health Insurance Program [SCHIP])[5] or other publicly funded programs at the state and local levels when their private insurance is exhausted. Evidence indicates that these benefit limits most often are reached by individuals with some of the most severe mental illness diagnoses, including depression, bipolar disorder, and psychoses. There is also evidence that other serious diagnoses appearing in childhood, such as autism, are excluded from coverage under certain private health benefit plans (Peele et al., 2002). The lesser availability of health insurance for severe mental illnesses and for substance-use treatment also helps explain the involvement of other public sectors (i.e., child welfare and juvenile justice) in the delivery of mental health care (as described below).

The federal Substance Abuse Prevention and Treatment (SAPT) and Community Mental Health Services (CMHS) Block Grant programs provide funds to states help fill these gaps. SAPT and CMHS grants to states support the planning, delivery, and evaluation of M/SU treatment services. SAPT funds can be used for individuals regardless of the severity of their substance-use problem or illness, while CMHS grant funds may be used only for individuals with serious mental illnesses and children with "serious

---

[5]The Medicaid and SCHIP programs also deliver mental health services to individuals for whom these programs are the primary source of health insurance as a result of low income.

emotional disturbances" (SAMHSA, undated). Some of these funds also are given to county and other local government units to use in the planning and delivery of care. In a number of states, major responsibility for mental health services rests with local government, and the extent of coordination between state and local governments is variable.

In addition, public mental health hospitals play a key role in the care of forensic patients—those charged with crimes and being evaluated for competence to stand trial or assume criminal responsibility, or for other issues; those found incompetent to stand trial and being treated to restore competence; those found not guilty by reason of insanity and being treated; those referred for presentencing evaluation; and those sent from prison for hospital-based treatment. In some states, these and related categories account for more than half of all inpatient beds in public mental hospitals. A growing number of people in each of these categories are also being treated in the public (or equivalent community mental health clinic–based) outpatient system. To a considerable extent, this is a function that the public sector has always served. But as other functions have shrunk or been transferred to the private sector (e.g., acute care in many states), forensic functions have come to account for a larger percentage of the public system.

Involvement of Non–Health Care Sectors in M/SU Health Care

M/SU problems and illnesses often are detected (sometimes for the first time) by agencies or organizations that are not part of the traditional health care sector, such as schools, employers, or the welfare and justice systems. These organizations often refer, arrange for, support, monitor, and sometimes deliver M/SU health services. School mental health services and the child welfare and juvenile justice systems provide access to mental health services for the majority of children (DHHS, 1999). The criminal justice system also plays a role in securing M/SU services for some adults. In the private sector, employee assistance programs play a key role in the identification, referral, and provision of services to individuals with M/SU problems and illnesses. Moreover, many other publicly funded entities, such as housing programs, programs for individuals who are homeless, income maintenance programs, and employment programs, provide services that are essential to the recovery of many individuals with severe and chronic M/SU illnesses. The involvement of this array of human service providers generally not considered to be part of the health care sector necessitates additional levels of care coordination. This coordination must be effected despite the inevitable difficulties of working with multiple bureaucracies and in systems with differing priorities, knowledge bases, and practices.

Schools

Most children and adolescents who receive health care for mental conditions receive that care through their schools, not from primary medical or specialty mental health care providers (Kessler et al., 2001). The approaches used by schools to deliver M/SU health care services are highly variable, ranging from (1) class-room based, teacher-implemented programs; to (2) multifaceted, schoolwide programs that employ multiple strategies, such as modification of school policies, classroom management strategies, curriculum changes, and facilitation of parent–school communications; to (3) therapy provided to an individual student, group, or family; to (4) other strategies, such as parent training and education, case management, and consultation. Some of these approaches are prevention-oriented, while others are designed to treat individuals with identified psychopathology. Service modality, intensity, and duration also vary according to individual needs (Rones and Hoagwood, 2000). Some programs rely primarily or exclusively on school-supported mental health professionals (e.g., school social workers, guidance counselors, school nurses), while others have varying degrees of linkage with community mental health agencies and providers (e.g., clinical psychologists, social workers, psychiatrists) who either provide the mental health services exclusively in the school or partner with school staff. In some cases, mental health providers from the school and/or community work on-site in school-based health centers in partnership with primary care providers (Weist et al., 2005).

A review of research on such school-based mental health services published between 1985 and 1999 found that although evidence exists for the effectiveness of a subset of strong programs across a range of emotional and behavioral problems, most school-based programs have no evidence to support their impact, and no programs are targeted to specific clinical syndromes such as anxiety, attention deficit hyperactivity disorder (ADHD), and depression. This same study also found that precisely what is provided by schools under the rubric of mental health services is largely unknown, as is whether those services are effective (Rones and Hoagwood, 2000).

To learn more about school-based mental health services, SAMHSA and Abt Associates recently conducted a national survey aimed at providing information on mental health services delivered in U.S. public schools, including:

• The types of mental health problems/issues encountered most frequently in the school setting.
• The types of mental health services delivered, and models and arrangements for their delivery in public elementary, middle, and secondary schools.

- Barriers to the provision and coordination of mental health services in school settings.
- The numbers, availability, and qualifications of mental health staff in public schools.

The final report is to be released during fall 2005.[6]

Experts on school-based mental health services note that (1) schools should not be viewed as responsible for meeting all the mental health needs of their students (in some cases they are already overburdened with demands that should be addressed elsewhere); and (2) connections between school-based mental health services and substance-use treatment services are nonexistent or tenuous (Weist et al., 2005). These two factors, plus the need to coordinate M/SU services with general health care, impose responsibilities on school-based M/SU providers to collaborate with other specialty and general health care providers serving the student, and for the other specialty and general health care providers to do the same.

Child Welfare Services

Almost half (47.9 percent) of a nationally representative, random sample of children aged 2–14 who were investigated by child welfare services in 1999–2000 had a clinically significant need for mental health care (Burns et al., 2004). Even higher rates have been observed in children placed in foster care arrangements (Landsverk, 2005). This is not surprising given that the circumstances of children who are the subject of reports of maltreatment and investigated by child welfare services are characterized by the presence of known risk factors for the development of emotional and behavioral problems, including abuse, neglect, poverty, domestic violence, and parental substance abuse (Burns et al., 2004). Moreover, substantial rates of substance use among adolescents in child welfare have been detected (Aarons et al., 2001).

Ensuring the well-being of children is typically considered part of the mandate of child welfare services, and the children served by these agencies also have very high rates of use of mental health services. However, the first nationally representative study examining the well-being of children and families that came to the attention of child welfare services (the National Survey of Child and Adolescent Well-Being [NSCAW]) found that three of four youths in child welfare who met a stringent criterion of need did not receive mental health care within 12 months of a child abuse and neglect investigation (Landsverk, 2005). States have traditionally used Medicaid to provide medical, developmental, and mental health services to children in

---

[6]Personal communication, Judith L. Teich, ACSW, Health Policy Analyst. Center for Mental Health Services/SAMHSA on July 15 and October 10, 2005.

foster care;[7] however, use of this resource requires that child welfare services first identify children in need of such services. Analysis of the NSCAW data found that although 94 percent of counties participating in the survey assessed all children entering foster care for physical health problems, only 47.8 percent had policies for assessing mental health problems (Leslie et al., 2003). Data from the NSCAW also indicate that underutilization of needed services can be alleviated when there is strong coordination between local child welfare and public mental health agencies (Hurlburt et al., 2004).

Justice Systems

Criminal justice system The proportion of U.S. citizens incarcerated has been increasing annually—from a rate of 601 persons in custody per 100,000 U.S. residents in 1995 to 715 persons in custody per 100,000 residents in 2003. As of mid-2003, the nation's prisons and jails[8] held 2,078,570 persons—one in every 140 U.S. residents (Harrison and Karberg, 2004). Corrections facilities increasingly must attend to M/SU treatment because of this growth in the proportion of the U.S. population that is incarcerated and the requirement that prisons and jails provide treatment to inmates with medical needs (Haney and Specter, 2003).

A rigorous epidemiologic study of the prevalence of mental and substance-use illnesses in correctional settings has not been undertaken.[9] According to the U.S. Bureau of Justice, however, approximately 16 percent of all persons in jails and state prisons reported having either a mental "condition" or an overnight stay in a psychiatric facility, as did 7 percent of those in federal prisons (Ditton, 1999). Consistent with the evidence in Chapter 3 indicating that those with mental illnesses are responsible for a small share of violence in society, this rate is not much higher than that among the U.S. population overall (13 percent of those over age 18 reported receiving mental health treatment in an inpatient or outpatient setting in 2003[10]) (SAMHSA, 2004). Also consistent with the evidence in

---

[7]Little information is available about the need for and use of mental health services for children whose families receive in-home services from the child welfare system (Landsverk, 2005).

[8]In general, prisons and jails differ by the inmates' length of sentence. Prisons hold those convicted of felonies and serving sentences longer than a year, while jails hold those awaiting adjudication, convicted of misdemeanors, and serving sentences of a year or less. Prisons are operated by the state; jails by counties and other localities (Wolff, 2004).

[9]A more rigorous epidemiologic study of the prevalence of mental and substance use illnesses in correctional settings, modeled on the prevalence studies of the general population in the United States (Kessler et al., 2001) and the correctional and general populations in the United Kingdom, has been called for (Wolff, 2004).

[10]This figure does not include treatment solely for substance use.

Chapter 3, substance use plays a larger role in incarceration. Over half of inmates in state prisons and local jails were under the influence of alcohol or other drugs at the time of their offense, as were 33 to 46 percent of federal prison inmates (Ditton, 1999). In an average year, moreover, approximately one-third of new admissions to prisons result from a violation of parole conditions, nearly 16 percent of which are for some type of drug-related violation, such as a positive test for drug use or possession of drugs (Hughes et al., 2001). Although the majority of prisons and jails screen, assess, and provide treatment for mental illnesses, far fewer prisoners receive treatment for their substance-use problems and illnesses. When they do, detoxification and self-help group/peer support counseling are most commonly provided (Wolff, 2004).

The police and courts also interact with systems providing treatment for M/SU illnesses as they exercise their judgment and license to divert individuals with such illnesses from criminal processing (Metzner, 2002). As discussed in Chapter 3, courts increasingly influence the receipt of treatment for M/SU illnesses through the use of specialty drug and mental health courts. Defendants in these courts have the option of treatment or incarceration. If they choose treatment, they may forgo criminal processing altogether, or undergo criminal processing but forgo sentencing. The court supervises compliance with treatment. Police also influence treatment; as the gatekeepers for the criminal justice process, they are charged with determining whether to "socialize, medicalize, or criminalize" the event. And probation and parole officers influence treatment in exercising their oversight over compliance with terms of probation and parole. All of these actors' decisions are influenced by their personal understanding of these issues, the culture of their agency, and their localities' enforcement policies and social norms (Wolff, 2004).

Appropriate decision making about diverting or prosecuting, exercising coercion into treatment in a way that preserves patient-centered care (see Chapter 3), and fulfilling the right of incarcerated persons to medical treatment requires policies and practices that reflect an understanding of M/SU problems and illnesses and their effective treatment, as well as knowledge of the availability of treatment in the local community. However, individual agents of the judicial system vary in their training on these issues, and the policies and practices of each locality vary according to local norms and the public's beliefs about M/SU illnesses[11] (Wolff, 2004). As a result, coordination with specialty M/SU providers, organizations, and systems is essential to the development of evidence-based criminal justice policies and

---

[11]Since the chief prosecutor in each jurisdiction is typically elected, the public's perception of M/SU illnesses and dangerousness, for example (see Chapter 3), even if erroneous, may shape policies and practices (Wolff, 2004).

practices and to the delivery of effective care to individuals in the criminal justice system.

However, numerous and sizable obstacles to coordination between M/SU health care and criminal justice systems have been documented. Several actions that are consistent with the *Quality Chasm* framework for redesigning health care have been recommended to overcome these obstacles. These include using performance measures of the coordination between M/SU health care and criminal justice systems at the system, agency, program, and individual levels; providing combined, interdisciplinary training in collaboration and coordination for personnel from both types of agencies and programs; incentivizing coordination through promotion, salary, and budget decisions; providing education and decision support to prosecutors and judges; and using information systems to facilitate the communication of information essential to responding appropriately to each individual (Wolff, 2004).

Juvenile justice system Primary components of the juvenile justice system include intake, detention centers, probation services, secure residential facilities, and aftercare programs (Cocozza, 2004). Although research on the prevalence and nature of M/SU illnesses in juvenile justice systems is limited (Cocozza, 2004), between 60 and 75 percent of youths in these systems are estimated to have a diagnosable mental health "disorder" (Cocozza 2004; Teplin et al., 2002; Wierson et al., 1992), and 20 percent are conservatively estimated to have a severe mental illness (Cocozza and Skowyra, 2000). Rates of co-occurring substance-use illnesses also are high (Cocozza, 2004; Grisso, 2004).

Moreover, in a 2003 survey of all (698) secure juvenile detention facilities in the United States,[12] two-thirds of the facilities reported holding youths (prior to, after, or absent any pending adjudication) because they were awaiting community mental health services. Further, like youths who are not abused or neglected but are placed in child welfare solely to obtain mental health services (discussed in Chapter 1), children who are not guilty of any offence are similarly placed in local juvenile justice systems and incarcerated solely to obtain mental health services not otherwise available. Although no formal counting and tracking of such children takes place, juvenile justice officials in 33 counties in the 17 states with the largest populations of children under age 18 estimated that approximately 9,000 such children entered their juvenile justice systems under these circumstances in 2001. County juvenile justice officials' estimates ranged from zero to 1,750, with a median of 140. Nationwide the number of children

---

[12]Response rate of 75 percent.

placed in juvenile justice systems is likely to be higher; 11 states reported to the Government Accountability Office (GAO) that they could not provide estimates even though they were aware that such placements occur (GAO, 2003).

Although the vast majority of juvenile justice facilities report providing some type of mental health service (Goldstrom et al., 2001), "numerous investigations suggest that many youth in the juvenile justice system do not receive needed mental health services and that available services are insufficient and inadequate." Most existing programs have not been evaluated, and some of the most popular and widely implemented programs have no evidence to support them and may actually be harmful. Juvenile justice systems, however, lack the training, service, and expertise to respond more effectively (Cocozza, 2004). Because many youths are in juvenile justice systems for relatively minor, nonviolent offenses, there also is a growing sentiment that whenever possible, youths with serious mental illnesses should be diverted from those systems. However, the limited amount of research on the efficacy of juvenile diversion programs has yielded mixed results. To achieve appropriate diversion and the provision of evidence-based care to children and youths in juvenile justice, coordination is crucial: "Almost every study and report that has focused on youth with mental health disorders who come in contact with the juvenile justice system has arrived at the same conclusion—that collaboration between mental health and juvenile justice (and other systems such as child welfare and education as well) at every level and at every stage is critical to any progress. The problem cannot be solved by any single agency" (Cocozza, 2004:35).

Employee Assistance Programs

An increasing number of individuals are covered by employee assistance programs (EAPs). An estimated 66.5 million employees were enrolled in such programs in 2000—a 245 percent increase since 1994 and a 13 percent increase over the year before (Fox et al., 2000). EAPs offered by employers[13] to their employees (and frequently employees' family members) vary in structure, types and qualifications of personnel, scope and length of services provided, location, and relationship to health plans providing M/SU and general health care services to the same employees. Although EAPs began as occupational programs to address alcohol-related problems in the workplace, they now typically offer consultation with personnel in identifying and resolving other job performance issues, and pro-

---

[13]Other organizations, such as labor organizations, unions, and professional associations, also sponsor EAPs.

vide further assessment, referral, and follow-up services. Additional services offered include assistance to employees experiencing stressful events, wellness training, assistance with work/life issues, legal assistance, and financial services. EAPs sometimes have a formal relationship with the M/SU services offered by a health plan and/or serve as a required gateway to M/SU services (Masi et al., 2004). Thus, an EAP's caseload can include individuals with severe M/SU problems and illnesses (Masi, 2004). EAPs are distinct in that their services are typically brief (an average of six counseling sessions) and often are provided via telephone or the Internet by a provider in a different location—perhaps several states away—and with round-the-clock access (Masi, 2004).

Linkages with Community and Other Human Services Resources

Individuals with M/SU problems and illnesses sometimes require additional services from a variety of community resources, such as self-help and support programs for individuals with specific diseases, housing services, income maintenance programs, and employment services, that are essential to the recovery of many individuals with severe and chronic M/SU illnesses. Appendix C contains a description of an array of such support services provided by the Veterans Health Administration to veterans with severe M/SU illnesses.

Discharge planning units or similar staff within inpatient facilities, as well as case management staff within outpatient treatment settings or programs, must assess patients for the need for these services, establish referral arrangements, and coordinate the services with the human service agencies providing them. Such coordination of care across inpatient and outpatient providers is essential to ensure timely access to these services. When discharge planning or outpatient care fails to ensure speedy access to these services and continuity of care within the community, patients are at risk for failure to implement their treatment plans, homelessness, incarceration, or other adverse outcomes.

Unclear Accountability for Coordination

Because patients receive care from multiple providers and delivery systems, there often is an unclear point (or points) of accountability for patients' treatment outcomes. When organizations or providers are reimbursed separately for the services they provide, each may perceive no responsibility for the services delivered by others and, as a result, for any patient outcomes likely to be affected by those services. Unless providers' accountability for sharing information or collaborating with other providers is explicitly identified in their agreements with purchasers, they may reasonably believe that those other providers have primary responsibility for initiating and maintaining ongoing communication and collaboration.

Moreover, the concept of collaboration has not been clearly defined (Schmitt, 2001). Thus, when providers do accept responsibility for collaborating with other providers, what constitutes "collaboration" is left to their own interpretation based on historical local practice patterns and limitations imposed by their current workload. This unclear accountability has been acknowledged and addressed in a conceptual model for coordinated care delivery developed by the National Association of State Mental Health Program Directors and the National Association of State Alcohol and Drug Abuse Directors. This model articulates a vision of coordinated care involving primary, mental health, substance-use, and other health and human service providers who share responsibility for delivering care to the full population in need of M/SU health care depending upon the predominance of medical, mental, or substance-use symptoms (SAMHSA, undated).

DIFFICULTIES IN INFORMATION SHARING

The sharing of patient information across providers treating the same patient so that care can be coordinated is widely acknowledged as necessary to effective and appropriate care. This need was acknowledged most recently in regulations governing the privacy of individually identifiable health information under the authority of the Health Insurance Portability and Accountability Act (HIPAA) of 1996. HIPAA's implementing regulations generally permit health care organizations to release—without requiring patient consent—individually identifiable information (except psychotherapy notes) about the patient to another provider or organization for treatment purposes.[14]

However, the HIPAA regulations are superseded by other federal and state statutory and regulatory provisions that may make it difficult for different providers or treatment organizations to share information. First, HIPAA itself (Section 264 (c)(2)) requires that regulations promulgated to implement its privacy provisions not supersede any contrary provisions of state law that impose more stringent requirements, standards, or implementation specifications pertaining to patient privacy. Each of the 50 states (and the District of Columbia) has a number of statutes governing the confidentiality of medical records, and specifically governing aspects of mental health records. Many of these statutes are more stringent than the HIPAA requirements, and the variation among them is great (see Appendix B for a detailed discussion of federal and state laws regarding confidential-

---

[14]45 CFR Part 164, Subpart E, § 164.502.

ity and the release of health care information pertaining to mental and substance-use conditions).

Second, regulations implementing HIPAA also permit health care organizations to implement their own patient consent policies for the release of patient information to other treating providers.[15] As a result, health care organizations may adopt even more stringent privacy protections that require participating providers to adhere to additional procedures before sharing patient information with other treatment providers or organizations.

Moreover, separate federal laws govern the release of information pertaining to an individual's treatment for drug or alcohol use. These laws do not permit sharing of records related to substance-use treatment or rehabilitation by organizations operated, regulated, or funded by the federal government without the patient's consent, except within a program or with an entity with administrative control over the program, between a program and organizations that provide support services such as billing and data processing, or in case of a "bona fide medical emergency." These federal laws are also superseded by any state laws that are more stringent (see Appendix B). The preamble to the HIPAA privacy regulations also recognizes the constraints of the substance-use confidentiality law and states that wherever one is more protective of privacy than the other, the more restrictive should govern (65 Fed. Reg. 82462, 82482–82483).

The bottom line is that clinicians providing treatment to individuals with M/SU illnesses must comply with multiple sets of rules governing the release of information: one prescribed federally and pertaining to information on treatment for alcohol or drug problems, state laws that pertain to information on health care for mental and substance-use conditions (depending upon whether they are more stringent than the federal rules), and other policies prescribed by the organization or multiple organizations under whose auspices patient care is provided.

STRUCTURES AND PROCESSES FOR COLLABORATION THAT CAN PROMOTE COORDINATED CARE

Because of the complexities described above, strategies to improve coordination of care need to be multidimensional (Gilbody et al., 2003; Pincus et al., 2003). A systematic review of studies of organizational and educational interventions to improve the management of depression in primary care settings found that initiatives with the most multidimensional approaches generally achieved positive results in their primary outcomes (Gilbody et al., 2003). Components of multidimensional strategies to im-

---

[15] 45 CFR Part 164 Subpart E § 164.506(b).

prove care coordination that can be used by providers and health care organizations at the locus of care include (1) screening for co-occurring conditions; (2) making a formal determination to either treat, or refer for treatment of, co-occurring conditions; (3) implementing more effective mechanisms for linking providers of different services to enable joint planning and coordinated treatment; and (4) providing organizational supports for collaboration between clinicians on- and off-site. Purchasers and quality oversight organizations can create incentives for providers to employ these strategies through their funding and accountability mechanisms and by exercising leadership within their spheres of influence.

Health Care Provider and Organization Strategies

Screening

Because of the high rates of comorbidity described above—especially among those seeking treatment—screening to detect the presence of co-morbid conditions is a necessary first step in care coordination. Screening enables a service provider to determine whether an individual with a substance-use problem or illness shows signs of a mental health problem or illness, and vice versa. If a potential problem is identified, a more detailed assessment is undertaken. Routine screening has been shown to improve rates of accurate mental health and substance-use diagnosis (Pignone et al., 2002; Williams et al., 2002).

The above-mentioned congressionally mandated study of the prevention and treatment of co-occurring substance-use and mental conditions (SAMHSA, undated) identified screening as critical to the successful treatment of comorbid conditions. Similarly, because of the high prevalence of emotional and behavioral problems among children served by child welfare services, screening has been recommended for children in the child welfare system overall (Burns et al., 2004) and especially for those placed in foster care (American Academy of Child & Adolescent Psychiatry and Child Welfare League of America, 2003). The U.S. Preventive Services Task Force also has recommended two types of screening in primary care settings:

- Screening for alcohol misuse by adults, including pregnant women, along with behavioral counseling interventions.
- Screening for depression in adults in clinical practices that have systems in place to ensure accurate diagnosis, effective treatment, and follow-up (AHRQ, 2002–2003).

The U.S. Preventive Services Task Force has not addressed the issue of screening for comorbid mental or substance-use conditions among individuals presenting with either condition. To facilitate the adoption of screening and treatment for comorbid mental and substance-use illnesses, the task force could include among its recommended guidelines screening for a co-occurring mental or substance-use problem at the time of an individual's initial presentation with either condition.

As discussed earlier, however, when screening is done, it often is not performed effectively (Friedmann et al., 2000b; Saitz et al., 2002). Effectiveness can be increased by use of any of a broad range of available and reliable instruments for screening for mental illnesses and co-occurring substance-use problems and illnesses (NIAAA, 2002; Pignone et al., 2002; Williams et al., 2002). An example is the Patient Health Questionnaire, a self-administered instrument designed to screen for depression, anxiety disorders, alcohol abuse, and somatiform and eating disorders in primary care (Spitzer et al., 1999). Other very brief, single-question screens have been evaluated for use in screening for alcohol-use problems (Canagasaby and Vinson, 2005). NIAAA has developed a single question (one for men and one for women) for screening for alcohol-use problems in primary care and other settings (NIAAA, 2005).

Anticipation of Comorbidity and Formal Determination to Treat or Refer

Again because of the high prevalence of co-occurring conditions, especially among individuals seeking treatment, the congressionally mandated study of the prevention and treatment of co-occurring substance-use and mental conditions (SAMHSA, undated) stated that individuals with co-occurring disorders should be the expectation, not the exception, in the substance-use and mental health treatment systems. SAMHSA and others have concluded that substance-use treatment providers should expect and be prepared to treat patients with mental illnesses, and similarly that mental health care providers should be prepared to treat patients with substantial past and current drug problems (Havassy et al., 2004; SAMHSA, undated). In its report to Congress, SAMHSA stated that one of the principles for effective treatment of co-occurring disorders is that "any door is the right door"; that is, people with co-occurring disorders should be able to receive or be referred to appropriate services whenever they enter any agency for mental health or substance-use treatment.

This same principle is applicable to general health problems and illnesses as well. A review of innovative state practices for treating comorbid M/SU conditions found that agency staff *expected* their clients to present with co-occurring general health problems. They screened and assessed for related conditions, including HIV/AIDS, physical and sexual abuse, brain disorders, and physical disabilities. Staff were cross-trained in both mental health and substance-use disciplines (although they did not work outside of their primary discipline) (NASMHPD and NASADAD, 2002). The congressionally mandated study also stated that with training and other supports, primary care settings can undertake diagnosis and treatment of these interrelated disorders (SAMHSA, undated). Alternatively, use of a systematic approach to referral to and consultation with a mental health specialist is often used in model programs for better care (Pincus et al., 2003).

Linking Mechanisms to Foster Collaborative Planning and Treatment

As discussed at the beginning of this chapter, the simple sharing of information, by itself, is insufficient to achieve care coordination. Care coordination is the result of collaboration, which exists when the sharing of information is accompanied by joint determination of treatment plans and goals for recovery, as well as the ongoing communication of changes in patient status and modification of treatment plans. Such collaboration requires structures and processes that enable, support, and promote it (IOM, 2004a).

Not surprisingly, available evidence indicates that referrals alone do not lead to collaboration or coordinated care (Friedmann et al., 2000a). Stronger approaches are needed to establish effective linkages among primary care, specialty mental health and substance-use treatment services, and other care systems that are involved in the delivery of M/SU treatment. These stronger linkage mechanisms vary in form and are theorized to exist along a continuum of efficacy. The extremes range from the ad hoc purchase of services from separate providers to on-site programs (see Figure 5-1) (D'Aunno, 1997; Friedmann et al., 2000a). Linkage mechanisms toward the right of the continuum are theorized to be stronger because they lower barriers or causes of "friction" (e.g., problems in identifying willing providers, clients' personal disorganization, and lack of transportation[16]) that prevent patients from receiving services.

Lowest		Certainty of Service Delivery			Highest
Informal Ad Hoc	Referral Agreement	Contractual Arrangement	Joint Program or Venture	Case Management/ Transportation	On Site Program

FIGURE 5-1   The continuum of linkage mechanisms.
SOURCE: Friedmann et al., 2000a. Reprinted, with permission, from Health Services Research, June 2000. Copyright 2000 by the Health Research and Educational Trust.

Approaches whose effectiveness in securing collaboration has some conceptual and/or empirical support include collocation and clinical integration of services, use of a shared patient record, case (or care) manage-

---

[16]These are in addition to the problems in insurance coverage discussed in Chapter 3.

ment, and formal agreements with external providers. Evidence to date also indicates that some of these approaches are more effective than others. Moreover, their successful implementation requires leadership within an organization, facilitating structures and processes within treatment settings, and often redesigned professional roles and training in these new roles.

Collocation and clinical integration of services Physical proximity of would-be collaborators facilitates collaboration (IOM, 2004a). This point is exemplified by the multiple studies of mental or substance-use health care showing that same-site delivery of both types of care or primary care is more effective in identifying comorbid conditions (Weisner et al., 2001), effectively links clients to the collocated services (Druss et al., 2001; Samet et al., 2001), and can improve treatment outcomes (Unutzer et al., 2001; Weisner et al., 2001). In a 1995 study of a nationally representative sample of all outpatient drug-use treatment units, same-site delivery of services was more effective than formal arrangements with external providers, referral agreements, or case management in ensuring that patients would utilize necessary services (a first step in collaborative care) (Friedmann et al., 2000a). For these reasons, the collocation of multiple services (mental, substance-use, and/or general health) at the same site is a frequently cited feature of many care collaboration programs. The congressionally mandated study of prevention and treatment of co-occurring substance-use and mental conditions (SAMHSA, undated) highlighted "integrated treatment" as an evidence-based approach for co-occurring disorders, defined, in part, as services delivered "in one setting." The report noted that such integrated treatment programs can take place in either the mental or substance-use treatment setting, but require that treatment and service for both conditions be delivered by appropriately trained staff "within the same setting."

Others have noted the benefits of integrating behavioral health specialists into primary settings, as well as the reciprocal strategy of including primary care providers at locations that deliver care to individuals with severe mental and substance-use illnesses. This type of collocation facilitates patient follow-through on a referrals, allows for face-to-face verbal communication in addition to or as an alternative to communicating in writing, and allows for informal sharing of the views of different disciplines and easy exchange of expertise (Pincus, 2003).

Such opportunities for face-to-face communication are important because multiple studies identify effective communication as a key feature of collaboration (Baggs and Schmitt, 1988; Knaus et al., 1986; Schmitt, 2001; Shortell et al., 1994). "Effective" communication is described as frequent and timely (Gittell et al., 2000; Shortell et al., 1994),[17] and is characterized

---

[17]As well as accurate, understandable, and satisfying.

by discussion with contributions by all parties, active listening, openness, a willingness to consider other ideas and ask for opinions, questioning (Baggs and Schmitt, 1997; Shortell et al., 1994), and the free flow of information among participants. This type of communication is less easily achieved through electronic, mail, and telephone communications. Nonetheless, when physical integration of services is not feasible, other efforts to promote effective collaboration (i.e., communication between providers by indirect means such as shared patient records or use of a case manager) may yield benefits.

Shared patient records Coordination of care provided by different providers can also be facilitated by shared patient records and documentation practices that promote interdisciplinary information exchange. Electronic health records (EHRs) are supported as an important mechanism for sharing such information and have been highlighted as one of the essential components of the developing National Health Information Infrastructure (NHII). EHRs allow (1) the longitudinal collection of electronic information pertaining to an individual's health and health care; (2) immediate electronic access—by authorized users only—to person- and population-level information; (3) provision of knowledge and decision support to enhance the quality, safety, and efficiency of patient care; and (4) support for efficient processes of health care delivery (IOM, 2003b). Although still in a minority, hospitals and ambulatory practices are increasingly investing in EHRs; these investments typically are being made by larger facilities, creating what is referred to as the "adoption gap" between large and small organizations (Brailer and Terasawa, 2003). Although sharing of patient information maintained in paper-based records can still take place, the capture and storage of patient information electronically is endorsed as a more thorough and efficient mechanism for timely access to needed information by the many providers serving a patient.

Case (care) management Case (or care) management refers to varying combinations of actions performed by a designated individual[18] (i.e., case manager) to arrange for, coordinate, and monitor health, psychological, and social services important to an individual's recovery from illness and the effects of these services on the patient's health. Although the services encompassed by case management often vary by the severity of the illness, the needs of the individual, and the specific model of case management

---

[18]We distinguish in this section between case management, provided by an additional resource *person* working with both the patient and the involved clinicians, and disease management *programs*. The latter often involve transfer of the overall medical and related health care management of a patient's specific disease to a separate organization or program, frequently through a contract. Disease management programs can also offer case management services by an individual as a part of their approach to disease management.

employed (Gilbody et al., 2003; Marshall et al., 2004), typical activities include assessment of the patient's need for supportive services; individual care planning, referral, and connection of the patient with other necessary services and supports; ongoing monitoring of the patients' care plan; advocacy; and monitoring of the patient's symptoms.

Although systematic reviews of the effectiveness of case management for individuals with serious mental illnesses have been conducted with different review strategies and produced conflicting findings (Marshall et al., 2004; Ziguras and Stuart, 2000) (perhaps in part because of the large number of different models of case management [Zwarenstein et al., 2000]), the approach continues to be a common component of many mental health treatment services for individuals with other than mild mental illnesses. A systematic review of studies of organizational and educational interventions to improve the management of depression in primary care settings found that although most initiatives used multiples strategies, case management was one of two approaches used most often in projects achieving positive outcomes and health-related quality of life[19] (Gilbody et al., 2003). More recently, within The Robert Wood Johnson Foundation's national program for depression treatment in primary care, all eight demonstration sites independently designed their interventions to incorporate case management, often with expanded roles for case managers that include ensuring that treatment guidelines and protocols are followed and that a depression registry is used by clinicians. Case managers also serve as intermediaries between patients' primary care providers and mental health specialists (Anonymous, 2004; Rollman et al., 2003). Case management is an essential element as well of the MacArthur Foundation's RESPECT—Depression Project for improving the treatment of depression in primary care, and of disease management programs such The John A. Hartford Foundation and California Health Care Foundation's Project IMPACT program for treating late-life depression (Unutzer et al., 2001).

Formal agreements with external providers Formal agreements with external providers also can influence patients' appropriate utilization of needed services (Friedmann et al., 2000a). Such agreements can include, for example, a substance-use treatment or mental health organization that contracts with a medical group practice to provide physical examinations and routine medical care for its patients. The advantages of this approach are

---

[19]In some studies, the case manger role was of low intensity and included follow-up phone calls to monitor medication adherence, providing brief patient education and medication counseling, or giving support over the phone. In other programs, nurse case managers took on additional roles that included, for example, ongoing support and monitoring of patient therapy and treatment response according to algorithms.

that it requires fewer organizational and physical plant resources than do collocated services, and it makes use of existing community resources (Samet et al., 2001). Specialty consultation with primary care providers is another frequently identified service that can be secured through a formal agreement with an external provider (Pincus et al., 2003). At a minimum, formal agreements with external providers should include not just the agreement to provide the referred service, but also provisions addressing information sharing, joint treatment planning, and monitoring of patient outcomes.

Organizational Support for Collaboration

Successfully implementing the above strategies for care coordination requires facilitating structures and processes within treatment settings. Collaboration also often requires changes in the design of work processes at treatment sites, in particular, flexibility in professional roles. Effective leadership is an overarching need to help health care providers successfully adopt, adapt to, and sustain these changes.

Facilitating structures and processes at treatment sites Structures and processes that encourage multidisciplinary providers to come together for joint treatment planning foster collaboration. For example, in acute, general inpatient care, there is evidence that using interdisciplinary rounds can be effective in improving patient care (Curley et al., 1998). Improvement in care can also be achieved by involving primary and mental health care providers in interdisciplinary team meetings (Druss et al., 2001; Unutzer et al., 2001) at which joint care planning takes place, or by providing case managers (see above) to facilitate patient education, monitoring, and communication between primary care providers and M/SU specialists (Feldman et al., 2005). In addition, a number of more general quality improvement strategies, such as medication algorithms, hold the potential to improve coordination of care by standardizing care processes and creating channels of communication. For instance, the Texas Medication Algorithm Project includes a clinical coordinator to help ensure appropriate coordination among clinicians, patients, and family members in promoting adherence to medication guidelines (Miller et al., 2004; Rush et al., 2003).

In a randomized controlled trial of the integration of medical care with mental health services, it was found that same-site location, common charting, enhanced channels of communication (including joint meetings and e-mail), and in-person contact facilitated the development of common goals and sharing of information between medical and mental health providers. Interdisciplinary team meetings involving primary and behavioral health care providers can do the same (Druss et al., 2001).

Heavy workloads can interfere with the formation of collaborative relationships. Collaboration requires that staff have the time to participate in such activities as interdisciplinary team meetings (Baggs and Schmitt, 1997). Illustrating this point, additional staff resources and reduced caseload were identified as two of several components of success in a randomized controlled trial of collocating and integrating medical care with mental health care (Druss et al., 2001). When staff are overwhelmed with caregiving responsibilities, they may not take the time to collaborate. Yet while unilateral decision making is easier in the short run, collaborative relationships are viewed as saving time in the long run (Baggs and Schmitt, 1997).

The committee also calls attention to the Chronic Care Model, used to improve the health care of individuals with chronic illnesses in primary care settings. This model has six components: (1) providing chronic illness self-management support to patients and their families (see Chapter 3); (2) redesigning care delivery structures and operations; (3) linking patients and their care with community resources to support their management of their illness (described above); (4) providing decision support to clinicians (see Chapter 4); (5) using computerized clinical information systems to support compliance with treatment protocols and monitor patient health indicators (see Chapter 6); and (6) aligning the health care organization's (or provider's) structures, goals, and values to support chronic care (discussed below) (Bodenheimer et al., 2002). The Chronic Care Model has been applied successfully to the treatment of a wide variety of general chronic illnesses, such as diabetes, asthma, and heart failure (The National Coalition on Health Care and The Institute for Healthcare Improvement, 2002), as well as to common mental illnesses such as depression (Badamgarev et al., 2003), and has been theorized to have the potential for improving the quality of care for persons with other M/SU illnesses (Watkins et al., 2003).

The Chronic Care Model also emphasizes the use of certain organizational structures and processes, including interdisciplinary practices in which a clear division of the roles and responsibilities of the various team members fosters their collaboration. Instituting such arrangements may necessitate new roles and divisions of labor among clinicians with differing training and expertise. In the Chronic Care Model, for example, physician team members are often responsible for the treatment of patients with acute conditions, intervene in stubbornly difficult chronic care problems, and train other team members. Nonphysician personnel support patients in the self-management of their illnesses and arrange for routine periodic health monitoring and follow-up. Providing chronic care consistent with this model requires support from health care organizations, health plans, purchasers, insurers, and other providers. Elements of the Chronic Care Model have been implemented in a variety of care settings, including private general medical practices, integrated delivery systems, and a community health center for general health care (Bodenheimer et al., 2002). The committee believes this model should be developed for use in the care of individuals with chronic M/SU illnesses as a mechanism for improving coordination of care, as well as other dimensions of quality.

Flexibility in professional roles As seen in the Chronic Care Model, collaboration sometimes requires revision in professional roles, including the shifting of roles among health care professionals and the expansion of roles to include new tasks (Gilbody et al., 2003; Katon et al., 2001). It also often requires participating as part of an interdisciplinary team with certain prescribed roles (Unutzer et al., 2001). Research findings and other empirical evidence show that health care workers of all types are capable of performing new tasks necessitated by advances in therapeutics, shortages in the health care workforce, and the pressures of cost containment. For example, the development of safer and more effective medications for mental and substance-use illnesses (e.g., selective serotonin reuptake inhibitors) has enabled the treatment of depression by primary care clinicians. Other medications, such as buprenorphine, may do the same. Other developments that are likely to require redefinition of professional roles include the use of peer support personnel (described in Chapter 3) and the delivery of more M/SU health care in primary care settings and by primary care providers (Strosahl, 2005).

However, new communication patterns and changes in roles, especially functioning as part of an interdisciplinary team, can at times be uncomfortable for health professionals. Role confusion and conflict are a frequent barrier to interdisciplinary collaboration (Rice, 2000). As a result, it may be necessary to provide training and development in collaborative practice behaviors, such as effective communication and conflict resolution (Disch et al., 2001; Strosahl, 2005). Collaboration is enhanced by a shared understanding of agreed-upon collective goals and new individual roles (Gittell et al., 2000).

Leadership Leadership is well known to be a critical factor in the success of any major change initiative or quality improvement effort (Baldridge National Quality Program, 2003; Davenport et al., 1998) and an essential feature of successful programs in care coordination (NASMHPD, NASADAD, 2002). Effective leadership in part models the behaviors that are expected at the clinical care level. For example, in The Robert Wood Johnson Foundation's *Initiative on Depression in Primary Care*, leadership was one of six component interventions to overcome barriers to the delivery of effective care for depression in primary care settings. Teams of primary care, mental health, and senior administrative personnel were responsible for securing needed resources, representing stakeholder interests, promoting adherence to practice standards, setting goals for key process measures and outcomes, and encouraging sustained efforts at continuous quality improvement (Pincus et al., 2003). Such activities ensure that the structures and processes that enable and nurture collaboration are in place at the locus of care.

Practices of Purchasers, Quality Oversight Organizations, and Public Policy Leaders

Clinicians and health care organizations will not be able to achieve full coordination of patient care without complementary and supporting activities on the part of federal and state governments, health care purchasers, quality oversight organizations, and other organizations that shape the environment in which clinical care is delivered. As noted earlier, care coordination has been identified by the IOM as one of 20 priority areas deserving immediate attention by all participants in the American health care system. Health care purchasers, quality oversight organizations, and public policy leaders can help give care coordination this immediate attention by (1) clarifying their expectations for information sharing, collaboration, and coordination in their purchasing agreements; (2) including the care coordination practices recommended above in their quality oversight standards and purchasing criteria; and (3) modeling collaborative practices across health care for general, mental, and substance-use health conditions in their policy-making and operational activities.

Purchaser Practices

Purchasers can stimulate and incentivize better coordination of care among general, mental, and substance-use health care by including care coordination as one of the quality-of-care parameters used to evaluate proposals and award contracts for the delivery of general, specialty M/SU, and comprehensive (general and M/SU) health care (see Chapter 8). In soliciting health plans and providers to deliver these health care services, purchasers can ask bidders to specify what care coordination practices they require of their clinicians, and how the organization supports clinicians and measures care coordination. When awarding contracts, purchasers can clarify in contracts with health care plans their expectations for information sharing, collaboration, and coordination. In addition, purchasers should allow primary care providers to bill for the M/SU treatment services they provide, a practice now under way in some MBHO settings (Feldman et al., 2005). Doing so will allow consumers and their primary care providers to determine jointly, as they do for other medical conditions, when specialty consultation and care are appropriate; enable coordination of care through the use of a single provider to treat general and M/SU conditions; and eliminate the adverse consequences that arise when primary care providers code visits related to M/SU problems and illnesses as being due to somatic complaints.

Quality Oversight Practices

Many purchasers delegate their attention to care coordination and other quality-related issues by accepting the quality-of-care determinations made by expert quality oversight organizations, such as accrediting bodies. Four main organizations accredit M/SU health care organizations (and sometimes individual providers). The National Committee for Quality Assurance (NCQA) accredits managed care organizations, MBHOs, and disease management programs and recognizes physician practices through other oversight programs. The Joint Commission on Accreditation of Healthcare Organizations (JCAHO) accredits hospitals and specialty behavioral health care organizations. The Commission on Accreditation of Rehabilitation Facilities accredits a wide variety of behavioral health programs and services. Finally, the Council on Accreditation for Children and Family Services, Inc. accredits a wide variety of counseling and other M/SU programs and services, as well as EAPs. These accrediting bodies generally perform their quality oversight activities either through review of an organization's structures and operational practices or through measurement of an organization's or provider's clinical care processes and outcomes. Clinical care processes and outcomes are generally evaluated through performance measures (discussed in Chapter 4). Organizational structures and processes such as the linking strategies recommended above are typically reviewed through evaluation of compliance with the established structural and procedural standards that make up an organization's accreditation standards.

Although the accreditation standards of each of the above four organizations address care coordination and collaboration to some extent (CARF, 2005; COA, 2001; JCAHO, 2004; NCQA, 2004), accreditation standards for care coordination could be improved. For example, NCQA's MBHO accreditation standards address care coordination between M/SU and general health care in Standard QI 10, "Continuity and Coordination between Behavioral Health and Medical Care," which states (NCQA, 2004:91):

> The organization collaborates with relevant medical delivery systems or primary care physicians to monitor and improve coordination between behavioral health and medical care.

However, the following note is appended to this standard:

Note: If the organization does not have any formal relationship with the medical delivery system through contracts, delegation, or otherwise, NCQA considers this standard NA. (NCQA, 2004:91). NCQA's customer support line clarifies that "NA" means "Not Applicable."[20]

Collaboration and Coordination in Policy Making and Programming

Throughout this report, the committee emphasizes the need for collaboration and coordination in mental, substance-use, and general health care policy making and programming that parallels desired collaboration and coordination at the care delivery level—for example, in the dissemination of information on innovations in new treatments (see Chapter 4), in the measurement of the quality of M/SU care (see Chapter 4), and in the development of information technology for M/SU care (see Chapter 6). Such attention to coordination and collaboration at the policy and programming represents an opportunity for federal, state, and local officials to model and promote the coordination and collaboration needed at the clinical level—across M/SU health care and across providers of these specialty health care services and general health care. The importance of seizing this opportunity is emphasized in the IOM report *Leadership by Example: Coordinating Government Roles in Improving Health Care Quality*. That report, commissioned by Congress to examine and recommend quality improvement activities in six major federal programs,[21] concluded that the federal government must assume a strong leadership role in quality improvement:

> By exercising its roles as purchaser, regulator, provider of health services, and sponsor of applied health services research, the federal government has the necessary influence to direct the attention and resources of the health care sector in pursuit of quality. There is no other stakeholder with such a combination of roles and influence. (IOM, 2002:*x*)

Because coordination of care is one dimension of quality, the federal government needs to exercise leadership and model coordination and collaboration in general, mental, and substance-use health care. This coordination and collaboration should be practiced across the separate Centers

---

[20]Conversation with NCQA Customer Support on July 22, 2005.

[21]Even this initiative represents a missed opportunity for collaboration and coordination. Congress charged the IOM with examining the roles of Medicare, Medicaid, the Indian Health Service, the State Children's Health Insurance Program, the Department of Defense's TRICARE program, and the program of the Veterans Health Administration in enhancing health care quality, but not the role of federal M/SU programs administered by SAMHSA.

for Substance Abuse Prevention and Treatment and Center for Mental Health Services within SAMHSA, across SAMHSA and other operating divisions of the Department of Health and Human Services (DHHS), across DHHS and other departments, and across the public and private sectors.

A strong example of such leadership in coordination and collaboration is found in the federal action agenda, *Transforming Mental Health Care in America,* formulated to implement the recommendations of the President's New Freedom Commission on Mental Health. This action agenda is the collaborative product of 12 DHHS agencies (the Administration on Aging, Administration for Children and Families, Agency for Healthcare Research and Quality, Centers for Disease Control and Prevention, Centers for Medicare and Medicaid Services, Health Resources and Services Administration, Indian Health Service, National Institutes of Health, Office for Disability, Office for Civil Rights, Office of Public Health and Science, and SAMHSA), five other departments (Education, Housing and Urban Development, Justice, Labor, and Veterans Affairs), and the Social Security Administration. To guide the implementation of this agenda, DHHS is leading an intra- and interagency Federal Executive Steering Committee composed of high-level representatives from DHHS agencies and other federal departments that serve individuals with mental illnesses (SAMHSA, 2005). This strong model of collaboration and coordination could be strengthened by including on the action agenda items addressing the substance-use problems and illnesses that so frequently accompany mental illnesses, and by including more explicitly in implementation activities the SAMHSA centers and state agencies responsible for planning and arranging for care for co-occurring substance-use illnesses. Similarly engaging key private-sector entities, especially those in the general health sector who deliver much care for mental illnesses, would strengthen this collaborative approach and help break down the separations discussed earlier in this chapter between mental and substance-use illnesses, between specialty M/SU and general health care, and between the public and private sectors.

New Mexico provides one example of processes now under way to achieve such coordination and collaboration at the state level (see Box 5-1). While the fruits of this initiative are not yet known, these efforts are testimony to the critical need for such coordination and collaboration at the policy level and the importance of high-level leadership in meeting this need.

BOX 5-1   New Mexico's Behavioral Health Collaborative:
A Case Study in Policy Coordination

In 2003 the Governor of New Mexico identified as a major policy issue the fact that New Mexico's behavioral health system (like others across the United States) reflected the problems cited in the report of the President's New Freedom Commission: insufficient and inappropriate services, uneven access and quality, failure to maximize resources across funding streams, duplication of effort, higher administrative costs for providers, and overall fragmentation that makes service systems difficult to access and manage effectively. After consultation with key cabinet secretaries, the governor announced a new approach to address these problems through the creation of a high-level policy collaborative. This executive-level body was charged specifically with achieving better access, better services, and better value for taxpayer dollars in mental and substance-use health care.

This group, consisting of 17 members including the heads of 15 agencies, was established in law by the New Mexico legislature effective May 2004 and charged with creating a single behavioral health (mental and substance-use treatment) delivery system across multiple state agencies and funding sources. The vision that guided this effort, based on months of public participation, was that this single system must support recovery and resiliency so that consumers can participate fully in the life of their communities. The agencies forming the collaborative reflected these broad goals and included those responsible for such areas as housing, corrections, labor, and education, as well as primary health and human services agencies.

To ensure that this broad perspective would be reflected in the collaborative's actions, the group decided that decisions would be made whenever feasible by consensus, but that if votes were required, each agency would have a single vote regardless of its budget or size. The group is cochaired by the secretary of Human Services and (in alternating years) the secretary of Children, Youth, and Families or the secretary of Health. Such a broad policy vision clearly also required that the collaborative develop coordinated structures for the efficient management of a broad range of funds and services. Therefore, a request for proposals was issued, and a contractor was selected as the single statewide entity to manage approximately $350,000,000 in cross-agency funds for the first phase of the change process. In addition, the collaborative has formed senior-level coordination teams, including one focused specifically on cross-cutting policy issues. A single Behavioral Health Planning Council has also been established to form an ongoing partnership with consumers, families, providers, and state agencies in keeping the system on track. In addition, local collaboratives are being formed with cross-agency state assistance across all of the state's 13 judicial districts, as well as in its Native American communities, to ensure strong feedback and coordination involving stakeholders at the local level as a guide for collaborative state policies and actions. The overall transformation also is being carefully evaluated by multiple groups to help guide future work of this broad policy nature.

SOURCE: Personal communication, Leslie Tremaine, Behavioral Health Coordinator, New Mexico BH Collaborative, on July 28, 2005.

Recommendations

To address the complex obstacles to care coordination and collaboration described above, the committee recommends a set of related actions to be undertaken by individual clinicians, health care organizations, health plans, health care purchasers, accrediting organizations, and policy officials.

Recommendation 5-1. To make collaboration and coordination of patients' M/SU health care services the norm, providers of the services should establish clinically effective linkages within their own organizations and between providers of mental health and substance-use treatment. The necessary communications and interactions should take place with the patient's knowledge and consent and be fostered by:

- Routine sharing of information on patients' problems and pharmacologic and nonpharmacologic treatments among providers of M/SU treatment.
- Valid, age-appropriate screening of patients for comorbid mental, substance-use, and general medical problems in these clinical settings and reliable monitoring of their progress.

Recommendation 5-2. To facilitate the delivery of coordinated care by primary care, mental health, and substance-use treatment providers, government agencies, purchasers, health plans, and accreditation organizations should implement policies and incentives to continually increase collaboration among these providers to achieve evidence-based screening and care of their patients with general, mental, and/or substance-use health conditions. The following specific measures should be undertaken to carry out this recommendation:

- Primary care and specialty M/SU health care providers should transition along a continuum of evidence-based coordination models from (1) formal agreements among mental, substance-use, and primary health care providers; to (2) case management of mental, substance-use, and primary health care; to (3) collocation of mental, substance-use, and primary health care services; and then to (4) delivery of mental, substance-use, and primary health care through clinically integrated practices of primary and M/SU care providers. Organizations should adopt models to which they can most easily transition from their current structure, that best meet the needs of their patient populations, and that ensure accountability.

- DHHS should fund demonstration programs to offer incentives for the transition of multiple primary care and M/SU practices along this continuum of coordination models.
- Purchasers should modify policies and practices that preclude paying for evidence-based screening, treatment, and coordination of M/SU care and require (with patients' knowledge and consent) all health care organizations with which they contract to ensure appropriate sharing of clinical information essential for coordination of care with other providers treating their patients.
- Organizations that accredit mental, substance-use, or primary health care organizations should use accrediting practices that assess, for all providers, the use of evidence-based approaches to coordinating mental, substance-use, and primary health care.
- Federal and state governments should revise laws, regulations, and administrative practices that create inappropriate barriers to the communication of information between providers of health care for mental and substance-use conditions and between those providers and providers of general care.

With respect to the need for purchasers to modify practices that preclude paying for evidence-based screening, treatment, and coordination of health care for mental and substance-use conditions, the committee calls particular attention to practices that prevent primary care providers from receiving payment for delivery of the M/SU health services they provide and the failure of some benefit plans to cover certain evidence-based treatments.

Recommendation 5-3. To ensure the health of persons for whom they are responsible, M/SU providers should:

- Coordinate their services with those of other human services and education agencies, such as schools, housing and vocational rehabilitation agencies, and providers of services for older adults.
- Establish referral arrangements for needed services.

Providers of services to high-risk populations—such as child welfare agencies, criminal and juvenile justice agencies, and long-term care facilities for older adults—should use valid, age-appropriate, and culturally appropriate techniques to screen all entrants into their systems to detect M/SU problems and illnesses.

Recommendation 5-4. To provide leadership in coordination, DHHS should create a high-level, continuing entity reporting directly to the secretary to improve collaboration and coordination across its mental, substance-use, and general health care agencies, including the Substance Abuse and Mental Health Services Administration; the Agency for Healthcare Research and Quality; the Centers for Disease Control and Prevention; and the Administration for Children, Youth, and Families. DHHS also should implement performance measures to monitor its progress toward achieving internal interagency collaboration and publicly report its performance on these measures annually. State governments should create analogous linkages across state agencies.

With respect to recommendation 5-4, the committee notes that this recommendation echoes the call made in the report *Leadership by Example: Coordinating Government Roles in Improving Health Care Quality* for Congress to consider directing the Secretary of DHHS to produce an annual progress report "detailing the collaborative and individual efforts of the various government programs to redesign their quality enhancement processes" (IOM, 2002:11).

REFERENCES

Aarons GA, Brown SA, Hough RL, Garland AF, Wood PA. 2001. Prevalence of adolescent substance use disorders across five sectors of care. *Journal of the American Academy of Child & Adolescent Psychiatry* 40(4):419–426.

Abraham HD, Degli-Esposti S, Marino L. 1999. Seroprevalence of hepatitis C in a sample of middle class substance abusers. *Journal of Addictive Diseases* 18(4):77–87.

AHRQ (Agency for Healthcare Research and Quality). 2002–2003. *U.S. Preventive Services Task Force Ratings: Strength of Recommendations and Quality of Evidence. Guide to Clinical Preventive Services.* Periodic updates, 2002–2003. Rockville, MD: AHRQ. [Online]. Available: http:www.ahrq.gov/clinic/3rduspstf/ratings.htm [accessed February 28, 2005].

Alter MJ. 1999. Hepatitis C virus infection in the United States. *Journal of Hepatology* 31 (Supplement 1):88–91.

American Academy of Child & Adolescent Psychiatry and Child Welfare League of America. 2003. *Policy Statement: AACAP/CWLA Policy Statement on Mental Health and Use of Alcohol and Other Drugs, Screening and Assessment of Children in Foster Care.* [Online]. Available: http://www.aacap.org/publications/policy/collab02.htm [accessed December 2, 2005].

American Diabetes Association, American Psychiatric Association, American Association of Clinical Endocrinologists, North American Association for the Study of Obesity. 2004. Consensus development conference on antipsychotic drugs and obesity and diabetes. *Journal of Clinical Psychiatry* 65(2):267–272.

Anonymous. 2004. *Depression in Primary Care—Linking Clinical & System Strategies.* [Online]. Available: http://www.wpic.pitt.edu/dppc [accessed December 23, 2004].

Badamgarev E, Weingarten S, Henning J, Knight K, Hasselblad V, Gano A Jr, Ofman J. 2003. *American Journal of Psychiatry* 160(12):2080–2090.

Baggs J, Schmitt M. 1988. Collaboration between nurses and physicians. *IMAGE: Journal of Nursing Scholarship* 20(3):145–149.

Baggs J, Schmitt M. 1997. Nurses' and resident physicians' perception of the process of collaboration in an MICU. *Research in Nursing & Health* 20(1):71–80.

Baggs J, Schmitt M, Mushlin A, Mitchell PH, Eldredge DH, Oakes D, Hutson AD. 1999. Association between nurse-physician collaboration and patient outcomes in three intensive care units. *Critical Care Medicine* 27(9):1991–1998.

Baldridge National Quality Program. 2003. *Criteria for Performance Excellence*. National Institute of Standards and Technology, U.S. Department of Commerce. [Online]. Available: http://www.quality.nist.gov/PDF_files/2003_Business_Criteria.pdf [accessed April 24, 2003].

Barry CL, Gabel JR, Frank RG, Hawkins S, Whitmore HH, Pickreign JD. 2003. Design of mental health benefits: Still unequal after all these years. *Health Affairs* 22(5):127–137.

Berwick DM. 1998. Keynote Address: Taking action to improve safety: How to increase the odds of success. *1998 Conference: Enhancing Patient Safety and Reducing Errors in Health Care*. National Patient Safety Foundation. Rancho Mirage, CA , on November 8–10, 1998. [Online]. Available: http://www.npsf.org/congress_archive/1998/html/keynote.html [accessed December 16, 2004].

Bodenheimer T, Wagner EH, Grumbach K. 2002. Improving primary care for patients with chronic illness. *Journal of the American Medical Association* 288(14):1775–1779.

Brailer DJ, Terasawa E. 2003. *Use and Adoption of Computer-Based Patient Records in the United States*. Presentation to IOM Committee on Data Standards for Patient Safety on January 23, 2003. [Online]. Available: http://www.iom.edu/file.asp?id=10988 [accessed October 17, 2004].

Brunette MF, Drake RE, Marsh BJ, Torrey WC, Rosenberg SD. 2003. Five-Site Health and Risk Study Research Committee. Responding to blood-borne infections among persons with severe mental illness. *Psychiatric Services* 54(6):860–865.

Burns BJ, Phillips SD, Wagner R, Barth RP, Kolko DJ, Campbel Y, Landsverk J. 2004. Mental health need and access to mental health services by youths involved with child welfare: A national survey. *Journal of the American Academy of Child and Adolescent Psychiatry* 43(8):960–970.

Bush DE, Ziegeldein RC, Patel UV, Thombs BD, Ford DE, Fauerbach JA, McCann UD, Stewart KJ, Tsilidis KK, Patel AL, Feuerstein CJ, Bass EB. 2005. *Post-Myocardial Infarction Depression. Summary*. AHRQ Publication Number 05-E018-1. Evidence Report/ Technology Assessment Number 123. Rockville, MD: Agency for Healthcare Research and Quality.

Canagasaby A, Vinson DC. 2005. Screening for hazardous or harmful drinking using one or two quantity-frequency questions. *Alcohol and Alcoholism* 40(3):208–213.

CARF (Commission on Accreditation of Rehabilitation Facilities). 2005. *Standards Manual with Survey Preparation Questions, July 2005–June 2006*. Washington, DC: CARF.

Carlsson S, Hammar N, Efendic S, Persson PG, Ostenson CG, Grill V. 2000. Alcohol consumption, Type 2 diabetes mellitus and impaired glucose tolerance in middle-aged Swedish men. *Diabetes Medicine* 17(11):776–781.

CDC (Centers for Disease Control and Prevention). 2001. HIV Prevention Strategic Plan through 2005. [Online]. Available: www.cdc.gov/nchstp/od/hiv_plan [accessed October 13, 2005].

COA (Council on Accreditation for Children and Family Services, Inc). 2001. *Standards and Self-Study Manual, 7th ed., version1.1*. New York: COA.

Cocozza JJ. 2004. *Juvenile Justice Systems: Improving Mental Health Treatment Services for Children and Adolescents*. Paper commissioned by the Institute of Medicine Committee on Crossing the Quality Chasm: Adaptation to Mental Health and Addictive Disorders. Available from the Institute of Medicine.

Cocozza JJ, Skowyra K. 2000. Youth with mental disorders: Issues and emerging responses. *Juvenile Justice* 7(1):3–13.

Conigliaro J, Gordon AJ, McGinnis KA, Rabeneck L, Justice AC. 2003. How harmful is hazardous alcohol use and abuse in HIV infection: Do health care providers know who is at risk? *JAIDS: Journal of Acquired Immune Deficiency Syndromes* 33(4):521–525.

Cook RI, Render M, Woods DD. 2000. Gaps in the continuity of care and progress on patient safety. *British Medical Journal* 320(7237):791–794.

Corrao G, Rubbiati L, Bagnardi V, Zanbon A, Poikolainen K. 2000. Alcohol and coronary heart disease: A meta-analysis. *Addiction* 95(10):1505–1523.

Curley C, McEachern JE, Speroff T. 1998. A firm trial of interdisciplinary rounds on the inpatient medical wards: An intervention designed using continuous quality improvement. *Medical Care* 36(8 Supplement):AS4–AS12.

D'Aunno TA. 1997. Linking substance abuse treatment and primary health care. In: Egertson JA, Fox DM, Leshman AI, eds. *Treating Drug Users Effectively*. Malden, MA: Blackwell. Pp. 311–351.

Davenport T, DeLong D, Beers M. 1998. Successful knowledge management projects. *Sloan Management Review* Winter(1):43–57.

De Alba I, Samet J, Saitz R. 2004. Burden of medical illness in drug- and alcohol-dependent persons without primary care. *The American Journal on Addiction* 13(1):33–45.

DHHS (U.S. Department of Health and Human Services). 1999. *Mental Health: A Report of the Surgeon General*. Rockville, MD: DHHS.

Dietrich AJ, Oxman TE, Williams JW Jr, Kroenke K, Schulberg HC, Bruce M, Barry SL. 2004. Going to scale: Re-engineering systems for primary care treatment of depression. *Annals of Family Medicine* 2(4):301–304.

Disch J, Beilmann G, Ingbar D. 2001. Medical directors as partners in creating healthy work environments. *AACN Clinical Issues* 12(3):366–377.

Ditton P. 1999. *Mental Health and Treatment of Inmates and Probationers*. Bureau of Justice Statistics, NCJ 174463. Washington, DC: Department of Justice.

Donohue J, Frank RG. 2000. Medicaid behavioral health carve-outs: A new generation of privatization decisions. *Harvard Review of Psychiatry* 8(5):231–241.

Druss B, Rohrbaugh R, Levinson C, Rosenheck R. 2001. Integrated medical care for patients with serious psychiatric illness: A randomized trial. *Archives of General Psychiatry* 58(9):861–868.

Edlund MJ, Unutzer J, Wells KB. 2004. Clinician screening and treatment of alcohol, drug, and mental problems in primary care: Results from Healthcare for Communities. *Medical Care* 42(12):1158–1166.

Fein G, Fletcher DJ, Di Sclafani V. 1998. Effect of chronic alcohol abuse on the CNS morbidity of HIV disease. *Alcoholism: Clinical and Experimental Research* 22(5 Supplement): 196S–200S.

Feldman MD, Ong MK, Lee DL, Perez-Stable EJ. 2005. Realigning economic incentives for depression care at UCSF. *Administration and Policy in Mental Health and Mental Health Services Research* 33(1):35–39.

Feldman S. 2003. Choices and challenges. In: Feldman S, ed. *Managed Behavioral Health Services: Perspectives and Practice*. Springfield, IL: Charles C. Thomas Publisher, Pp. 3–23.

Fox A, Oss M, Jardine E. 2000. *OPEN MINDS Yearbook of Managed Behavioral Health Market Share in the United States 2000-2001*. Gettysburg, PA: OPEN MINDS.

Friedmann PD, D'Aunno TA, Jin L, Alexander J. 2000a. Medical and psychosocial services in drug abuse treatment: Do stronger linkages promote client utilization? *HSR: Health Services Research* 35(2):443–465.

Friedmann PD, McCulloch D, Chin MH, Saitz R. 2000b. Screening and intervention for alcohol problems: A national survey of primary care physicians and psychiatrists. *Journal of General Internal Medicine* 15(2):84–91.

Friedmann PD, McCullough D, Saitz R. 2001. Screening and intervention for illicit drug abuse: A national survey of primary care physicians and psychiatrists. *Archives of Internal Medicine.* 161(2):248–251.

Fronstin P. 2003. *Sources of Health Insurance and Characteristics of the Uninsured: Analysis of the March 2003 Current Population Survey.* Washington, DC: Employee Benefit Research Institute.

GAO (U.S. General Accounting Office). 2003. *Child Welfare and Juvenile Justice: Federal Agencies Could Play a Stronger Role in Helping States Reduce the Number of Children Placed Solely to Obtain Mental Health Services.* GAO-03-397. [Online]. Available: http:// www.gao.gov/new.items/d03397.pdf [accessed October 25, 2004].

Garfein RS, Vlahov D, Galai N, Doherty MC, Nelson KE. 1996. Viral infections in short-term injection drug users and the prevalence of the hepatitis C, hepatitis B, human immunodeficiency, and human T-lymphotropic viruses. *American Journal of Public Health* 86(5):655–661.

Gilbody S, Whitty P, Grimshaw J, Thomas R. 2003. Educational and organizational interventions to improve the management of depression in primary care: A systematic review. *JAMA* 289(23):3145–3151.

Gittell J, Fairfield K, Bierbaum B, Head W, Jackson R, Kelly M, Laskin R, Lipson S, Siliski J, Thornhill T, Zuckerman J. 2000. Impact of relational coordination on quality of care, postoperative pain and functioning, and length of stay. *Medical Care* 38(8):807–819.

Goff DC, Cather C, Evins AE, Henderson DC, Freudenreich O, Copeland PM, Bierer M, Duckworth K, Sacks FM. 2005. Medical morbidity and mortality in schizophrenia: Guidelines for psychiatrists. *Journal of Clinical Psychiatry* 66(2):183–194.

Goldstrom I, Jaiquan F, Henderson M, Male A, Mandersheid R. 2001.The Availability of Mental Health Services to Young People in Juvenile Justice Facilities: A National Survey. In: Manderscheid RW, Henderson MJ, eds. *Mental Health, United States 2000.* (SMA) 01-3537. Washington, DC: U.S. Government Printing Office.

Graber M, Bergus G, Dawson J, Wood G, Levy B, Levin I. 2000. Effect of a patient's psychiatric history on physicians' estimation of probability of disease. *Journal of General Internal Medicine* 15(3):204–206.

Grant BF, Stinson FS, Dawson DA, Chou P, Dufour MC, Compton W, Pickering RP, Kaplan K. 2004a. Prevalence and co-occurrence of substance use disorders and independent mood and anxiety disorders: Results from the National Epidemiologic Survey on Alcohol and Related Conditions. *Archives of General Psychiatry* 61(8):807–816.

Grant BF, Stinson FS, Dawson DA, Chou SP, Ruan WJ, Pickering RP. 2004b. Co-occurrence of 12-month alcohol and drug use disorders and personality disorders in the United States: Results from the National Epidemiologic Survey on Alcohol and Related Conditions. *Archives of General Psychiatry* 61(4):361–368.

Grazier KL, Eselius LL. 1999. Mental health carve-outs: Effects and implications. *Medical Care Research and Review* 56 (Supplement 2):37–59.

Green AI, Canuso CM, Brenner MJ, Wojcik JD. 2003. Detection and management of comorbidity in patients with schizophrenia. *Psychiatric Clinics of North America* 26(1):115–138.

Grisso T. 2004. *Double Jeopardy: Adolescent Offenders with Mental Disorders.* Chicago, IL: University of Chicago Press.

Haney C, Specter D. 2003. Treatment rights in uncertain legal times. In: Ashford JB, Sales BD, Reid WH, eds. *Treating Adult and Juvenile Offenders with Special Needs.* Washington, DC: American Psychological Association. Pp. 51–80.

Harrison PM, Karberg JC. 2004. *Prison and Jail Inmates at Midyear 2003.* Bureau of Justice Statistics Bulletin, Office of Justice Programs, NCJ 203947. Washington, DC: U.S. Department of Justice. [Online]. Available: http://www.ojp.usdoj.gov/bjs/pub/pdf/pjim03.pdf [accessed August 4, 2004].

Harter MC, Conway KP, Merikangas KR. 2003. Associations between anxiety disorders and physical illness. *European Archives of Psychiatry and Clinical Neurosciences* 253(6): 313–320.

Havassy BE, Alvidrez J, Own KK. 2004. Comparisons of patients with comorbid psychiatric and substance use disorders. Implications for treatment and service delivery. *American Journal of Psychiatry* 161(1):139–145.

Henningsen P, Zimmerman T, Sattel H. 2003. Medically unexplained physical symptoms, anxiety, and depression: A meta-analytic review. *Psychosomatic Medicine* 65(4):528–533.

Hogan MF. 1999. Public-sector mental health care: New challenges. *Health Affairs* 18(5): 106–111.

Hughes TA, Wilson DJ, Beck AJ. 2001. *Trends in State Parole, 1990–2000*. Bureau of Justice Statistics, NCJ 184735. Washington, DC: Department of Justice. [Online]. Available: http://www.Ojp.Usdoj.Gov/Bjs/Pub/Pdf/Tsp00.Pdf [accessed July 31, 2005].

Hurlburt MS, Leslie LK, Landsverk J, Barth RP, Burns BJ, Gibbons RD, Slymen DJ, Zhang J. 2004. Contextual predictors of mental health service use among children open to child welfare. *Archives of General Psychiatry* 61(12):1217–1224.

Hutchinson AB, Foster EM. 2003. The effect of Medicaid managed care on mental health care for children: A review of the literature. *Mental Health Services Research* 5(1): 39–54.

IOM (Institute of Medicine). 1997. Edmunds M, Frank, R, Hogan M, McCarty D, Robinson-Beale R, Weisner C, eds. *Managing Managed Care—Quality Improvement in Behavioral Health*. Washington, DC: National Academy Press.

IOM. 2001. *Crossing the Quality Chasm: A New Health System for the 21st Century*. Washington, DC: National Academy Press.

IOM. 2002. Eden J, Smith BM, eds. *Leadership by Example: Coordinating Government Roles in Improving Health Care Quality*. Washington, DC: The National Academies Press.

IOM. 2003a. Corrigan JM, Adams K, eds. *Priority Areas for National Attention: Transforming Health Care Quality*. Washington, DC: The National Academies Press.

IOM. 2003b. *Key Capabilities of an Electronic Health Record System*. Washington, DC: The National Academies Press.

IOM. 2004a. Fostering interdisciplinary collaboration. *Keeping Patients Safe: Transforming the Work Environment of Nurses*. Washington, DC: The National Academies Press. Pp. 212–217.

IOM. 2004b. Page A, ed. *Keeping Patients Safe: Transforming the Work Environment of Nurses*. Washington, DC: The National Academies Press.

Jaycox LH, Morral AR, Juvonen J. 2003. Mental health and medical problems and service use among adolescent substance users. *Journal of the American Academy of Child & Adolescent Psychiatry* 42(6):701–719.

JCAHO (Joint Commission for the Accreditation of Healthcare Organizations). 2004. *Comprehensive Accreditation Manual for Behavioral Health Care 2004–2005*. Oakbrook Terrace, IL: Joint Commission Resources.

Katon W. 2003. Clinical and health services relationships between major depression, depressive symptoms, and general medical illness. *Biological Psychiatry* 54(3):216–226.

Katon W, Von Korff M, Lin E, Simon G. 2001. Rethinking practitioner roles in chronic illness: The specialist, primary care physician, and the practice nurse. *General Hospital Psychiatry* 23(3):138–144.

Kessler RC. 2004. The epidemiology of dual diagnosis. *Biological Psychiatry* 56(10): 730–737.

Kessler RC, Nelson CB, McGonagle KA, Edlund MJ, Frank, RG, Leaf PJ. 1996. The epidemiology of co-occurring addictive and mental disorders: Implications for prevention and service utilization. *American Journal of Orthopsychiatry* 66(1):17–31.

Kessler RC, Costello EJ, Merikangas KR, Ustun TB. 2001. Psychiatric epidemiology: Recent advances and future directions. In: Manderscheid RW, Henderson MJ, eds. *Mental Health, United States, 2000*. DHHS Publication Number: (SMA) 01-3537. Washington, DC: U.S. Government Printing Office. Pp. 29–42.

Knaus W, Draper E, Wagner D, Zimmerman J. 1986. An evaluation of outcome from intensive care in major medical centers. *Annals of Internal Medicine* 104(3):410–418.

Kroenke K. 2003. Patients presenting with somatic complaints: Epidemiology, psychiatric comorbidity and management. *International Journal of Methods in Psychiatric Research* 12(1):34–43.

Kroenke K, Taylor-Vaisey A, Dietrich AJ, Oxman TE. 2000. Interventions to improve provider diagnosis and treatment of mental disorders in primary care: A critical review of the literature. *Psychosomatics* 41(1):39–52.

Landsverk J. 2005. *Improving the Quality of Mental Health and Substance Use Treatment Services for Children Involved in Child Welfare*. Paper commissioned by the Institute of Medicine Committee on Crossing the Quality Chasm: Adaptation to Mental Health and Addictive Disorders.

Leslie LK, Hurlburt MS, Landsverk J, Rolls JA, Wood PA, Kelleher KJ. 2003. Comprehensive assessments for children entering foster care: A national perspective. *Pediatrics* 112(1): 134–142.

Marshall M, Gray A, Lockwood A, Green R. 2004. *Case Management for People with Severe Mental Disorders (Cochrane Review)*. Chichester, UK: John Wiley & Sons. Issue 4.

Masi D. 2004. *Issues in Delivering Mental Health and Substance Abuse Services through Employee Assistance Programs (EAPs)*. Testimony to the Institute of Medicine Committee on Crossing the Quality Chasm: Adaptation to Mental Health and Addictive Disorders on November 15, 2004. Irvine, California.

Masi D, Altman L, Benayon C, Healy H, Jorgensen DG, Kennish R, Keary D, Thompson C, Marsden B, McCann B, Watkins G, Williams C. 2004. Employee assistance programs in the year 2002. In: Manderscheid RW, Henderson MJ, eds. *Mental Health, United States, 2002*. DHHS Publication Number: SMA 3938. Rockville, MD: Substance Abuse and Mental Health Services Administration.

Mertens JR, Lu YW, Parthasarathy S, Moore C, Weisner CM. 2003. Medical and psychiatric conditions of alcohol and drug treatment patients in an HMO: Comparison with matched controls. *Archives of Internal Medicine* 163(20):2511–2517.

Metzner JL. 2002. Class action litigation in correctional psychiatry. *Journal of the American Academy of Psychiatry and the Law* 30(1):19–29.

Mickus M, Colenda CC, Hogan AJ. 2000. Knowledge of mental health benefits and preferences for type of mental health providers among the general public. *Psychiatric Services* 51(2):199–202.

Miller AL, Crismon ML, Rush AJ, Chiles J, Kashner TM, Toprac M, Carmody T, Biggs M, Shores-Wilson K, Chiles J, Witte B, Bow-Thomas C, Velligan DI, Trivedi M, Suppes T, Shon S. 2004. The Texas medication algorithm project: Clinical results for schizophrenia. *Schizophrenia Bulletin* 30(3):627–647.

Miller CL, Druss BG, Dombrowski EA, Rosenheck RA. 2003. Barriers to primary medical care at a community mental health center. *Psychiatric Services* 54(8):1158–1160.

Moore RD, Keruly JC, Chaisson RE. 2004. Differences in HIV disease progression by injecting drug use in HIV-infected persons in care. *JAIDS Journal of Acquired Immune Deficiency Syndromes* 35(1):46–51.

NASMHPD, NASADAD (National Association of State Mental Health Program Directors and National Association of State Alcohol and Drug Abuse Directors). 2002. Final report of the NASMHPD-NASADAD Task Force on Co-Occurring Mental Health and Substance Use Disorders. *Exemplary Methods of Financing Integrated Service Programs for Persons with Co-Occurring Mental Health and Substance Use Disorders.* Alexandria, VA and Washington, DC: NASMHPD, NASADAD. [Online]. Available: http://www.nasmhpd.org/general_files/publications/NASADAD%20NASMHPD%20PUBS/Exemplary%20methods_3.pdf [accessed August 14, 2005].

NCQA (National Committee for Quality Assurance). 2004. *Standards and Guidelines for the Accreditation of MBOs.* Washington, DC: NCQA.

New Freedom Commission on Mental Health. 2003. *Achieving the Promise: Transforming Mental Health Care in America. Final Report.* DHHS Publication Number SMA-03-3832. Rockville, MD: U.S. Department of Health and Human Services.

NIAAA (National Institute on Alcohol Abuse and Alcoholism). 2000. *10th Special Report to the U.S. Congress on Alcohol and Health.* [Online]. Available: http://www.niaaa.nih.gov/publications/10 report [accessed May 6, 2005].

NIAAA. 2002. *Screening for Alcohol Problems: An Update.* Alcohol Alert. 56. [Online]. Available: http://pubs.niaaa.nih.gov/publications/aa56.htm [accessed October 13, 2005].

NIAAA. 2005. *Helping Patients Who Drink Too Much: A Clinician's Guide.* [Online]. Available: http://pubs.niaaa.nih.gov/publications/Practitioner/Clinicians Guide2005/guide.pdf [accessed October 12, 2005].

Palepu A, Tyndall M, Yip P, Shaughnessy MV, Hogg RS, Montaner JSG. 2003. Impaired virologic response to highly active antiretroviral therapy associated with ongoing injection drug use. *JAIDS Journal of Acquired Immune Deficiency Syndromes* 32(5): 522–526.

Peele PB, Lave JR, Kelleher KJ. 2002. Exclusions and limitations in children's behavioral health care coverage. *Psychiatric Services* 53(5):591–594.

Pignone MP, Gaynes BN, Rushton JL, Burchell CM, Orleans TC, Mulrow CD, Lohr KN. 2002. Screening for depression in adults: A summary of the evidence for the U.S. Preventive Services Task Force. *Annals of Internal Medicine* 136(10):765–776.

Pincus HA. 2003. The future of behavioral health and primary care: Drowning in the mainstream or left on the bank? *Psychosomatics* 44(1):1–11.

Pincus HA, Hough L, Houtsinger JK, Rollman BL, Frank R. 2003. Emerging models of depression care: Multi-level ('6P') strategies. *International Journal of Methods in Psychiatric Research* 12(1):54–63.

Rice A. 2000. Interdisciplinary collaboration in health care: Education, practice, and research. *National Academies of Practice Forum: Issues in Interdisciplinary Care* 2(1): 59–73.

Rollman BL, Belnap BH, Reynolds CF, Schulberg HC, Shear MK. 2003. A contemporary protocol to assist primary care physicians in the treatment of panic and generalized anxiety disorders. *General Hospital Psychiatry* 25(2):74–82.

Rones M, Hoagwood K. 2000. School-based mental health services: A research review. *Clinical Child and Family Psychology Review* 3(4):223–241.

Rosenberg SD, Goodman LA, Osher FC, Swartz MS, Essock SM, Butterfield MI, Constantine NT, Wolford GL, Salyers MP. 2001. Prevalence of HIV, hepatitis B, and hepatitis C in people with severe mental illness. *American Journal of Public Health* 91(1):31–37.

Rost K, Smith R, Matthews DB, Guise B. 1994. The deliberate misdiagnosis of major depression in primary care. *Archives of Family Medicine* 3(4):333–337.

Rush AJ, Crismon ML, Kashner TM, Toprac MG, Carmody TJ, Trivedi MH, Suppes T, Miller AL, Biggs MM, Shores-Wilson K, Witte BP, Shon SP, Rago WV, Altshuler KZ, TMAP Research Group. 2003. Texas Medication Algorithm Project, phase 3 (TMAP-3): Rationale and study design. *Journal of Clinical Psychiatry* 64(4):357–369.

Saitz R, Mulvey KP, Plough A, Samet JH. 1997. Physician unawareness of serious substance abuse. *American Journal of Drug and Alcohol Abuse* 23(3):343–354.

Saitz R, Friedman PD, Sullivan LM, Winter MR, Lloyd-Travaglini C, Moskowitz MA, Samet J. 2002. Professional satisfaction experienced when caring for substance-abusing patients: Faculty and resident physician perspectives. *Journal of General Internal Medicine* 17(5):373–376.

Samet JH, Friedmann P, Saitz R. 2001. Benefits of linking primary medical care and substance abuse services: Patient, provider, and societal perspectives. *Archives of Internal Medicine* 161(1):85–91.

Samet JH, Horton NJ, Meli S, Freedberg KA, Palepu A. 2004. Alcohol consumption and antiretroviral adherence among HIV-infected persons with alcohol problems. *Alcoholism: Clinical and Experimental Research* 28(4):572–577.

SAMHSA (Substance Abuse and Mental Health Services Administration). 2004. *Results from the 2003 National Survey on Drug Use and Health: National Findings.* DHHS Publication Number SMA 04-3964. NSDUH Series H-25. Rockville, MD: SAMHSA.

SAMHSA. 2005. *Transforming Mental Health Care in America. The Federal Action Agenda: First Steps.* [Online]. Available: http://www.samhsa.gov/Federalactionagenda/NFC_TOC.aspx [accessed July 23, 2005].

SAMHSA. undated. *Report to Congress on the Prevention and Treatment of Co-Occurring Substance Abuse Disorders and Mental Disorders.* [Online]. Available: http://www.samhsa.gov/reports/congress2002/CoOccurringRpt.pdf [accessed April 25, 2004].

Schmitt M. 2001. Collaboration improves the quality of care: Methodological challenges and evidence from U.S. health care research. *Journal of Interprofessional Care* 15(1):47–66.

Shortell S, Zimmerman J, Rousseau D, Gillies RR, Wagner DP, Draper EA, Knaus WA, Duffy J. 1994. The performance of intensive care units: Does good management make a difference? *Medical Care* 32(5):508–525.

Shortell SM, Gillies RR, Anderson DA, Erickson KM, Mitchell JB. 2000. *Remaking Health Care in America: The Evolution of Organized Delivery Systems* 2nd ed. San Francisco, CA: Jossey-Bass.

Sokol J, Messias E, Dickerson FB, Kreyenbuhl J, Brown CH, Goldberg RW, Dixon LB. 2004. Comorbidity of medical illnesses among adults with serious mental illness who are receiving community psychiatric services. *Journal of Nervous and Mental Diseases* 192(6):421–427.

Spitzer RL, Kroenke K, Williams JBW. 1999. Validation and utility of a self-report version of PRIME-MD: The PHQ Primary Care Study. *Journal of the American Medical Association* 282(18):1737–1744.

Strosahl KD. 2005. Training behavioral health and primary care providers for integrated care: A core competencies approach. In: O'Donohue WT, Byrd M, Cummings N, Henderson D, eds. *Behavioral Integrative Care: Treatments That Work in the Primary Care Setting.* New York: Brunner-Routledge.

Sullivan G, Koegel P, Kanouse DE, Cournos F, McKinnon K, Young AS, Bean D. 1999. HIV and people with serious mental illness: The public sector's role in reducing HIV risk and improving care. *Psychiatric Services* 50(5):648–652.

Teplin L, Abram K, McClelland G, Dulcan M, Mericle A. 2002. Psychiatric disorders in youth in juvenile detention. *Archives of General Psychiatry* 59(12):1133–1143.

The National Coalition on Health Care, The Institute for Healthcare Improvement. 2002. *Curing the System: Stories of Change in Chronic Illness Care.* [Online]. Available: http://www.improvingchroniccare.org/ACT_Report_May_2002_Curing_The_System_.pdf [accessed July 24, 2005].

Tyor WR, Middaugh LD. 1999. Do alcohol and cocaine abuse alter the course of HIV-associated dementia complex? *Journal of Leukocyte Biology* 65(4):475–481.

Unutzer J, Katon W, Williams JW Jr, Callahan CM, Harpole L, Hunkeler EM, Hoffing M, Arean P, Hegel MT, Schoenbaum M, Oishi SM, Langston CA. 2001. Improving primary care for depression in late life. *Medical Care* 39(8):785–799.

Upshur CC. 2005. Crossing the divide: Primary care and mental health integration. *Administration and Policy in Mental Health* 32(4):341–355.

Watkins KE, Burnam A, Kung F-Y, Paddock S. 2001. A national survey of care for persons with co-occurring mental and substance use disorders. *Psychiatric Services* 52(8):1062–1068.

Watkins K, Pincus HA, Tanielian TL, Lloyd J. 2003. Using the chronic care model to improve treatment of alcohol use disorders in primary care settings. *Journal of Studies on Alcohol* 64(2):209–218.

Weisner C, Mertens J, Parthasarathy S, Moore C, Lu Y. 2001. Integrating primary medical care with addiction treatment: A randomized controlled trial. *Journal of the American Medical Association* 286(14):1715–1723.

Weist MD, Paternite CE, Adelsheim S. 2005. *School-Based Mental Health Services.* Paper commissioned by the Institute of Medicine Committee on Crossing the Quality Chasm: Adaptation to Mental Health and Addictive Disorders. Available from Institute of Medicine.

Wierson M, Forehand R, Frame C. 1992. Epidemiology and treatment of mental health problems in juvenile delinquents. *Advances in Behavior Research and Therapy* 14:93–120.

Williams JW, Pignone M, Ramirez G, Perez SC. 2002. Identifying depression in primary care: A literature synthesis of case-finding instruments. *General Hospital Psychiatry* 24(4):225–237.

Wolff NP. 2004. *Law and Disorder: The Case Against Diminished Responsibility.* Paper commissioned by the Institute of Medicine Committee on Crossing the Quality Chasm: Adaptation to Mental Health and Addictive Disorders. Center for Mental Health Services & Criminal Justice Research and Edward J. Bloustein School of Planning and Public Policy, Rutgers, the State University of New Jersey. Available from the author.

Zarski JP, Bohn B, Bastie A, Pawlotsky JM, Baud M, Bost-Bezeaux F, Tran van Nhieu J, Seigneurin JM, Buffet C, Dhumeaux D. 1998. Characteristics of patients with dual infection by hepatitis B and C viruses. *Journal of Hepatology* 28(1):27–33.

Ziguras SJ, Stuart GW. 2000. A meta-analysis of the effectiveness of mental health case management over 20 years. *Psychiatric Services* 51(11):1410–1421.

Zwarenstein M, Stephenson B, Johnston L. 2000. Case management: Effects on professional practice and health care outcomes. (Protocol) *The Cochrane Database of Systematic Reviews* 2000, Issue 4. Art. No.: CD002797. DOI: 10.1002/14651858.CD002797.

6

Ensuring the National Health Information Infrastructure Benefits Persons with Mental and Substance-Use Conditions

Summary

Health care providers' ability to obtain information quickly on a patient's health, health care, and potential treatments and to share this information in a timely manner with other providers caring for the patient is essential to the delivery of safe, patient-centered, coordinated, and effective health care. To meet this need, major public- and private-sector collaborations are under way to develop three essential components of a National Health Information Infrastructure (NHII): (1) electronic health record (EHR)[1] systems with decision support for clinicians, (2) a secure platform for the exchange of patient information across health care settings, and (3) data standards that will make shared information understandable to all users (IOM, 2004). Efforts also are under way in the public sector to create information systems for mental and substance-use health care. Ensuring that the developing NHII serves consumers of health care for mental and/or substance use (M/SU) conditions as well as it does those with general health care needs is essential to improving the quality of M/SU health care.

However, M/SU health care currently is not well addressed by NHII initiatives, nor are separate public-sector efforts aimed

---

[1]EHRs have a variety of names, including automated medical record, computer-based patient record, electronic medical record, electronic patient record, and others (Brailer and Terasawa, 2003).

at creating information systems for M/SU health care well coordinated with NHII initiatives. M/SU health care also lags behind general health care in its use of information technology (IT). To realize the potential of the NHII for consumers of M/SU health care, NHII initiatives and public-sector efforts to develop specialized information systems for M/SU health care need to take advantage of each other's expertise and capabilities. Doing so will ensure that the NHII provides relevant information to M/SU health care consumers, providers, payers, and oversight organizations, and that providers serving in both the public and private sectors do not face redundant or conflicting information demands. The committee recommends actions to (1) coordinate the activities of the NHII and public-sector M/SU IT initiatives, (2) bring M/SU expertise to the development of the NHII, and (3) support individual M/SU clinicians in their use of IT.

A STRONG INFORMATION INFRASTRUCTURE IS VITAL TO QUALITY

Crossing the Quality Chasm (IOM, 2001) and several preceding and subsequent reports from the Institute of Medicine (IOM), the federal government, and leading private-sector organizations (IOM, 2004; National Committee on Vital and Health Statistics, 2001; Thompson and Brailer, 2004) emphasize the vital role of information technology (IT) in the safety, effectiveness, patient-centeredness, timeliness, efficiency, and equity of health care. These organizations and many others find that a strong IT infrastructure is crucial to:

- Supporting consumers in illness self-management and marketplace choices.
- Supporting providers in the delivery of evidence-based clinical care.
- Coordinating care across clinicians, settings, and time.
- Facilitating performance and outcome measurement.
- Educating clinicians.

An example of the role of IT in achieving improved quality of care is presented in Box 6-1.

In addition to its uses in coordinating care, IT has begun to be used to support the delivery of treatment for mental and substance-use conditions—over the World Wide Web, by e-mail, and through other technology-mediated interactions (Flanagan and Needham, 2003) (see Chapter 7). Determination of research priorities and public policy decisions about the best allocation of scarce public dollars also can be facilitated through

BOX 6-1   Improving Care Using Information Technology

Mark is a 38-year-old veteran with schizophrenia who receives health care at a Veterans Administration (VA) medical center. He lived with his parents until they died 2 years ago and has since lived with his brother Sam and Sam's family. He has not worked recently, but he volunteers at a local library and lives off his military pension. Recently he enrolled in EQUIP, a project aimed at improving care for people with schizophrenia by applying illness management principles effective in treating other chronic illnesses. EQUIP uses the VA's electronic health record (EHR) enhanced by an information system that supports management of care, structured psychiatric evaluations, and secure messaging between clinicians. As a result, Mark's treatment team was alerted to several emerging problems that might have been missed with the old paper chart system.

The old paper charts included handwritten notes that were sometimes illegible and typically did not include useful psychiatric assessment data. The charts often arrived after a scheduled appointment, or not at all, and whether Mark had scheduled or kept medical appointments was unknown to his treatment team. With the enhanced EHR, Mark's psychiatrist was able to review Mark's full, up-to-date record, including the team nurse's routine assessments of Mark's symptoms and other problems. These assessments indicated chronic medical problems, including diabetes, a heart problem, a possible seizure disorder, obesity, and smoking. Several problems needing immediate attention were highlighted.

With the EHR and information system, the team received a list of previously scheduled and upcoming appointments. It was clear that Mark had missed multiple visits and was at risk for severe medical complications. The information system also indicated serious problems at home. With the previous paper charts, contact information and Mark's preferences regarding family contact were not documented. Now, this information was easily at hand, and his brother was called. He told the team that Mark was having daytime sleepiness that led to his missed appointments and that Mark was awake late at night, disturbing the family, and overeating. Most disturbing was that he was irritable and combative when confronted by Sam about these problems. Sam wanted to help Mark and had promised their parents to care for him. But he did not know what to do.

Previously, communication among the team took place only when someone remembered to bring a patient up at the weekly team meeting. Now, team members received a regular report on the clinical status of each of the patients under their care. They used a secure electronic messaging system to discuss Mark's problems. The team implemented a comprehensive behavioral program addressing sleep scheduling, caloric intake, exercise, and missed visits. Clinicians used the messaging system to update each other and ensure that their advice and instructions to Mark were consistent at each visit. The computer screen displayed updated messages when each clinician looked at Mark's medical record. A clinician also reviewed a weekly EQUIP-automated appointment report and used it to remind the family about upcoming appointments.

Mark began making it to his appointments regularly. Sam was included in medication change decisions. He ensured that the new medications were taken correctly and reported any changes to the team. With time, Mark began to express an interest in living more independently and working for pay. By the end of the project,

(continued on next page)

BOX 6-1 continued

he had moved to a residential group home, developed a better relationship with his family, improved his sleep habits, lost 10 pounds, and cut down his smoking. He was attending to his chronic medical problems through regular appointments and considering joining a vocational rehabilitation program.

SOURCE: Personal communication, Alexander S. Young and Amy N. Cohen, Greater Los Angeles Veterans Healthcare Center EQUIP project, on August 9, 2005.

---

technology-supported information systems. *Crossing the Quality Chasm* (IOM, 2001:165) found that IT "must play a central role in the design of health care systems if a substantial improvement in health care quality is to be achieved" and recommended that:

> Congress, the executive branch, leaders of health care organizations, public and private purchasers, and health informatics associations and vendors should make a renewed national commitment to building an information infrastructure to support health care delivery, consumer health, quality measurement and improvement, public accountability, clinical and health services research, and clinical education. This commitment should lead to the elimination of most handwritten clinical data by the end of the decade.

The remaining sections of this chapter address (1) activities under way to build the National Health Information Infrastructure (NHII), (2) the need for attention to mental and/or substance-use (M/SU) conditions in the NHII, (3) health information infrastructure and technologies under development for M/SU health care in the public sector, (4) issues affecting the adoption of IT by individual M/SU clinicians, and (5) recommendations for integrating health care for M/SU conditions into the NHII.

ACTIVITIES UNDER WAY TO BUILD A NATIONAL HEALTH INFORMATION INFRASTRUCTURE

Strong commitment has emerged in both the public and private sectors to working together to develop an NHII for the United States. The NHII will consist of (1) electronic health record (EHR) systems with decision support for clinicians, (2) a secure platform for the exchange of patient information across health care settings, and (3) data standards that will make shared information understandable to all users (IOM, 2004).

There also is consensus that although creating the NHII requires a partnership of public- and private-sector leaders, the federal government needs to play a leadership role in several ways, including promulgating certain data and other IT standards (IOM, 2004; Thompson and Brailer, 2004). The federal government also needs to provide financial support in three main areas. First, federal funds should support the development of critical components of the NHII that are unlikely to receive support from private-sector stakeholders. These include the establishment of a secure platform for the exchange of data across all providers and maintenance of a process for ongoing promulgation of national data standards. Second, the federal government should provide financial incentives to stimulate private-sector investment in EHR systems through the use of special loans, payment incentives to providers, or other mechanisms. Finally, federal funding of safety net providers is needed to support their adoption of IT (IOM, 2004).

Development of the NHII is expected to take many years, perhaps as long as a decade (Thompson and Brailer, 2004).[2] To jump-start the process, in 2004 the President established the Office of the National Coordinator for Health Information Technology (ONCHIT), charged with the following (DHHS, 2005b):

- Serving as the senior advisor to the President and the Secretary of the Department of Health and Human Services (DHHS) on all health IT programs and initiatives.
- Developing and maintaining a strategic plan to guide the nation-wide implementation of interoperable EHRs in both the public and private health care sectors.
- Coordinating the spending of approximately $4 billion for health IT programs and initiatives across the federal government.
- Coordinating all outreach activities to private industry and serving as the catalyst for health industry change.

Three months later, ONCHIT's National Coordinator put forth a framework for strategic action, *The Decade of Health Information Technology: Delivering Consumer-centric and Information-rich Health Care,* which included a 10-year plan to develop the NHII in partnership with the private sector. This plan addresses the development of EHRs, data standards, and interoperable technologies for the exchange of patient data across providers and settings of care (Thompson and Brailer, 2004).

---

[2]In this regard, the NHII is not unlike other ground-breaking health care initiatives, such as the mapping of the human genome.

Subsequently, in June 2005, DHHS announced the establishment of the American Health Information Community (AHIC), a commission of members from the public and private sectors, to advise the Secretary concerning efforts to develop IT standards and achieve interoperability for health IT. In particular, the AHIC is expected to develop recommendations for the following:

- Protecting health information through appropriate privacy and security practices.
- Achieving ongoing harmony of industrywide health IT standards.
- Achieving a nationwide, Internet-based health information network that includes information tools, specialized network functions, and security protections for interoperable exchange of health information.
- Accelerating the adoption of interoperable EHRs across the broad spectrum of health care providers.
- Developing compliance certification and inspection processes for EHRs, including the infrastructure components through which EHRs can interoperate.
- Identifying health IT standards for use by the National Institute of Standards and Technology (NIST) in an information processing standards-setting process relevant to federal agencies.
- Identifying and prioritizing specific uses for which health IT is valuable, beneficial, and feasible.
- Transitioning the work of the AHIC to a private-sector health information initiative (DHHS, 2005a).

Electronic Health Records[3]

An EHR system encompasses (1) the longitudinal collection of electronic information pertaining to an individual's health and health care; (2) immediate electronic access—by authorized users only—to person- and population-level information; (3) provision of knowledge and decision support to enhance the quality, safety, and efficiency of patient care; and (4) support for efficient processes of health care delivery (IOM, 2003).

As noted in Chapter 5, although still a minority, increasing numbers of hospitals and ambulatory practices are investing in EHRs, although this

---

[3]In addition to the development of EHRs, architects of the NHII are calling for the establishment of personal health records (PHRs)—an electronic, lifelong resource of health information needed by consumers to make health decisions. Consumers/patients own and manage the information in their PHR, which comes from health care providers and the patient. The PHR is maintained in a secure and private environment, with the patient determining who has the right to access it. The PHR does not replace the legal record of any provider (AHIMA e-HIM Personal Health Record Work Group, 2005).

typically occurs in larger and "more wired" facilities—referred to as the "adoption gap" between large and small organizations (Brailer and Terasawa, 2003). Many hospitals have made progress in adopting certain EHR components, such as automated laboratory results. Use of EHRs is higher in ambulatory settings—approximately 5 to 10 percent of physician offices—but there is much variation in their content and functionality (IOM, 2004). The federal strategic framework identifies the total cost of EHRs (purchase price + implementation costs + maintenance costs + impact on operations) as the primary impediment to their more widespread adoption (Thompson and Brailer, 2004).

The federal government's NHII strategic framework calls for the adoption of interoperable EHRs within 10 years (Thompson and Brailer, 2004). Several activities are under way to help achieve this goal. The IOM has provided a framework that should prove useful to accreditation organizations in establishing standards for EHR systems, as well as to providers in selecting vendors to design such systems (IOM, 2004). Standards for EHRs are under development by Health Level 7, the leading private-sector standards-setting organization (Thompson and Brailer, 2004). Three leading associations in health care information management and technology—the American Health Information Management Association, the Healthcare Information and Management Systems Society, and the National Alliance for Health Information Technology—have jointly launched the Certification Commission for Healthcare Information Technology to create a mechanism for the certification of health care information technology products, in particular EHRs (CCHIT, 2004).

The Veterans Health Administration has used an EHR system (VistA) for over two decades for its physicians, clinics, and hospitals. VistA is in the public domain, and in September 2005 Medicare released an evaluation version of the system (Vista-Office) for use by private physicians' offices in computerizing their medical practices. This evaluation version will be assessed to determine the extent to which physician offices can implement the software effectively. The evaluation phase will also allow software vendors to improve upon the system and develop a version that meets any standards for EHRs (CMS, 2005). Medicare will provide doctors with lists of companies that have been trained to install and maintain the system. Because so many doctors participate in Medicare, the distribution of Vista-Office is viewed as a significant development in the advancement of EHRs (Kolata, 2005).

Data Standards

In addition to cost factors, efforts of both the public and private sectors to invest in IT are hampered by the lack of nationwide standards for the collection, coding, classification, and exchange of clinical and administrative data. In particular, standards are needed in three areas:

- *Terminologies*—the terms and concepts used to describe, classify, and code health care data and the processes that describe the relationships among the terms and concepts (see the discussion of needed improvements to coding for M/SU health care in Chapter 4).
- *Data interchange*—standard formats for electronically encoding health care data elements and structuring the data elements as they are exchanged, and information models that define the relationships among data elements. Several standards for electronic data interchange have been endorsed by the Secretary of DHHS, including those for the exchange of clinical and administrative data. However, there remains a need to update these standards and create implementation guides, tests for conformance, and certification procedures to ensure that the standards actually work and are being used as intended (IOM, 2004).
- *Knowledge representation*—methods for electronically representing health care literature, clinical guidelines, and similar sources of information for decision support so that they can be called upon automatically for the practitioner in response to triggers embedded in the EHR or other electronic clinical or administrative document (IOM, 2004).

Standardizing these data and processes requires not just a one-time effort, but an ongoing, permanent process for updating the standards as scientific knowledge, clinical practices, and information needs change. In October 2001, the federal government established the Consolidated Health Informatics interagency initiative to adopt interoperability data standards for federally operated and funded health care providers. Given that the federal government represents more than 40 percent of health care expenditures in the United States, this action is viewed as a powerful means of establishing such standards nationally across the public and private health care sectors (IOM, 2004). As of May 2004, the Consolidated Health Informatics initiative had approved 20 standards for adoption by the federal Departments of Defense, Veterans Affairs, Health and Human Services, State, Education, Energy, and Justice, as well as the Social Security Administration, General Services Administration, Office of Management and Budget, and Environmental Protection Agency (Anonymous, 2004).

In response to a request from the federal government to undertake a study of standards for health care safety reporting systems, the IOM (2004:12) made the following recommendation:

Congress should provide clear direction, enabling authority, and financial support for the establishment of national standards for data that support patient safety. Various government agencies will need to assume major new responsibilities, and additional support will be required. Specifically:

- The Department of Health and Human Services (DHHS) should be given the lead role in establishing and maintaining a public–private partnership for the promulgation of standards for data that support patient safety.
- The Consolidated Health Informatics (CHI) initiative, in collaboration with the National Committee on Vital and Health Statistics (NCVHS), should identify data standards appropriate for national adoption and gaps in existing standards that need to be addressed. The membership of NCVHS should continue to be broad and diverse, with adequate representation of all stakeholders, including consumers, state governments, professional groups, and standard-setting bodies.
- The Agency for Healthcare Research and Quality (AHRQ) in collaboration with the National Library of Medicine and others should (1) provide administrative and technical support for the CHI and NCVHS efforts; (2) ensure the development of implementation guides, certification procedures, and conformance testing for all data standards; (3) provide financial support and oversight for developmental activities to fill gaps in data standards; and (4) coordinate activities and maintain a clearinghouse of information in support of national data standards and their implementation to improve patient safety.
- The National Library of Medicine should be designated as the responsible entity for distributing all national clinical terminologies that relate to patient safety and for ensuring the quality of terminology mappings.

The IOM also recommended that, after allowing a reasonable time for health care organizations to comply with national standards identified by the Consolidated Health Informatics initiative, the major government health care programs, including those operated by DHHS, the Veterans Administration, and the Department of Defense, should immediately incorporate these data standards into their contractual and regulatory requirements (e.g., Medicare conditions of participation).

A Secure Interoperable Platform for Exchange of Patient Information Across Health Care Settings

Sharing patient data across providers and settings of care requires an interoperable infrastructure to provide clinicians with access to critical health care information at the time of care delivery. To meet this need, the strategic framework for the NHII calls for (1) fostering of regional collaborations; (2) a set of common national communication tools, such as web services architecture, security technologies, and a national health information network, that can provide low-cost and secure data movement; and (3) coordination of existing federal health information systems consistent with the NHII.

Several initiatives are now under way to develop regional collaborations for the creation of this interoperable infrastructure. First, the Health Resources and Services Administration (HRSA) has a cooperative agreement with the Foundation for eHealth Initiative to administer the Connecting Communities for Better Health program. The $2.3 million program provides seed funding and support to multistakeholder collaboratives within communities (both geographic and nongeographic) for the implementation of health information exchanges, including the formation of regional health information organizations (Thompson and Brailer, 2004). Second, in October 2004, the Agency for Healthcare Research and Quality (AHRQ) awarded $139 million in grants and contracts to promote the use of health information technology through the development of networks for sharing clinical data, as well as to support projects for planning, implementing, and demonstrating the value of IT (AHRQ, 2004). Finally, Connecting for Health, a public–private collaborative of more than 100 diverse organizations, has launched a prototype electronic national health information exchange based on common, open standards that will allow authorized users of three very different health information networks located in California, Massachusetts, and Indiana to share health information both within and among their local regions and communities. Teams in Mendocino, Boston, and Indianapolis will work with one another and with Connecting for Health to launch prototype networks that will connect the diverse technologies within each region's health network and accommodate the differing social and economic profiles of the various communities (Markle Foundation, 2005).

In general, however, the committee finds that information needs pertaining to health care for M/SU conditions have not been well addressed in these initiatives.

NEED FOR ATTENTION TO MENTAL AND SUBSTANCE-USE CONDITIONS IN THE NHII

There is evidence that health care for M/SU conditions could be better addressed in the many efforts under way to develop the NHII. For example, in the "comprehensive catalogue of identifiable federal health information technology programs" included in the framework for strategic action submitted to the President by the National Coordinator for Health Information Technology, the listing of IT initiatives by DHHS agencies identifies those of AHRQ, the Centers for Medicare and Medicaid Services (CMS), the Food and Drug Administration (FDA), the National Institutes of Health (NIH), the Indian Health Service (IHS), HRSA, and the Centers for Disease Control and Prevention (CDC), among others. There is no listing for the Substance Abuse and Mental Health Services Administration (SAMHSA) and its IT initiatives (Thompson and Brailer, 2004). A subsequent July 2005 update still contained no listing of SAMHSA's IT initiatives (ONCHIT, 2005). Moreover, although SAMHSA is listed as a partner in the federal government's Consolidated Health Informatics initiative, it is not listed as a member of any of the work groups consisting of staff from many federal agencies, including CMS, ARHQ, IHS, CDC, NIH, the Department of Defense, the National Library of Medicine, the National Aeronautics and Space Administration, the Social Security Administration, the Environmental Protection Agency, the U.S. Agency for International Development, and the National Center for Health Statistics, that have established vocabularies and standards for demographic, diagnosis and problem list, encounter, medication, interventions and procedures, billing, and other types of data (OMB, undated).

In addition, health care for M/SU conditions was not strongly represented among either the applicants or awardees in AHRQ's 2004 awards of $139 million in grants and contracts to promote the use of health IT through the development of networks for sharing clinical data, as well as to support projects for planning, implementing, and demonstrating the value of IT. Of the nearly 600 applications for funding, only "a handful" had any substantial behavioral health content, and of the 103 grants awarded, only 1 specifically targeted M/SU health care.[4]

Finally, leaders of SAMHSA's predominantly public-sector Mental Health Statistics Improvement Project (MHSIP) initiative (discussed below) note that MHSIP has not been "at the table" when broader data initiatives have been developed (Smith et al., 2004). Moreover, SAMHSA has identified important features of health care for mental conditions that are not captured in datasets approved under the Health Insurance Portability and Accountability Act (HIPAA). SAMHSA plans to address these issues through its Decision Support 2000+ (DS 2000+) initiative (Manderscheid and Henderson, 2003). Alternatively, these issues could be brought before the standards-setting groups referenced in the HIPAA legislation and used to inform the development of HIPAA-approved datasets that would serve both the private and public sectors. Moreover, because primary care providers are increasingly providing care for mental conditions, these impor-

---

[4]Conversation with Scott Young, MD, Director of Health Information Technology, Agency for Healthcare Research and Quality, November 1, 2004.

tant features of mental health care need to be identified and considered with respect to data standards intended for primary care as well.

The committee concludes that mental and substance-use health care systems and treatment providers in both the public and private sectors should have a strong voice in efforts to create the NHII, including the creation of data standards, regional and community health information networks, and EHRs. Their participation will ensure that the characteristics of mental health and substance-use services with unique implications for the NHII will be addressed in its design, and that the benefits of the NHII will accrue to consumers of M/SU health care. Substantial expertise exists with regard to the clinical data needs for quality M/SU health care and the information systems required for M/SU clinical care, performance measurement, policy planning, and research. This expertise should be brought to bear in the various initiatives to build the NHII.

INFORMATION TECHNOLOGY INITIATIVES FOR HEALTH CARE FOR MENTAL/SUBSTANCE-USE CONDITIONS

Efforts to create components of an information infrastructure for mental and substance-use health care have been under way for some time—predominantly in the public sector under the auspices of SAMHSA. The knowledge and networks of experts generated by these activities should be invaluable resources in the development of the NHII. This section reviews these initiatives, as well as two issues pertinent to development of the NHII with respect to M/SU health care: the need to balance privacy concerns with data access, and the delivery of care for M/SU conditions by non–health care sectors, which may also be users of the NHII.

Information Infrastructure Initiatives for Health Care for M/SU Conditions

SAMHSA Initiatives

Mental health Decision Support 2000+ and statistics improvement program SAMHSA's Decision Support 2000+ (DS 2000+) initiative is developing an integrated set of mental health data standards and information infrastructure to collect data on community health and population characteristics, enrollment in insurance programs, clients' utilization of services and encounters, providers' use of evidence-based practices, patient outcomes, and other performance measures. Work is nearly complete on core data standards for enrollment and encounter data; drafts of core datasets exist for the other data domains; and three parallel stakeholder-specific datasets are being developed for state mental health systems, providers, and consumers/families. SAMHSA envisions that most of the data elements in the core person/enrollment, encounter, and financial datasets will be based on required HIPAA data elements; those not based on the HIPAA data elements will be "value added" DS 2000+ data elements. SAMHSA plans to implement these standards by embedding them into web-based software, which will be made available to the industry. SAMHSA has partnered with the Software and Technology Vendors' Association (SATVA), which serves behavioral health and human services organizations, to implement the DS 2000+ data standards and develop a national online decision-support infrastructure. DS 2000+ will differ from the NHII in that it is envisioned to contain no individually identifiable data; instead, aggregate data will be deidentified at the provider or state level (Manderscheid and Henderson, 2003; Smith et al., 2004).

DS 2000+ is in part a product of the long-standing and ongoing activities of MHSIP. Sponsored initially by the National Institute of Mental Health and now by SAMHSA, MHSIP's structure consists of an ad hoc policy group that provides national leadership, direction, and consensus development around issues related to mental health data collection, and of regional users groups that include all 50 states, the District of Columbia, and 6 U.S. territories. Over the past 25 years, MHSIP has produced data standards and standardized tools such as report cards and consumer surveys that are in wide use across all states' public mental health systems. MHSIP's FN-10 data standards serve as the foundation for many state mental health data systems. Various aspects of its Consumer-Oriented Mental Health Report Card are being implemented by more than 45 states and territories. The MHSIP Consumer Survey also is widely used in the public sector. This instrument served as part of the basis for the Experience of Care and Health Outcomes Survey developed by Harvard University and adapted by the National Committee for Quality Assurance (NCQA) for use as part of the Healthplan Employer Data and Information Set (HEDIS) performance measure set. Implementation of MHSIP's standards and products is facilitated by the voluntary participation of staff from all state mental health agencies and by states' receipt of federal grants that have promoted the development of their data system infrastructures (Smith et al., 2004).

State data infrastructure grants SAMHSA has supported states in applying IT to improve health care for mental conditions through its State Data Infrastructure Grant program. Through this program, states are adopting common data and information technology standards, with a focus on improving information from local providers so that states can report data on the characteristics and performance of their mental health systems. As of 2005, 58 states and territories had received these grants, and the resulting data are being reported to the federal government (SAMHSA, 2005a).

Behavioral Health Data Standards Workgroup (BHDSW) SAMHSA recently convened an ad hoc work group to develop consensus on issues related to data standards for behavioral health. The work group shares its topical expertise on data standards in behavioral health care, apprises relevant groups in the behavioral health care field of activities and trends in national data standards, facilitates and coordinates efforts to influence national data standards, and supports the implementation of data standards in the behavioral health care field.

Uniform Reporting System (URS) for block grant reporting under performance partnership grants SAMHSA's Center for Mental Health Services (CMHS), in collaboration with state mental health agencies, developed the URS—a set of 23 performance measures for the states derived from administrative data and consumer surveys. Through the State Data Infrastructure Grants, the infrastructure needed to report these performance measures is being built. The 10 national outcome measures (see Chapter 5) defined by SAMHSA as critical performance measures for all agency grantees are a subset of the URS measures.[5]

EHRs and personal health records CMHS is currently implementing a contract to develop prototypes of an EHR and a personal health record (PHR) for consumers of mental health services. As an initial phase of this work, the contractor is reviewing work already under way in the field in both the public and private sectors. The direction of the EHR work is toward a core set of common data standards and interoperability among ongoing systems. The PHR work will center on consumer-operated websites for negotiating and evaluating local systems of care, as well as on collaboration with consumer and family groups to develop the content for a PHR. The contractor is also examining examples of the local health information infrastructure necessary to operate such systems.[6]

Substance abuse information system The Services Accountability Improvement System (SAIS) of SAMHSA's Center for Substance Abuse Treatment (CSAT) is an online, web-based information system used by all of SAMHSA's substance abuse treatment grantees to input data about their projects that can be used for improved project oversight. In addition, training and technical assistance are provided to grantees on the collection of Government Performance and Results Act (GPRA) data, with SAIS serving as a data

---

[5]Personal communication, Ronald Manderscheid, Chief, Survey and Analysis Branch, CMHS, SAMHSA, on July 27, 2005.
[6]Personal communication, Ronald Manderscheid, Chief, Survey and Analysis Branch, CMHS, SAMHSA, on July 27, 2005.

entry point for GPRA data collection. Moreover, SAIS currently serves as a data repository for more than 600 grantees, giving CSAT the capacity to report on populations served; types and locations of activities supported; effectiveness across programs for particular populations; and the characteristics and effectiveness across programs of activities related to national, subpopulation, and geographic area data and trends. The SAIS data also help improve clinical treatment programs and inform decisions on the intensity of monitoring, technical assistance needs, and funding requests. The feedback grantees receive from the system helps them evaluate and enhance their performance. In addition, the system is able to report on employment, involvement in the criminal justice system, and living situation among substance users; social, behavioral, and psychological consequences of drug and alcohol use; and other, related performance data.[7]

Drug Evaluation Network System (DENS) DENS (Carise et al., 1999), initially funded through the Office of National Drug Control Policy, was designed to serve as a national electronic treatment-information system, providing practical and timely clinical and administrative information on patients entering into substance-use treatment throughout the nation. The system also was designed to serve individual treatment programs by performing an electronic, standardized clinical admission assessment on every client entering treatment at the site. The questions within DENS are from the Addiction Severity Index (ASI), since it has been well tested and validated in many settings, and it is in the public domain and available without charge or restriction. Program staff administer the ASI interview and record the answers given on a lap-top computer. The raw ASI data are automatically transformed into a Joint Commission on Accreditation of Healthcare Organizations (JCAHO)-approved assessment, biopsychosocial narrative, and treatment plan for use by the program counselors (saving about 3 hours of work), and the raw data are automatically transmitted (without personal identifiers) to a server. Program-level summary reports are also available for directors on a quarterly basis. DENS has been in continuous operation at more than 100 experimental sites since 2003 and is now operational in more than 250 other sites. The Department of Veterans Affairs and many state and city systems use DENS.

Nationwide summit on behavioral health information management and the NHII SAMHSA and SATVA held a working summit in September 2005 to define a strategy for behavioral health information management and its role within the NHII. This summit provided an initial opportunity

---

[7]Personal communication, Mady Chalk, PhD, Director, Division of Services Improvement, CSAT, SAMHSA, on July 28, 2005.

for leaders of major stakeholder groups and national organizations to discuss such a strategy. The National Coordinator of Health Information Technology delivered the keynote address, thus beginning work on one of the summit's aims—incorporating behavioral health data and policy concerns into the NHII.

Private-Sector Initiatives

Mental Health Corporations of America This industry trade association for more than 100 leading community behavioral health organizations nationwide is working with SATVA in a joint effort to develop best-practice guidelines for selecting software, contracting with software vendors, and implementing information systems and EHRs.

The Davies Award This award is given annually by the Health Information Management Systems Society to a small number of organizations in recognition of their outstanding efforts to implement EHRs. In 2000, the award was extended to include behavioral health care organizations. Since that time, one such organization has received an honorable mention and another has won the award.

Unique Characteristics of M/SU Services with Implications for the NHII

As discussed in Chapter 2, M/SU health care has several features that distinguish it from general health care. Two of these features have implications for the development of the NHII: the particular importance of privacy concerns (discussed more fully in Chapter 5) and the fact that much care for M/SU conditions is delivered by or through the auspices of entities that are not primarily health care organizations, such as schools and child welfare agencies (also discussed in Chapter 5).

Need to Balance Privacy Concerns with Data Access

The privacy of M/SU treatment data is a sensitive issue, in part because of the stigma and discrimination described in Chapter 3. More broadly, this issue is grounded in people's common inclination to regard their most personal and intimate experiences, thoughts, and feelings as private and not readily shared outside of trusted relationships. Consequently, and as discussed more fully in Chapter 5, consumer data pertaining to M/SU treatment services are more protected than most general and other specialty health care data. These protections are reflected in federal and state regulations governing the disclosure of information related to health care for mental or substance-use conditions (detailed in Appendix B). While these regulations help assure consumers of M/SU services that their privacy will be protected, they also can create barriers to accessing data and complicate coordination of care, especially with respect to the use of EHRs and electronic networks. Public policy must balance the sometimes competing priorities of respect for data privacy and facilitation of appropriate data access to support care coordination.

Many privacy regulations address the exchange of paper-based information, although some, such as those contained in HIPAA, address data in electronic formats. However, none of these regulations explicitly address the more recently proposed and innovative components of the NHII, such as:

- Regional health information organizations (RHIOs) that will provide electronic networks containing data elements essential to care coordination and accessible by diverse participating health care organizations in a defined geographic region.
- PHRs that are consumer controlled, incorporate selected data elements from existing health records, and include data a consumer may choose to add for service providers' attention.

Work is under way on formulating, developing, and implementing RHIOs (such as the Connecting for Health Initiative discussed above) and PHRs as components of the NHII. The National Committee on Vital and Health Statistics has received testimony on the new types of privacy challenges that will be generated by the NHII and on how these challenges should be addressed (Newman, 2005).

Care Delivered by or Through Non–Health Care Sectors

As discussed in Chapter 5, much M/SU health care is delivered by or through agencies not typically considered part of the health care sector. In particular, the education system delivers the majority of mental health services to children. The welfare and criminal justice systems also are involved in the delivery of much M/SU health care. How are services delivered in schools to be captured in the NHII? Will the NHII capture data only on services that generate a claim or encounter form? Should schools have access to the clinical information on the NHII about their students? What special confidentiality provisions might apply to children served through the welfare system? Can or should the welfare system have access to data on the NHII? These and similar questions need to be addressed in the design of the NHII so it will capture the data needed for effective care coordination while protecting patient privacy.

BUILDING THE CAPACITY OF CLINICIANS TREATING MENTAL AND SUBSTANCE-USE CONDITIONS TO PARTICIPATE IN THE NHII

The utility to the M/SU health care field of the above system-level initiatives to build information infrastructure will ultimately depend upon the capacity of M/SU health care clinicians and organizations to fully utilize the NHII and accompanying technologies as they develop. The less well developed IT infrastructure among M/SU health care clinicians and organizations, the small size of many M/SU clinicians' practices, the more diverse M/SU workforce, and financial considerations are likely to impede the ability of these providers to participate in the NHII and must be addressed.

Less Use of Information Technology Among M/SU Providers

M/SU health care generally has less well developed information systems compared with general health care (Trabin and Maloney, 2003). SATVA testified to the committee that more complex billing, reimbursement, and regulatory reporting requirements for M/SU health care have required treatment providers (individual clinicians, group practices, community mental health centers, and treatment facilities) to focus the use of IT on billing and other functions unrelated to quality of care (Paton, 2004).

With respect to substance-use treatment providers, telephone interviews conducted in 2003 with a random sample of 175 directors of inpatient/residential, outpatient, and methadone maintenance programs across the nation revealed that approximately 20 percent of programs had no information services of any type, e-mail, or even voice mail for their phone systems. Fifty percent had some form of computerized administrative information system for billing or administrative record keeping, but their information services were typically available only to administrative staff. Thirty percent of the programs—mostly those that were part of a larger hospital or health systems—had seemingly well-developed information systems; however, only 3 of the 175 treatment programs had an integrated clinical information system for use by the majority of their treatment staff (McLellan et al., 2003). Part of the problem is the many M/SU clinicians practicing independently or as part of small group practices, as discussed below. The size of health care provider organizations has been shown to be related to the uptake of IT. As noted earlier, for example, use of EHRs is typically found in larger health care organizations (Brailer and Terasawa, 2003).

Many Mental Health and Substance-Use
Clinicians in Solo or Small Practices

Many mental health clinicians report that "individual practice" is either their primary or secondary[8] employment setting (Duffy et al., 2004) (see Chapter 7). This has substantial implications for these clinicians' uptake and use of IT. A 2000–2001 nationally representative telephone survey of physicians involved in direct patient care in the continental United States, for example, found wide variation in IT adoption across physician practices, with practice setting, especially size, being a much more important determinant of adoption than age of provider, practice location (metropolitan or nonmetropolitan area), or type of specialty. In examining IT adoption for five clinical functions—obtaining treatment guidelines, exchanging clinical data with other physicians, accessing patient notes, generating treatment reminders for physicians, and writing prescriptions—the survey found that the vast majority of patients were treated in physician practices lacking significant IT support for patient care. One-quarter of all physicians were in practices with no computer or other form of IT support for any of the five functions, and another quarter had IT support for just one function. Among the five functions examined, physicians were most likely to report that IT was used in their practice to access treatment guidelines (53 percent) (Reed and Grossman, 2004).

The survey further found that nearly 60 percent of physicians in traditional practice settings—solo, small groups with up to 50 physicians, or practices owned by hospitals—reported that their practice used IT for no more than one of the five clinical functions. Highest levels of IT support for patient care were found in staff- and group-model health maintenance organization (HMO) practices, followed by medical school faculty practices and large group practices. IT support varied to a lesser extent among primary care and medical and surgical specialists; some differences remained after controlling for practice setting, location, and physician age.

Psychiatrists as a group had statistically significant lower rates of IT support for patient care compared with all physicians, although psychiatrists practicing in hospitals, in staff/group HMOs, in medical schools, or as part of large (>50) group practices had significantly higher IT support than those in traditional practice settings.[9] The authors theorize that the differ-

---

[8]Many mental health practitioners work in multiple settings. For example, 60 percent of full-time psychiatrists reported working in two or more settings in 1998, as did 50 percent of psychologists, 20 percent of full-time counselors, and 29 percent of marriage/family therapists in 2002. Rates were higher for part-time counselors (Duffy et al., 2004).

[9]E-mail communication, Joy Grossman, PhD, Center for Studying Health System Change, on November 4, 2005.

ences in adoption by practice setting can be explained by larger groups' and HMOs' readier access to capital and administrative support staff, the ability to spread acquisition and implementation costs among more physicians, and active physician leadership in IT adoption (Reed and Grossman, 2004).

Data and observations from experts in the use of information systems among managed behavioral health care organizations support this premise. With respect to administrative (as opposed to clinical) IT applications, smaller providers in behavioral health care have lagged behind in use of electronic claims submission (Trabin and Maloney, 2003). Consistent with this observation, the survey of substance-use treatment providers described above found that although approximately 20 percent of surveyed programs had no information services of any type, e-mail, or even voice mail for their phone system, most of those that were part of larger hospital or health systems (approximately 30 percent of the sample) had access to well-developed clinical information systems, e-mail, and Internet services (McLellan et al., 2003).

The Center for Studying Health System Change has suggested that because barriers to IT adoption appear to be greatest for smaller practices, policy incentives for the uptake of IT may need to pay particular attention to those barriers. According to the center, direct grants or loans to acquire IT and strategies to lower the cost of IT may be especially successful approaches for smaller practices; some have advocated a government-sponsored funding mechanism, similar to the Hill-Burton Act for hospitals, to provide capital for IT to physicians and other providers (Reed and Grossman, 2004).

Diverse Types of Health Care Providers

Crossing the Quality Chasm notes that the health care workforce overall is highly variable in terms of IT-related knowledge and experience, and probably also in terms of receptivity to learning or acquiring these new skills (IOM, 2001). This is likely to be equally or more so the case with respect to M/SU clinicians because of their greater variability in education and training (see Chapter 7). Information system executives at six major managed behavioral health organizations and one HMO interviewed in 1999 reported a wide gap between their organization's interest in and readiness to adopt IT and that of their providers, as well as low acceptance of various technologies among clinical providers. For example, the managed behavioral health organizations and HMO reported that they could not require electronic transmission of claims and other forms because too few providers had the necessary skills and equipment to comply (Trabin and Maloney, 2003).

Varied Reimbursement and Reporting Requirements

Treatment providers, many of whom, as noted, are in solo or small group practices, must respond to varied and complex reimbursement and reporting requirements. With respect to substance-use treatment providers, for example, the telephone interviews conducted in 2003 with a random sample of 175 directors of inpatient/residential, outpatient, and methadone maintenance programs across the nation found that most of the programs had contracts with multiple managed care organizations and state agencies (e.g., justice, welfare), each requiring different data. Several programs reported that the data requirements of all these agencies required 2–4 hours of data collection per admission, and these administrative data were the only information collected by 30 percent of programs. Programs further indicated that "almost none" of these administrative data were clinically useful or employed in program planning. Staff described their collection as "just paperwork" (McLellan et al., 2003).

Simplifying these requirements will necessitate action across states—by insurers and/or by multiple state agencies. The committee calls attention to the need for a mechanism to examine variations in billing and reporting requirements and for efforts to reduce this variation to the extent possible across states and localities.

Financial Issues

Crossing the Quality Chasm (IOM, 2001) notes that deployment of IT requires a significant financial investment. Capital is needed by providers to purchase and install new technology (typically accompanied by temporary disruptions in patient care); specialized training and education are needed as well. With respect to EHRs, in two recent reports (IOM, 2003, 2004) the IOM has recommended that both public- and private-sector purchasers consider linking provider incentives to the acquisition of EHRs that possess the capabilities outlined by the IOM.

The strategic framework developed by the federal government also proposes three strategies for countering financial barriers to the adoption of EHRs: incentivizing the adoption of EHRs, reducing the risk of EHR investment, and supporting EHR diffusion in rural and underserved areas. Potential incentive mechanisms identified in the framework include incorporating support for EHRs in grants or contracts to regions, states, and communities for local IT infrastructure; making available low-interest loans for IT adoption; reimbursing for the use of EHRs; and incorporating EHR use in pay-for-performance projects (Thompson and Brailer, 2004).

INTEGRATING HEALTH CARE FOR MENTAL AND SUBSTANCE-USE CONDITIONS INTO THE NHII

The committee concludes that strong actions are needed to involve M/SU health care organizations, systems of care, and treatment providers quickly and directly in efforts to create the NHII, including initiatives to (1) develop EHR systems with decision-support capabilities, (2) design a secure platform for the exchange of patient information across health care settings, and (3) develop data standards that will make shared information understandable to all users. To this end, the committee makes the following recommendations.

Recommendation 6-1. To realize the benefits of the emerging National Health Information Infrastructure (NHII) for consumers of M/SU health care services, the secretaries of DHHS and the Department of Veterans Affairs should charge the Office of the National Coordinator of Health Information Technology and the Substance Abuse and Mental Health Services Administration to jointly develop and implement a plan for ensuring that the various components of the emerging NHII—including data and privacy standards, electronic health records, and community and regional health networks—address M/SU health care as fully as general health care. As part of this strategy:

- DHHS should create and support a continuing mechanism to engage M/SU health care stakeholders in the public and private sectors in developing consensus-based recommendations for the data elements, standards, and processes needed to address unique aspects of information management related to M/SU health care. These recommendations should be provided to the appropriate standards-setting entities and initiatives working with the Office of the National Coordinator of Health Information Technology.
- Federal grants and contracts for the development of components of the NHII should require and use as a criterion for making awards the involvement and inclusion of M/SU health care.
- The Substance Abuse and Mental Health Services Administration should increase its work with public and private stakeholders to support the building of information infrastructure components that address M/SU health care and coordinate these information initiatives with the NHII.
- Policies and information technology infrastructure should be used to create linkages (consistent with all privacy requirements) among patient records and other data sources pertaining to M/SU services received from health care providers and from education, social, criminal justice, and other agencies.

Recommendation 6-2. Public- and private-sector individuals, including organizational leaders in M/SU health care, should become involved in, and provide for staff involvement in, major national committees and initiatives working to set health care data and information technology standards to ensure that the unique needs of M/SU health care are designed into these initiatives at their earliest stages.

Recommendation 6-3. National associations of purchasers—such as the National Association of State Mental Health Program Directors, the National Association of State Alcohol and Drug Abuse Directors, the National Association of State Medicaid Directors, the National Association of County Behavioral Health Directors, the American Managed Behavioral Healthcare Association, and the national Blue Cross and Blue Shield Association—should decrease the burden of variable reporting and billing requirements by standardizing requirements at the national, state, and local levels.

Recommendation 6-4. Federal and state governments, public- and private-sector purchasers of M/SU health care, and private foundations should encourage the widespread adoption of electronic health records, computer-based clinical decision-support systems, computerized provider order entry, and other forms of information technology for M/SU care by:

- Offering financial incentives to individual M/SU clinicians and organizations for investments in information technology needed to participate fully in the emerging NHII.
- Providing capital and other incentives for the development of virtual networks to give individual and small-group providers standard access to software, clinical and population data and health records, and billing and clinical decision-support systems.
- Providing financial support for continuing technical assistance, training, and information technology maintenance.
- Including in purchasing decisions an assessment of the use of information technology by clinicians and health care organizations for clinical decision support, electronic health records, and other quality improvement applications.

With regard to recommendation 6-1, calling for the implementation of a plan to ensure that the emerging NHII will address health care for mental and substance-use conditions as fully as it does general health care, the committee again (see Chapter 5) calls attention to the diverse confidentiality laws created by states pertaining to the sharing of patient information on mental health care and to federal laws governing the sharing of information on substance-use diagnosis and treatment. These laws have substantial implications for the sharing of electronic information, just as they do for the sharing of information in other media. The committee therefore underscores the importance of its recommendations in Chapter 5 regarding the sharing of information on the part of providers of M/SU health care and the importance of eliminating inappropriate legal, regulatory, and administrative barriers to such communications:

> **Recommendation 5-1.** To make collaboration and coordination of patients' M/SU health care services the norm, providers of the services should establish clinically effective linkages within their own organizations and between providers of mental health and substance-use treatment. The necessary communications and interactions should take place with the patient's knowledge and consent and be fostered by:
>
> - Routine sharing of information on patients' problems and pharmacologic and nonpharmacologic treatments among and between providers of M/SU treatment. . . .
>
> **Recommendation 5-2.** To facilitate the delivery of coordinated care by primary care, mental health, and substance-use treatment providers, government agencies, purchasers, health plans, and accreditation organizations should implement policies and incentives to continually increase collaboration among these providers to achieve evidence-based screening and care of their patients with general, mental, and/or substance-use health conditions. The following specific measures should be undertaken to carry out this recommendation: . . .
>
> - Federal and state governments should revise laws, regulations, and administrative practices that create inappropriate barriers to the communication of information between providers of health care for mental and substance-use conditions and between those providers and providers of general care.

The committee also emphasizes that developing an effective mechanism to engage M/SU treatment stakeholders in the public and private sectors in the development of consensus recommendations for the entities and initiatives working with ONCHIT will require an ongoing commitment of resources from DHHS. This commitment will enable an ongoing process whereby the M/SU field can identify informatics needs pertaining to M/SU health care whose inclusion in the evolving IT initiative is important. Some of this work may already be under way. Following up on the President's New Freedom Commission on Mental Health, in July 2005 SAMHSA announced plans to develop a strategy for implementing innovative technology in the mental health field. SAMHSA plans to convene a consensus development work group, including ONCHIT and other public- and private-sector experts and stakeholders, to review the current status of telemedicine, information technology, Internet technology, and electronic decision-support tools in health care; examine the current status of implementation of these tools in mental health; and prepare key recommendations for immediate next steps in technology support for mental health services. SAMHSA also plans to explore the creation of a Capital Investment Fund for Technology to work with states in the design and implementation of an EHR and information system (SAMHSA, 2005b). These efforts should ensure the inclusion of both public- and private-sector issues and substance-use as well as mental health care in the ongoing IT initiative.

With respect to the recommendation that public- and private-sector individual and organizational leaders in health care for M/SU conditions become involved in national initiatives to set health care data and information technology standards, the committee notes that several public- and private-sector organizations and initiatives could illuminate key information and technology needs for M/SU health care that should be incorporated in the NHII. The 25 years of experience of the MHSIP and its regional users groups is an invaluable resource that can inform the NHII initiative.

REFERENCES

AHIMA e-HIM Personal Health Record Work Group. 2005. *Defining the Personal Health Record*. [Online]. Available: http://library.ahima.org/xpedia/groups/public/documents/ahima/pub_bok1_027351.html [accessed July 26, 2005].

AHRQ (Agency for Healthcare Research and Quality). 2004. *Health Information Technology Programs: State and Regional Demonstrations in Health Information Technology; Transforming Healthcare Quality Through Health Information Technology (THQIT); National Health Information Technology Resource Center (National HITRC). Fact Sheet*. Rockville, MD: AHRQ. [Online]. Available: http://www.ahrq.gov/research/hitfact.htm [accessed October 29, 2004].

Anonymous. 2004. *Consolidated Health Informatics*. [Online]. Available: http://www.whitehouse.gov/onb/egov/gtob/health_informatics.htm [accessed October 31, 2004].

Brailer DJ, Terasawa E. 2003. *Use and Adoption of Computer-Based Patient Records in the United States*. Presentation to IOM Committee on Data Standards for Patient Safety on January 23, 2003. [Online]. Available: http://www.iom.edu/file.asp?id=10988 [accessed October 17, 2004].

Carise D, McLellan AT, Gifford L, Kleber H. 1999. Developing a national addiction treatment information system: An introduction to the Drug Evaluation Network System. *Journal of Substance Abuse Treatment* 17(1–2):67–77.

CCHIT (Certification Commission for Healthcare Information Technology). 2004. *About CCHIT—A Certification Commission for Healthcare Information Technology: A Voluntary, Private-Sector Initiative to Certify HIT Products*. [Online]. Available: http://www.cchit.org/about.htm [accessed July 26, 2005].

CMS (Centers for Medicare and Medicaid Services). 2005. *CMS Delivers Electronic Health Record Software to Physician Offices*. Evaluation version of Vista-Office expected to improve quality of care and stem costs. Press release. [Online]. Available: http://www.cms.hhs.gov/media/press/release.asp?Counter =1563 [accessed October 13, 2005].

DHHS (U.S. Department of Health and Human Services). 2005a. *American Health Information Community (the Community)*. [Online]. Available: http://www.hhs.gov/healthit/ahic. html [accessed July 25, 2005].

DHHS. 2005b. *Office of the National Coordinator for Health Information Technology (ONCHIT): Mission*. [Online]. Available: http://www.os.dhhs.gov/healthit/mission.html [accessed April 5, 2005].

Duffy FF, West JC, Wilk J, Narrow WE, Hales D, Thompson J, Regier DA, Kohout J, Pion GM, Wicherski MM, Bateman N, Whitaker T, Merwin EI, Lyon D, Fox JC, Delaney KR, Hanrahan N, Stockton R, Garbelman J, Kaladow J, Clawson TW, Smith SC, Bergman DM, Northey WF, Blankertz L, Thomas A, Sullivan LD, Dwyer KP, Fleischer MS, Woodruff CR, Goldsmith HF, Henderson MJ, Atay JJ, Manderscheid RW. 2004. Mental health practitioners and trainees. In: Manderscheid RW, Henderson MJ, eds. *Mental Health, United States, 2002*. DHHS publication Number: (SMA) 3938. Rockville, MD: U.S. Department of Health and Human Services. Pp. 327–368.

Flanagan RD, Needham SL. 2003. The internet. In: Feldman S, ed. *Managed Behavioral Health Services: Perspectives and Practice*. Springfield, IL: Charles C. Thomas, Publisher Pp. 307–325.

IOM (Institute of Medicine). 2001. *Crossing the Quality Chasm: A New Health System for the 21st Century*. Washington, DC: National Academy Press.

IOM. 2003. *Key Capabilities of an Electronic Health Record System*. Washington, DC: The National Academies Press.

IOM. 2004. Aspden P, Corrigan JM, Wolcott J, Erickson SM, eds. *Patient Safety: Achieving a New Standard for Care*. Washington, DC: The National Academies Press.

Kolata G. 2005, July 21. In unexpected Medicare benefit U.S. will offer doctors free electronic records system. *New York Times*. p. A14.

Manderscheid RW, Henderson MJ. 2003. A progress report on Decision Support 2000+. *Behavioral Health Management* 23(2):46–47.

Markle Foundation. 2005. *Prototype for a Nationwide Health Information Exchange Launched by Connecting for Health*. [Online]. Available: http:www.connectingforhealth.org/news/pressrelease_060105.html [accessed July 25, 2005].

McLellan TA, Carise D, Kleber HD. 2003. Can the national addiction treatment infrastructure support the public's demand for quality care? *Journal of Substance Abuse Treatment* 25(2):117–121.

National Committee on Vital and Health Statistics. 2001. *Information for Health: A Strategy for Building the National Health Information Infrastructure*. [Online]. Available: http://ncvhs.hhs.gov/nhiilayo.pdf [accessed October 15, 2004].

Newman R. 2005. Testimony to the Subcommittee on Privacy and Confidentiality of the National Committee on Vital and Health Statistics on March 30, 2005. American Psychological Association. [Online]. Available: http://www.apapractice.org/apo/press/whatshot/testimony.

OMB (Office of Management and Budget). Undated. *E-GOV—Presidential Initiatives—Consolidated Health Informatics*. [Online]. Available: http://www.whitehouse.gov/omb/egov/c-3-6-chi.htm [accessed April 5, 2005].

ONCHIT (Office of the National Coordinator for Health Information Technology). 2005. *Directory of Federal HIT Programs*. [Online]. Available: http://www.os.dhhs.gov/healthit/federalprojectlist.html [accessed April 5, 2005].

Paton JA. 2004.Testimony before the Institute of Medicine Committee, Crossing the Quality Chasm: Adaptation for Mental Health and Addictive Disorders. September 14, 2004. Available from the Institute of Medicine.

Reed MC, Grossman JM. 2004. *Limited Information Technology for Patient Care in Physician Offices*. No. 89. Issue Brief. Washington, DC: Center for Studying Health System Change. [Online]. Available: http://www.hschange.org/CONTENT/708/708.pdf [accessed November 1, 2004].

SAMHSA (Substance Abuse and Mental Health Services Administration). 2005a. *Fiscal Year 2006 Justification of Estimates for Appropriations Committees*. [Online]. Available: http://www.samhsa.gov/budget/FY2006/FY2006Budget.doc [accessed March 26, 2005].

SAMHSA. 2005b. *Transforming Mental Health Care in America. The Federal Action Agenda: First Steps*. [Online]. Available: http://www.samhsa.gov/Federalactionagenda/NFC_TOC.aspx [accessed July 23, 2005].

Smith ME, Davis S, Ganju V, Tremaine L, Adams N, Felton HC, Gonzalez O, Hall J, Hopkins C, Lutterman T, Smith M, Tracy B, Manderscheid RW. 2004. *Twenty-Five Years of the Mental Health Statistics Improvement Program: Past, Present, and Future—Where Have We Been and Where Are We Going?* DHHS Publication Number: (SMA) 3938. Rockville, MD: Center for Mental Health Services, Substance Use and Mental Health Services Administration.

Thompson TG, Brailer DJ. 2004. *The Decade of Information Technology: Delivering Consumer-Centric and Information-Rich Health Care Framework for Strategic Action*. [Online]. Available: http://www.hhs.gov/onchit/hitframework.pdf [accessed October 24, 2004].

Trabin T, Maloney W. 2003. Information systems. In: Feldman S, ed. *Managed Behavioral Health Services: Perspectives and Practices*. Springfield, IL: Charles C. Thomas Publisher. Pp. 326–370.

7

Increasing Workforce Capacity for Quality Improvement

Summary

The health care workforce treating mental and/or substance-use (M/SU) conditions is not equipped uniformly and sufficiently in terms of knowledge and skills, cultural diversity and understanding, geographic distribution, and numbers to provide the access to and quality of M/SU services needed by consumers. This has long been the case and has been persistently resistant to change despite recurring acknowledgments of the problems and repeated recommendations for major improvements to address them.

Although similar to those that afflict the general health care workforce, these problems require special attention in the M/SU workforce not only because of the high prevalence and serious consequences of M/SU problems and illnesses (see Chapter 1), but also because of the great variation in the types of clinicians licensed to diagnose and treat M/SU conditions and substantial variations in their training. In contrast to general health care, in which the diagnosis and treatment of medical conditions are typically provided by physicians, individuals licensed to diagnose and treat M/SU problems and illnesses include a wide range of practitioners—psychologists, psychiatrists, primary care and specialist physicians, social workers, psychiatric nurses, marriage and family therapists, addiction therapists, and a wide variety of counselors (e.g., psychosocial rehabilitation, school, addiction, and pastoral counselors), many of whom are licensed to provide M/SU services in independent

286

practice. These practitioners are trained apart from each other— in different schools by different faculties, with curriculums encompassing few if any core competencies and little interdisciplinary training. Further, despite the wide variety of theories and therapies that have been developed to deal with M/SU problems and illnesses (see Chapter 4), there are no mechanisms in place to ensure that any given clinician has been adequately educated and trained to offer any specific therapy. Such a process is essential to the provision of safe, effective, and efficient care. The wide variety of provider types and treatments makes it difficult to provide consumers of M/SU health care with information on the competencies of any particular practitioner and to assist them in finding the right clinician for help, a key element of patient-centered care. Variations in state licensing requirements further complicate efforts to reduce inappropriate variations in care.

There is a long history of short-lived and unheeded commissions, expert panels, reports, and recommendations to improve the capacity and quality of the M/SU workforce. Reports dealing with the general health care workforce typically have failed to address the unique issues in M/SU health care. Those that have done so have addressed either mental health or substance use, but not both. Substance use, despite its magnitude and high rate of comorbidity with mental health problems, is often neglected in the professional training of all the major mental health disciplines and the training received by primary health care practitioners as well. Training does not sufficiently emphasize the advances made in evidence-based practice for treatment of mental and substance-use conditions, nor does it include enough content on self-help groups, community systems of support, and social services. Teaching methods across all the schools in which the M/SU disciplines are trained vary substantially as well, reflecting little cognizance of the advances that have been made in evidence-based teaching methods and lifelong learning.

Past recommendations calling for changes in the curriculums and methods for educating and training M/SU practitioners have typically been ignored. As a result, there continues to be a large gap between what is known, what is taught, and therefore what is done in practice. Sustained, multiyear attention and resources have been applied successfully to the education and training of physicians and nurses through the Council on Graduate Medical Education and the National Advisory Council on Nurse Education and Practice. A similar sustained, multiyear strategy, as well as action by institutions of higher education, licensing boards, accrediting bodies, the federal government, and purchasers, is needed to increase the M/SU workforce's competencies to deliver high-quality care.

CRITICAL ROLE OF THE WORKFORCE AND LIMITATIONS TO ITS EFFECTIVENESS

Previous reports of the Institute of Medicine (IOM) and other authoritative bodies have documented the critical roles played by the health care workforce in the delivery of high-quality health care. *Crossing the Quality Chasm* identifies the health care workforce as the health system's most important resource, and critical to improving the quality of care (IOM, 2001). All of the recommendations of the previous chapters—providing patient-centered, safe, effective, and coordinated care and taking advantages of the opportunities offered by information technology—require a workforce sufficient in numbers, with the necessary competencies, and enabled by the environments in which they practice to deliver care consistent with these competencies. However, the entire health care workforce—including those who provide care for mental and substance-use conditions—faces numerous obstacles to delivering high-quality care. These include a shortage and geographic maldistribution of workers (see Box 7-1), work environments that thwart clinicians' delivery of quality health care (AHRQ, 2003; IOM, 2004b), a lack of ethnic diversity and cultural expertise (IOM, 2004a) (see Box 7-2), outdated education and training content and methods (IOM, 2003), state-to-state variation in scopes of practice and assurance of competency, and concerns about legal liability (IOM, 2001).

Although the M/SU health care workforce faces all of the same problems as the health care workforce overall, building its capacity to deliver higher-quality care for M/SU conditions is particularly problematic because of the greater variety of types of M/SU health care providers and an even greater variation in how they are educated, licensed, and certified/credentialed for practice. While recognizing the importance of such problems as workforce shortages, geographic maldistribution, and insufficient diversity that afflict the M/SU and general health care workforces alike, this chapter focuses on the special problems resulting from the greater diversity of the M/SU health care workforce, their varying education and training, and the difficulties of delivering high-quality patient care in the solo practices that are more typical among those who treat M/SU conditions.

GREATER VARIATION IN THE WORKFORCE TREATING M/SU CONDITIONS

Caregivers who provide care to individuals with M/SU problems and illnesses, like those who care for those with general health care problems

---

BOX 7-1   Workforce Shortages and Geographic Maldistribution

Shortages and maldistribution of M/SU treatment professionals, as in the general health care workforce, are a major and long-recognized problem. In 1999, the Surgeon General's report on mental health stated: "The supply of well-trained mental health professionals is inadequate in many areas of the country, especially in rural areas. Particularly keen shortages are found in the numbers of mental health professionals serving children and adolescents with serious mental disorders, and older people" (DHHS, 1999:455). Echoing this statement, in 2003 the President's New Freedom Commission on Mental Health reported: "In rural and other geographically remote areas, many people with mental illnesses have inadequate access to care [and] limited availability of skilled care providers. . ." (New Freedom Commission on Mental Health, 2003:51).

Despite recognition of the problem and various attempts to motivate people to work in underserved areas, however, little progress has been made. In the east south central region of the United States (Alabama, Kentucky, Mississippi, and Tennessee), for example, there are 8.2 psychiatrists per 100,000 population, compared with 22.1 per 100,000 in the mid-Atlantic region (New Jersey, New York, and Pennsylvania). Similarly, there are 53.0 psychologists per 100,000 people in New England, compared with 14.4 per 100,000 in the west south central states, such as Arkansas, Oklahoma, and Texas (Duffy et al., 2004). Shortages of clinicians with expertise in caring for certain groups, such as children and adolescents (Koppelman, 2004) and older adults (New Freedom Commission on Mental Health, 2003), also persist nationwide. This variation reflects the historical tendency of highly skilled professionals to locate in urban areas (Morris et al., 2004).

Similar problems in the substance-use treatment workforce have been documented. Low salaries are accompanied by high turnover rates in both managerial and clinical positions (McLellan et al., 2003). This situation can compromise continuity of care for patients and also threatens to leave the field without a leadership infrastructure through which advances in care can be infused. Moreover, the stigma experienced by individuals with substance-use illnesses is sometimes felt by their treatment providers (Kaplan, 2003).

---

and illnesses, include licensed clinicians; unlicensed, paid providers (both certified and uncertified); volunteers; and the patient's family and informal supports. The roles of patients and their families in care and illness management, as well as those of individuals in recovery who offer peer and recovery support services, are addressed in Chapter 3. In this chapter we focus on the role of the licensed M/SU treatment workforce.[1]

---

[1]Although the role of unlicensed and voluntary care providers is substantial and important, the committee focuses here on licensed caregivers because the education and oversight structures for unlicensed voluntary caregivers are less well developed at present. Moreover, the committee believes that a well-trained and -educated licensed and credentialed workforce, through its leadership and modeling of best-care practices such as patient-centered care, can do much to strengthen the knowledge, skills, and abilities of the unlicensed workforce and volunteer supports.

BOX 7-2   Insufficient Workforce Diversity

Like the health care workforce overall (IOM, 2004a), the M/SU workforce does not reflect the increasing ethnic and cultural diversity of the population it serves. At the beginning of the 1900s, only one of every eight Americans identified himself or herself as a race other than "white." At the end of the century, one of four did so, as the white population grew more slowly than every other racial/ethnic group. Increasing diversity accelerated in the latter half of the century. From 1970 to 2000, the population of races other than "white" or "black" grew considerably, and by 2000 was comparable in size to the black population. The black population represented a slightly smaller share of the total U.S. population in 1970 than in 1900, while the Hispanic population more than doubled from 1980 to 2000. The racial/ethnic composition of the U.S. population according to the 2000 census was as follows: 75.1 percent white, 12.3 percent black, 3.6 percent Asian or Pacific Islander, 0.9 percent American Indian or Alaska Native, 5.5 percent claiming a race other than those already cited, and 2.4 percent claiming two or more races. Individuals (of any race) claiming Hispanic origin constituted 12.5 percent of the U.S. population (Hobbs and Stoops, 2002).

Despite this increasing diversity and decades of concern about the failure of the health care workforce to reflect it, there are still far too few minority M/SU professionals. The 2001 supplement to the Surgeon General's report on mental health, *Mental Health: Culture, Race, and Ethnicity*, stated: "Racial and ethnic minorities continue to be badly underrepresented, relative to their proportion of the U.S. population, within the core mental health professions—psychiatry, psychology, and social work, counseling, and psychiatric nursing" (DHHS, 2001:167). The President's New Freedom Commission on Mental Health echoed that observation: "Racial and ethnic minorities are seriously under-represented in the core mental health professions [and] . . . many providers are inadequately prepared to serve culturally diverse populations, and investigators are not trained in research on minority populations" (New Freedom Commission on Mental Health, 2003:50). Similarly, members of the substance-use treatment workforce do not reflect the gender, racial, and ethnic composition of those they treat (Mulvey et al., 2003).

As noted above, clinicians licensed to diagnose and treat M/SU problems and illnesses are uniquely varied. Although the diagnosis and treatment of general health conditions are typically limited to physicians, advanced practice nurses, and physician assistants,[2] M/SU health care clinicians include psychologists, psychiatrists, other specialty or primary care physicians, social workers, psychiatric nurses, marriage and family therapists, addiction therapists, psychosocial rehabilitation therapists, sociologists, and a variety of counselors with different education and certifications

---

[2]Dentists, chiropractors, and podiatrists also are licensed to diagnose and treat, but typically within prescribed domains.

(e.g., school counselors, pastoral counselors, guidance counselors, and drug and alcohol counselors), each with differing education and training.

The effect on clinical practice of this variation in provider types and in the corresponding education and training is unknown; however, variation in the education and training of different types of physicians who deliver care for mental illnesses has been shown to result in variations in the quality of care (Young et al., 2001). Also, although many different therapies have been developed for M/SU problems and illnesses (see Chapter 4), there is no mechanism in place to ensure that any given clinician has been adequately educated and trained to offer any specific therapy. Such a process is essential to the delivery of safe, effective, and efficient care. The wider variety of provider types also has implications for the ability to provide consumers with the information they need to select a clinician to help them—a key element of patient-centered care—as it is difficult to provide consumers with information on the competencies of any individual practitioner and to guarantee a uniform, safe level of abilities across all types of clinicians.

In spite of this, no mechanisms exist for routinely capturing adequate information on the characteristics of the M/SU workforce comparable to, for example, the National Sample Survey of Registered Nurses regularly conducted by the National Advisory Council on Nurse Education and Practice. Moreover, administrative data routinely collected as part of health care claims or billing do not include a code for provider type. Although it may not be necessary to capture this information in general health care, in which the great majority of billing clinicians are physicians, the failure to do so for M/SU services neglects a substantial opportunity to learn about the M/SU workforce and its patterns of care. The Substance Abuse and Mental Health Services Administration (SAMHSA) has organized periodic efforts to collect data on mental health practitioners (see Table 7-1) (Duffy et al., 2004), but the information collected is incomplete, collected inconsistently across professions, and insufficient for policy and workforce analysis. This and the few other available data sources provide only limited information about specialty and general health care clinicians providing M/SU treatment services.

Specialty Mental Health Providers

Specialty mental health providers include psychiatrists, psychologists, and psychiatric nurses possessing formal graduate degrees in mental health. They also include social workers, counselors, nurses, and therapists who either have received additional, specialized training in treating mental problems and illnesses prior to their professional practice, or have chosen to practice in a mental health care setting and gained advanced knowledge in treating mental problems and illnesses through experience (West et al.,

TABLE 7-1   Estimated Number of Clinically Active (CA) or Clinically Trained (CT) Mental Health Personnel and Rate per 100,000 Civilian Population in the United States, by Discipline and Year

Discipline	Number	Rate per 100,000 U.S. Civilian Population	Reporting Year
Counseling	111,931 (CA)	49.4	2002
Psychosocial Rehabilitation	100,000 (CT)	37.7	1996
Social Work	99,341 (CA)	35.3	2002
Psychology	88,491 (CT)	31.1	2002
Marriage and Family Therapy	47,111 (CA)	16.7	2002
Psychiatry[a]	38,436 (CT)	13.7	2001
School Psychology	31,278 (CT)	11.4	2003
Psychiatric Nursing	18,269 (CT)	6.5	2000
Pastoral Counseling	Data not available		

[a]Based on clinically active psychiatrists in the private sector; excludes residents and fellows.
SOURCE: Duffy et al., 2004.

2001). Individuals with more severe mental illnesses are more likely to receive care from specialty mental health providers (Wang et al., 2000). Psychiatrists, for example, are likely to treat individuals with illnesses such as schizophrenia and bipolar disorder (West et al., 2001). SAMHSA's most recent estimates of the numbers of clinically trained and clinically active[3] mental health personnel are shown in Table 7-1.

Specialty Substance-Use Treatment Providers

Data on the specialty substance-use treatment workforce overall are sparse; no database systematically collects such data (Kaplan, 2003). SAMHSA's 1996–1997 Alcohol and Drug Services study (Phase I) published in 2003 (SAMHSA, 2003) collected data on the credentials of staff working in a national inventory of hospital, residential, and outpatient substance-use treatment facilities and programs (Mulvey et al., 2003). However, subsequent national surveys of substance-use treatment services have not collected data on staff licensure and certification (SAMHSA, 2004), and in studies of the health care workforce overall, "the addiction treatment workforce is generally overlooked" (McCarty, 2002:1). Experts also note the paucity of data on the preparation of this workforce (Morris et al., 2004).

---

[3]"Clinically trained" personnel include those who, because of formal training and experience, could provide direct clinical care for mental health conditions, whether or not they do so. "Clinically active" personnel are those actively providing such care.

It is known, however, that the specialty substance-use treatment workforce includes individuals from all of the above mental health professions (IOM, 1997) but is predominantly composed of counselors (McLellan et al., 2003). In 1998 approximately half of the staff delivering substance-use treatment services in about 13,000 outpatient clinics was licensed as substance-abuse counselors. The remainder were about equally composed of unlicensed counselors and "other" professionals who were predominantly master's-level social workers, mental health counselors, marriage and family therapists, and psychologists with no certification or licensure as substance-use treatment providers; these "other" professionals also included psychiatrists and specialty-certified primary care physicians and nurses (Harwood, 2002). A more recent 2003 survey of 175 directors of inpatient/residential, outpatient, and methadone maintenance programs across the nation also found that apart from counselors, very few professional disciplines were represented among the treatment staff of these programs. With respect to program directors, 15 percent had no college degree; 58 percent had a bachelor's degree, and 20 percent had a master's degree. One program was under the direction of a physician (McLellan et al., 2003).

General Medical/Primary Care Providers

M/SU problems and illnesses are also treated by general internists, family medicine physicians, pediatricians, other medical specialists, and advanced practice nurses who have not been certified as mental health or substance-use treatment specialists and are delivering primary or specialty health care in office-based practices, clinics, acute general hospitals, and nursing homes. These providers are often the first point of contact for many adults with mental problems or illnesses. There is also some evidence that they are consumers' preferred point of first contact for care: the majority of consumers initially turn to their primary care providers for mental health services (Mickus et al., 2000), and use of general medical providers for treatment of M/SU problems and illnesses increased more than 150 percent between 1990–1992 and 2001–2003—a significant shift away from other sectors of care (Kessler et al., 2005). An equal (DHHS, 1999) or greater (Wang et al., 2000) number of adults with M/SU problems and illnesses receive care from general medical providers relative to specialty mental health providers in a given year. Primary care physicians and physician specialists other than psychiatrists also prescribe the majority of psychotropic medications (Pincus et al., 1998). However, there also is evidence that the care provided by general, primary care physicians is less often consistent with clinical practice guidelines than that provided by psychiatrists (Friedmann et al., 2000; Young et al., 2001).

The diversity of professions and disciplines within the M/SU workforce has implications for quality of care. First, it is difficult for consumers to know which type of clinician has the best knowledge and skills to provide them with the safest, most effective, and most efficient care. This might not be a problem if all types of practitioners had a minimum level of competency and the special added competencies of the different types of clinicians were reliably known. This however, is not the case, as discussed in the next section. Professional licensure and ongoing assurance of competencies in specific therapies involve many different bodies. Experts in the education of the M/SU workforce report that prelicensure education is uneven, as are licensure standards and the use of postlicensure competency evaluation mechanisms (Daniels and Walter, 2002; Hoge, 2002; Hoge et al., 2002).

PROBLEMS IN PROFESSIONAL EDUCATION AND TRAINING[4]

Providers in the above multiple disciplines, many of whom are licensed to practice independently, differ in the amounts of education and training they receive prior to professional practice. The content of the education they receive and the places in which they are educated also differ. This section reviews these variations, as well as deficiencies in the professional education of the M/SU workforce overall.

Variation in Amounts and Types of Education

Psychiatry

Eligibility for board certification in psychiatry requires 4 years of college, 4 additional years of medical education leading to a medical degree, followed by a minimum of 4 years of residency training.

Psychology

Although the doctoral degree in psychology is the standard educational path for independent clinical practice, individuals with a master's degree in psychology also can practice under the direction of a doctorally prepared

---

[4]This section incorporates content from a paper commissioned by the committee on "Workforce Issues in Behavioral Health," by John A. Morris, MSW, Professor of Clinical Neuropsychiatry and Behavioral Science at the University of South Carolina School of Medicine; Eric N. Goplerud, PhD, Research Professor at the School of Public Health and Health Services at George Washington University Medical Center; and Michael A. Hoge, PhD, Professor of Psychology (in Psychiatry) at Yale University School of Medicine.

psychologist, or independently as school psychologists or counselors (American Psychological Association, 2003; Duffy et al., 2004). To become a licensed clinical psychologist, graduates from doctoral programs also must complete supervised postdoctoral training (Olvey and Hogg, 2002). Practicing as a school psychologist requires a minimum of a master's degree, followed by additional training leading toward certification or licensure at the state level or nationally by the National Association of School Psychologists (Morris et al., 2004).

Social Work

Although social workers can practice with a bachelor's, master's, or doctoral degree, the Master of Social Work (MSW) is considered the routine degree for practitioners and is the most common academic requirement for licensure. Obtaining an MSW degree usually requires 2 years of postundergraduate study and field placements/practica (Morris et al., 2004).

Psychiatric Nursing

Individuals may become a registered nurse (RN) through three different educational pathways: a 2-year program leading to an associate's degree (AD) in nursing, a 3-year program (usually hospital-based) leading to a diploma in nursing, or a 4-year college or university program leading to a bachelor's degree in nursing. Those completing all of these programs are eligible to take the RN licensing examination after graduation. Psychiatric nurses may have this basic level of education or a graduate degree. Specialty certification for psychiatric nurses at all levels is provided by the American Nurses Credentialing Center. Psychiatric nurses are certified at both the basic ("C" after RN) and advanced ("CS" or "BC" after RN) levels. The majority of psychiatric nurses are prepared at the basic level of education; advanced-level certification requires that the nurse have either a master's or doctoral degree. Many nurses working in psychiatric settings do not have advanced certification in psychiatric nursing (Morris et al., 2004).

Counseling

The master's degree is the most common practice degree in counseling and enables licensure as a counselor. Accredited graduate programs require a minimum of 72 quarter hours or 48 semester hours of postundergraduate study leading to a master's degree. Doctoral degree programs usually require a minimum of 2 additional years of study (Morris et al., 2004).

Marriage and Family Therapy

Marriage and family therapists are trained in three different ways: master's degree (requiring 2–3 years of postundergraduate training); doctoral program (requiring 3–5 years of postundergraduate training); or a postgraduate clinical training program following training in psychology, psychiatry, social work, nursing, pastoral counseling, or education (Morris et al., 2004).

Pastoral Counseling

Persons credentialed as clinical pastoral counselors are either ordained or otherwise recognized by identified groups of religious faith and have completed a course of study approved by the Association for Clinical Pastoral Counseling. There are only 2,812 certified pastoral counselors nationwide, making them one of the smallest specialty provider groups in mental health (Morris et al., 2004).

Psychosocial Rehabilitation

Psychosocial rehabilitation is an approach to working with individuals with severe mental illnesses to teach them the skills they need to achieve their goals for living in the community. This type of care typically includes some combination of residential services, training in community living skills, socialization services, crisis services, case management, vocational rehabilitation, and other related services. Educational options for psychosocial rehabilitation workers are diverse and range from training following high school to an associate's, bachelor's, master's, or doctoral degree in psychosocial rehabilitation. Recent statistics indicate that 2 percent of these workers have a doctoral degree, 24 percent a master's degree, 13 percent some college or an associate's degree, and 22 percent a high school diploma (Duffy et al., 2004).

Substance-Use Treatment Counseling

As described above, most of the substance-use treatment workforce consists of counselors. The composition of this workforce is shifting from those whose expertise is experience-based (from their personal experience with substance-use problems or illnesses and recovery) to those with more formal education at the graduate level (McCarty, 2002). However, a representative survey of all state-recognized substance-use treatment programs found that 26 percent of counselors did not have a bachelor's degree, 32 percent possessed a bachelor's degree only, and 42 percent possessed a master's degree (none possessed a doctoral degree). And 39 percent of these counselors were clinically supervised by individuals who themselves lacked a graduate degree. This survey did not distinguish between counselors with and without a license/certification (Mulvey et al., 2003). A 1998 survey of staff delivering substance-use treatment services in approximately 13,000 outpatient clinics nationally found that 54 percent of unlicensed counselors had fewer than 4 years of college; in contrast, a master's degree was possessed by 56 percent of licensed counselors and 82 percent of "other behavioral health professionals" (Harwood, 2002). This higher level of formal education may not necessarily provide greater knowledge and expertise in providing effective care, however. Graduate programs in social work and psychology, for example, often do not provide specialized training in treatment of alcohol- and other drug-use problems and illnesses (Straussner and Senreich, 2002) and have a number of other limitations.

Deficiencies in Professional Education

The education of all health professionals is deficient in a number of areas and has not kept pace with advances in knowledge and changes in the delivery of health care (IOM, 2001, 2003), despite an IOM call that:

> All health professionals should be educated to deliver patient-centered care as members of an interdisciplinary team, emphasizing evidence-based practice, quality improvement approaches, and informatics (IOM, 2003:3).

Leaders in the education of clinicians to treat M/SU conditions testify that the educational preparation of this workforce does not address many of these areas adequately. For example, not all M/SU clinicians are educated about evidence-based care or receive training in the use of evidence-based clinical practice guidelines (Manderscheid et al., 2001). Without education in the use of such guidelines, these clinicians may be more committed to schools of practice than to providing the best therapy for a given patient (Jackim, 2003). The varying education of the different provider types discussed above results in differences in clinicians' theoretical orientations and therapeutic approaches, as well as in the professional journals they read and the professional organizations to which they belong. The result is little cross-fertilization of knowledge and skills across provider types, and few common standards of care and agreed-upon core competencies that transcend the borders of the separate schools of thought in which M/SU health care clinicians are trained.

Experts in the education of M/SU clinicians also report that graduate education is inadequately grounded in the scientific evidence base for treatments and that some professional education and training programs have been reluctant to incorporate clinical practice guidelines in traditional classroom content as well as clinical education placements (Hoge et al., 2002). Moreover, quality improvement strategies have received little attention in M/SU education (Morris et al., 2004). Similarly, despite the need for interprofessional collaboration described in Chapter 5, graduate training in M/SU health care continues to be conducted in single-discipline silos with little interdisciplinary coordination. Multispecialty training, such as that involving both mental health and primary care providers, also remains infrequent (Hoge et al., 2002).

Further, available information shows that there is no agreed-upon level of competency within any profession (or across professions) with respect to providing M/SU health care. Graduate training has not kept pace with changes in health care delivery, and the achievement of expected educational outcomes has not been demonstrated (Hoge et al., 2002). Recent changes in the licensing examination for nurses have decreased the content devoted to psychosocial issues, which some fear will encourage nursing schools to weaken mental health content in their curriculums (Poster, 2004). There also is strong evidence that education of all clinicians inadequately addresses substance-use problems and illnesses despite their high rates of co-occurrence with mental problems and illnesses.

Little Assurance of Competencies in Discipline-Specific and Core Knowledge

A primary concern regarding M/SU clinicians' education and training is the general absence of clearly specified competencies that students are to develop and a process for routinely assessing whether those competencies have actually been achieved. Leaders in the education of M/SU health care clinicians cite a historical reluctance in some professional education and training programs to require students to demonstrate competence in specific treatments, and note that general M/SU graduate education does not guarantee competence in advanced or specialized skills. As a result, it is recommended that training programs specify the minimum competencies expected of their graduates and verify that these competencies have been achieved (Hoge et al., 2002).

Multiple organizations are in various (mainly early) stages of developing discipline-specific, population-specific, or subject matter-specific competencies for clinicians providing health care for mental or substance-use conditions. However, these competencies have not yet been adopted as standards of professional practice, and together represent a not-yet-finished "patchwork quilt" of competencies. Moreover, still less attention has been directed to developing and implementing strategies for assessing the extent to which students and current members of the workforce possess or practice these competencies (Hoge et al., 2005a).

Leaders in M/SU education and clinical care also have called for certain knowledge, skills, and attitudes (i.e., core competencies) to be addressed by the education of *all* clinicians providing M/SU health care. Such competencies include, for example, detecting co-occurring mental and substance-use problems and illnesses, and avoiding the stigmatizing attitudes and practices of health care providers that obstruct patients' self-management of their illness and recovery, as described in Chapter 3. Several initiatives have been undertaken to develop and implement core competencies, including two for those treating substance use and one for those treating mental conditions. But these initiatives (described below) have not yet fully taken hold.

Addiction Counseling Competencies: The Knowledge, Skills, and Attitudes of Professional Practice In 1995, the National Curriculum Committee of the Addiction Technology Transfer Center program, a nationwide training system supported by SAMHSA's Center for Substance Abuse Treatment (CSAT), reached agreement on core competencies for addiction counseling across professional groups that may treat people with substance-use problems and illnesses. The resulting document, *Addiction Counseling Competencies: The Knowledge, Skills, and Attitudes of Professional Practice,* identifies the basic knowledge and attitudes required for all disciplines in the addiction field, as well as those necessary for the professional practice of addiction counseling (clinical evaluation; treatment planning; referral; service coordination; counseling; client, family, and community education; documentation; and professional and ethical responsibilities, each with its own set of competencies). The goal is for every addiction counselor and every specialty treatment facility to possess every competency, regardless of setting or treatment model (Addiction Technology Transfer Centers National Curriculum Committee, 1998; Hoge et al., 2005a).

Interdisciplinary Project to Improve Health Professional Education in Substance Abuse This 5-year cooperative project of the Health Resources and Services Administration (HRSA), the Association for Medical Education and Research in Substance Abuse (AMERSA), and CSAT produced (1) a strategic plan for interdisciplinary faculty development to prepare the general health professions workforce to provide care for substance-use problems and illnesses, (2) an interdisciplinary faculty development program to improve the educational curriculums for general health care professionals, and (3) an infrastructure to support faculty development in substance-use treatment. The initiative also produced a set of core and discipline-specific knowledge, attitudes, and competencies needed by health professionals to effectively identify, intervene with, and refer patients with substance-use problems and illnesses (Haack and Adger, 2002). Transmission of this set of knowledge, attitudes, and competencies to the workforce was initiated by the Multi-Agency INitiative on Substance abuse TRaining and Education for AMerica (Project MAINSTREAM), which provided trainers to train interdisciplinary faculty (Samet et al., 2006). The students trained by these faculty enter the workforce with the knowledge and skills needed to provide care for individuals and communities dealing with substance-use problems and illnesses.

Annapolis Coalition on Behavioral Health Workforce Education The Annapolis Coalition on Behavioral Health Workforce Education (Annapolis Coalition) grew out of a 2001 conference convened by the American College of Mental Health Administration and the Academic Behavioral Health Consortium, with funding from SAMHSA and the Agency for Healthcare Research and Quality (AHRQ). The Annapolis Coalition distilled recommendations from a substantial number of peer-reviewed publications addressing the need for training reform in the M/SU treatment field and subjected those recommendations to further vetting by experts in the field by preparing and distributing for comment of a series of review papers (Daniels and Walter, 2002; Hoge et al., 2002), as well as discussing the recommendations at a national summit of experts on workforce development (Hoge and Morris, 2002). The result was a series of 10 recommended best practices for improving the quality and relevance of workforce education (Hoge et al., 2005a).

Paucity of Content on Substance-Use Care

Despite the frequency of co-occurrence of general medical, mental, and substance-use problems and illnesses, many providers in each of these areas receive little or no education in the others and their effects on the presenting condition. According to the congressionally mandated study of the prevention and treatment of co-occurring substance-use and mental conditions (SAMHSA, undated:15), "Perhaps one of the most significant program-level barriers, noted by consumers and family members as well as by providers. . .is the lack of staff trained in treating co-occurring disorders." The limited content of substance-use education in most health professions is evidence of this.

Physician education Medical students can be educated about substance-use problems and illnesses in a variety of settings. During the first 2 years of medical school, however, the subject is often integrated into standard coursework; and separate courses on addiction medicine are rarely taught.

During the final 2 years of medical school, students also may have some experience with substance-use health care during required or elective clinical rotations in internal medicine, family medicine, neurology, or psychiatry. Overall, however, dedicated training in substance-use problems and illnesses is rarely offered in medical schools. A 1998–1999 survey of the Liaison Committee on Medical Education found that of the 125 accredited U.S. medical schools, 95 percent provided training in substance-use health care as part of a larger required course, 8 percent had a separate required course, and 36 percent offered an elective course (Haack and Adger, 2002). This current level of exposure of medical students to substance-use health care issues has not given recent medical school graduates the confidence to screen, assess, or provide needed interventions for these patients (Miller et al., 2001; Saitz et al., 2002; Vastag, 2003).

With respect to residency training, a 1997 national survey of residency program directors found that the percentage of programs with required training in care for substance-use problems and illnesses ranged from 32 percent in pediatrics to 95 percent in psychiatry, with an average of 56 percent across all emergency medicine, family medicine, internal medicine, obstetrics/gynecology, osteopathic medicine, pediatrics, and psychiatry residency programs. However, the survey found that even when there was required curriculum content in substance-use health care, the median number of curriculum hours dedicated to the subject varied greatly, ranging from 3 (emergency medicine and obstetrics/gynecology) to 12 (family medicine). Psychiatry residency programs reported an average of 8 hours devoted to substance-use health care in their curriculums (Isaacson et al., 2000). Even in preventive medicine residency training, most of the alcohol-, tobacco-, and other drug-use training focuses solely on tobacco (Abrams Weintraub et al., 2003).

Psychologist education Psychologists typically receive very little training in or preparation for dealing with substance-use problems and illnesses. Results of a 1994 survey indicated that although 91 percent of psychologists encountered substance-use problems or illnesses in their daily work, 74 percent had received no formal undergraduate or graduate coursework in the subject, and slightly more than half (54 percent) had received no training in substance-use conditions during their internships. Although few had received such training as part of their formal education, 86 percent subsequently acquired training in substance-use conditions through workshops, supervision, and other sources (Aanavai et al., 1999).

Social work education The Interdisciplinary Project to Improve Health Professional Education in Substance Abuse found that most schools of social work failed to provide students with a basic knowledge of alcohol-

and drug-use issues. Moreover, when graduate schools of social work offered a concentration or elective courses in the treatment of alcohol- and drug-use problems and illnesses, most students did not take these courses, and only a few schools of social work offered postgraduate training programs covering services for substance use. A significant factor contributing to this is that the Council on Social Work Education, the national policy-making body for social work education, does not mandate that curriculums contain substance-use content (Straussner and Senreich, 2002).

Nursing education Data on the amount of education in substance-use health care provided to nurses use are highly limited. The report of the Interdisciplinary Project to Improve Health Professional Education in Substance Abuse (Naegle, 2002) includes only information from two surveys conducted in 1987. The first found that undergraduate nursing curriculums typically offered 1–5 hours of instruction in substance-use problems and illnesses over 2–4 years of study, usually combined with other course content, and focused primarily on definitions and descriptions of the phenomena surrounding substance use and their health consequences. The second study likewise found little content on substance-use problems and illnesses incorporated into psychiatric nursing programs. A systematic review of studies of chemical dependency training within schools of nursing, covering the period 1966–1996, also found only a small number of studies, which frequently were methodologically flawed. Despite these shortcomings, the investigators concluded from the available data that schools of nursing generally provided minimal exposure to important concepts related to alcohol and drug dependence. Few classroom hours were dedicated to alcohol and drug issues, and individual courses devoted to substance-use problems and illnesses were rare. Clinical training also was neglected. "Neither the scope nor intensity of clinical instruction was sufficient to ensure that graduating nurses could effectively intervene with chemically dependent patients" (Howard et al., 1997:54).

Counselor education Even among substance-use treatment counselors, the duration and content of preprofessional training received by certified substance-use counselors varies widely. A large proportion of alcohol and other drug treatment counselors report receiving their counseling education through associate's degree and certificate programs at 2-year community colleges. Little information exists on the quality of these programs, or on programs offering higher levels of education. These programs typically operate with little or no external review and accreditation (McCarty, 2002). However, a 2000–2001 review of undergraduate programs based on published catalogues and Internet sites found 260 programs listed on the website of the National Association of Alcohol and Drug Abuse Counselors

(NAADAC) as offering formal education in preparation for working as a substance-use treatment practitioner. Approximately 55 percent of these programs were at the community college or 2-year level, 13 percent at the bachelor's degree level, and 32 percent at the graduate level. Undergraduate programs varied in their titles, the types of degrees awarded, the numbers of credits and courses required for a degree, and in whether program graduates are prepared to function as counselors and be certified by states (Edmundson, 2002).

Inadequate Faculty Development

Training health professionals to provide them with the knowledge and skills needed to treat M/SU problems and illnesses requires not just strong curriculum content, but also high-quality faculty to present that curriculum who are well trained and knowledgeable about current effective M/SU therapies, contemporary practice, and interdisciplinary care (Haack and Adger, 2002; Hoge et al., 2002). Yet past deficiencies in the education of those serving in faculty positions, particularly generalist clinicians (e.g., physicians, nurses), have resulted in insufficient numbers of qualified generalist faculty to teach about M/SU health care issues even when curriculums concerning these issues exist.

The Career Teachers Program (1972–1982), sponsored by the National Institute on Alcohol Abuse and Alcoholism and the National Institute on Drug Abuse, was one of the first multidisciplinary faculty development programs in substance use health care for health professionals (Galanter, 1980). Over the course of this program's existence, 59 career teachers (faculty in medical and public health schools) were challenged to enhance substance-use treatment education within their own professional schools. This program was followed by faculty development programs sponsored by federal agencies for medical, nursing, social work, public health, and psychology faculty. Projects associated with these programs enriched the curriculums of their respective schools and demonstrated that training providers, either community clinicians or emergency medicine residents, could increase the extent to which they addressed patients' unhealthy alcohol use (D'Onofrio et al., 2002; Saitz et al., 2000). The continuing need for faculty training programs is evident in the ongoing faculty development efforts of the Association for Medical Education and Research in Substance Abuse (Samet et al., 2006).

Summary

The above discussion illustrates that even when well-developed sets of competencies (such as those of the Interdisciplinary Project to Improve

Health Professional Education in Substance Abuse) exist, they often are not incorporated into education programs. Licensing and credentialing are two mechanisms used to assure the public that health care professionals are competent to deliver services once they have completed their preprofessional education. However, many of the core and discipline-, subject matter-, or population-specific professional competencies discussed above have not been adopted or incorporated into training programs, licensing standards, or certification requirements. Until this happens, the promulgation of competencies is likely to have limited impact (Hoge et al., 2005a). The variation in competencies resulting from differences in preprofessional education is compounded by state-to-state variation in licensing and credentialing, discussed next.

VARIATION IN LICENSURE AND CREDENTIALING REQUIREMENTS

Licensing standards for the health professions are set by the states and typically specify minimum standards for competency. In addition, the different health professional associations, such as NAADAC—the Association for Addiction Professionals, and the American Nurses Association, frequently establish independent certification or credentialing processes that formally recognize an individual's knowledge or competency in a specialized area. The latter standards often go beyond the requirements for state licensure, although there is some overlap as some states mandate credentialing as a part of licensure for certain professions (IOM, 2003).

Taking psychologists as an example, all but four states require a doctoral degree to practice clinical psychology independently; Alaska, Oregon, Vermont, and West Virginia also license master's-level clinicians to practice independently. All states except California and Pennsylvania require degrees to be from schools accredited by regional accrediting bodies; the two exceptions accept degrees recognized by state law. Mississippi and Oklahoma require the degrees to be from programs accredited by the American Psychological Association. All states further require supervised experience prior to independent practice, but the number of hours required varies. Most states require 1,500–2,000 postdoctoral hours, but Delaware requires 3,000 and Michigan and Washington 4,000 (Olvey and Hogg, 2002). Moreover, there are variations in how individuals with a master's degree in psychology can practice across states. Twenty-six states and the District of Columbia do not license master's-level psychologists to practice independently. In the other states, licensed master's-level psychologists are variably restricted in their scope of practice and amount of required supervision. Titles used in the states for these licensed and master's-prepared clinicians also vary; they include psychological associate, psychological technician, psychological assistant, registered psychological assistant, licensed master's-level psychologist, certified psychological associate, psychological examiner, licensed psychological practitioner, psychologist associate, and others. The amount of supervision required varies from none to supervision of all practice activity. Requirements for supervised experience pre- and postlicensure also vary (Association of State and Provincial Psychology Boards, 2000).

Considerable variation exists as well in the certification of specializations provided by professional associations. Only a few state certification boards, for example, use SAMHSA's addiction counseling competencies as the basis for their education and training requirements (Hoge et al., 2005a). Although a number of states (e.g., New York, New Mexico, Arizona) are moving toward the establishment of a required basic level of competency for M/SU treatment providers who are offering integrated services, there remain no uniform standards of competency across states.

The above variations in licensure standards and credentialing processes contribute to the varying capacity of the M/SU workforce to deliver high-quality health care.

INADEQUATE CONTINUING EDUCATION

Beyond the variations in education, licensing, and credentialing discussed above, the rapidly expanding evidence base and broad range of specialized populations and treatment settings make it unlikely that all clinicians (especially those newly licensed) will come to their place of employment possessing the knowledge and skills needed to practice at a high level of expertise (Hoge et al., 2002). Prelicensure or preemployment education cannot provide sufficient frequency and diversity of experience (and sometimes offer no experience) in the performance of every therapeutic intervention appropriate for every clinical condition seen in patients, especially as the breadth of knowledge and technology expands. Practitioners, therefore, come to their initial place of employment as novices without certain skills and knowledge—their limited skill and expertise reflecting the limitations of time and experience in their academic education and the sheer number of effective therapies. Moreover, it is obviously impossible for prelicensure education to teach students about diagnostic and therapeutic advances not yet invented (IOM, 2004b). Many of the health professions are thus grappling with the need to ensure the continuing competency of licensed health professionals (IOM, 2003). Like professional practice education, however, continuing education for health professionals has been found lacking in content, methods, financing, and organizational support.

Content

Continuing education focuses on refining existing and developing new skills, as well as mastering changes in the knowledge base and treatment approaches. Unlike preservice education, which is organized around a formal curriculum, continuing education is commonly self-directed by the practitioner, who selects areas of interest to pursue (Daniels and Walter, 2002).

Few standards or guidelines govern the continuing education content that providers choose to study. Continuing education requirements are set principally by licensing and certification bodies, many of which are controlled by the states. These requirements are generally nonspecific, outlining only the number of hours of continuing education that must be completed during a specified number of years in order to maintain licensure or certification. While some states and disciplines mandate continuing education in specific content areas, such as professional ethics (Daniels and Walter, 2002), "the general absence of standards or guidelines regarding content raises concern that many practitioners may never become educated about critical, emerging issues in the field, such as patient safety" (Morris et al., 2004:18), illness self-management (see Chapter 3), or the Chronic Care Model (see Chapter 5).

A 2001 survey of the continuing education requirements for M/SU disciplines set by the states for licensure renewal found a striking lack of consistency in the requirements for a given professional discipline across states, as well as in the requirements for different mental health disciplines within states. The requirements for psychologists, for example, range from zero hours of continuing education (11 states), to 12 hours per year (Alabama), to 50 hours per year (Kansas) (Daniels and Walter, 2002).

Methods

As usually provided (i.e., in single-session events such as conferences, lectures, workshops, and dissemination of written materials), continuing education has been found to have little effect in changing clinical practice (Davis et al., 1999). Teaching adult learners clearly requires different approaches; moreover, research has shown that not everyone learns the same way. While many individuals learn well through reading, for example, others learn better through approaches that allow them to use their motor skills. Clinicians also can benefit from being taught individually, rather than in a group, at a pace suited to their particular learning style (Lazear, 1991). Empirical support exists as well for education strategies such as interactive sessions (role playing, discussion groups, and experiential problem solving); academic detailing, in which trained experts meet with providers in their practice setting; audit and feedback (Morris et al., 2004); use of information technology (IT) (IOM, 2003); and learning through decision support at the point of care delivery.

The IOM's report on health professions education (IOM, 2003) identifies utilizing information technology to communicate, manage knowledge, mitigate error, and support decision making as a core competency that should be possessed by all health professionals. Proficiency in using IT can also be an effective vehicle for continuing education. CD-ROM–based and text-based programs can be used to provide individualized learning during times when the clinician is not involved in direct patient care. Online learning also presents new opportunities for continuing education, and many state licensing boards accept completion of online courses as satisfying at least part of the continuing education requirements for license renewal (Flanagan and Needham, 2003).

Learning can take place as well through clinical decision-support software that integrates information on individual patients with a computerized knowledge base to generate patient-specific assessments or recommendations, thereby helping clinicians or patients make clinical decisions. In general health care, clinical decision-support systems assist clinicians in applying new information to patient care through the analysis of patient-specific clinical variables. These systems vary in complexity, function, and application; some but not all are computer based. According to AHRQ's evidence-based report *Making Health Care Safer: A Critical Analysis of Patient Safety Practices*, the preponderance of evidence suggests that these systems are at least somewhat effective, especially with respect to the prevention of medical errors (Trowbridge and Weingarten, 2001). Although such software is common in general health care, however, it is not highly developed or widely available in M/SU health care (Morris et al., 2004). Other decision supports (some "low tech") include using memory/cognition aids, such as protocols and checklists, and clinical pathways.

Financing

The financing of continuing education for M/SU practitioners has been identified as a critical issue (Daniels and Walter, 2002). Pharmaceutical companies have been a major source of funding for continuing education in M/SU health care, but that support is being curtailed. Provider organizations, which historically have financed a large share of the continuing education for their employees, also have substantially scaled back their training departments, staff, and programs, as well as travel support for continuing education conferences, as a result of severe budgetary pressures (IOM, 2004b; Morris et al., 2004).

The IOM report *Keeping Patients Safe: Transforming the Work Environment of Nurses* shows that the issue of continuing worker education and training is not unique to the health care industry. In many industries, the ongoing acquisition and management of knowledge by employees is increasingly recognized as an essential responsibility of the employing organization. Organizations need to play an active role in managing their learning process and transferring knowledge quickly and efficiently to their employees. This organizational role is critical to supporting the continuing growth of clinicians' knowledge and skills (IOM, 2004b).

In general health care, for example, hospitals with high retention of nurses in the face of nursing shortages ("magnet hospitals") are characterized by the provision of high levels of postemployment training and education of nursing staff, beginning with orientation and lasting several weeks to months (McClure et al., 2002). Developing and managing human skills and intellect—more than managing physical and capital assets—is increasingly recognized as a dominant concern of managers in successful companies (Quinn, 1992). Given the career-long need for clinicians to maintain competency through the acquisition of new knowledge and skills and the essential role of health care organizations in helping to meet this need, *Keeping Patients Safe* recommends that all health care organizations routinely dedicate a defined portion of budgetary resources to support for staff in their ongoing acquisition and maintenance of knowledge and skills (IOM, 2004b).

Organizational Support

Extensive research has demonstrated that an individual's possession of required competencies by itself is not sufficient for safe and effective performance in the workplace (IOM, 2004b). When the organization in which an individual works does not support and reward competency, the worker is not likely to display competency on an ongoing basis (Hoge et al., 2005b; IOM, 2004b). In patient care, what matters is the clinician's *performance*, rather than the *possession* of necessary competencies. In the performance of clinical competencies, organizational characteristics are equally or more influential than individual education, training, and other characteristics (IOM, 2004b). Advances in education for M/SU clinicians therefore need to be coupled with efforts to help the organizations in which they work provide the culture and other practice supports that allow and promote competent performance (Hoge et al., 2005b).

In addition to the many problems discussed above, M/SU clinicians' ability to provide high-quality care is compromised by their frequent isolation from their peers and colleagues from other disciplines as a result of working in individual, or solo, practices (discussed next). Solo practice does not facilitate building the infrastructure needed to take up new knowledge and store, collect, and share the clinical information required to deliver high-quality collaborative patient care.

TABLE 7-2   Percentage of Clinically Trained Specialty Mental Health Personnel Reporting Individual Practice as Their Primary or Secondary Place of Employment

Discipline	Primary Employment	Secondary Employment	Reporting Year
Psychiatry	37.0	18.0	1998
Psychology	38.0	28.0	2002
Social work	18.5	27.1	2000
Counseling	15.1	21.6	2002
Marriage/family therapy	34.9	28.5	2000

SOURCE: Duffy et al., 2004.

MORE SOLO PRACTICE

Many mental health clinicians report that individual practice is either their primary or secondary[5] employment setting (Duffy et al., 2004) (see Table 7-2).

Solo practice may impede the uptake of evidence-based practices and other changes needed in treatment settings. For example, as discussed in Chapter 6, the size of health care organizations has been shown to be related to the uptake of IT. Use of electronic health records (EHRs), for instance, is typically found in larger health care organizations (Brailer and Terasawa, 2003), and the size of a practice has been found to be the main determinant of IT adoption for five clinical functions—obtaining treatment guidelines, exchanging clinical data with other physicians, accessing patient notes, generating treatment reminders for physicians, and writing prescriptions. Indeed, physicians in solo or two-person practices are more than three times likelier to have limited IT support for patient care compared with large group practices of more than 50 physicians (Reed and Grossman, 2004). Observations from experts in the use of information systems by managed behavioral health care organizations support this conclusion.

With respect to administrative (as opposed to clinical) IT applications, smaller M/SU providers lag behind in the use of electronic claims submission (Trabin and Maloney, 2003). Likewise, a random sample of 175 directors of inpatient/residential, outpatient, and methadone maintenance pro-

---

[5]Many mental health practitioners work in multiple settings. For example, 60 percent of full-time psychiatrists reported working in two or more settings in 1998, as did 50 percent of psychologists, 20 percent of full-time counselors, and 29 percent of marriage/family therapists in 2002. Rates were higher for part-time counselors (Duffy et al., 2004).

grams across the nation found that approximately 20 percent of the programs had no information systems of any type, e-mail, or even voice mail for their phone system. In contrast, most of those that were part of larger hospital or health systems had access to well-developed clinical information systems, e-mail, and Internet services (McLellan and Meyers, 2004). Most public and private substance-use treatment programs are outside the purview of medical facilities where such technology might be more available. To the extent that other M/SU clinicians also provide care in solo or small group practices, low adoption of IT to support clinical care may also be present. Differences in IT uptake are theorized to reflect differences in provider size: larger groups and health maintenance organizations (HMOs) have readier access to capital and administrative support staff and the ability to spread acquisition and implementation costs among more providers (Reed and Grossman, 2004).

Knowledge uptake and application require other resources for timely identification of scientific advances and innovations. For example, as described in Chapter 4, SAMHSA's National Registry of Evidence-based Programs and Practices contains such information, but if no one in the care delivery organization has the time or responsibility to review this registry of effective practices and provide the information to the organization, improvements in care delivery are less likely to occur. Large organizations may have more capital resources and greater ability to create mechanisms for carrying out such activities; solo or smaller practices may need to band together to achieve the economies of scale required for this purpose (Berwick, 2003). In a study of the adoption of clinical practice guidelines for treatment of attention deficit hyperactivity disorder (ADHD), for example, having a solo practice was found to be associated with a reduced likelihood of adopting the practice guidelines (Rushton et al., 2004).

Evidence shows that an organization will assimilate innovations more readily if it is large, mature, functionally differentiated (i.e., divided into semiautonomous departments and units), and specialized, with foci of professional knowledge; if it has flexible resources to channel into new projects; and if it has decentralized decision-making structures. Size is almost certainly a proxy for these characteristics (Greenhalgh et al., 2004).

USE OF THE INTERNET AND OTHER COMMUNICATION TECHNOLOGIES FOR SERVICE DELIVERY

In addition to the telephone, communication technologies such as video conferencing and the Internet are increasingly being used to evaluate, diagnose, and provide M/SU services to people who lack face-to-face access to such services (Benderly, 2005) or prefer these other approaches. At a minimum, advances in use of Internet-mediated and other communication technologies require research on their effectiveness, specialized training of clinicians in their use, additional protection of consumer information, and mechanisms for ensuring the competencies of those who provide such forms of care.

Like consumers of general health care services (Baker et al., 2003), many consumers of M/SU health care are already turning to the Internet to obtain information and support from peers to help them manage their M/SU problems and illnesses (Lamberg, 2003). Indeed, the Internet may be especially useful to consumers of M/SU health care as a source of clinical treatment. As some assert, "while face-to-face contact with patients is certainly desirable, the primary medium of treatment, psychotherapy, requires no direct physical contact; many assessment and treatment services could potentially be delivered, at least in part, over the Internet" (Flanagan and Needham, 2003:312).

However, use of the Internet to deliver M/SU health care carries several risks. One is the issue of the privacy and confidentiality of information transmitted by patients over the Internet—information that, when transmitted face to face and incorporated into the patient's health record, is subject to greater privacy protections than exist for general health care (see Chapter 5 and Appendix B). Other concerns relate to questions about the safety and effectiveness of Internet-based therapy compared with traditional face-to-face therapy, especially since the practitioner is unable to observe the physical behaviors of the patient, which can inform experienced clinicians. Moreover, practitioners providing face-to-face care must be licensed by the state in which they practice—typically the same state in which the patient resides. If a counselor in California delivers care to an individual in Mississippi over the Internet, how is such a provider to be credentialed—by the state in which he or she resides, in which the patient resides, or both? The Internet makes delivery of services by a single practitioner to individuals in all 50 states feasible. Should licensing be required in all 50 states (Copeland and Martin, 2004; Flanagan and Needham, 2003)? At present, "consumers are able to find licensed, and for that matter unlicensed, professionals offering therapy. . .online" (Flanagan and Needham, 2003:313).

Despite these issues, there is no question that the communication technology exists to provide M/SU care and that people are willing to use it. For the Internet, as for the telephone and video conferencing, providing care that is clinically appropriate, therapeutically productive, and socially supportive requires that practitioners address issues of the technological parameters of electronic service delivery, requisite systems for credentialing and credential verification, and the appropriate balance between face-to-face and electronic communications.

LONG HISTORY OF WELL-INTENTIONED BUT
SHORT-LIVED WORKFORCE INITIATIVES

Most of the issues discussed above are not new; they have been acknowledged for many years—some for decades. They have also been the
subject of many short-lived, ad hoc initiatives that overall have failed to
provide the sustained leadership, attention, resources, and collaboration
necessary to resolve them. A chronology of these efforts is provided below.
In the next section, the committee calls for a sustained, multiyear, collaborative initiative to address these issues, modeled after those created for the
physician and nursing workforces.

1956. The American Psychiatric Association Committee on Medical
Education proposes a curriculum for teaching psychiatry in medical schools
and recommends that physician training develop "well-rounded physicians,
who, in their relationships with all patients, recognize the importance of
unconscious motivation, the role of emotional maladjustment in the ideol-
ogy and chronicity of illness, the emotional and personality problems en-
gendered by various illnesses; and who habitually see the patient in his
family and general environmental setting" (APA Committee on Medical
Education, 1956:128). The committee also recommends that during the
first 2 years, all medical students be exposed to themes of personality
growth, development, structure, and integration; adaptive needs; social and
cultural forces affecting personality and behavior; the role of language
and mentation; the role played by emotions and physiological functioning;
and psychopathology.

1961. In the final report of the Joint Commission on Mental Illness
and Health, titled *Action for Mental Health*, the commission makes the
following recommendation: "Child specialists offer a considerable potential for helping emotionally disturbed children, but in many cases lack
sufficient psychiatric orientation to capitalize on this potential. The National Institute of Mental Health should provide support for resident training programs in pediatrics that make well-designed efforts to incorporate
adequate psychiatric information as a part of the pediatrician's graduate
training. It should also provide stipends for pediatricians who wish to take
post-graduate courses in psychiatry. The aim is not to convert pediatricians
into psychiatrists, but to increase the mental patient care resources of the
community in which the pediatrician practices" (Joint Commission on
Mental Illness and Health, 1961:*xiii*).

1972. The National Association of Alcohol and Drug Abuse Counselors is founded, in part to begin a national credentialing/certification program for addiction counselors (NAADAC, 2005).

1972–1982. The Career Teachers Program is sponsored by the National Institute on Alcohol Abuse and Alcoholism (NIAAA) and the Na-

tional Institute on Drug Abuse (NIDA) as one of the first multidisciplinary health professional faculty development programs in substance-use education (Galanter, 1980).

1976. The Association for Medical Education and Research in Substance Abuse (AMERSA) is created to expand education in substance-use health care for all health care professionals (Samet et al., 2006).

1976–1982. The National Institute of Mental Health Staff College is created to enhance the effectiveness of the leaders of federally funded community mental health centers across the United States. It closes with a change in administrations in Washington.

1978. The President's Commission on Mental Health points out problems in the M/SU workforce and recommends several actions to address them, including more systematic training for all mental health professions in the social structures, beliefs, value systems, and patterns of various subcultures, and how to work with individuals from these subcultures in therapy. The commission also recommends multidisciplinary training to address what it identifies as "problems of role-blurring, rivalries, and turf battles" (President's Commission on Mental Health, 1978:459). In addition, the commission reaffirms the need to provide training in administration in both the basic and continuing education curriculums of all mental health professionals.

1978–1986. A 5-year doctorate in mental health at the University of California-Berkeley and the University of California-San Francisco Medical School is initiated. The program aims to develop a new profession combining three main areas of knowledge—biological science, psychological science, and social science—in a clinical curriculum, with the goal of unifying the way behavioral health professionals are trained (Wallerstein, 1991).

1979. NIAAA initiates a State Manpower Development Program to provide categorical grant funding to each of the state alcoholism authorities for the development of a manpower plan and training of treatment providers. The program ends in 1982 when its funding is incorporated into block grants to states (IOM, 1990).

1984. NIAAA publishes core competencies and credentialing standards for counselors treating alcohol dependence (Birch and Davis Associates, 1984).

1990. The IOM documents the "serious lack of accurate, timely data at the national level" on the workforce treating alcohol-use problems and illnesses and notes: "This lack of data compromises efforts to plan for future training and professional needs. Fundamental questions for each of the disciplines involved cannot be answered. . . .As a consequence it is not possible to formulate a forward-looking workforce training policy" (IOM, 1990:131).

1993. SAMHSA issues *Workforce Training and Development for Mental Health Systems.*

1999. *Mental Health: A Report of the Surgeon General* again documents the inadequate supply of well-trained mental health professionals, especially those serving children and adolescents and individuals with severe mental illnesses, and those providing specific forms of psychotherapy effective for many types of mental illnesses (DHHS, 1999).

2000. SAMHSA's National Treatment Plan Initiative for Improving Substance Abuse Treatment calls for a National Workforce Development Office to secure valid, nationwide workforce data to guide policy making and support development of the substance-use treatment workforce at the national level. That office's efforts would address the implementation of core competency guidelines, credentialing standards, and other education and training activities (SAMHSA, 2000).

2001–2002. The American College of Mental Health Administration (ACMHA) and the Academic Behavioral Health Consortium (ABHC) initiate the Annapolis Coalition on Behavioral Health Workforce Education to build national consensus on the nature of the problems facing the M/SU treatment workforce and improve the quality and relevance of their education and training. The coalition's findings and recommendations are published in 2002 (Adams and Daniels, 2002; Daniels and Walter, 2002; Hoge, 2002; Hoge and Morris, 2002; Hoge et al., 2002).

2002. The HRSA–AMERSA–SAMHSA/CSAT Interdisciplinary Project to Improve Health Professional Education in Substance Abuse issues a strategic plan to enable the nation's health professions workforce to care for individuals with substance-use problems and illnesses. The plan makes 12 recommendations for the Secretary of DHHS, the U.S Surgeon General, other federal agencies, and agencies and organizations in the public and private sectors, calling for, in part, the creation of a Secretary's Advisory Committee on Health Professions Education on Substance-Use Disorders; a Surgeon General's report on the state of substance abuse prevention and treatment, similar to the Surgeon General's report on mental health; the convening of a national forum on health professions education on substance-use disorders; the creation of national centers of excellence for leadership in interdisciplinary faculty development; and other mechanisms to strengthen workforce competencies in substance-use health care (Haack and Adger, 2002).

2003. In its report *Health Professions Education: A Bridge to Quality*, the IOM makes 10 recommendations for improving all health professions education to support improvements in health care quality (IOM, 2003).

2003. The President's New Freedom Commission on Mental Health (2003) reports that "the Commission heard consistent testimony from consumers, families, advocates, and public and private providers about the 'workforce crisis' in mental health care. Today, not only is there a shortage of providers, but those providers who are available are not trained in evidenced-based and other innovative practices. This lack of education, training, or supervision leads to a workforce that is ill-equipped to use the latest breakthroughs in modern medicine" (p. 70). The commission further states that the mental health field needs "a comprehensive strategic plan to improve workforce recruitment, retention, diversity, and skills training" and calls on DHHS to "initiate and coordinate a public-private partnership to undertake such a strategy" (p. 75).

2004. The Annapolis Coalition on Behavioral Health Workforce Education convenes a national meeting that generates 10 consensus recommendations to guide the development of M/SU health care workforce competencies (Hoge et al., 2005a).

2005. SAMHSA contracts with the Annapolis Coalition on the Behavioral Health Workforce to develop a national strategic plan on workforce development by December 2005.

NEED FOR A SUSTAINED COMMITMENT TO BRING ABOUT CHANGE

Some changes have taken place as result of the initiatives described above. In general, however, M/SU health care professionals are trained the way they have been for many years, and problems such as maldistribution and the lack of representation of minorities in the workforce have improved only slightly, if at all. Despite significant efforts, attempts to train non-psychiatric physicians to do a better job of caring for people with M/SU problems and illnesses have not been particularly effective. Broader efforts to bring about similar changes in the M/SU treatment workforce overall have had similar results.

The committee finds, as others have before, that without a properly trained, culturally relevant, and appropriately distributed M/SU health care workforce, significant improvements in the quality of care are not likely. The committee further finds that the problems that attenuate the effectiveness of the M/SU health workforce in America are so complex that they require an ongoing, priority commitment of attention and resources, as opposed to the short-term, ad hoc initiatives that have often characterized responses to the problem in the past. As noted above, the committee recommends that the approach used to educate and train other key providers (physicians and nurses) in the health care workforce, as described below, be employed to marshal the sustained attention, collaboration, and resources needed to produce a stronger M/SU health care workforce.

Council on Graduate Medical Education

The Council on Graduate Medical Education (COGME) was authorized by Congress in 1986 to "provide an ongoing assessment of physician workforce trends, training issues and financing policies, and to recommend appropriate federal and private sector efforts to address identified needs" (HRSA, 2002). Council members include "representatives of practicing primary care physicians, national and specialty physician organizations, international medical graduates, medical student and house staff associations, schools of medicine and osteopathy, public and private teaching hospitals, health insurers, business, and labor. Federal representation includes the Assistant Secretary for Health, the U.S. Department of Health and Human Services (DHHS); the Administrator of the Centers for Medicare and Medicaid Services; and the Chief Medical Director of the Veterans Administration." COGME advises and makes recommendations to the Secretary of DHHS; the Senate Committee on Health, Education, Labor and Pensions; and the House of Representatives Committee on Commerce.

The charge to COGME is broader than its name implies. Its authorizing legislation requires its advice and recommendations to address the following (HRSA, 2002):

- The supply and distribution of physicians in the United States.
- Current and future shortages or excesses of physicians in specialties and subspecialties.
- Related federal policies, including the financing of undergraduate and graduate medical education programs and the types of medical education and training in the latter programs.
- Efforts to be carried out by hospitals, educational institutions, and accrediting bodies with respect to these matters, including changes in undergraduate and graduate medical education programs.
- Improvements needed in databases concerning the supply and distribution of, and postgraduate training programs for, physicians in the United States and steps that should be taken to eliminate those deficiencies.

COGME periodically studies and issues reports on these issues that have been influential in health care policy arenas. While these reports have sometimes been controversial (Phillips et al., 2005), they have been successful in focusing national attention on the issues and stimulating policy responses.

National Advisory Council on Nurse Education and Practice

The National Advisory Council on Nurse Education and Practice (NACNEP) was established as the Advisory Council on Nurse Training in 1964 and renamed in 1988. It similarly advises the Secretary of DHHS and the U.S. Congress on policy issues related to the nursing programs administered by HRSA's Bureau of Health Professions Division of Nursing, including nurse workforce supply, education, and practice improvement. Among its reports are the following: *Basic Registered Nurse Workforce, National Informatics Agenda for Nursing Education and Practice, Collaborative Education to Ensure Patient Safety, A National Agenda for Nursing Workforce Racial/Ethnic Diversity, Federal Support for the Preparation of the Nurse Practitioner Workforce through Title VIII,* and *Federal Support for the Preparation of the Clinical Nurse Specialist Workforce through Title VIII.*

The efforts of COGME and NACNEP have resulted in a number of accomplishments in workforce development. With respect to furthering interdisciplinary education and practice, for example, the two worked together to produce the report *Collaborative Education to Ensure Patient Safety* (COGME and NACNEP, 2000), which makes recommendations pertaining to faculty development, quality improvement, interdisciplinary collaboration, and competency development. These recommendations fostered cooperative agreements with public and private nonprofit entities that were cosponsored by HRSA's nursing and medicine divisions (NACNEP, 2002).

Recommendations

To secure sustained attention and resources for the development of the M/SU treatment workforce similar to what has been accomplished for the physician and nurse workforces, the committee makes the following recommendations:

Recommendation 7-1. To ensure sustained attention to the development of a stronger M/SU health care workforce, Congress should authorize and appropriate funds to create and maintain a Council on the Mental and Substance-Use Health Care Workforce as a public–private partnership. Recognizing that the quality of M/SU services is dependent upon a highly competent professional workforce, the council should develop and implement a comprehensive plan for strengthening the quality and capacity of the workforce to improve the quality of M/SU services substantially by:

- **Identifying the specific clinical competencies that all M/SU professionals must possess to be licensed or certified and the competencies that must be maintained over time.**
- **Developing national standards for the credentialing and licensure of M/SU providers to eliminate differences in the standards now**

used by the states. Such standards should be based on core competencies and should be included in curriculums and education programs across all the M/SU disciplines.

- Proposing programs to be funded by government and the private sector to address and resolve such long-standing M/SU workforce issues as diversity, cultural relevance, faculty development, and continuing shortages of the well-trained clinicians and consumer providers needed to work with children and the elderly; and of programs for training competent clinician administrators.
- Providing a continuing assessment of M/SU workforce trends, issues, and financing policies.
- Measuring the extent to which the plan's objectives have been met and reporting annually to the nation on the status of the M/SU workforce.
- Soliciting technical assistance from public–private partnerships to facilitate the work of the council and the efforts of educational and accreditation bodies to implement its recommendations.

Recommendation 7-2. Licensing boards, accrediting bodies, and purchasers should incorporate the competencies and national standards established by the Council on the Mental and Substance-Use Health Care Workforce in discharging their regulatory and contracting responsibilities.

Recommendation 7-3. The federal government should support the development of M/SU faculty leaders in health professions schools, such as schools of nursing and medicine, and in schools and programs that educate M/SU professionals, such as psychologists and social workers. The aim should be to narrow the gaps among what is known through research, what is taught, and what is done by those who provide M/SU services.

Recommendation 7-4. To facilitate the development and implementation of core competencies across all M/SU disciplines, institutions of higher education should place much greater emphasis on interdisciplinary didactic and experiential learning and should bring together faculty and trainees from their various education programs.

The committee calls particular attention to two components of recommendation 7-1. First, the recommendation calls for a public–private partnership to address the problems plaguing the M/SU workforce. Federal leadership can provide sustained national policy attention to these problems and unique influence with the educational institutions and their accreditors, licensing bodies, health professions associations, and health care organizations that need to be engaged in resolving the issues involved. At the same time, private-sector organizations such as AMERSA (Samet et al., 2006) and, more recently, the Annapolis Coalition on Behavioral Health Workforce Education can offer the expertise, collaboration, and flexibility necessary to collect and analyze additional evidence that needs to be brought to bear on these issues. Therefore, the committee strongly recommends that the council seek out AMERSA and the Annapolis Coalition as partners in this process.

Second, with respect to the portion of recommendation 7-1 that calls for the Council on the Mental and Substance-Use Health Care Workforce to provide "an ongoing assessment of M/SU workforce trends, issues, and financing policies," the committee underscores the paucity of comprehensive and reliable data on the M/SU workforce that it encountered in conducting this study. Thus the committee strongly recommends the inclusion of a mechanism or mechanisms for collecting better data on the M/SU workforce as a part of the process for assessing workforce trends and issues.

REFERENCES

Aanavai MP, Taube DO, Ja DY, Duran EF. 1999. The status of psychologists' training about and treatment of substance-abusing clients. *Journal of Psychoactive Drugs* 31(4):441–444.

Abrams Weintraub T, Saitz R, Samet JH. 2003. Education of preventive medicine residents: Alcohol, tobacco, and other drug abuse. *American Journal of Preventive Medicine* 24(1):101–105.

Adams N, Daniels AS. 2002. Sometimes a great notion...a common agenda for change. *Administration and Policy in Mental Health* 29(4–5):319–324.

Addiction Technology Transfer Centers National Curriculum Committee. 1998. *Addiction Counseling Competencies: The Knowledge, Skills and Attitudes of Professional Practice.* DHHS Publication No. (SMA)98-3171. Technical Assistance Publication Series 21. Rockville, MD: U.S. Department of Health and Human Services. [Online]. Available: http://www.nattc.org/pdf/accksa.pdf [accessed June 28, 2005].

AHRQ (Agency for Healthcare Research and Quality). 2003. *The Effect of Health Care Working Conditions on Patient Safety: Summary.* AHRQ Publication Number/ 03-E024. [Online]. Available: http://www.ahrq.gov/clinic/epcsums/worksum.pdf [accessed July 1, 2005].

American Psychological Association (APA). 2003. *Psychology: Scientific Problem Solvers—Careers for the 21st Century.* [Online]. Available: www.apa.org/students/brocure/brochurenew. pdf [accessed June 28, 2005]. Washington, DC: American Psychological Association.

APA Committee on Medical Education. 1956. An outline for a curriculum for teaching psychiatry in medical schools. *Journal of Medical Education* 31(2):115–128.

Association of State and Provincial Psychology Boards. 2000. *Handbook of Licensing and Certification Requirements for Psychologists in the U.S. and Canada.* Montgomery, AL: Association of State and Provincial Psychology Boards.

Baker L, Wagner TH, Singer S, Bundorf MK. 2003. Use of the Internet and e-mail for health care information: Results from a national survey. *Journal of the American Medical Association* 289(18):2400–2406.

Benderly BL. 2005. Conference explores high-tech treatments. *SAMHSA NEWS* 13(1):1–4.

Berwick DM. 2003. Dissemination innovations in health care. *Journal of the American Medical Association* 289(15):1969–1975.

Birch and Davis Associates, Inc. 1984. *Development of Model Professional Standards for Counselor Credentialling. Prepared for the National Institute on Alcohol Abuse and Alcoholism.* Reprinted in 1986. Dubuque, IA and Washington, DC: Kendall/Hunt Publishing.

Brailer DJ, Terasawa E. 2003. *Use and Adoption of Computer-Based Patient Records in the United States.* Presentation to IOM Committee on Data Standards for Patient Safety on January 23, 2003. [Online]. Available: http://www.iom.edu/file.asp?id=10988 [accessed October 17, 2004].

COGME, NACNEP (Council on Graduate Medical Education, National Advisory Council on Nurse Education and Practice). 2000. *Collaborative Education to Ensure Patient Safety.* [Online]. Available: ftp://ftp.hrsa.gov/bhpr/nursing/patientsafety/safetyreport.pdf [accessed November 16, 2005].

Copeland J, Martin G. 2004. Web-based interventions for substance use disorders: A qualitative review. *Journal of Substance Abuse Treatment* 26(2):109–116.

D'Onofrio G, Nadel ES, Degutis LC, Sullivan LM, Casper K, Bernstein E, Samet JH. 2002. Improving emergency medicine residents' approach to patients with alcohol problems: A controlled educational trial. *Annals of Emergency Medicine* 40(1):50–62.

Daniels AS, Walter DA. 2002. Current issues in continuing education for contemporary behavioral health practices. *Administration and Policy in Mental Health* 29(4/5):359–376.

Davis D, O'Brien M, Freemantle N, Wolf F, Mazmanian P, Taylor-Vaisey A. 1999. Impact of formal continuing medical education: Do conferences, workshops, rounds, and other traditional continuing education activities change physician behavior or health care outcomes? *Journal of the American Medical Association* 282(9):867–874.

DHHS (U.S. Department of Health and Human Services). 1999. *Mental Health: A Report of the Surgeon General.* Rockville, MD: DHHS.

Duffy FF, West JC, Wilk J, Narrow WE, Hales D, Thompson J, Regier DA, Kohout J, Pion GM, Wicherski MM, Bateman N, Whitaker T, Merwin EI, Lyon D, Fox JC, Delaney KR, Hanrahan N, Stockton R, Garbelman J, Kaladow J, Clawson TW, Smith SC, Bergman DM, Northey WF, Blankertz L, Thomas A, Sullivan LD, Dwyer KP, Fleischer MS, Woodruff CR, Goldsmith HF, Henderson MJ, Atay JJ, Manderscheid RW. 2004. Mental health practitioners and trainees. In: Manderscheid RW, Henderson MJ, eds. *Mental Health, United States, 2002.* DHHS publication Number: (SMA) 3938. Rockville, MD: DHHS Substance Abuse and Mental Health Services Administration. Pp. 327–368.

Edmundson E. 2002. Significant variation in undergraduate training programs *Frontlines: Linking Alcohol Services Research and Practice.* Washington, DC: National Institute on Alcohol Abuse and Alcoholism in conjunction with AcademyHealth.

Flanagan RD, Needham SL. 2003. The internet. In: Feldman S, ed. *Managed Behavioral Health Services: Perspectives and Practice.* Springfield, IL: Charles C. Thomas, Publisher Pp. 307–325.

Friedmann PD, McCulloch D, Chin MH, Saitz R. 2000. Screening and intervention for alcohol problems: A national survey of primary care physicians and psychiatrists. *Journal of General Internal Medicine* 15(2):84–91.

Galanter M. 1980. *Alcohol and Drug Abuse in Medical Education.* Washington, DC: U.S. Government Printing Office.

Greenhalgh T, Robert G, MacFarlane F, Bate P, Kyriakidou O. 2004. Diffusion of innovations in service organizations: Systematic review and recommendations. *The Milbank Quarterly* 82(4):581–629.

Haack MR, Adger H, eds. 2002. *Strategic Plan for Interdisciplinary Faculty Development: Arming the Nation's Health Professional Workforce for a New Approach to Substance Use Disorders.* Dordrecht, the Netherlands: Kluwer Academic/Plenum Publishers.

Harwood HJ. 2002. Survey on behavioral health workplace. *Frontlines: Linking Alcohol Services Research and Practice.* Washington, DC: National Institute on Alcohol Abuse and Alcoholism in conjunction with AcademyHealth. P. 3.

Hobbs F, Stoops N, Census Bureau, U.S. Department of Commerce. 2002. *Demographic Trends in the 20th Century.* Washington, DC: U.S. Government Printing Office. Census 2000 Special Reports. Series CENSR-4. [Online]. Available: http://landview.census.gov/prod/2002pubs/censr-4.pdf [accessed October 4, 2003].

Hoge MA. 2002. The training gap: An acute crisis in behavioral health education. *Administration and Policy in Mental Health* 29(4-5):305–317.

Hoge MA, Morris JA. 2002. Guest editors' introduction. *Administration and Policy in Mental Health* 29(4/5):297–303.

Hoge MA, Jacobs S, Belitsky R, Migdole S. 2002. Graduate education and training for contemporary behavioral health practice. *Administration and Policy in Mental Health* 29(4/5):335–357.

Hoge MA, Morris JA, Daniels AS, Huey LY, Stuart GW, Adams N, Paris M Jr, Goplerud E, Horgan CM, Kaplan L, Storti SA, Dodge JM. 2005a. Report of recommendations: The Annapolis Coalition conference on behavioral health work force competencies. *Administration and Policy in Mental Health* 32(5):651–663.

Hoge MA, Tondora J, Marrelli AF. 2005b. The fundamentals of workforce competency: Implications for behavioral health. *Administration and Policy in Mental Health* 32(5):509–531.

Howard MO, Walker RD, Walker PS, Suchinsky RT. 1997. Alcohol and drug education in schools of nursing. *Journal of Alcohol and Drug Education* 42(3):54–80.

HRSA (Health Resources and Services Administration). 2002. *COGME: About the Council.* [Online]. Available: http://www.cogme.gov/whois.htm [accessed July 1, 2005].

IOM (Institute of Medicine). 1990. *Broadening the Base of Treatment for Alcohol Problems.* Washington, DC: National Academy Press.

IOM. 1997. Edmunds M, Frank R, Hogan M, McCarty D, Robinson-Beale R, Weisner C, eds. *Managing Managed Care: Quality Improvement in Behavioral Health.* Washington, DC: National Academy Press.

IOM. 2001. *Crossing the Quality Chasm: A New Health System for the 21st Century.* Washington, DC: National Academy Press.

IOM. 2003. Greiner AC, Knebel E, eds. *Health Professions Education: A Bridge to Quality.* Washington, DC: The National Academies Press.

IOM. 2004a. *In the Nation's Compelling Interest: Ensuring Diversity in the Health-Care Workforce.* Washington, DC: The National Academies Press.

IOM. 2004b. Page A, ed. *Keeping Patients Safe: Transforming the Work Environment of Nurses.* Washington, DC: The National Academies Press.

Isaacson JH, Fleming M, Kraus M, Kahn R, Mundt M. 2000. A national survey of training in substance use disorders in residency programs. *Journal of Studies on Alcohol* 61(6):912–915.

Jackim LW. 2003. Is all the evidence in? Range of popular treatments subsist despite lack of science base. Is that damaging? *Behavioral Healthcare Tomorrow* 12(5):21–26.

Joint Commission on Mental Illness and Health. 1961. *Action for Mental Health: Final Report of the Joint Commission on Mental Illness and Health.* New York: John Wiley and Sons.

Kaplan L. 2003. *Substance Abuse Treatment Workforce Environmental Scan.* Contract #282-98-0006, Task Order #29. Bethesda, MD. Abt Associates, Inc.

Kessler RC, Demler O, Frank RG, Olfson M, Pincus HA, Walters EE, Wang P, Wells KB, Zaslavsky AM. 2005. Prevalence and treatment of mental disorders, 1990 to 2003. *New England Journal of Medicine* 352(24):2515–2523.

Koppelman J. 2004. The provider system for children's mental health: Workforce capacity and effective treatment. NHPF Issue Brief No. 801. Washington, DC: The George Washington University National Health Policy Forum.

Lamberg L. 2003. Online empathy for mood disorders: Patients turn to internet support groups. *Journal of the American Medical Association* 289(23):3073–3077.

Lazear D. 1991. *Seven Ways of Knowing: Teaching to Multiple Intelligences.* Palatine, IL: Skylight Publishing.

Manderscheid RW, Henderson MJ, Brown DY. 2001. Status of national accountability efforts at the millenium. In: Manderscheid RW, Henderson MJ, eds. *Mental Health, United States, 2000.* DHHS Publication number: (SMA) 01-3537. Washington DC: U.S. Government Printing Office. Pp. 43–52.

McCarty D. 2002. The alcohol and drug abuse treatment workforce. *Frontlines: Linking Alcohol Services Research and Practice.* Washington, DC: National Institute on Alcohol Abuse and Alcoholism in conjunction with AcademyHealth.

McClure M, Poulin M, Sovie M, Wandelt M. 2002. Magnet hospitals: Attraction and retention of professional nurses (The Original Study). In: McClure M, Hinshaw A, eds. *Magnet Hospitals Revisited.* Washington, DC: American Nurses Publishing. Pp. 1–24.

McLellan AT, Carise D, Kleber HD. 2003. Can the national addiction treatment infrastructure support the public's demand for quality care? *Journal of Substance Abuse Treatment* 25(2):117–121.

McLellan AT, Meyers K. 2004. Contemporary addiction treatment: A review of systems problems for adults and adolescents. *Biological Psychiatry* 56(10):764–770.

Mickus M, Colenda CC, Hogan AJ. 2000. Knowledge of mental health benefits and preferences for type of mental health providers among the general public. *Psychiatric Services* 51(2):199–202.

Miller NS, Sheppard LM, Colenda CC, Magen J. 2001. Why physicians are unprepared to treat patients who have alcohol- and drug-related disorders. *Academic Medicine* 76(5):410–418.

Morris JA, Goplerud EN, Hoge MA. 2004. *Workforce Issues in Behavioral Health.* Paper commissioned by the IOM Committee on Crossing the Quality Chasm—Adaptation to Mental Health and Addictive Disorders. Available from the Institute of Medicine.

Mulvey KP, Hubbard S, Hayashi S. 2003. A national study of the substance abuse treatment workforce. *Journal of Substance Abuse Treatment* 24(1):51–57.

NAADAC (National Association of Alcohol and Drug Abuse Counselors). 2005. *About NAADAC.* [Online]. Available: http://naadac.org/documents/index.php?CategoryID=1 [accessed October 16, 2005].

NACNEP (National Advisory Council on Nurse Education and Practice). 2002. *Nurse Education and Practice: Second Report to the Secretary of Health and Human Services and the Congress.* [Online]. Available: ftp://ftp.hrsa.gov/bhpr/nursing/secondreport.pdf [accessed October 16, 2005].

Naegle M. 2002. Nursing education in the prevention and treatment of SUD. In: Haack MR, Adger H, eds. *Strategic Plan for Interdisciplinary Faculty Development: Arming the Nation's Health Professional Workforce for a New Approach to Substance Use Disorders*. AH Dordrecht, The Netherlands: Kluwer Academic/Plenum Publishers.

New Freedom Commission on Mental Health. 2003. *Achieving the Promise: Transforming Mental Health Care in America. Final Report*. DHHS Publication Number: SMA-03-3832. Rockville, MD: U.S. Department of Health and Human Services.

Olvey CDV, Hogg A. 2002. Licensure requirements: Have we raised the bar too far? *Professional Psychology: Research and Practice* 33(3):323–329.

Phillips RL, Dodoo M, Jaen CR, Green LA. 2005. COGME's 16th report to Congress: Too many physicians could be worse than wasted. *Annals of Family Medicine* 3(3):268–270.

Pincus HA, Tanielian TL, Marcus SC, Olfson M, Zarin DA, Thompson J, Zito JM. 1998. Prescribing trends in psychotropic medications: Primary care, psychiatry, and other medical specialties. *Journal of the American Medical Association* 279(7):526–531.

Poster EC. 2004. Psychiatric nursing at risk: The new NCLEX-RN test plan. *Journal of Child and Adolescent Psychiatric Nursing* 17(2):47–48.

President's Commission on Mental Health. 1978. *Report of the President's Commission on Mental Health, Vol. II*. Washington, DC: U.S. Government Printing Office.

Quinn J. 1992. *Intelligent Enterprise: A Knowledge and Service Based Paradigm for Industry*. New York: The Free Press.

Reed MC, Grossman JM. 2004. *Limited Information Technology for Patient Care in Physician Offices*. No. 89. Washington, DC: Center for Studying Health System Change. Issue Brief. [Online]. Available: http://www.hschange.org/CONTENT/708/708.pdf [accessed November 1, 2004].

Rushton JL, Fant K, Clark SJ. 2004. Use of practice guidelines in the primary care of children with Attention-Deficit Hyperactivity Disorder. *Pediatrics* 114(1):e23–e28. [Online]. Available: http://www.pediatrics.aappublications.org/cgi/reprint/114/1/e23 [accessed on September 1, 2005].

Saitz R, Sullivan LM, Samet JH. 2000. Training community-based clinicians in screening and brief intervention for substance abuse problems: Translating evidence into practice. *Substance Abuse* 21(1):21–31.

Saitz R, Friedman PD, Sullivan LM, Winter MR, Lloyd-Travaglini C, Moskowitz MA, Samet J. 2002. Professional satisfaction experienced when caring for substance-abusing patients: Faculty and resident physician perspectives. *Journal of General Internal Medicine* 17(5):373–376.

Samet JH, Galanter M, Bridden C, Lewis DC. 2006. Association for Medical Education and Research in Substance Abuse. *Addiction* 101(1):10–15.

SAMHSA (Substance Abuse and Mental Health Services Administration). 2000. *Changing the Conversation: Improving Substance Abuse Treatment: The National Treatment Plan Initiative*. DHHS Publication No. (SMA) 00-3479. U.S. Department of Health and Human Services.

SAMHSA. 2003. *Alcohol and Drug Services Study (ADSS): The National Substance Abuse Treatment System: Facilities, Clients, Services, and Staffing*. Rockville, MD: Office of Applied Studies. [Online]. Available: http://www.oas.samhsa.gov/ADSS/ADSSorg.pdf [accessed June 30, 2005].

SAMHSA. 2004. *National Survey of Substance Abuse Treatment Services (N-SSATS): 2003— Data on Substance Abuse Treatment Facilities*. DASIS Series: S-24. DHHS Publication Number: (SMA) 04-3966. Rockville, MD: U.S. Department of Health and Human Services.

SAMHSA. undated. *Report to Congress on the Prevention and Treatment of Co-Occurring Substance Abuse Disorders and Mental Disorders*: U.S. Department of Health and Human Services. [Online]. Available: http://www.samhsa.gov/reports/congress2002/CoOccurringRpt.pdf [accessed April 25, 2004].

Straussner SLA, Senreich E. 2002. Educating social workers to work with individuals affected by substance use disorders. In: Haack MR, Adger H Jr, eds. *Strategic Plan for Interdisciplinary Faculty Development: Arming the Nation's Health Professional Workforce for a New Approach to Substance Use Disorders* 23:319–340. Dordrecht, the Netherlands: Kluwer Academic/Plenum Publishers.

Trabin T, Maloney W. 2003. Information systems. In: Feldman S, ed. *Managed Behavioral Health Services: Perspectives and Practices*. Springfield, IL: Charles C. Thomas Publisher. Pp. 326–370.

Trowbridge R, Weingarten S. 2001. Clinical decision support systems. In: Shojania K, Duncan B, McDonald K, Wachter R, eds. *Making Health Care Safer: A Critical Analysis of Patient Safety Practices*. Evidence Report/Technology Assessment Number 43. AHRQ Publication No. 01-E058. Rockville, MD: Agency for Healthcare Research and Quality.

Vastag B. 2003. Addiction poorly understood by clinicians: Experts say attitudes, lack of knowledge hinder treatment. *Journal of the American Medical Association* 290(10): 1299–1303.

Wallerstein R, ed. 1991. *The Doctorate in Mental Health: An Experiment in Mental Health Professional Education*. Lanham, MD: University Press of America.

Wang PS, Berglund P, Kessler RC. 2000. Recent care of common mental disorders in the United States: Prevalence and conformance with evidence-based recommendations. *Journal of General Internal Medicine* 15(5):284–292.

West J, Kohout J, Pion GM, Wicherski MM, Vandivort-Warren RE, Palmiter ML, Merwin EI, Lyon D, Fox JC, Clawson TW, Smith SC, Stockton R, Nitza AG, Ambrose JP, Blankertz L, Thomas A, Sullivan LD, Dwyer KP, Fleischer MS, Goldsmith HF, Henderson MJ, Atay JE, Manderscheid RW. 2001. Mental health practitioners and trainees. In: Manderscheid RW, Henderson MJ, eds. *Mental Health, United States, 2000*. DHHS Publication No. (SMA) 01-3537.Washington, DC: U.S. Government Printing Office. Pp. 279–315.

Young AS, Klap R, Sherbourne C, Wells KB. 2001. The quality of care for depressive and anxiety disorders in the United States. *Archives of General Psychiatry* 58(1):55–61.

8

Using Marketplace Incentives to Leverage Needed Change

Summary

The previous chapters identify areas in which change is needed on the part of federal and state governments, health care organizations, and individual clinicians, among others. The feasibility of many of these changes depends on how accommodating the marketplace is to them, particularly with respect to the ways in which purchasers of mental and/or substance-use (M/SU) health care exercise their marketplace roles.

The M/SU health care marketplace has some unique features that distinguish it from the general health care marketplace. These include the dominance of government (state and local) purchasers, the frequent purchase of insurance for M/SU health care separately from that for other health care (i.e., the use of "carve-out" arrangements), the tendency of the private insurance marketplace to avoid covering or to offer more-limited coverage to individuals with M/SU illnesses, and government purchasers' greater use of direct provision and purchase of care rather than insurance arrangements. Attending to these differences is essential if the marketplace is to promote quality improvement in M/SU health care. The committee recommends four ways of strengthening the marketplace to this end.

KEY FEATURES OF THE MARKETPLACE FOR MENTAL AND SUBSTANCE-USE HEALTH CARE

People with mental and/or substance-use (M/SU) problems and illnesses receive care from a range of provider organizations and individual clinicians—most often from private providers operating in market settings. However, while the majority of *individuals* have their general and mental health care paid for by private insurance, most *payments* for M/SU treatments are made by government, either in the form of payments from public insurance (Medicare and Medicaid) or through states' direct purchase of services from providers. This section reviews the key features of the marketplace for M/SU health care that distinguish it from that for other types of care.

Dominance of Government Purchasing

Recent estimates suggest that payment for roughly 63 percent of mental health care and 76 percent of substance-use treatment is made by public sources (Mark et al., 2005). Figure 8-1 shows the distribution of spending for M/SU care by major sources of payment as of 2001. In the case of mental health care, the majority (54 percent) of all public spending (direct public purchasing and public insurance) makes use of health insurance

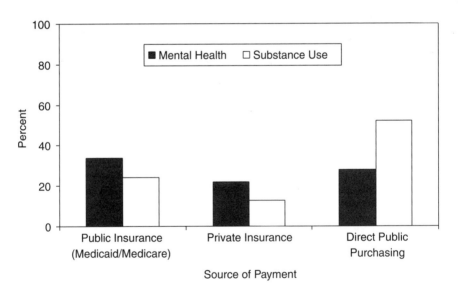

FIGURE 8-1   Financing methods for mental health/substance-use care in 2001.
SOURCE: Mark et al., 2005.

mechanisms; public health insurance consists primarily of the Medicaid and Medicare programs. For substance-use treatment, a larger majority (68 percent) of spending is on direct government grants and contracts with providers. The implication is that payments for substance-use services are most frequently allocated outside of markets. When private spending is also considered, approximately 56 percent of all payments for mental health care are made through insurance mechanisms, as opposed to out-of-pocket payments, grants, donations, and other sources of private financing. In contrast, only 27 percent of private payments for substance-use treatment flows through insurance arrangements. Again, this suggests a somewhat lesser impact of insurance market failure on substance-use care.

The implication of these figures is that choices about the level and composition of spending on M/SU health care are affected by a mix of market and political forces and that these forces differ for health care for mental and substance-use conditions. The willingness to pay for treatment for M/SU problems and illnesses is expressed through private markets for health insurance; political decisions about the design of public insurance; and the categorical program budgets of federal, state, and local agencies charged with providing such treatment.

Purchase of M/SU Health Insurance Separately from General Health Insurance

Insurance for M/SU health care is governed by a distinctive set of arrangements. Although the proportion has been declining in recent years, most Americans (64 percent in 2002) under the age of 65 continue to receive health care through insurance provided by either their own employer or that of a family member (Fronstin, 2003). The terms under which individuals choose insurance and under which health plans compete to provide it are defined by organizations that purchase the insurance in the marketplace. Employers, state governments as administrators of Medicaid programs, and the federal government through the Medicare program all define the rules under which markets for health insurance operate.

Larger employers allow employees and their dependents to choose among a number of insurers and products (e.g., preferred provider organization, health maintenance organization) in competitive insurance markets. Smaller employers frequently offer only a single insurance plan to their employees. Some large employers focus special attention on M/SU coverage and spending. In these cases, employers separate the insurance risk for M/SU treatment from that for other health insurance, and create what have become known as managed behavioral health care organization (MBHO) carve-out contracts (Frank and McGuire, 2000). Under such circumstances, an employee has no choice of coverage for M/SU health care since the benefit is managed by a single organization, regardless of the options available for general health care. Approximately 20 percent of privately insured people are covered under such a carve-out arrangement. For most of the remaining 80 percent, their private general health plan enters into a subcontract with a carve-out MBHO to manage its M/SU care benefit. In this case, employees and their dependents can choose among both general and M/SU health care benefits across a set of health plans. Finally, some health plans offer M/SU coverage that is integrated with the rest of the health insurance risk; such plans represent a modest share of the private market.

Medicaid, the federal–state government program that focuses on the poor and disabled, includes managed care arrangements and insurance that follows the principles of fee-for-service–indemnity health insurance. Under Medicaid managed care, the use of MBHO carve-outs mirrors the approach taken by private insurance. Roughly 16 states have direct payer carve-out contracts with MBHOs (CMS, 2004). Most Medicaid managed care plans not operating in environments where the Medicaid program has a direct carve-out have subcontracts with carve-out vendors.

More Limited Insurance Coverage

While nearly all private insurance plans offer some coverage for treatment of M/SU illnesses, the coverage is often substantially more limited than that for other medical conditions (Barry et al., 2003). In 2002, 96 percent of people with employer-based coverage had inpatient M/SU coverage, and 98 percent had outpatient coverage; these figures represent a small increase over the proportion of insured covered for these treatments in 1991. M/SU services are typically subject to limits on the number of annual reimbursable outpatient visits and inpatient days. Approximately 74 percent of covered employees have limits on outpatient visits and 65 percent limits on inpatient days.

The fee-for-service component of Medicaid pays for a range of mental health services. Because there is little reliance on consumer cost sharing, however, rationing of supply is common. This is a side effect of below-market payment rates for providers, especially providers of ambulatory care. The result is low participation rates in Medicaid among office-based clinicians, such as psychiatrists and psychologists. Coverage for substance-use care under Medicaid is considerably more limited than that for mental health services (McCarty et al., 1999). Inpatient care for mental illnesses in adults under the age of 65 is limited to general hospitals under the so-called Institutions for Mental Disease (IMD) exclusion provisions of the original enabling Medicaid legislation. Thus the breadth of providers available is limited to a subset of those that supply inpatient psychiatric and substance-use treatment (for a detailed discussion and history of the IMD provisions, see HCFA, 1992).

Medicare offers a fee-for-service indemnity insurance type of benefit. A small portion (about 14 percent) of Medicare beneficiaries are enrolled in managed care plans that contract with the Medicare program to offer services to Medicare beneficiaries (CMS, 2005). Traditional Medicare (the indemnity component) covers M/SU care. Outpatient coverage carries relatively high cost sharing (50 percent), except for medication management (20 percent). Inpatient coverage is largely on the same basis as that for other medical conditions, with one exception: treatment in specialty psychiatric hospitals is limited to 190 days over an individual recipient's lifetime. Also, psychiatric care is covered under a form of prospective payment that differs from the case-based diagnosis-related group (DRG) system used in Medicare generally.

Frequent Direct Provision and Purchase of Care by State and Local Governments

A unique feature of the structure of service delivery for M/SU health care is the large role assigned to public hospitals and clinics and to non–insurance-based purchase of services by state and local governments. In the United States, state and local governments directly deliver or purchase the bulk of M/SU services. Thus, financing relies on state and local tax revenues instead of individual consumer premiums or federal government funding, although the federal government plays a larger role in funding the direct purchase of substance-use treatment services through the federal block grants to states. Further, nearly all states operate under balanced-budget statutes. As a result, the political competition for funding of public services is intense. Funding for M/SU services is frequently pitted against that for roads, schools, and prisons in state budgeting processes. State and local governments pay for direct provision of M/SU services through networks of community-based providers that commonly serve a catchment area with a defined population. These community-based providers are most often private nonprofit organizations and are generally long-time incumbents in their service delivery role. Public M/SU services therefore resemble a monopoly arrangement whereby state and local governments grant a franchise to a nonprofit care provider agency.

Thus, the delivery of M/SU care in the United States is organized and financed through a patchwork of insurance and direct provision of services. In some cases, markets play a prominent role in resource allocation; in others, government and administrative practices are central in shaping what services are delivered and which people are served. In all cases, powerful institutions are involved in the purchase of the services. Understanding how these approaches to purchasing operate and what effects they have on the marketplace may help in identifying ways to facilitate improvements in the quality of care for people with M/SU problems and illnesses.

CHARACTERISTICS OF DIFFERENT PURCHASING STRATEGIES

M/SU health care delivery systems encompass a diverse array of purchasing arrangements, market structures, and government participation, each with differing effects on access to and the quality and cost of care.

Purchase Through Competitive Insurance Markets: Competition for Enrollees

One common approach to the purchase of insurance is for an employer or a state Medicaid program to select a group of health plans that will be permitted to compete for its enrollees. The payer first establishes a set of criteria that plans wishing to compete for its enrollees must meet. Such criteria typically address benefit design, performance, and cost. Programs that meet these criteria are then permitted to compete for enrollees, who are offered information on benefit structure and some quality indicators for each plan offered. In most cases, enrollees face premiums that are subsidized (zero in the case of Medicaid). In theory, payments made by the payer to the plan create incentives for efficient provision of services. Competition for enrollees should be less oriented toward price because of the subsidy and thus should promote consumer choice based on quality. The combination of capitation payments and quality competition among plans should lead to a reasonable balance between cost and quality.

However, competition for enrollees in the presence of risk-based premiums (e.g., capitation) also has some well-known drawbacks (Cutler and Zeckhauser, 2000; IOM, 1993). This type of purchasing creates financial incentives for health plans to adopt policies that discourage high-cost individuals from enrolling. These incentives also may result in uneven coverage across therapeutic areas and potentially uneven quality.

Ideally, health plans would ration care so that the incremental contributions to health of spending on each type of service (e.g., cancer care, heart disease treatment, and mental health) would be equal. This approach would guarantee the maximum level of health for a population given a fixed budget (as is implied by capitation payments). Under a fixed-payment arrangement, however, competitive health plans have incentives to depart from such an ideal allocation strategy. Specifically, since people with M/SU illnesses are more costly to insure and payments to health plans do not recognize those differences, plans have an incentive to avoid enrolling persons with such illnesses. An example comes from recent analyses of the Medical Expenditure Panel Survey (Anderson and Knickman, 2001; Druss et al., 2001) showing that per capita health spending for people with mood disorders is more than four times that for individuals without such illnesses.

Incentives to avoid enrolling these people create a serious threat to quality of care through health insurance.

In insurance markets where M/SU services are part of the general risk pool, competition is reoriented to avoiding "bad risks." One result is that plans limit coverage for conditions, such as M/SU illnesses, that attract high-cost enrollees. Low-cost individuals gravitate toward health plans offering limited insurance coverage at a lower premium, leaving the sickest enrollees in plans with relatively generous coverage. If premiums do not reflect differences in the enrolled population, plans offering more generous coverage will lose money; the result can be a so-called "death spiral" in coverage for treatment of M/SU illnesses. The Federal Employees Health Benefit Program (FEHBP) during the 1980s and 1990s offers an important case study of this phenomenon. In 1980, the FEHBP was viewed as model for mental health coverage; at that time, 7.8 percent of the program's spending was devoted to treatment of mental illnesses. By 1997, the coverage offered had deteriorated to involve high levels of cost sharing and strict limits on inpatient days and outpatient visits. Observed spending on mental health as a share of total health spending had declined to 1.9 percent (Foote and Jones, 1999; Padgett et al., 1993).

Quality of care can be affected by the same market dynamics as those associated with selection incentives. In the era of managed care and its offshoots, those same competitive incentives can result in markets for health insurance supplying insufficient levels of service and quality of care for M/SU illnesses. The hallmark of the modern health plan is that a variety of new rationing mechanisms—including provider payment strategies, prior authorization programs, and the design of provider networks—are substituted for traditional demand-side cost-sharing features. Miller and Luft (1997:20) highlight this point:

> Under the simple capitation payment arrangements that now exist, plans and providers face strong financial disincentives to excel in the care for the sickest and most expensive patients. Plans that develop a strong reputation for excellence in quality of care for the sickest will attract new higher-cost enrollees. . . .

The implication is that health plans can use administrative mechanisms to compete to avoid "bad risks." Rationing so as not to offer the best quality of M/SU health care in a market represents one method of trying to avoid a group of high-cost enrollees. Nothing in the modern market for health insurance has diminished the incentives to avoid enrolling high-cost individuals. Moreover, the evidence of market outcomes consistent with selection incentives for people with M/SU illnesses is strong (Cao, 2003; Cao and McGuire, 2003; Deb et al., 1996; Ellis, 1985; Frank et al., 2000; Normand et al., 2003).

There are two means by which a health plan can affect the intensity of rationing of M/SU health care when it (rather then the employer or other group purchaser) carves out behavioral health care: through the level at which it sets the carve-out health plan's budget (via the capitation rate) and through the performance requirements specified in a contract. It is common to see capitation rates of $2.00 or less per member per month, a figure generally viewed as being consistent with a minimal level of care.

Direct Purchase of Carve-Out Services by Group Payers

A second prominent approach to purchasing insurance coverage for M/SU health care is for the payer to purchase carve-out services directly. This approach involves separating the risks associated with care for these illnesses from general health care risks and entering into specific contracts for coverage of M/SU care. Such direct purchase of carve-out services is used by approximately one-third of large employers (5,000 employees or more), 5 percent of midsized employers, and about 16 state Medicaid programs (Hodgkin et al., 2000; CMS, 2004). This method of purchasing removes M/SU health care from competition for enrollees, thereby attenuating the selection incentives concerning coverage and quality discussed above. However, use of such carve-out arrangements has implications for care coordination (see Chapter 5).

Direct purchase of carve-out M/SU services by group health care payers uses competition as the means of awarding contracts for these services. That is, a payer will frequently solicit proposals and bids from MBHO carve-out vendors to manage the M/SU health care for a defined population. The requests for proposals specify the areas of performance on which the contract will be awarded. The most common areas of performance are costs, responses of the utilization management system (e.g., speed of telephone response to member calls, speed of referral to a provider), and plan member satisfaction. There is, of course, considerable variation in the specifics, with some payers developing relatively elaborate measures of access and quality. However, the typical contract specifies few indicators of clinical quality, such as depression medication measures.

State Medicaid programs typically operate under state procurement regulations that place great emphasis on pursuing the lowest-cost bid if it is "technically acceptable" to reviewers of the proposal. It should be noted that many states include consumers of M/SU services as advisers to the state in the procurement of MBHO carve-out services. Private payers commonly use consultants as advisers in their procurement process.

The market for MBHO carve-out services consists of several large national vendors (e.g., United Behavioral Health, Magellan, and Value-

Options), several smaller national firms (e.g., CIGNA Behavioral Health, PacifiCare Behavioral Health), and numerous smaller regional vendors (e.g., Beacon Health Strategies in the northeast). Competition for contracts is very intense, resulting in aggressively priced bids. In both the public and private sectors, disproportionate weight is usually placed on the cost portion of the proposal. States in particular are reluctant to deviate from awarding contracts to organizations other than the lowest-cost bidder. While private purchasers have greater flexibility in selecting vendors, they, too, commonly place heavy emphasis on price in awarding a contract. This emphasis on price, together with the limited use of quality measures in most procurements, creates an incentive for MBHO carve-out vendors to gear their care management practices to meet cost goals, possibly at the expense of quality. Payers are left to rely on complaints and highly visible indicators of quality deficits to identify a quality-of-care problem.

Widespread evidence shows that MBHO carve-out programs reduce spending on both mental health and substance-use treatment (Frank and Lave, 2003; Frank et al., 1995; Sturm, 1999), although the evidence to date on the impact on quality of care is limited and mixed (Barry et al., 2003; see Frank and Lave, 2003, for a recent review). Studies of early programs typically showed no differences in quality (Busch, 2002; Dickey et al., 1998; Merrick, 1998). Findings of two more recent studies, however, suggest that people with severe mental illnesses may be especially disadvantaged under MBHO carve-out arrangements in the context of state Medicaid programs. Manning and colleagues (1999) compared outcomes for patients with schizophrenia enrolled in a capitated carve-out program with those for similar patients whose care was paid for under fee-for-service arrangements. They found that people with schizophrenia in the carve-out program showed less improvement than those in fee-for-service arrangements (Manning et al., 1999). Busch and colleagues used data from one state Medicaid program to study indicators of the quality of care based on the schizophrenia Patient Outcomes Research Team (PORT) recommendations. Their comparison of a capitated MBHO carve-out and a primary care case management system found comparable quality of medication management under the two approaches, but substantially lower quality of psychosocial treatment under the capitated carve-out arrangement (Busch et al., 2004).

The above evidence suggests how MBHO carve-out arrangements alter the quality of care relative to fee-for-service arrangements. The more general question is whether existing levels of quality of care are sufficient. The evidence from several studies is that levels of care under both arrangements are lower than desired (Lehman and Steinwachs, 1998; McGlynn et al., 2003; Young et al., 2001).

Purchase of Services by Carve-Out Organizations

Carve-out vendors operate under very specific contracts. These contracts specify the benefit structure within which the MBHO carve-out has responsibility for managing care. They also specify the responsibilities of the carve-out vendor with respect to the services being managed. Payment arrangements, risk bearing, and performance standards are all established, as is the structure of the provider network. Virtually all carve-out contracts exclude prescription drugs from the services managed by the MBHO, as well as from the budget that is to be managed. The implication is that carve-out contracts are not "economically neutral"; that is, there are economic incentives favoring the use of medications over other components of treatment. In effect, psychotropic drugs are "free" to carve-out vendors, while they must pay market prices for hospital care and professional services.

Indeed, empirical analyses of treatment patterns show that patients treated for particular illnesses (e.g., depression) under a carve-out arrangement are more likely to be treated with medication—and medication alone—than are otherwise similar patients whose care is not managed under such a contract (Berndt et al., 1997; Busch, 2002). Other studies have shown that following implementation of a carve-out arrangement, spending on psychotropic drugs has increased, other factors being held constant (Ling et al., 2003; Norton et al., 1999). The result is that savings from carve-out programs come from reduced use of inpatient and outpatient specialty M/SU care. Increases in prescription drug spending serve to reduce some of the savings otherwise realized by the group purchaser.

In modern health care markets, it is rare for a single health plan to cover 30 percent of insured patients in a market. When individual health plans account for 5–20 percent of patients, a typical provider or professional may literally do business with dozens of plans. Thus, a physician may face a dozen formulary arrangements, many sets of clinical guidelines, an array of compensation arrangements, and numerous reporting requirements for any particular condition. In such cases, the impact on provider behavior of financial incentives or other directives specified in any one health plan will be quite diluted. Research has shown that physician practices appear to manage their operations in a manner that is responsive to the overall composition of their payer arrangements (e.g., the most frequent incentive scheme). This means that in general, an individual health plan has little ability to influence provider behavior if its approach differs from that commonly encountered in a practice (Glied and Zivin, 2002).

The MBHO carve-out market has consolidated notably since the early 1990s. At that time, there were nearly a dozen significant national vendors; today there are three or four. The implication is that in local markets for M/SU health care, individual carve-out companies may account for a larger share of patients than is common in health care generally. It is relatively common for a carve-out vendor to account for 30–50 percent of a market. This means carve-out vendors have the potential to affect the delivery of M/SU health care in a manner that health plans alone cannot. The consolidation of the carve-out marketplace serves to increase the potential bargaining power of the larger carve-out vendors. That bargaining power is achieved because a carve-out vendor can direct patients away from providers that offer prices or other dimensions of performance not consistent with the vendor's economic and clinical aims. The result is a considerable amount of power not only in setting prices, but also potentially in establishing standards of care.

To date, the MBHO carve-out industry has used its power to (1) increase access to care (as measured by utilization rates), (2) reduce utilization of inpatient care for both mental health and substance-use care, (3) reduce provider payments, and (4) reduce the duration of some ambulatory episodes of treatment. The exertion of pricing power on the one hand contributes to cost control. However, excessive price reductions can decrease the effective supply of providers that are willing to participate in managed behavioral health care networks. This in turn creates the appearance of a shortage for enrollees and managers of those plans, even though there is no shortage in the aggregate. Low prices can result as well in an undersupply of quality (to be discussed further in the context of Medicaid). Yet the consolidation of the market also creates an opportunity to influence provider behavior in the service of quality improvement. The possession of market power with respect to providers means that efforts to improve quality will be less diluted than is typical in the health sector generally. Some managed behavioral health care initiatives have used this market power to both reduce costs and improve quality. When the Massachusetts Medicaid program instituted a managed behavioral health care carve-out program in the early 1990s, the number of inpatient providers supplying care to Medicaid enrollees with M/SU illnesses was reduced by about 30 percent. Hospitals were eliminated from the program based in part on historical performance on quality, as well as price (Callahan et al., 1995; Frank and McGuire, 1997). The result was reduced inpatient spending and constant or improved quality of inpatient care. The implication is that network design can be used to exert economic power not only to control spending, but also to improve quality.

Purchase of Services in Traditional Medicaid Programs

State Medicaid programs typically cover and pay for a wide range of services for the treatment of mental illnesses. Coverage for treatment of substance-use illnesses is far less consistent across the states (McCarty et al.,

1999). On the mental health side, the array of services covered by Medicaid is consistent with the provision of evidence-based treatment. This is often not the case for treatment of substance-use illnesses. Traditional Medicaid programs purchase ambulatory services on a fee-for-service basis. States use a variety of arrangements to pay for hospital services. These range from prospective per diem rates, to per case prospective payment, to the occasional use of prospective budgets. Prescription drugs are paid for under a "most favored nation" arrangement, whereby Medicaid is guaranteed the best private price (Scott-Morton, 1997). Under the traditional Medicaid structure, a state's ability to use cost sharing to control costs and utilization is minimal. Thus traditional Medicaid relies on setting prices for ambulatory services at rates below market levels. Those prices reduce provider willingness to accept reimbursement and participate in the program. Payment levels are therefore low, and the quantity of care is constrained by the available supply. Data from the mid-1990s show that among physicians, psychiatrists had the lowest rate of Medicaid participation (Perloff et al., 1995). Only about 28 percent of psychiatrists were full participants in Medicaid, compared with 56 percent of all specialists and 36 percent of primary care physicians. These low rates of payment and participation are generally thought to be consistent with lower-quality care (Rowland and Tallon, 2003). Hospital payment rates have also tended to be somewhat lower than market rates; as a result of congressional action and litigation, however, the differential is smaller than is the case for ambulatory services (MEDPAC, 2003).

Publicly Budgeted Systems of Care

The ways in which publicly budgeted M/SU services are organized and funded varies greatly across the 50 states (Lutterman and Hogan, 2001). Substance-use treatment services are far more reliant on direct funding through state and local government than is mental health care (Figure 8-1). Yet while there is tremendous variation in the details of how intergovernmental transfers are designed and organized within both the public mental health and substance-use treatment systems, some common features germane to the analysis of quality are found with considerable frequency.

First, organizations that receive funds directly from state and local government for the treatment of substance use are frequently responsible for geographic catchment areas that serve a defined population. In the case of community mental health centers, nearly 60 percent of revenues represent direct grants and contracts from federal, state, and local government (DHHS, 2002). This figure tends to be even higher for agencies that supply primarily substance-use treatment (Tabulations from the National Drug Abuse Treatment System Survey). Within a defined population, these agencies typically serve individuals with low incomes. Some are "insured" by Medicaid, but many are uninsured (e.g., 20 percent of people with severe mental illness [McAlpine and Mechanic, 2000]).

State and local mental health budgets have been under great pressure for some time. In the first years of the new century, a recession and state budget crises forced cuts in most social service programs. A longer-term problem on the mental health front is that an increasing share of state general fund allocations for mental health services is being allocated to the states' Medicaid matching obligations (Frank et al., 2003). In the substance-use area, modest growth rates in the funding of the federal block grants to states have further stressed states' abilities to fund local agencies serving poor people with substance-use illnesses. For example, from 2003 to 2004, the Substance Abuse Prevention and Treatment Block Grant grew by just 1.4 percent (www.samhsa.gov/budget/B2005/spending/cj_12.aspx).

The fact that publicly funded M/SU treatment providers typically are (1) well-established nonprofit agencies with exclusive responsibility for providing treatment for low-income, uninsured populations and (2) funded through grant mechanisms or prospectively set budgets with volume requirements (Alexander et al., 2002; Frank and Goldman, 1989) creates incentives that can conflict with the provision of high-quality care. In effect, these agencies commonly face fixed budgets, excess demand for services (as evidenced by waiting lines), and no competition. Moreover, because agencies are responsible for serving defined populations, there tend to be consumer-based and political pressures to minimize waiting lists and serve as many people as possible (see Lindsay [1976] and Michael [1980] for examples of economic models of public provision of general and mental health care). The result is that economic and political forces reinforce an emphasis on maximizing the number of people served, possibly at the expense of investments in quality. State and local governments have little leverage in such cases even if their goals differ because the agencies are in effect monopoly franchises. Thus, state and local governments concerned about quality levels cannot easily direct consumers to other providers.

PROCUREMENT AND THE CONSUMER ROLE

The purchasing arrangements described above shape the role of the consumer of M/SU treatment services. They also affect the market outcomes stemming from active consumerism.

The modern consumer movement in health care dates back to the 1960s, when President Kennedy set forth a consumer bill of rights in his "Consumer Message" of 1962 (Tomes, 1999). This action coincided with the deinstitutionalization movement in mental health and widespread dissatisfaction with institutional psychiatry. The result was an energized patient advocacy movement and successful litigation by public interest lawyers on behalf of psychiatric patients. It was during the 1960s and 1970s that people who used M/SU treatment services began to call themselves consumers (Chu and Trotter, 1972). Yet the notion of consumerism in the M/SU sector went beyond that of individuals empowered to exercise choice in the marketplace; rather, it involved the exercise of "voice." That is, through the strategic use of lawsuits and active lobbying, federal and state governments began to directly address the concerns of patients and their families (Tomes, 1999). In recent years, however, the fragmentation of financing for treatment of M/SU illnesses has made it more difficult to focus the consumer's voice. For example, the state mental health agency is no longer the primary payer and regulator of mental health services in most states; Medicaid now has that responsibility (Frank et al., 2003).

The consumer role also involves a more commercial or market-oriented set of activities whereby consumers seek to obtain services that offer the mix of price and quality that best suits their needs. This role typically involves obtaining and processing information on the cost and quality of various health care services, including health insurance.

Privately insured people frequently have a choice of health insurance plans. However, evidence to date suggests that consumers make little use of information on quality and frequently focus primarily on price. In the case of those with M/SU illnesses, the selection incentives described earlier lead to the troubling result that greater choice and consumerism tend to compromise the coverage and quality of services offered by health plans. This holds true for Medicaid managed care arrangements that rely on health plans competing for enrollees. The presence of payer carve-outs diminishes consumer choice in coverage for M/SU treatment coverage and focuses choice on providers. In traditional Medicaid programs, there is no insurance choice as is the case in traditional Medicare (Parts A and B).

Insured consumers of treatment for M/SU problems and illnesses (and those covered by Medicare) commonly have a good deal of choice among providers. Like all health care consumers, however, those seeking help for M/SU illnesses must choose among a large number of providers that are highly heterogeneous with respect to training, therapeutic orientation, technical capabilities, and expertise in specific types of problems (see Chapter 7), and there is little consistent information on provider performance in a typical consumer's choice set. Furthermore, these choices must be made in the context of complex coverage and payment arrangements. It is common for a privately insured person to have coverage for mental health care that involves a deductible, coinsurance, and then a limit on coverage after a specific number of visits or days of care. In addition, some providers are "in network" while others are "out," which means that coinsurance rates will differ. Also, as discussed previously, consumers of M/SU treatment services face more-limited coverage—and as a result, higher prices and greater financial risks—relative to other health care consumers, while the economic circumstances of insurance coverage generally make using services considerably more expensive to the household. Finally, M/SU illnesses can affect a consumer's outlook and attitude toward treatment (e.g., pessimism among those with depression), thereby influencing the ability to exercise commercial aspects of the consumer role.

Consumers who rely on traditional Medicaid or providers that are directly funded by state and local governments have very limited choices of providers. Because budgeted systems are most often organized as franchises that cover catchment areas, consumerism does not play a role in determining the quality or price of services. These are the types of providers that have been the focus of lobbying by advocacy groups and lawsuits by public interest lawyers. Thus consumerism in this subsector has come to mean the exercise of voice. Without fundamental change in the organization of care delivery, the existing consumer role will persist for these individuals. The Medicaid program in theory allows for a broad choice of providers; however, rationing by paying providers fees that are below market rates results in a limited supply of providers willing to treat Medicaid recipients with M/SU illnesses. The end result is that most Medicaid recipients have a very limited choice of providers for M/SU treatment.

EFFECTS OF MARKET AND POLICY STRUCTURES ON QUALITY

The above discussion identifies several key forces that affect the quality of M/SU care according to the main types of funding arrangements (competitive insurance, direct carve-out), under differing methods of organizing the financing of services (carve-out networks, traditional Medicaid), and with differing sources of payment (direct government, Medicaid, private insurance). Each of the main structures identified offers a potential target for policy intervention.

Quality Distortions in the Purchase of Health Plan Services Through Competition for Enrollees

When a group purchaser offers its enrollees more than one health plan from which to choose, most private insurance and many state Medicaid programs create competitive markets in which health plans compete to enroll members. In these cases, incentives to avoid enrolling high-cost individuals may cause distortions in insurance coverage for and the quality of M/SU care. These incentives arise because people with M/SU illnesses generally incur higher health care costs that persist over time relative to other segments of an insured population. Such distortions in private insurance coverage can be addressed by mandating minimum levels of coverage for M/SU care. "Parity" legislation is an example of such measures. As noted earlier, however, managed care tactics can substitute for demand-side cost-sharing policies (e.g., copayments, limits) to control costs. Under parity laws, health plans continue to have an incentive to avoid enrolling high-cost individuals. By applying the tools of managed care to M/SU services more stringently, plans can affect aspects of the quality of care they provide (e.g., convenience and availability of providers) and make themselves less attractive to potential enrollees who anticipate availing themselves of M/SU treatment services. Thus parity laws appear to be necessary but not sufficient to address selection incentives that distort coverage and quality of care (Frank et al., 2001).

Two approaches to stemming adverse selection incentives in M/SU care are currently in use. The first is payer carve-out of M/SU health care services, whereby the employer or other group purchaser separates M/SU health care from the remainder of insurance risk and eliminates its management as a competitive strategy (see the discussion earlier in this chapter). Coverage and rationing for M/SU health care are arranged directly by the payer with the carve-out vendor through a contract. The payer's procurement process and the terms of the contract thus become the determinants of rationing (as discussed below). Carve-outs carry their own disadvantages, including relatively high administrative costs, potential difficulties in coordination of care between general medical care and specialty behavioral health providers, and incentives to shift costs and responsibility for care across insurance segments (e.g., pharmacy benefits). It is important to note as well that most carve-out arrangements in private health insurance are not payer carve-outs but are implemented by an individual health plan; these arrangements do not affect selection-related incentives. There is also anecdotal evidence suggesting that some large insurers are shifting away from the carve-out approach to managing M/SU care, as exemplified by Aetna's recent decision to "carve back in" M/SU health care instead of contracting out for these services.

The second approach to reducing selection incentives is risk adjustment, a strategy consistent with either integration of the risk associated with M/SU health services with other medical risks or a health plan carve-out structure. The idea behind risk adjustment is that if health plans are paid more for enrolling high-cost individuals, they will be less inclined to try to avoid doing so. Most risk adjustment systems rely on patient demographics and clinical information, such as diagnoses, to create clusters of potential enrollees according to the intensity and complexity of past treatment (Weiner et al., 1996). These clusters are used to predict costs. If individuals choose plans based in part on predictable expenses, the risk adjustment approach can be used to adjust plan payments so as to diminish the selection incentive. However, risk adjustment systems in general explain only about 7 percent of variations in spending. Ettner and colleagues compared the performance of several risk adjustment systems for M/SU services in private insurance and Medicaid. They found that no existing risk adjustment classification system displayed strong predictive ability for spending on M/SU care (Ettner, 2001; Ettner et al., 1998). Thus existing risk adjustment approaches appear to be limited in their ability to stem selection-driven distortions in quality affecting those at risk for using M/SU treatment services. Organizational strategies can also be used to address selection incentives.

Direct Public Purchase of Behavioral Carve-out Services in Medicaid

Currently, approximately 16 states and territories (or substate units) contract directly with carve-out vendors for some M/SU health care services. As discussed earlier, this approach to the purchase of coverage and managed care for M/SU treatment offers the advantage of attenuating distortions in quality of care that may result from selection-related incentives. Yet the procurement process for these contracts is frequently structured so that performance with respect to contract costs may be overemphasized relative to performance on quality of care. If costs and quality are positively correlated, the implication of this procurement structure is that there will be a tendency to choose lower-cost, lower-quality contract proposals. One is reminded of the remarks of astronaut Allen Shepard, who just prior to being launched into space expressed concern that he would be aboard the spacecraft that had been built by the lowest-cost bidder.

One approach to addressing this concern would be to reorient the procurement process toward a two-step procedure. In the first step, states would engage in a rate-finding process. They would collect information on the outcomes of contracting processes in other states and in the private sector and interview potential vendors concerning the costs of their services. They would then analyze these data to determine the "reasonable" costs of providing MBHO services to the state's Medicaid population. A level of reasonable costs would be selected and announced as the contract "price." In the second stage of the procurement, interested vendors would submit competing proposals. The proposals would be judged solely on the proposed quality of services, access to care, and ability to coordinate with other systems of care (general medical care, social services, housing, and income support). With the procurement process structured in this way, competition would be reoriented toward offering innovative approaches to improving the quality of clinical services and developing mechanisms for coordination of care with relevant components of the health and human service sectors that offer complementary services. The incentive would be for vendors to propose the highest-quality program consistent with the announced budget (price(s) times the size of the population(s)).

Private Payer Direct Procurement of Carve-Out Services

Private direct purchasers of carve-out services operate in a somewhat different economic and regulatory environment relative to public direct purchasers. First, private payers are not usually as constrained to choose the lowest-cost bidder. In addition, the Employee Retirement Income Security Act (ERISA) constrains the use of risk-based payments to vendors. Second, employers compete in labor markets for employees; one important dimension of this competition is the nature and value of the fringe benefits package. Thus, there are typically weaker incentives driving employers to select vendors solely on the basis of the lowest price. Nevertheless, cost pressures in American business are strong, so that some of the same principles noted in the Medicaid case above could be applied to private purchasers.

Traditional Medicaid Programs

Two core features of traditional Medicaid programs impede high-quality M/SU health care. One is the reliance on setting prices for services below market rates to constrain supply; the result is low participation rates by providers and lower-quality service. The other is extremely limited coverage for substance-use treatment services by some state Medicaid programs. While raising the prices of ambulatory M/SU treatment services would likely serve to increase quality, it is impractical to expect such change under current fiscal conditions in the states. Thus there is little opportunity to ameliorate matters in the context of a system of disaggregated office-based providers. Instead, the best option within the Medicaid program is to create contracts with organizations that can manage budgets for treating groups of patients (the underlying presumption being that a substantial volume of services is currently being allocated ineffectively). These contracts in the extreme might expand use of managed care. Alternatively, specific disease management contracts for illnesses such as depression, schizophrenia, or heroin dependence might be procured. Specialty clinics might also receive contracts for organizing care for particular patient groups. In each case, the ability to reorganize services and manage care might permit sufficient funds to be aimed at treating individual cases so as to improve the quality of care.

Budgeted Systems of Care

It is difficult to introduce change into budgeted systems of care from the top down. The basic economics of the public system are at odds with shifts from well-established practices. The grant-based financing system and the franchise nature of most local public delivery systems for M/SU health care tend to inhibit change. Given existing budget levels, introducing competition appears to be impractical. A more practical candidate for policy attention is the content of the grant-based financing system. Pay-for-performance principles could be introduced into such an environment without creating undue disruption. For example, to ensure some financial stability, the majority of funding could continue to be guaranteed via contracts or grants; however, performance criteria would be used to allocate the remainder (e.g., 25–30 percent) of historical funding levels, along with future increases (distribution of inflation or other budgetary increases).

There are, however, numerous challenges to implementing pay for performance in public M/SU treatment systems. First is the primitive state of performance measurement with respect to both the development of measures and the ability of states to implement such measures (Lutterman et al., 2004). In addition, there is concern that pay for performance would distort quality improvement efforts to focus only on those areas in which measures have been developed and payments are made (teaching to the test). There is also little understanding of how such payment might be structured to maximize quality improvement across, say, a state substance-use treatment system. Finally, it was found that in the substance-use sector, use of treatment outcome as a performance indicator created an incentive to treat the least problematic clients presenting for care (Lu, 1999).

CONCLUSIONS AND RECOMMENDATIONS

The incentives created by competitive insurance arrangements, whereby health plans compete to enroll individuals, can be especially deleterious to insurance coverage for and quality of M/SU health care. Because people with M/SU illnesses are more costly to care for than other types of enrollees and because the costs of treating these illnesses persist over time, health plans have economic incentives to avoid enrolling these individuals—a phenomenon known as adverse selection. These selection incentives result in distorted terms of insurance coverage for M/SU services, as well as distortions in the quality of care. The end result is that competitive insurance markets (private or public) tend to generate quality levels for M/SU care that are too low.

The committee recognizes that none of the measures recommended below will fully address the powerful incentives to avoid enrolling people with M/SU illnesses in competitive health plans and that each measure involves a unique set of costs, benefits, and practical considerations that may make it more or less attractive to an individual purchaser. However, the committee is persuaded by the strength of existing evidence that addressing selection-related incentives is central to improving the quality of care for M/SU illnesses in the context of competitive health insurance markets.

> **Recommendation 8-1. Health care purchasers that offer enrollees a choice of health plans should evaluate and select one or more available tools for use in reducing selection-related incentives to limit the coverage and quality of M/SU health care. Risk adjustment, payer "carve-outs," risk-sharing or mixed-payment contracts, and benefit standardization across the health plans offered can partially address selection-related incentives. Congress and state legislatures should improve coverage by enacting a form of benefit standardization known as parity for coverage of M/SU treatment.**

The committee also believes that special attention must be given to state procurement processes, as states are the funders of most M/SU health care. State government procurement regulations typically emphasize choosing the lowest-cost of those contractors submitting proposals that are technically acceptable. Currently, about 16 states choose to purchase behavioral health care carve-out services directly from specialty managed behavioral health care vendors on behalf of their Medicaid programs. Among these states are some that delegate procurement to substate authorities (e.g., counties, regions). A review of state requests for proposals indicates infrequent use of performance measures related to clinical quality in state procurement processes, in part because of the limited availability of well-constructed performance indicators. Performance measures that are specified in requests for proposals frequently focus on administrative services such as telephone response times, claims payment speed, and network size. Taken together, the emphasis on choosing the lowest-cost vendor and the limited use and availability of performance indicators result in an almost exclusive focus on price in the competitive selection of specialty managed behavioral health care carve-out vendors. The result is that vendors have powerful incentives to offer products and services that permit attractive price offers and little counterbalancing incentive to offer high-quality services.

> **Recommendation 8-2. State government procurement processes should be reoriented so that the greatest weight is given to the quality of care to be provided by vendors.**

The committee notes that a number of approaches could be taken to implement this recommendation. A few states have recently adopted approaches that give greater weight to quality. Such a reorientation can likely be accomplished with little risk of incurring "runaway costs" because there is now abundant experience with state procurement of managed behavioral health care services. The range of prices is well known, so that price bids can to some extent be bound in the procurement process. Promising examples of reoriented procurement approaches include assigning relatively low weight to price-related dimensions of a bid and relatively higher weight to proposal features that address quality of care and other aspects of service. A second approach is to engage in a rate-finding process for proposals that sets a price for bids and then focus the competition on the quality and service dimensions of performance.

The committee recognizes that procurement processes in which price is overemphasized at the expense of quality considerations are not limited to public-sector purchasing of managed behavioral health care services, although approaches to purchasing in the private sector are more heterogeneous. Nevertheless, we believe the principles set forth in recommendation 8-2 apply to a substantial segment of private-sector purchasers.

Moreover, a substantial proportion of public M/SU treatment services are purchased through government grants to local providers. These providers are frequently private nonprofit organizations that serve the population of a particular geographically defined catchment area, and are typically well-established organizations having long-standing relationships with state and local governments. Services are purchased most commonly through a system of grants. The grants are awarded subject to the provider's meeting licensing standards and achieving specified service levels. Funding is frequently set at levels that result in patient queues—indicating excess demand for services. There are few quality-of-care standards forming a basis for accountability for these organizations. Moreover, pressures from excess demand create incentives for local providers to expand the volume of treatment even if doing so results in reduced quality.

The committee recognizes the difficult circumstances within which providers that receive the bulk of their funding directly from state and local budgets operate. Health care for substance-use conditions is especially reliant on these purchasing methods and will be affected more strongly. At the same time, we note that there are currently few inducements for these provider organizations to focus on improving quality of care and adopting evidence-based practices.

Recommendation 8-3. Government and private purchasers should use M/SU health care quality measures (including measures of the coordination of health care for mental, substance-use, and general health conditions) in procurement and accountability processes.

Recommendation 8-4. State and local governments should reduce the emphasis on the grant-based systems of financing that currently dominate public M/SU treatment systems and should increase the use of funding mechanisms that link some funds to measures of quality.

The committee acknowledges the underdeveloped state of performance measurement in M/SU health care (see Chapter 4). However, there is an adequate knowledge base to permit state and local governments to redesign grant-based financing systems incrementally so as to incorporate some simple and meaningful performance indicators. The Washington Circle Group measures for substance-use health care are a case in point. The committee envisions that initial efforts in this regard would tie either new funds or a small percentage of existing budgets to performance indicators as a means of reorienting the management of public M/SU treatment provision toward quality improvement. In this way, the refocusing of accountability would not result in budgetary instability. Over time, as performance measures improved and providers altered their management practices, performance measures might be given greater weight in budget allocations.

REFERENCES

Alexander JA, Lemak CH, Campbell CI. 2002. Changes in managed care activity in outpatient substance abuse treatment organizations 1995-2000. University of Michigan School of Public Health. Unpublished manuscript.

Anderson G, Knickman JR. 2001. Changing the chronic care system to meet people's needs. *Health Affairs* 20(6):146–160.

Barry CL, Gabel JR, Frank RG, Hawkins S, Whitmore HH, Pickreign JD. 2003. Design of mental health benefits: Still unequal after all these years. *Health Affairs* 22(5):127–137.

Berndt E, Frank RG, McGuire TG. 1997. Alternate insurance arrangements and the treatment of depression: What are the facts? *American Journal of Managed Care* 3(2): 243–252.

Busch SH. 2002. Specialty health care, treatment patterns, and quality: The impact of a mental health carve-out on care for depression. *Health Services Research* 37(6):1583–1601.

Busch A, Frank R, Lehman A. 2004. The effect of a managed behavioral health carve-out on quality of care for Medicaid patients diagnosed as having schizophrenia. *Archives of General Psychiatry* 61(5):442–448.

Callahan JJ, Shepard DS, Beinecke RH, Larson MJ, Cavanaugh D. 1995. Mental health/substance abuse treatment in managed care: The Massachusetts Medicaid experience. *Health Affairs* 14(3):173–184.

Cao Z. 2003. *Comparing the Pre HMO Enrollment Costs Between Switchers and Stayers: Evidence from Medicare Working Paper.* Cambridge, MA: Cambridge Health Alliance Center for Multicultural Studies.

Cao Z, McGuire TG. 2003. Service-level selection by HMOs in Medicare. *Journal of Health Economics* 22(6):91–931.

Chu FB, Trotter S. 1972. The fires of irrelevancy. *MH* Fall 56 (4):6:passim.

CMS (Centers for Medicare and Medicaid Services). 2004. Medicaid Managed Care Program Summary. [Online]. Available: http://www.cms.hhs.gov/medicad/managedcare/er04net.pdf [accessed December 2, 2005].

CMS. 2005. 2005 CMS Statistics. [Online]. Available: http://www.cms.hhs.gov/MedicareMedicaidStatSupp/downloads/2005_CMS_Statistics.pdf [accessed January 13, 2006].

Cutler D, Zeckhauser R. 2000. The anatomy of health insurance. In: Cuyler AJ, Newhouse JP, eds. *Handbook of Health Economics*. Amsterdam, the Netherlands: Elsevier. Pp. 563–1644.

Deb P, Wilcox-Gok V, Holmes A, Rubin J. 1996. Choice of health insurance by families of the mentally ill. *Health Economics* 5(1):61–76.

DHHS (Department of Health and Human Services). 2002 *Mental Health, United States 2002*, DHHS Publication number (SMA) 3938: Rockville, MD: U.S. Department of Health and Human Services, Substance Abuse and Mental Health Services Administration.

Dickey B, Hermann RC, Eisen SV. 1998. Assessing the quality of psychiatric care: Research methods and application in clinical practice. *Harvard Review of Psychiatry* 6(2):88–96.

Druss BG, Marcus SC, Olfson M, Taniellan T, Elinsin C, Pincus HA. 2001. Comparing the national economic burden of five chronic conditions. *Health Affairs* 20(6):233–241.

Ellis RP. 1985. The effect of prior-year health expenditures on health coverage plan choice. In: Scheffler, R, Rossiter, L, eds. *Advances in Health Economics and Health Services Research*. Greenwich, CT: JAI Press

Ettner SL. 2001. The setting of psychiatric care for Medicare recipients in general hospitals with specialty units. *Psychiatric Services* 52(2):237–239.

Ettner SL, Frank RG, McGuire TG, Newhouse JP, Notman EH. 1998. Risk adjustment of mental health and substance abuse payments. *Inquiry* 35(2):223–239.

Foote SM, Jones SB. 1999. Consumer-choice markets: Lessons from FEHBP mental health coverage. *Health Affairs* 18(5):125–130.

Frank RG, Goldman HH. 1989. Financing care of the severely mentally ill: Incentives, contracts, and public responsibility. *Journal of Social Issues* 45(3):131–144.

Frank RG, Lave J. 2003. Economics. In: Feldman S, ed. *Managed Behavioral Health Services*. Springfield, IL: Charles C. Thomas Publisher. Pp. 146–165.

Frank RG, McGuire TG. 1997. Savings from a carve-out program for mental health and substance abuse in Massachusetts Medicaid. *Psychiatric Services* 48(9):1147–1152.

Frank RG, McGuire TG. 2000. Economics and mental health. In: Cuyler AJ, Newhouse JP, eds. *Handbook of Health Economics*. Vol. 1B, No. 17. Amsterdam, the Netherlands: Elsevier Science. Pp. 893–954.

Frank RG, Glazier J, McGuire TG. 2000. Measuring adverse selection in managed health care. *Journal of Health Economics* 19(6):829–854.

Frank RG, Goldman HH, McGuire TG. 2001. Will parity in coverage result in better mental health care? *New England Journal of Medicine* 345(23):1701–1704.

Frank RG, Goldman HH, Hogan M. 2003. Medicaid and mental health: Be careful what you ask for. *Health Affairs* 22(1):101–113.

Frank RG, McGuire TG, Newhouse JP. 1995. Risk contracts in managed mental health care. *Health Affairs* 14(3):50–64.

Fronstin P. 2003. *Sources of Health Insurance and Characteristics of the Uninsured: Analysis of the March 2003 Current Population Survey*. Washington, DC: Employee Benefit Research Institute.

Glied S, Zivin JG. 2002. How do doctors behave when some (but not all) of their patients are in managed care? *Journal of Health Economics* 21(2):337–353.

HCFA (Health Care Financing Administration). 1992. HCFA Pub. No. 03339, Report to Congress: Medicaid and Institutions for Mental Diseases. Washington, DC: U.S. Department of Health and Human Services.

Hodgkin D, Hogan CM, Garnick DW, Merrick EL, Goldin D. 2000. Why carve-out? Determinants of behavioral carve-out choice among large US employers. *Journal of Behavioral Health Services and Research* 27(2):178–193.

IOM (Institute of Medicine). 1993. Field MJ, Shapiro HT, eds. *Employment and Health Benefits: A Connection at Risk.* Washington, DC: National Academy Press.

Lehman AF, Steinwachs DM. 1998. Translating research into practice: The schizophrenia Patient Outcomes Research Team (PORT) treatment recommendations. *Schizophrenia Bulletin* 24(1):1–10.

Lindsay CM. 1976. A theory of government enterprise. *Journal of Political Economy* 84(5): 1061–1078.

Ling DC, Berndt EB, Frank RG. 2003. General purpose technologies, capital-skill complementarity, and the diffusion of new psychotropic medications among Medicaid populations. unpublished data. Department of Health Care Policy, Harvard University Working Paper.

Lu M. 1999. Separating the true effect from gaming in incentive-based contracts in health care. *Journal of Economics and Management Strategy* 8(3):383–432.

Lutterman T, Hogan M. 2001. State mental health agency controlled expenditures and revenues for mental health services, FY 1981 to FY 1997. In: Manderscheid R, Henderson M, eds. *Mental Health, United States 2000.* DHHS Publication number (SMA) 01-3537. Rockville, MD: U.S. Department of Health and Human Services, Substance Abuse and Mental Health Services Administration.

Lutterman T, Ganju V, Schact L, Shaw R, Higgins K, Bottger R, Brunk M, Koch RJ, Callahan N, Colton C, Geertsen D, Hall J, Kupfer D, Letourneau J, McGrew J, Mehta S, Pandiani J, Phelan B, Smith M, Onken S, Stimpson DC, Rock AE, Wackwitz J, Danforth M, Gonzalez O, Thomas N, Manderscheid R. 2004. Sixteen state study on mental health performance measures. In: Manderscheid R, Henderson M, eds. *Mental Health, United States 2002.* DHHS Publication Number (SMA) 3938. Rockville, MD: U.S. Department of Health and Human Services, Substance Abuse and Mental Health Services Administration.

Manning WG, Liu CF, Stoner TJ, Gray DZ, Lurie N, Popkin M, Christianson JB. 1999. Outcomes for Medicaid beneficiaries with schizophrenia under a prepaid mental health carve-out. *Journal of Behavioral Health Services and Research* 26(4):442–450.

Mark TL, Coffey RM, Vandivort-Warren R, Harwood HJ, King EC, the MHSA Spending Estimates Team. 2005. U.S. spending for mental health and substance abuse treatment, 1991–2001. *Health Affairs Web Exclusive* W5-133–W5-142.

McAlpine DD, Mechanic D. 2000. Utilization of specialty mental health care among persons with severe mental illness: The roles of demographics, need, insurance, and risk. *Health Services Research* 35(1 Pt 2):277–292.

McCarty D, Frank RG, Denmead G. 1999. Methadone maintenance and state Medicaid managed care programs. *Milbank Quarterly* 77(3):341–362.

McGlynn EA, Asch SM, Adams J, Keesey J, Hicks J, DeCristofaro A, Kerr EA. 2003. The quality of health care delivered to adults in the United States. *New England Journal of Medicine* 348(26):2635–2645.

MEDPAC (Medicare Payment Advisory Commission) 2003. Report to Congress: Medicare Payment Policy. Washington, DC: MEDPAC.

Merrick E. 1998. Treatment of major depression before and after implementation of a behavioral health carve-out plan. *Psychiatric Services* 49(11):1563–1567.

Michael RJ. 1980. Bureaucrats, legislators, and the decline of the state mental hospital. *Journal of Economics and Business* 32(3):198–205.

Miller RH, Luft HS. 1997. Does managed care lead to better or worse quality of care? *Health Affairs* 16(5):7–25.

Normand SL, Belanger AJ, Frank RG. 2003. Evaluating selection out of plans for Medicaid beneficiaries with substance abuse. *Journal of Behavioral Health Services & Research* 30(1):78–92.

Norton EC, Lindrooth RC, Dickey B. 1999. Cost-shifting in managed care. *Mental Health Services Research* 1(3):185–196.

Padgett DK, Patrick C, Burns BJ, Schlesinger HJ, Cohen J. 1993. The effect of insurance benefit changes and use of child and adolescent outpatient mental health services. *Medical Care* 31(2):96–110.

Perloff JD, Kletke P, Fossett JW. 1995. Which physicians limit their Medicaid participation, and why. *Health Services Research* 30(1):7–26.

Rowland D, Tallon JR. 2003. Medicaid: Lessons from a decade. *Health Affairs* 22(1): 138–144.

Scott-Morton F. 1997. The strategic response by pharmaceutical firms to the Medicaid most favored customer rules. *RAND Journal of Economics* 28(2):269–290.

Sturm R. 1999. Tracking changes in behavioral health services: How have carve-outs changed care? *Journal of Behavioral Health Services & Research* 26(4):360–371.

Tomes N. 1999. From patients' rights to consumer rights: Historical reflections on the evolution of a concept. In: *Making History: Shaping the Future.* Proceedings of the 8th Annual MHS Conference September 7–9, 1999 in Hobart, Tasmania, Australia. Australia and New Zealand: The Mental Health Services Conference Inc.

Weiner JP, Dobson A, Maxwell SL, Coleman K, Starfield B, Anderson GF. 1996. Risk-adjusted capitation rates using ambulatory and inpatient diagnoses. *Health Care Financing Review* 17(3):77–99.

Young AS, Klap R, Sherbourne C, Wells KB. 2001. The quality of care for depressive and anxiety disorders in the United States. *Archives of General Psychiatry* 58(1):55–61.

9

An Agenda for Change

Summary

Much is known about ways to improve the quality of health care for mental and substance-use conditions. Nonetheless, as discussed throughout this report, gaps remain in our knowledge—for example, with regard to providing care in some clinical situations and for some populations, as well as ensuring that the treatments produced by research are actually received by and effective for the people who need them. In particular, as discussed in Chapter 4, research that has identified the efficacy of specific treatments under rigorously controlled conditions has been accompanied by almost no research identifying how to make these same treatments effective when delivered in usual settings of care and in the presence of common confounding problems, such as comorbid conditions and social stressors, and when administered by service providers without specialized education in the therapy. In addition, there are many gaps in knowledge about effective treatment, especially for children and adolescents. Also noted in Chapter 4 is the paucity of information about the most effective ways of ensuring the consistent application of research findings in routine clinical practice. To fill these knowledge gaps, the committee recommends the formulation of a coordinated research agenda for quality improvement in M/SU health care, along with the use of more-diverse research approaches.

Implementing these research recommendations, as well as undertaking the multiple actions recommended in previous chapters, will require concerted efforts on the part of participants at every level of the health care system—clinicians; health care organizations; health plans and payers; regulators, lawmakers, and other policy makers; accrediting organizations; educational institutions; and all those who shape the environment in which care is delivered. The preceding chapters present recommendations for all these parties organized according to the problems addressed. This chapter concludes by presenting those recommendations separately for each party. From this latter perspective, the recommendations form an agenda that can be pursued at each level of the health care system to improve the quality of M/SU health care.

KNOWLEDGE GAPS IN TREATMENT, CARE DELIVERY, AND QUALITY IMPROVEMENT

Previous chapters of this report have identified gaps in our knowledge about how best to treat certain mental and/or substance-use (M/SU) problems and illnesses; how best to treat these conditions when the patient's and treating provider's resources and environments do not match those of the researchers developing the treatment; and how to ensure that evidence-based practices identified through research are applied uniformly to all those patients for whom they are appropriate. Filling these knowledge gaps will require that the finite available research dollars be used strategically and coordinated across funders. Also necessary will be a thoughtful approach to the more rapid generation of valid and reliable evidence of practical use to treating clinicians in their usual settings of care.

Gaps in Treatment Knowledge

The numerous gaps in our knowledge about how to treat M/SU problems and illnesses encompass effective treatments, effective delivery of known treatments, and ways to improve care quality. A few examples of each of these knowledge gaps are discussed below.

Gaps in Knowledge About Effective Treatments

Treatment of multiple conditions Despite the high degree of comorbidity of mental and substance-use conditions, as described in Chapter 5, and the great strides made in understanding the relationship between co-occurring mental and substance-use problems and illnesses, little is known about the etiology and temporal ordering of these comorbidities (SAMHSA, undated). There also is a substantial lack of knowledge about effective treatment for individuals with certain complex comorbidities, such as schizophrenia and concurrent mood disorders (Kessler, 2004) and comorbid general health conditions (Kane et al., 2003).

Optimal pharmacotherapy for psychosis Unanswered questions include which antipsychotic medication should be the first line of therapy, what constitutes a sufficient period of time to determine whether a new medication is effective, how to handle poor response to the initial prescribed medication (Kane et al., 2003), and how the dosing of combination antipsychotics should be managed in the presence of increased symptoms or side effects. Moreover, multiple antipsychotic medications are used in the absence of evidence on their combined efficacy (Miller and Craig, 2002).

Medication treatments for certain substance dependencies No medications have yet shown effectiveness in the treatment of amphetamine or marijuana dependence.

The prevention and treatment of posttraumatic stress disorder (PTSD) Although PTSD has been recognized for centuries as a frequent consequence among those engaged in warfare (often under different names, such as "shell shock"), high rates of trauma and its adverse mental health sequelae also are experienced by significant portions of the general population—for example, as a result of childhood neglect and abuse; rape and other physical assaults or acts of personal violence; life-threatening or other serious accidents; and mass trauma affecting populations, such as through acts of terrorism, war, and natural disasters (Mueser et al., 2002; National Center for Post Traumatic Stress Disorder, 2005). Some types of psychotherapy (i.e., trauma-focused cognitive behavioral/exposure therapy for individuals and groups, and stress management) have been found to be effective in treating PTSD (Bisson and Andrew, 2005), as have some medications (Stein et al., 2005). Nonetheless, gaps remain in our knowledge of how to prevent PTSD from developing after trauma, what the risk factors are for PTSD (Rose et al., 2005; Work Group on ASD and PTSD, 2004), and how to treat the condition once it develops. With respect to treatment, for example, more knowledge is needed about what drugs and drug classes are most effective; which patients will respond best to medication (Stein et al., 2005); how best to combine pharmacotherapy and psychotherapy; and how to relieve some specific symptoms, such as insomnia or nightmares, by themselves and in the presence of other symptoms requiring medication (Work Group on ASD and PTSD, 2004). Moreover, although cognitive and behavioral therapies have demonstrated efficacy in treating victims of sexual assault, interpersonal violence, and industrial or vehicular accidents, their effectiveness in treating PTSD in combat veterans and victims of mass violence requires further study (Work Group on ASD and PTSD, 2004).

Therapies for high-prevalence childhood conditions While there has been an impressive increase in the number and quality of studies of effective therapies for children, major gaps remain in our knowledge in this area. For example, despite the increasing use of psychotropic medications, little is known about the effect of multiple medications on children's outcomes or about the efficacy of different therapies for severe conditions (e.g., bipolar disorder, childhood depression) (Kane et al., 2003). Insufficient evidence exists to guide follow-up and long-term management of attention deficit hyperactivity disorder (ADHD), despite its being considered a chronic condition (Stein, 2002). There also is very limited knowledge about treatments for co-occurring conditions in childhood.

Therapies for other population subgroups There is little evidence on the effectiveness of treatment modalities for certain subgroups of patients, such as racial and ethnic minorities, as well as the frail elderly (Borson et al., 2001).

Relative effectiveness of different treatments (alone and in combination) More than 550 psychotherapies are currently in use for children and adolescents, but little helpful information exists for clinicians or consumers on their *comparative* effectiveness (Kazdin, 2004). As in other areas of health care, the Food and Drug Administration's drug approval rules offer little incentive for head-to-head clinical trials (Pincus, 2003), and there is a lack of substantial capital investment in the development and testing of psychosocial approaches. Moreover, our knowledge about the optimal use of combination treatments (e.g., medications and psychotherapies) is limited.

Prevention studies Large gaps remain in our knowledge about how to prevent M/SU illnesses.

Gaps in Knowledge About Effective Care Delivery

In addition to the above gaps in our knowledge of effective treatments, there is a profound lack of knowledge on the effective delivery of treatments already known to be efficacious. Chapter 4 describes the efficacy–effectiveness gap that exists in M/SU health care. That discussion demonstrates that there has been more research on the *efficacy* of specific treatments than on how to make these treatments *effective* when delivered in usual settings of care (Essock et al., 2003; Kazdin, 2004). Other chapters of this report identify gaps in our knowledge about additional health care delivery issues that affect the ability to make effective use of what is already known, as well as the ability to meet the quality aims and apply the rules for care set forth in the *Quality Chasm* report (IOM, 2001) (see Chapter 2).

Providing patient-centered care Knowledge is lacking about what factors contribute to patient recovery; how to prevent discrimination in health care and related social programs; how best to support patients' decision-making abilities; and how best to implement illness self-management programs for individuals with M/SU conditions (see Chapter 3).

Preventing unintentional discrimination by health care providers Research is needed on practitioner attitudes toward patient-centered care, how to nurture supportive attitudes in professional training, and how language and wording used to describe M/SU illnesses may contribute to stigmatizing attitudes (see Chapter 3).

Potential modification of certain public policies Research is needed to evaluate the effectiveness of polices such as those that restrict access to student loans and impose a potential lifetime ban on food stamps and Temporary Assistance for Needy Families (TANF) benefits as a result of drug convictions, in particular their effect on patient recovery and subsequent drug use (see Chapter 3).

Coercion into treatment Research is needed on how determinations of competence and dangerousness are made, and on how best to minimize the use of coercion and use it most effectively when it is unavoidable. In mental health care, "little hard information exists on the pervasiveness of the various forms of mandated treatment for people with mental disorders, how leverage is imposed, or what the measurable outcomes of using leverage actually are" (Monahan et al., 2003:37). With respect to the use of coercion in substance-use treatment, research is likewise needed to determine the effects, both positive and negative, of various mechanisms of coercion, of drug courts, and of the use of treatment conditions in probation and parole. Empirical data will not answer questions about the legitimacy of these approaches, but to the extent that their consequences are known, such data can inform normative discussions. Data may also be useful in identifying means of avoiding involuntary interventions, whether by improving services that can be accessed voluntarily or working collaboratively with patients to identify acceptable alternative interventions (see Chapter 3).

Understanding decisional capacity among people with substance-use illnesses The available data on decisional capacity among persons suffering from substance-use illnesses are meager; however, recent years have seen a move to reverse that trend. There is a need for research using standardized instruments, such as the Mac-CAT-T, that take into account the possible effects of associated physical and mental (e.g., depression, delirium) illnesses and involve repeat assessments during periods of sobriety. A careful evaluation of decisional capacity to consent to treatment is warranted in these patients.

Demonstrations of illness self-management programs Demonstrations of programs for illness self-management for individuals with M/SU illnesses are needed (see Chapter 3).

Gaps in Knowledge About How to Improve Quality

As discussed in Chapter 4, many published reports on successful quality improvement initiatives clearly show that it is possible for organizations to improve the quality of their health care (Shojania and Grimshaw, 2005). Yet little evidence exists about the most effective ways to ensure the consistent application of research findings in routine clinical practice (Shojania et al., 2004). Still less evidence exists about how to do so across the diverse clinicians, organizations, and systems delivering M/SU health care.

Shortcomings in Public Policy

Gaps in knowledge about treatment, the effectiveness of care delivery, and mechanisms and processes for improving quality all lead to shortcomings in public policy for the management of M/SU care. These shortcomings are reflected throughout this report and need to be redressed. Thus research to fill the knowledge gaps described above must result in an agenda that supports and informs policy.

Improved treatment models that support patient-centered care by involving patients in treatment choices (see Chapter 3) will necessitate changes in the structure and delivery of M/SU care. Purchasing decisions that are based on established and common outcomes, guided by market incentives, and driven by quality measures (see Chapters 4 and 8) will also serve as leverage for the needed changes. The structure of public policy will be impacted as well by efforts to address the M/SU workforce issues discussed in Chapter 7.

Thus while the committee recommends a coordinated research agenda and a diversity of research approaches (see below), a central theme must also be the impact on public policy. In addition, research must continually address the shortcomings in public policy noted above and inform the purchasing, management, and delivery of systems of care. This need is applicable at all levels, including patients and families, microsystems of care, health care organizations, and the larger health care environment (Berwick, 2002).

STRATEGIES FOR FILLING KNOWLEDGE GAPS

The committee concludes that a coordinated and broadened program of research is needed to fill the gaps in knowledge and inform public policy with regard to M/SU health care. Many public and private funders of research on M/SU health care have their own research portfolios and priority-setting processes. Unless these efforts are coordinated, important knowledge gaps and policy shortcomings may persist. A similar problem was addressed by the National Institutes of Health (NIH) when the incoming director convened a series of meetings in 2002 to chart a roadmap for medical research in the 21st century. The purpose was to identify major opportunities and gaps in biomedical research that no single institute at NIH could tackle by itself, but that required coordinated action by multiple institutes to best improve the progress of medical research. The resulting roadmap for research provides a framework of the priorities NIH as a whole must address to optimize its entire research portfolio and sets forth a vision for a more efficient and productive system of medical research (NIH, undated). A similar process cutting across health services and translational research conducted by the multiple public and private funders of M/SU research efforts could also be beneficial.

Concern has been raised that much of the research on M/SU that is funded, while methodologically pure, may be minimally relevant to those who shape much of M/SU health care delivery (Feldman, 1999). Funded research is at risk of continuing to generate more and more knowledge about efficacious treatments, but failing to examine implementation strategies for facilitating the delivery of these treatments to patients. While practical clinical trials have been encouraged in some of the NIH institutes, they often have focused on a limited set of conditions, rather than addressing the broader issues of quality improvement for a range of M/SU conditions. As a result, public policy practices, reimbursement arrangements, and other environmental factors that influence how care is delivered are not aligned so as to promote the delivery of effective care.

Thus in addition to clinical research, translational research and demonstration projects and activities are needed, for example, to:

- Synthesize, develop, and demonstrate *effective* clinical practices for use in usual settings of care delivery on the basis of known *efficacious* treatments identified through clinical trials.
- Explore and develop processes for providing M/SU expertise in general health specialist settings (e.g., cancer, cardiac, geriatric centers) to address general health and M/SU comorbidities.
- Demonstrate and evaluate processes and procedures for providing appropriately coordinated and comprehensive care involving M/SU health care specialists; general health care specialists; patients and family members; and representatives of related social, educational, criminal justice, and other systems.

•   Test effective and reliable processes for disseminating to the broader health care field findings on practice guidelines, processes, and procedures that result from translational research activities.

•   Inform public policy; continually examine the overall impact of research findings on the purchasing, management, and delivery of care; and monitor fidelity with the findings of this report and the principles of the *Quality Chasm* report.

The committee believes the timely and efficient production of the evidence needed to address such a broad range of issues will require a research agenda that makes appropriate use of experimental, quasi-experimental, and observational approaches.

Research Designs

As discussed in Chapter 4, while well-designed, randomized controlled trials are recognized as the gold standard for generating sound clinical evidence, the sheer number of possible pharmacological and nonpharmacological treatments for many M/SU illnesses makes relying solely on such trials to identify evidence-based care infeasible (Essock et al., 2003). Moreover, some features of mental health care make the use of such trials methodologically problematic (Tanenbaum, 2003). For these reasons, behavioral and social science research has often used quasi-experimental as well as qualitative research designs (National Academy of Sciences, undated); indeed, some assert that quasi-experimental studies often are more useful in generating practical information about how to provide effective mental health interventions in some clinical areas (Essock et al., 2003). Consistent with this point of view, the U.S. Preventive Services Task Force notes that a well-designed cohort study may be more compelling than a poorly designed or weakly powered randomized controlled trial (Harris et al., 2001). Observational studies also have been identified as a valid source of evidence useful in determining aspects of better quality of care (West et al., 2002). However, others note the comparative weakness of these study designs in controlling for bias and other sources of error and exclude them from systematic reviews of evidence for the determination of evidence-based practices. Many researchers and methodologists already are considering strategies for addressing these difficult issues (Wolff, 2000).

As this study was under way, the National Research Council had established a planning committee to oversee the development of a broad, multiyear effort—the Standards of Evidence–Strategic Planning Initiative—to identify critical issues affecting the quality and utility of research in the behavioral and social sciences and education (National Academy of Sciences, undated). The committee believes such discussions are critical to strengthening the appropriate use of all of the above types of research in building the evidence base on effective treatments for M/SU illnesses. However, the committee also believes that the methodologically sound use of these different research designs can produce empirical evidence useful for guiding initiatives to improve the delivery of M/SU care. The committee notes that care will continue to be delivered even in the absence of empirical evidence on the best (or better) ways of doing so; until further funding is made available for more rigorous (and more expensive) research designs, quasi-experimental and observational studies in usual settings of care can help inform improvements in care and its delivery.

Consistent with these conclusions, the committee makes the following recommendations.

> **Recommendation 9-1.** The secretary of DHHS should provide leadership, strategic development support, and additional funding for research and demonstrations aimed at improving the quality of M/SU health care. This initiative should coordinate the existing quality improvement research efforts of the National Institute of Mental Health, National Institute on Drug Abuse, National Institute on Alcohol Abuse and Alcoholism, Department of Veterans Affairs, Substance Abuse and Mental Health Services Administration, Agency for Healthcare Research and Quality, and Centers for Medicare and Medicaid Services, and it should develop and fund cross-agency efforts in necessary new research. To that end, the initiative should address the full range of research needed to reduce gaps in knowledge at the clinical, services, systems, and policy levels and should establish links to and encourage expanded efforts by foundations, states, and other nonfederal organizations.

> **Recommendation 9-2.** Federal and state agencies and private foundations should create health services research strategies and innovative approaches that address treatment effectiveness and quality improvement in usual settings of care delivery. To that end, they should develop new research and demonstration funding models that encourage local innovation, that include research designs in addition to randomized controlled trials, that are committed to partnerships between researchers and stakeholders, and that create a critical mass of interdisciplinary research partnerships involving usual settings of care. Stakeholders should include consumers/patients, parents or guardians of children, clinicians and clinical teams, organization managers, purchasers, and policy makers.

With respect to the above recommendation for the creation of research partnerships between researchers and stakeholders, the committee took note of some research–community partnerships already under way that can serve as models. Two such partnerships are described below.

Agency for Healthcare Research and Quality's Integrated Delivery System Research Network

In 2000, the Agency for Healthcare Research and Quality (AHRQ) initiated the Integrated Delivery Systems Research Network (IDSRN) as a field-based research strategy to link the nation's top researchers with some of the largest health care systems for the conduct of research on cutting-edge issues in health care on an accelerated timetable. IDSRN was developed to capitalize on the research capacity of and opportunities occurring within integrated delivery systems. The network creates, supports, and disseminates scientific evidence on what does and does not work in terms of data and measurement systems, organizational best practices related to care delivery, and diffusion of research results. It also provides a cadre of delivery-affiliated researchers and sites to test ways of adapting and applying existing knowledge. Each of the nine IDSRN partners has three unique attributes that make it particularly suited for time-sensitive research projects:

- **Data availability**—IDSRN partners collect and maintain administrative, claims, encounter, and other data on large populations that are clinically, demographically, and geographically diverse.
- **Research expertise**—IDSRN partners include some of the country's leading health services researchers, with proficiency in quantitative and qualitative methodologies and expertise in emerging delivery system issues.
- **Management authority to implement a health care intervention**—IDSRN partners have responsibility for managing delivery systems and are in a position to implement financial and organizational strategies with an evaluation component.

From 2000 through 2004, AHRQ's commitment totaled nearly $20 million for 75 IDSRN projects (AHRQ, 2002). Although IDSRN is a model of a research network involving large, technologically rich health care organizations, it is instructive in considering how to develop a research network for M/SU health care. Many managed behavioral health care organizations have similar capacity with regard to data availability, research expertise, and management authority. Some already engage in partnerships with research organizations to address questions pertaining to such issues as utilization, the parity of M/SU benefits, and the effects of integrated treatment of clinical care (Feldman, 1999).

Network for the Improvement of Addiction Treatment

The Network for the Improvement of Addiction Treatment, described in Chapter 4, is a university–treatment provider consortium that involves smaller and less technologically rich organizations. This model also could be replicated as a community laboratory for the conduct of translational research on M/SU care.

REVIEW OF ACTIONS NEEDED FOR QUALITY IMPROVEMENT AT ALL LEVELS OF THE HEALTH CARE SYSTEM

The committee's recommendations call for action on the part of clinicians, health care organizations, purchasers, health plans, educational institutions, federal and state legislators and executive agencies, and many others. These recommendations are organized according to the entities charged with their implementation in Tables 9-1 through 9-8. Note that because many of the recommendations are relevant to multiple parties, they appear in more than one table. Also identified are the aims and rules from the *Quality Chasm* report supported by each recommendation.

TABLE 9-1 Recommendations for Clinicians

Action to Be Taken	Relevant *Quality Chasm* Aims and Rules
Overarching Recommendation 1. Health care for general, mental, and substance-use problems and illnesses must be delivered with an understanding of the inherent interactions between the mind/brain and the rest of the body.	**Rule 5. Evidence-based decision making**—Patients should receive care based on the best available scientific knowledge. Care should not vary illogically from clinician to clinician or from place to place. **Rule 8. Anticipation of needs**—The health system should anticipate patient needs, rather than simply reacting to events.
Overarching Recommendation 2. The aims, rules, and strategies for redesign set forth in *Crossing the Quality Chasm* should be applied throughout M/SU health care on a day-to-day operational basis, but tailored to reflect the characteristics that distinguish care for these problems and illnesses from general health care.	**All six aims and ten rules.**
Recommendation 3-1.[a] Clinicians providing M/SU treatment services should support the decision-making abilities, and preferences for treatment and recovery, of individuals with M/SU problems and illnesses by: • Incorporating informed, patient-centered decision making throughout their practices, including active patient participation in the design and revision of patient treatment and recovery plans, the use of psychiatric advance directives, and (for children) informed family decision making. To ensure informed decision making, information on the availability and effectiveness of M/SU treatment options should be provided.	**Aim of patient-centered care**—Providing care that is respectful of and responsive to individual patient preferences, needs, and values and ensuring that patient values guide all clinical decisions. **Rule 2. Customization based on patient needs and values**—The system of care should be designed to meet the most common types of needs, but have the capability to respond to individual patient choices and preferences.

(continued on next page)

TABLE 9-1 continued

Action to Be Taken	Relevant *Quality Chasm* Aims and Rules
• Adopting recovery-oriented and illness self-management practices that support patient preferences for treatment (including medications), peer support, and other elements of the wellness recovery plan. • Maintaining effective, formal linkages with community resources to support patient illness self-management and recovery.	**Rule 3. The patient as the source of control**—Patients should be given the necessary information and the opportunity to exercise the degree of control they choose over health care decisions that affect them. The health system should be able to accommodate differences in patient preferences and encourage shared decision making.
Recommendation 3-2. Coercion should be avoided whenever possible. When coercion is legally authorized, patient-centered care is still applicable and should be undertaken by: • Making the policies and practices used for determining dangerousness and decision-making capacity transparent to patients and their caregivers. • Obtaining the best available comparative information on safety, effectiveness, and availability of care and providers, and using that information to guide treatment decisions. • Maximizing patient decision making and involvement in the selection of treatments and providers.	**Aim of patient-centered care, and Rules 2** (customization based on patient needs and values) **and 3** (the patient as the source of control) (see above). **Rule 7. The need for transparency**—The health care system should make available to patients and their families information that allows them to make informed decisions when selecting a health plan, hospital, or clinical practice, or choosing among alternative treatments. This should include information describing the system's performance on safety, evidence-based practice, and patient satisfaction.
Recommendation 4-2. Clinicians providing M/SU services should : • Increase their use of valid and reliable patient questionnaires or other patient-assessment instruments that are feasible for routine use to assess the progress and outcomes of treatment systematically and reliably. • Use measures of the processes and outcomes of care to continuously improve the quality of the care provided.	**Aim of effectiveness**—Providing services based on scientific knowledge to all who could benefit and refraining from providing services to those not likely to benefit (avoiding underuse and overuse, respectively). Also the other five aims (safety, patient-centeredness, timeliness, efficiency, and equity) and multiple rules.

Recommendation 5-1. To make collaboration and coordination of patients' M/SU health care services the norm, providers of the services should establish clinically effective linkages within their own organizations and between providers of mental health and substance-use treatment. The necessary communications and interactions should take place with the patient's knowledge and consent and be fostered by:

- Routine sharing of information on patients' problems and pharmacologic and nonpharmacologic treatments among providers of M/SU treatment.
- Valid, age-appropriate screening of patients for comorbid mental, substance-use, and general medical problems in these clinical settings and reliable monitoring of their progress.

Recommendation 5-2. To facilitate the delivery of coordinated care by primary care, mental health, and substance-use treatment providers:

- Primary care and specialty M/SU health care providers should transition along a continuum of evidence-based coordination models from (1) formal agreements among mental, substance-use, and primary health care providers; to (2) case management of mental, substance-use, and primary health care; to (3) collocation of mental, substance-use, and primary health care services; and then to (4) delivery of mental, substance-use, and primary health care through clinically integrated practices of primary and M/SU care providers. Organizations should adopt models to which they can most easily transition from their current structure, that best meet the needs of their patient populations, and that ensure accountability.

Rule 4. Shared knowledge and the free flow of information—Patients should have unfettered access to their own medical information and to clinical knowledge. Clinicians and patients should communicate effectively and share information.

Rule 8. Anticipation of needs (see above).

Rule 10. Cooperation among clinicians—Clinicians and institutions should actively collaborate and communicate to ensure an appropriate exchange of information and coordination of care.

Rules 4 (shared knowledge and the free flow of information) **and 10** (cooperation among clinicians) (see above).

(continued on next page)

TABLE 9-1 continued

Action to Be Taken	Relevant *Quality Chasm* Aims and Rules
Recommendation 5-3. To ensure the health of persons for whom they are responsible, M/SU providers should: • Coordinate their services with those of other human services and education agencies, such as schools, housing and vocational rehabilitation agencies, and providers of services for older adults. • Establish referral arrangements for needed services.	**Rules 4 (shared knowledge and the free flow of information) and 10 (cooperation among clinicians)** (see above).
Recommendation 6-2. Public- and private-sector individuals, including organizational leaders in M/SU health care, should become involved in, and provide for staff involvement in, major national committees and initiatives working to set health care data and information technology standards to ensure that the unique needs of M/SU health care are designed into these initiatives at their earliest stages.	**Aim of efficiency**—avoiding waste, including waste of equipment, supplies, ideas, and energy.

*a*The committee's recommendations for quality improvement are numbered according to the chapter of the main text in which they appear. Thus, for example, recommendation 3-1 is the first recommendation in Chapter 3.

TABLE 9-2 Recommendations for Organizations Providing M/SU Health Care

Overarching Recommendation 1. Health care for general, mental, and substance-use problems and illnesses must be delivered with an understanding of the inherent interactions between the mind/brain and the rest of the body.

Overarching Recommendation 2. The aims, rules, and strategies for redesign set forth in *Crossing the Quality Chasm* should be applied throughout M/SU health care on a day-to-day operational basis, but tailored to reflect the characteristics that distinguish care for these problems and illnesses from general health care.

Recommendation 3-1.[a] To promote patient-centered care, organizations providing M/SU treatment services should support the decision-making abilities and preferences for treatment and recovery of persons with M/SU problems and illnesses by:

- Having in place policies that implement informed, patient-centered participation and decision making in treatment, illness self-management, and recovery plans.
- Involving patients and their families in the design, administration, and delivery of treatment and recovery services.
- Incorporating informed, patient-centered decision making throughout their practices, including active patient participation in the design and revision of patient treatment and recovery plans, the use of psychiatric advance directives, and (for children) informed family decision making.

Rule 5. Evidence-based decision making—Patients should receive care based on the best available scientific knowledge. Care should not vary illogically from clinician to clinician or from place to place.

Rule 8. Anticipation of needs—The health system should anticipate patient needs, rather than simply reacting to events.

All six aims and ten rules.

Aim of patient-centered care—Providing care that is respectful of and responsive to individual patient preferences, needs, and values and ensuring that patient values guide all clinical decisions.

Rule 2. Customization based on patient needs and values—The system of care should be designed to meet the most common types of needs, but have the capability to respond to individual patient choices and preferences.

Rule 3. The patient as the source of control—Patients should be given the necessary information and the opportunity to exercise the degree of control they

(continued on next page)

TABLE 9-2 continued

To ensure informed decision making, information on the availability and effectiveness of M/SU treatment options should be provided.

- Adopting recovery-oriented and illness self-management practices that support patient preferences for treatment (including medications), peer support, and other elements of the wellness recovery plan.
- Maintaining effective, formal linkages with community resources to support patient illness self-management and recovery.

choose over health care decisions that affect them. The health system should be able to accommodate differences in patient preferences and encourage shared decision making.

Recommendation 3-2. Coercion should be avoided whenever possible. When coercion is legally authorized, patient-centered care is still applicable and should be undertaken by:

- Making the policies and practices used for determining dangerousness and decision-making capacity transparent to patients and their caregivers.
- Obtaining the best available comparative information on safety, effectiveness, and availability of care and providers, and using that information to guide treatment decisions.
- Maximizing patient decision making and involvement in the selection of treatments and providers.

Recommendation 4-2. Organizations providing M/SU services should:

- Increase their use of valid and reliable patient questionnaires or other patient-assessment instruments that are feasible for routine use to assess the progress and outcomes of treatment systematically and reliably.
- Use measures of the processes and outcomes of care to continuously improve the quality of the care provided.

Aim of effectiveness—Providing services based on scientific knowledge to all who could benefit and refraining from providing services to those not likely to benefit (avoiding underuse and overuse, respectively).

Also the other five aims (safety, patient-centeredness, timeliness, efficiency, and equity) and multiple rules.

Recommendation 5-1. To make collaboration and coordination of patients' M/SU health care services the norm, providers of the services should establish clinically effective linkages within their own organizations and between providers of mental health and substance-use treatment. The necessary communications and interactions should take place with the patient's knowledge and consent and be fostered by:

- Routine sharing of information on patients' problems and pharmacologic and nonpharmacologic treatments among providers of M/SU treatment.
- Valid, age-appropriate screening of patients for comorbid mental, substance-use, and general medical problems in these clinical settings and reliable monitoring of their progress.

Recommendation 5-2. To facilitate the delivery of coordinated care by primary care, mental health, and substance-use treatment providers:

- Primary care and specialty M/SU health care providers should transition along a continuum of evidence-based coordination models from (1) formal agreements among mental, substance-use, and primary health care providers; to (2) case management of mental, substance-use, and primary health care; to (3) collocation of mental, substance-use, and primary health care services; and then to (4) delivery of mental, substance-use, and primary health care through clinically integrated practices of primary and M/SU care providers. Organizations should adopt models to which they can most easily transition from their current structure, that best meet the needs of their patient populations, and that ensure accountability.

Rule 4. Shared knowledge and the free flow of information—Patients should have unfettered access to their own medical information and to clinical knowledge. Clinicians and patients should communicate effectively and share information.

Rule 8. Anticipation of needs (see above).

Rule 10. Cooperation among clinicians—Clinicians and institutions should actively collaborate and communicate to ensure an appropriate exchange of information and coordination of care.

Rules 4 (shared knowledge and the free flow of information) and 10 (cooperation among clinicians) (see above).

(continued on next page)

TABLE 9-2 continued

Recommendation 5-3. To ensure the health of persons for whom they are responsible, M/SU providers should: • Coordinate their services with those of other human services and education agencies, such as schools, housing and vocational rehabilitation agencies, and providers of services for older adults. • Establish referral arrangements for needed services.	**Rules 4 (shared knowledge and the free flow of information) and 10 (cooperation among clinicians)** (see above).
Providers of services to high-risk populations—such as child welfare agencies, criminal and juvenile justice agencies, and long-term care facilities for older adults—should use valid, age-appropriate, and culturally appropriate techniques to screen all entrants into their systems to detect M/SU problems and illnesses.	
Recommendation 6-2. Public- and private-sector individuals, including organizational leaders in M/SU health care, should become involved in, and provide for staff involvement in, major national committees and initiatives working to set health care data and information technology standards to ensure that the unique needs of M/SU health care are designed into these initiatives at their earliest stages.	**Aim of efficiency**—avoiding waste, including waste of equipment, supplies, ideas, and energy.

aThe committee's recommendations for quality improvement are numbered according to the chapter of the main text in which they appear. Thus, for example, recommendation 3-1 is the first recommendation in Chapter 3.

TABLE 9-3 Recommendations for Health Plans and Purchasers of M/SU Health Care

Overarching Recommendation 1. Health care for general, mental, and substance-use problems and illnesses must be delivered with an understanding of the inherent interactions between the mind/brain and the rest of the body.	Rule 5. Evidence-based decision making—Patients should receive care based on the best available scientific knowledge. Care should not vary illogically from clinician to clinician or from place to place. Rule 8. Anticipation of needs—The health system should anticipate patient needs, rather than simply reacting to events.
Overarching Recommendation 2. The aims, rules, and strategies for redesign set forth in *Crossing the Quality Chasm* should be applied throughout M/SU health care on a day-to-day operational basis, but tailored to reflect the characteristics that distinguish care for these problems and illnesses from general health care.	All six aims and ten rules.
Recommendation 3-1. To promote patient-centered care, health plans and direct payers of M/SU treatment services should: • For persons with chronic mental illnesses or substance-use dependence, pay for peer support and illness self-management programs that meet evidence-based standards. • Provide consumers with comparative information on the quality of care provided by practitioners and organizations, and use this information themselves when making their purchasing decisions. • Remove barriers to and restrictions on effective and appropriate treatment that may be created by copayments, service exclusions, benefit limits, and other coverage policies.	Rule 5. Evidence-based decision making (see above). Rule 7. The need for transparency—The health care system should make information available to patients and their families that allows them to make informed decisions when selecting a health plan, hospital, or clinical practice, or choosing among alternative treatments. This should include information describing the system's performance on safety, evidence-based practice, and patient satisfaction.

(continued on next page)

TABLE 9-3 continued

Recommendation 4-3. To measure quality better, DHHS, in partnership with the private sector, should charge and financially support an entity similar to the National Quality Forum to convene government regulators, accrediting organizations, consumer representatives, providers, and purchasers exercising leadership in quality-based purchasing for the purpose of reaching consensus on and implementing a common, continuously improving set of M/SU health care quality measures for providers, organizations, and systems of care. Participants in this consortium should commit to:

- Requiring the reporting and submission of the quality measures to a performance measure repository or repositories.
- Requiring validation of the measures for accuracy and adherence to specifications.
- Ensuring the analysis and display of measurement results in formats understandable by multiple audiences, including consumers, those reporting the measures, purchasers, and quality oversight organizations.
- Establishing models for the use of the measures for benchmarking and quality improvement purposes at sites of care delivery.
- Performing continuing review of the measures' effectiveness in improving care.

Recommendation 5-2. To facilitate the delivery of coordinated care by primary care, mental health, and substance-use treatment providers, . . . purchasers and health plans should implement policies and incentives to continually increase collaboration among these providers to achieve evidence-based screening and care of their patients with general, mental, and/or substance-use health conditions and by:

- Modifying policies and practices that preclude paying for evidence-based screening, treatment, and coordination of M/SU care.

Rule 7. The need for transparency (see above).

Aim of safety—avoiding injuries to patients from the care that is intended to help them.

Aim of timeliness—reducing waits and sometimes harmful delays for both those who receive and those who give care.

Aim of efficiency—avoiding waste, including waste of equipment, supplies, ideas, and energy.

- Requiring (with patients' knowledge and consent) all health care organizations with which they contract to ensure appropriate sharing of clinical information essential for coordination of care with other providers treating their patients.

Recommendation 6-2. Public- and private-sector individuals, including organizational leaders in M/SU health care, should become involved in, and provide for staff involvement in, major national committees and initiatives working to set health care data and information technology standards to ensure that the unique needs of M/SU health care are designed into these initiatives at their earliest stages.

Recommendation 6-3. National associations of purchasers—such as the National Association of State Mental Health Program Directors, the National Association of State Alcohol and Drug Abuse Directors, the National Association of State Medicaid Directors, the National Association of County Behavioral Health Directors, the American Managed Behavioral Healthcare Association, and the national Blue Cross and Blue Shield Association—should decrease the burden of variable reporting and billing requirements by standardizing requirements at the national, state, and local levels.

Recommendation 6-4. Public- and private-sector purchasers of M/SU health care should encourage the widespread adoption of electronic health records, computer-based clinical decision-support systems, computerized provider order entry, and other forms of information technology for M/SU care by:

- Offering financial incentives to individual M/SU clinicians and organizations for investments in information technology needed to participate fully in the emerging NHII.
- Providing capital and other incentives for the development of virtual networks to give individual and small-group providers standard access to software, clinical and population data and health records, and billing and clinical decision-support systems.

Rule 10. Cooperation among clinicians—Clinicians and institutions should actively collaborate and communicate to ensure an appropriate exchange of information and coordination of care.

Aim of efficiency—avoiding waste of equipment, supplies, ideas, and energy.

Aim of efficiency (see above).

Aim of safety (see above).

Aim of efficiency (see above).

Rule 10. Cooperation among clinicians (see above).

(continued on next page)

TABLE 9-3 continued

- Providing financial support for continuing technical assistance, training, and information technology maintenance.
- Including in purchasing decisions an assessment of the use of information technology by clinicians and health care organizations for clinical decision support, electronic health records, and other quality improvement applications.

Recommendation 8-1. Health care purchasers that offer enrollees a choice of health plans should evaluate and select one or more available tools for use in reducing selection-related incentives to limit the coverage and quality of M/SU health care. Risk adjustment, payer "carve-outs," risk-sharing or mixed-payment contracts, and benefit standardization across the health plans offered can partially address selection-related incentives. Congress and state legislatures should improve coverage by enacting a form of benefit standardization known as parity for coverage of M/SU treatment.

Recommendation 8-2. State government procurement processes should be reoriented so that the greatest weight is given to the quality of care to be provided by vendors.

Recommendation 8-3. Government and private purchasers should use M/SU health care quality measures (including measures of the coordination of health care for mental, substance-use, and general health conditions) in procurement and accountability processes.

Recommendation 8-4. State and local governments should reduce the emphasis on the grant-based systems of financing that currently dominate public M/SU treatment systems and should increase the use of funding mechanisms that link some funds to measures of quality.

All six aims (safety, effectiveness, patient-centeredness, timeliness, efficiency, and equity).

TABLE 9-4 Recommendations for State Policy Makers

Overarching Recommendation 1. Health care for general, mental, and substance-use problems and illnesses must be delivered with an understanding of the inherent interactions between the mind/brain and the rest of the body.	**Rule 5. Evidence-based decision making**—Patients should receive care based on the best available scientific knowledge. Care should not vary illogically from clinician to clinician or from place to place.
	Rule 8. Anticipation of needs—The health system should anticipate patient needs, rather than simply reacting to events.
	Aim of patient-centered care—Providing care that is respectful of and responsive to individual patient preferences, needs, and values and ensuring that patient values guide all clinical decisions.
Recommendation 3-2. Coercion should be avoided whenever possible. When coercion is legally authorized, patient-centered care is still applicable and should be undertaken by:	**Rule 2. Customization based on patient needs and values**—The system of care should be designed to meet the most common types of needs, but have the capability to respond to individual patient choices and preferences.
• Making the policies and practices used for determining dangerousness and decision-making capacity transparent to patients and their caregivers.	**Rule 3. The patient as the source of control**—Patients should be given the necessary information and the opportunity to exercise the degree of control they choose over health care decisions that affect them. The health system should be able to accommodate differences in patient preferences and encourage shared decision making.
• Obtaining the best available comparative information on safety, effectiveness, and availability of care and providers, and using that information to guide treatment decisions.	
• Maximizing patient decision making and involvement in the selection of treatments and providers.	**Rule 7. The need for transparency**—The health care system should make information available to patients and their families that allows them to make informed

(continued on next page)

TABLE 9-4 continued

Recommendation 5-2. To facilitate the delivery of coordinated care by primary care, mental health, and substance-use treatment providers, government agencies . . . should implement policies and incentives to continually increase collaboration among these providers to achieve evidence-based screening and care of their patients with general, mental, and/or substance-use health conditions.	decisions when selecting a health plan, hospital, or clinical practice, or choosing among alternative treatments. This should include information describing the system's performance on safety, evidence-based practice, and patient satisfaction. **Rule 4. Shared knowledge and the free flow of information**—Patients should have unfettered access to their own medical information and to clinical knowledge. Clinicians and patients should communicate effectively and share information.
• Federal and state governments should revise laws, regulations, and administrative practices that create inappropriate barriers to the communication of information between providers of health care for mental and substance-use conditions and between those providers and providers of general care.	
Recommendation 5-4. . . . State governments should create . . . high-level, continuing linkage mechanisms . . . to improve collaboration and coordination across their mental, substance use, and general health care agencies,	**Aim of timeliness**—reducing waits and sometimes harmful delays for both those who receive and those who give care. **Aim of efficiency**—avoiding waste, including waste of equipment, supplies, ideas, and energy. **Rule 10. Cooperation among clinicians**—Clinicians and institutions should actively collaborate and communicate to ensure an appropriate exchange of information and coordination of care.

Recommendation 6-2. Public- and private-sector individuals, including organizational leaders in M/SU health care, should become involved in, and provide for staff involvement in, major national committees and initiatives working to set health care data and information technology standards to ensure that the unique needs of M/SU health care are designed into these initiatives at their earliest stages.

Aim of efficiency—avoiding waste of equipment, supplies, ideas, and energy.

Recommendation 6-4. . . . state governments, (and) public-sector . . . purchasers of M/SU health care . . . should encourage the widespread adoption of electronic health records, computer-based clinical decision-support systems, computerized provider order entry, and other forms of information technology for M/SU care by:

- Offering financial incentives to individual M/SU clinicians and organizations for investments in information technology needed to participate fully in the emerging NHII.
- Providing capital and other incentives for the development of virtual networks to give individual and small-group providers standard access to software, clinical and population data and health records, and billing and clinical decision-support systems.
- Providing financial support for continuing technical assistance, training, and information technology maintenance.
- Including in purchasing decisions an assessment of the use of information technology by clinicians and health care organizations for clinical decision support, electronic health records, and other quality improvement applications.

Aim of safety—avoiding injuries to patients from the care that is intended to help them.

Aim of efficiency (see above).

Rule 10. Cooperation among clinicians (see above).

Recommendation 8-1. . . . state legislatures should improve coverage by enacting a form of benefit standardization known as parity for coverage of M/SU treatment.

Aim of effectiveness—providing services based on scientific knowledge to all who could benefit and refraining from providing services to those not likely to benefit (avoiding underuse and overuse, respectively).

(continued on next page)

TABLE 9-4   continued

Recommendation 8-2. State government procurement processes should be reoriented so that the greatest weight is given to the quality of care to be provided by vendors.	**All six aims** (safety, effectiveness, patient-centeredness, timeliness, efficiency, and equity).
Recommendation 8-3. Government . . . purchasers should use M/SU health care quality measures (including measures of the coordination of health care for mental, substance-use, and general health conditions) in procurement and accountability processes.	
Recommendation 8-4. State and local governments should reduce the emphasis on the grant-based systems of financing that currently dominate public M/SU treatment systems and should increase the use of funding mechanisms that link some funds to measures of quality.	

TABLE 9-5 Recommendations for Federal Policy Makers

Overarching Recommendation 1. Health care for general, mental, and substance-use problems and illnesses must be delivered with an understanding of the inherent interactions between the mind/brain and the rest of the body.

Rule 5. Evidence-based decision making—Patients should receive care based on the best available scientific knowledge. Care should not vary illogically from clinician to clinician or from place to place.

Rule 8. Anticipation of needs—The health system should anticipate patient needs, rather than simply reacting to events.

Aim of effectiveness—providing services based on scientific knowledge to all who could benefit and refraining from providing services to those not likely to benefit (avoiding underuse and overuse, respectively).

Rule 5. Evidence-based decision making (see above).

Recommendation 4-1. To better build and disseminate the evidence base, the Department of Health and Human Services (DHHS) should strengthen, coordinate, and consolidate the synthesis and dissemination of evidence on effective M/SU treatments and services by the Substance Abuse and Mental Health Services Administration; the National Institute of Mental Health; the National Institute on Drug Abuse; the National Institute on Alcohol Abuse and Alcoholism; the National Institute of Child Health and Human Development; the Agency for Healthcare Research and Quality; the Department of Justice; the Department of Veterans Affairs; the Department of Defense; the Department of Education; the Centers for Disease Control and Prevention; the Centers for Medicare and Medicaid Services; the Administration for Children, Youth, and Families; states; professional associations; and other private-sector entities.

To implement this recommendation, DHHS should charge or create one or more entities to:

• Describe and categorize available M/SU preventive, diagnostic, and therapeutic interventions (including screening, diagnostic, and symptom-monitoring tools) and develop individual procedure codes and definitions for these interventions and tools for their use in administrative datasets approved under the Health Insurance Portability and Accountability Act.

(continued on next page)

TABLE 9-5 continued

Aim of effectiveness (see above).

Rule 5. Evidence-based decision making (see above).

Rule 7. The need for transparency—The health care system should make information available to patients and their families that allows them to make informed decisions when selecting a health plan, hospital, or clinical practice, or choosing among alternative treatments. This should include information describing the system's performance on safety, evidence-based practice, and patient satisfaction.

- Assemble the scientific evidence on the efficacy and effectiveness of these interventions, including their use in varied age and ethnic groups; use a well-established approach to rate the strength of this evidence, and categorize the interventions accordingly; and recommend or endorse guidelines for the use of the evidence-based interventions for specific M/SU problems and illnesses.
- Substantially expand efforts to attain widespread adoption of evidence-based practices through the use of evidence-based approaches to knowledge dissemination and uptake. Dissemination strategies should always include entities that are commonly viewed as knowledge experts by general health care providers and makers of public policy, including the Centers for Disease Control and Prevention, the Agency for Healthcare Research and Quality, the Centers for Medicare and Medicaid Services, the Office of Minority Health, and professional associations and health care organizations.

Recommendation 4-3. To measure quality better, DHHS, in partnership with the private sector, should charge and financially support an entity similar to the National Quality Forum to convene government regulators, accrediting organizations, consumer representatives, providers, and purchasers exercising leadership in quality-based purchasing for the purpose of reaching consensus on and implementing a common, continuously improving set of M/SU health care quality measures for providers, organizations, and systems of care. Participants in this consortium should commit to:

- Requiring the reporting and submission of the quality measures to a performance measure repository or repositories.
- Requiring validation of the measures for accuracy and adherence to specifications.
- Ensuring the analysis and display of measurement results in formats understandable by multiple audiences, including consumers, those reporting the measures, purchasers, and quality oversight organizations.

- Establishing models for the use of the measures for benchmarking and quality improvement purposes at sites of care delivery.
- Performing continuing review of the measures' effectiveness in improving care.

Recommendation 4-4. To increase quality improvement capacity, DHHS, in collaboration with other government agencies, states, philanthropic organizations, and professional associations, should create or charge one or more entities as national or regional resources to test, disseminate knowledge about, and provide technical assistance and leadership on quality improvement practices for M/SU health care in public- and private-sector settings.

All six aims and ten rules.

Recommendation 5-2. To facilitate the delivery of coordinated care by primary care, mental health, and substance-use treatment providers, government agencies, . . . should implement policies and incentives to continually increase collaboration among these providers to achieve evidence-based screening and care of their patients with general, mental, and/or substance-use health conditions. The following specific measures should be undertaken to carry out this recommendation:

- DHHS should fund demonstration programs to offer incentives for the transition of multiple primary care and M/SU practices along a continuum of coordination models.
- Purchasers should modify policies and practices that preclude paying for evidence-based screening, treatment, and coordination of M/SU care and require (with patients' knowledge and consent) all health care organizations with which they contract to ensure appropriate sharing of clinical information essential for coordination of care with other providers treating their patients.

Rule 10. Cooperation among clinicians—Clinicians and institutions should actively collaborate and communicate to ensure an appropriate exchange of information and coordination of care.

(continued on next page)

TABLE 9-5 continued

- The Federal . . . government should revise laws, regulations, and administrative practices that create inappropriate barriers to the communication of information between providers of health care for mental and substance-use conditions and between those providers and providers of general care.

  Rule 10. Cooperation among clinicians (see above).

Recommendation 5-4. To provide leadership in coordination, DHHS should create a high-level, continuing entity reporting directly to the secretary to improve collaboration and coordination across its mental, substance-use, and general health care agencies, including the Substance Abuse and Mental Health Services Administration; the Agency for Healthcare Research and Quality; the Centers for Disease Control and Prevention; and the Administration for Children, Youth, and Families. DHHS also should implement performance measures to monitor its progress toward achieving internal interagency collaboration and publicly report its performance on these measures annually.

All six aims and ten rules.

Recommendation 6-1. To realize the benefits of the emerging National Health Information Infrastructure (NHII) for consumers of M/SU health care services, the secretaries of DHHS and the Department of Veterans Affairs should charge the Office of the National Coordinator of Health Information Technology and the Substance Abuse and Mental Health Services Administration to jointly develop and implement a plan for ensuring that the various components of the emerging NHII—including data and privacy standards, electronic health records, and community and regional health networks—address M/SU health care as fully as general health care. As part of this strategy:

- DHHS should create and support a continuing mechanism to engage M/SU health care stakeholders in the public and private sectors in developing consensus-based recommendations for the data elements, standards, and processes needed to address unique aspects of information management related to M/SU health care. These recommendations should be provided to the appropriate standards-setting entities and initiatives working with the Office of the National Coordinator of Health Information Technology.

- Federal grants and contracts for the development of components of the NHII should require and use as a criterion for making awards the involvement and inclusion of M/SU health care.
- The Substance Abuse and Mental Health Services Administration should increase its work with public and private stakeholders to support the building of information infrastructure components that address M/SU health care and coordinate these information initiatives with the NHII.
- Policies and information technology infrastructure should be used to create linkages (consistent with all privacy requirements) among patient records and other data sources pertaining to M/SU services received from health care providers and from education, social, criminal justice, and other agencies.

Recommendation 6-4. (The) Federal . . . government . . . should encourage the widespread adoption of electronic health records, computer-based clinical decision-support systems, computerized provider order entry, and other forms of information technology for M/SU care by:

- Offering financial incentives to individual M/SU clinicians and organizations for investments in information technology needed to participate fully in the emerging NHII.
- Providing capital and other incentives for the development of virtual networks to give individual and small-group providers standard access to software, clinical and population data and health records, and billing and clinical decision-support systems.

All six aims and ten rules.

(continued on next page)

TABLE 9-5 continued

- Providing financial support for continuing technical assistance, training, and information technology maintenance.
- Including in purchasing decisions an assessment of the use of information technology by clinicians and health care organizations for clinical decision support, electronic health records, and other quality improvement applications.

Recommendation 7-1. To ensure sustained attention to the development of a stronger M/SU health care workforce, Congress should authorize and appropriate funds to create and maintain a Council on the Mental and Substance-Use Health Care Workforce as a public–private partnership. Recognizing that the quality of M/SU services is dependent upon a highly competent professional workforce, the council should develop and implement a comprehensive plan for strengthening the quality and capacity of the workforce to improve the quality of M/SU services substantially by:

- Identifying the specific clinical competencies that all M/SU professionals must possess to be licensed or certified and the competencies that must be maintained over time.
- Developing national standards for the credentialing and licensure of M/SU providers to eliminate differences in the standards now used by the states. Such standards should be based on core competencies and should be included in curriculums and education programs across all the M/SU disciplines.
- Proposing programs to be funded by government and the private sector to address and resolve such long-standing M/SU workforce issues as diversity, cultural relevance, faculty development, and continuing shortages of the well-trained clinicians and consumer providers needed to work with children and the elderly, and of programs for training competent clinician administrators.
- Providing a continuing assessment of M/SU workforce trends, issues, and financing policies.

All six aims and ten rules.

All six aims and ten rules.

- Measuring the extent to which the plan's objectives have been met and reporting annually to the nation on the status of the M/SU workforce.
- Soliciting technical assistance from public–private partnerships to facilitate the work of the council and the efforts of educational and accreditation bodies to implement its recommendations.

Recommendation 7-3. The federal government should support the development of M/SU faculty leaders in health professions schools, such as schools of nursing and medicine, and in schools and programs that educate M/SU professionals, such as psychologists and social workers. The aim should be to narrow the gaps among what is known through research, what is taught, and what is done by those who provide M/SU services.

Recommendation 9-1. The secretary of DHHS should provide leadership, strategic development support, and additional funding for research and demonstrations aimed at improving the quality of M/SU health care. This initiative should coordinate the existing quality improvement research efforts of the National Institute of Mental Health, National Institute on Drug Abuse, National Institute on Alcohol Abuse and Alcoholism, Department of Veterans Affairs, Substance Abuse and Mental Health Services Administration, Agency for Healthcare Research and Quality, and Centers for Medicare and Medicaid Services, and it should develop and fund cross-agency efforts in necessary new research. To that end, the initiative should address the full range of research needed to reduce gaps in knowledge at the clinical, services, systems, and policy levels and should establish links to and encourage expanded efforts by foundations, states, and other nonfederal organizations.

TABLE 9-6   Recommendations for Accreditors of M/SU Health Care Organizations

Overarching Recommendation 1. Health care for general, mental, and substance-use problems and illnesses must be delivered with an understanding of the inherent interactions between the mind/brain and the rest of the body.

Recommendation 3-1. Accrediting bodies should adopt accreditation standards that require the following practices by organizations providing M/SU treatment services:

- Policies that implement informed, patient-centered participation and decision making in treatment, illness self-management, and recovery plans.
- The involvement of patients/consumers and families in the design, administration, and delivery of treatment and recovery services.
- The incorporation of informed, patient-centered decision making throughout their care, including active patient participation in the design and revisions of patient treatment and recovery plans, the use of psychiatric advance directives, and (for children) informed family decision making. To ensure informed decision making, information on the availability and effectiveness of M/SU treatment options should be provided.
- Recovery-oriented and illness self-management practices that support patient preferences for treatment (including medications), peer support, and other elements of the wellness recovery plan.
- Effective, formal linkages with community resources to support patient illness self-management and recovery.

Rule 5. Evidence-based decision making—Patients should receive care based on the best available scientific knowledge. Care should not vary illogically from clinician to clinician or from place to place.

Rule 8. Anticipation of needs—The health system should anticipate patient needs, rather than simply reacting to events.

Aim of patient-centered care—Providing care that is respectful of and responsive to individual patient preferences, needs, and values and ensuring that patient values guide all clinical decisions.

Rule 2. Customization based on patient needs and values—The system of care should be designed to meet the most common types of needs, but have the capability to respond to individual patient choices and preferences.

Rule 3. The patient as the source of control—Patients should be given the necessary information and the opportunity to exercise the degree of control they choose over health care decisions that affect them. The health system should be able to accommodate differences in patient preferences and encourage shared decision making.

Recommendation 5-2. To facilitate the delivery of coordinated care by primary care, mental health, and substance use treatment providers; organizations that accredit mental, substance-use, or primary health care organizations should use accrediting practices that assess, for all providers, the use of evidence-based approaches to coordinating mental, substance-use, and primary health care.

Rule 10. Cooperation among clinicians—Clinicians and institutions should actively collaborate and communicate to ensure an appropriate exchange of information and coordination of care.

TABLE 9-7 Recommendations for Institutions of Higher Education

Overarching Recommendation 1. Health care for general, mental, and substance-use problems and illnesses must be delivered with an understanding of the inherent interactions between the mind/brain and the rest of the body.	**Rule 5. Evidence-based decision making**—Patients should receive care based on the best available scientific knowledge. Care should not vary illogically from clinician to clinician or from place to place.
	Rule 8. Anticipation of needs—The health system should anticipate patient needs, rather than simply reacting to events.
Recommendation 7-1. (Facilitating and assisting the work of the). . . Council on the Mental and Substance Use Health Care Workforce as a public–private partnership. . .	**All six aims and ten rules.**
Recommendation 7-4. To facilitate the development and implementation of core competencies across all M/SU disciplines, institutions of higher education should place much greater emphasis on interdisciplinary didactic and experiential learning and should bring together faculty and trainees from their various education programs.	**All six aims and ten rules, but especially rule 10, Cooperation among clinicians**—Clinicians and institutions should actively collaborate and communicate to ensure an appropriate exchange of information and coordination of care.

TABLE 9-8 Recommendations for Funders of M/SU Health Care Research

Recommendation 4-4. To increase quality improvement capacity, DHHS, in collaboration with other government agencies, states, philanthropic organizations, and professional associations, should create or charge one or more entities as national or regional resources to test, disseminate knowledge about, and provide technical assistance and leadership on quality improvement practices for M/SU health care in public- and private-sector settings.	**All six aims and ten rules.**
Recommendation 4-5. Public and private sponsors of research on M/SU and general health care should include the following in their research funding priorities: • Development of reliable screening, diagnostic, and monitoring instruments that can validly assess response to treatment and that are practicable for routine use. These instruments should include a set of M/SU "vital signs": a brief set of indicators—measurable at the patient level and suitable for screening and early identification of problems and illnesses and for repeated administration during and following treatment—to monitor symptoms and functional status. The indicators should be accompanied by a specified standardized approach for routine collection and reporting as part of regular health care. Instruments should be appropriate as to age and culture. • Refinement and improvement of these instruments, procedures for categorizing M/SU interventions, and methods for providing public information on the effectiveness of those interventions. • Development of strategies to reduce the administrative burden of quality monitoring systems and to increase their effectiveness in improving quality.	**All six aims and ten rules.**

(continued on next page)

TABLE 9-8 continued

Recommendation 9-2. Federal and state agencies and private foundations should create health services research strategies and innovative approaches that address treatment effectiveness and quality improvement in usual settings of care delivery. To that end, they should develop new research and demonstration funding models that encourage local innovation, that include research designs in addition to randomized controlled trials, that are committed to partnerships between researchers and stakeholders, and that create a critical mass of interdisciplinary research partnerships involving usual settings of care. Stakeholders should include consumers/patients, parents or guardians of children, clinicians and clinical teams, organization managers, purchasers, and policy makers.	**All six aims and ten rules.**

REFERENCES

AHRQ (Agency for Healthcare Research and Quality). 2002. *Integrated Delivery System Research Network (IDSRN): Field Partnerships to Conduct and Use Research. Fact Sheet.* AHRQ Publication Number: 03-P002. Rockville, MD: AHRQ. [Online]. Available: http://www.ahrq.gov/research/idsrn.htm [accessed July 30, 2005].

Berwick DM. 2002. A user's manual for the IOM's "Quality Chasm" report. *Health Affairs* 21(3):80–90.

Bisson J, Andrew M. 2005. Psychological treatment of post-traumatic stress disorder (PTSD). *The Cochrane Collaboration* 3.

Borson S, Bartels SJ, Colenda CC, Gottlieb G. 2001. Geriatric mental health services research: Strategic plan for an aging population. *American Journal of Geriatric Psychiatry* 9(3): 191–204.

Essock SM, Drake RE, Frank RG, McGuire TG. 2003. Randomized controlled trials in evidence-based mental health care: Getting the right answer to the right question. *Schizophrenia Bulletin* 29(1):115–123.

Feldman S. 1999. Strangers in the night: Research and managed mental health care. *Health Affairs* 18(5):48–51.

Harris RP, Helfand M, Woolf SH, Lohr KN, Mulrow CD, Teutsch SM, Atkins D. 2001. Current methods of the U.S. Preventive Services Task Force: A review of the process. *American Journal of Preventive Medicine* 20(3S):21–35.

IOM (Institute of Medicine). 2001. *Crossing the Quality Chasm: A New Health System for the 21st Century.* Washington, DC: National Academy Press.

Kane JM, Leucht S, Carpenter D, Docherty JP. 2003. Optimizing pharmacologic treatment of psychotic disorders. *Journal of Clinical Psychiatry* 64(Supplement 12):5–19, quiz 1–100.

Kazdin AE. 2004. Evidence-based treatments: Challenges and priorities for practice and research. *Child and Adolescent Psychiatric Clinics of North America* 13(4):923–940.

Kessler RC. 2004. Impact of substance abuse on the diagnosis, course, and treatment of mood disorders: The epidemiology of dual diagnosis. *Biological Psychiatry* 56(10):730–737.

Miller AL, Craig CS. 2002. Combination antipsychotics: Pros, cons, and questions. *Schizophrenia Bulletin* 28(1):105–109.

Monahan J, Swartz M, Bonnie RJ. 2003. Mandated treatment in the community for people with mental disorders. *Health Affairs* 22(5):28–38.

Mueser KT, Rosenberg SD, Goodman LA, Trumbetta SL. 2002. Trauma, PTSD, and the course of severe mental illness: An interactive model. *Schizophrenia Research* 53(1–2): 123–143.

National Academy of Sciences. undated. *Standards of Evidence: Strategic Planning Initiative.* [Online]. Available: http://www7.nationalacademies.org/dbasse/Standards%20of%20 Evidence%20Description.html [accessed March 2, 2005].

National Center for Post Traumatic Stress Disorder. 2005. *What Is Posttraumatic Stress Disorder?* [Online]. Available: http://www.ncptsd.va.gov/facts/general/fs_what_is_ptsd. html [accessed September 24, 2005].

NIH (National Institutes of Health). undated. *Overview of the NIH Roadmap.* [Online]. Available: http://nihroadmap.nih.gov/overview.asp [accessed July 30, 2005].

Pincus HA. 2003. Psychiatric diagnosis, drug development and ethics. *BMJ USA* 3:468–472. [Online]. Available: http://bmjjournals.com/cgi/content/full/bmjusa.03090002v1.

Raich PC, Plomer KD, Coyne, C.A. 2001. Literacy, comprehension, and informed consent in clinical research. *Cancer Investigation* 19:437–445.

Rose S, Bisson J, Churchill R, Wessely S. 2005. Psychological debriefing for preventing post traumatic stress disorder. *The Cochrane Database of Systematic Reviews* 2.(Date of most recent update: 28-February 2005. Date of most recent substantive update: 03-December-2001):[electronic].

SAMHSA (Substance Abuse and Mental Health Services Administration). undated. *Report to Congress on the Prevention and Treatment of Co-Occurring Substance Abuse Disorders and Mental Disorders.* [Online]. Available: http://www.samhsa.gov/reports/congress 2002/CoOccurringRpt.pdf [accessed April 25, 2004].

Shojania KG, Grimshaw JM. 2005. Evidence-based quality improvement: The state of the science. *Health Affairs* 24(1):138–150.

Shojania KG, McDonald KM, Wachter RM, Owens DK. 2004. *Closing the Quality Gap: A Critical Analysis of Quality Improvement Strategies, Volume 1—Series Overview and Methodology.* AHRQ Publication Number: 04-0051-1. Rockville, MD: Agency for Healthcare Research and Quality.

Stein MT. 2002. The role of attention-deficit/hyperactivity disorder diagnostic and treatment guidelines in changing practices. *Pediatric Annals* 31(8):496–504.

Stein DJ, Zungu-Dirwayi N, van der Linden G, Seedat S. 2005. Pharnacotherapy for post traumatic stress disorder (PTSD). *The Cochrane Collaboration* 3. (Date of most recent update: 26-February-2005. date of most recent substantive update: 20-July-2000): [electronic—no page numbers].

Tanenbaum S. 2003. Evidence-based practice in mental health: Practical weaknesses meet political strengths. *Journal of Evaluation in Clinical Practice* 9(2):287–301.

West S, King V, Carey TS, Lohr K, McKoy N, Sutton S, Lux L. 2002. *Systems to Rate the Strength of Scientific Evidence.* AHRQ Publication No. 02-E016. Evidence Report/Technology Assessment No. 47. Rockville, MD: Agency for Healthcare Research and Quality.

Wolff N. 2000. Using randomized controlled trials to evaluate socially complex services: Problems, challenges, and recommendations. *Journal of Mental Health Policy and Economics* 3(2):97–109.

Work Group on ASD and PTSD. 2004. *Practice Guideline for the Treatment of Patients with Acute Stress Disorder and Posttraumatic Stress Disorder.* [Online]. Available: http:// www.psych.org/psych_prac/treatg/pg/PTSD-PG-PartsA-B-CNew.pdf [accessed June 6, 2005].

Appendix A

Study Process and Committee Membership

STUDY PROCESS

The Committee on Crossing the Quality Chasm: Adaptation to Mental Health and Addictive Disorders was formed by the Institute of Medicine in March 2004. The committee gathered evidence and conducted its analyses between April 2004 and June 2005. During the seven meetings it held during this period, the committee received testimony from people with mental or substance-use illnesses and their advocates; health care providers and organizations; health plans; purchasers; professional associations; researchers; federal, state, and local governments; and others presenting evidence about the quality of mental and substance-use health care and recommendations for its improvement. (See the acknowledgements section in the front of this report for a listing of those providing testimony.)

During this period, the committee also reviewed leading reports in the mental health and substance-use fields, such as the 1999 Surgeon General's report on mental health, the 2003 report of the President's New Freedom Commission on Mental Health, and the Substance Abuse and Mental Health Services Administration's (SAMHSA) report *Changing the Conversation— Improving Substance Abuse Treatment: The National Treatment Plan Initiative*. The committee also relied on the efforts of several experts in health care for mental and substance-use conditions who prepared commissioned papers providing the committee with in-depth reviews of several key issues:

- The impact of mental and substance-related illnesses on decision-making capacity

- Consumer-directed mental health services
- Statutory, regulatory, administrative, and other barriers to consumer-directed mental health care
- Issues in measuring the quality of care for adults and children with mental and substance-use problems and illnesses
- The experience of the Veterans Health Administration in measuring the quality of care for mental and substance-use conditions
- The safety of health care for mental and substance-use conditions
- Legal, policy, and programmatic considerations in patient-centered and self-directed care
- School-based mental health services
- Treatment services for mental and substance-use conditions for children involved in child welfare
- Health care for mental and substance-use conditions and the criminal justice system
- Improving treatment services for mental and substance-use conditions for children and adolescents in juvenile justice systems
- Workforce issues in health care for mental and substance-use conditions
- Constraints on sharing information on treatment for mental and substance-use conditions imposed by federal and state medical records privacy laws

The authors of these papers are listed in the acknowledgements section in the front of this report.

During this time, the committee also performed additional evidence review and analysis pertaining to its charge. Some of the extensive evidence reviewed by the committee came from the specialty mental health and substance-use health care fields, some from health services research and other empirical evidence from general health care, and some from other disciplines. The committee's interdisciplinary review of the evidence was completed in June 2005. A draft report containing the committee's recommendations was completed in July 2005 and was sent for external review in August 2005. The committee finalized the report in October 2005.

With respect to the organization of this report, although the committee used the aims and rules of the *Quality Chasm* report as its analytic framework, it was not possible to fully organize this report according to those aims or rules, for several reasons. First, there is a great deal of overlap among the aims and rules, as would be expected. The aims are the goals to be achieved; the rules are recommended strategies for achieving those goals. As a result, the rules were often more useful as an analytic approach than were the aims. For example, the aims are silent on the issue of care coordination, whereas care coordination and collaboration are explicitly discussed in the rules.

Second, many of the problems that the committee members identified, which became the focus of the report, fit equally well under more than one aim (e.g., lack of care coordination affects the effectiveness, safety, timeliness, efficiency, and even patient-centeredness of care—five of the six aims). Although it was relatively easy to separate out the issues most closely related to patient-centered care (as the committee did in a separate chapter), this did not hold true for the rest of the issues addressed by the committee. More problematic, the solutions to the problems also often addressed more than one aim or rule (e.g., better dissemination of evidence affects effective care, as well as safe and timely care). As a result, organizing the report's chapters by the rules or aims would have resulted in a great deal of redundancy.

COMMITTEE MEMBERSHIP

Mary Jane England, MD (*Chair*), graduated from Regis College and Boston University with a medical degree, and began a national and international career as a child psychiatrist, a Harvard University dean, and corporate executive and CEO. She served as commissioner of the Massachusetts Department of Social Services from 1979 to 1983, and later as associate dean and director of the Lucius N. Littauer Master in Public Administration Program at the John F. Kennedy School of Government at Harvard University (1983–1987), and then as president of the Washington Business Group on Health. In 2001 she returned to Regis College to become its ninth and first lay president. Recipient of numerous honors and awards, including honorary degrees from Boston University, the Massachusetts School of Professional Psychology, and the University of Texas, Dr. England is past president of the American Psychiatric Association and the American Women's Medical Association. In 2002 she served as a member of the blue-ribbon task force of professional experts in the new Commission for the Protection of Children in the troubled Archdiocese of Boston. During 2003, she received an ABCD (Action for Boston Community Development) award in Boston for her community service and outstanding contributions to protecting at-risk children and families. In 2004 she received the annual Elizabeth Blackwell Award for a distinguished American woman physician from the American Women's Medical Association.

Paul S. Appelbaum, MD, is A. F. Zeleznik distinguished professor of psychiatry, chairman of the Department of Psychiatry, and director of the Law and Psychiatry Program at the University of Massachusetts Medical School. He is the author of many articles and books on law and ethics in clinical practice, including four that were awarded the Manfred S. Guttmacher Award from the American Psychiatric Association and the American Academy of Psychiatry and the Law. He is past president of the American Psychiatric Association, past president of the American Academy of Psychiatry and the Law, and past president of the Massachusetts Psychiatric Society, and has served as chair of the Council on Psychiatry and Law and of the Commission on Judicial Action for the American Psychiatric Association and as a member of the MacArthur Foundation Research Network on Mental Health and the Law. He is currently a member of the MacArthur Foundation Network on Mandatory Outpatient Treatment. He has received the Isaac Ray Award of the American Psychiatric Association for "outstanding contributions to forensic psychiatry and the psychiatric aspects of jurisprudence," was Fritz Redlich fellow at the Center for Advanced Study in the Behavioral Sciences, and is a member of the Institute of Medicine (IOM) of the National Academy of Sciences. Dr. Appelbaum is a graduate of Columbia College, received his MD from Harvard Medical School, and completed his residency in psychiatry at the Massachusetts Mental Health Center in Boston.

Seth Bonder, PhD, has an international reputation in the field of systems, policy, and operations analysis. He was a full-time faculty member in the Department of Industrial and Operations Engineering at the University of Michigan until December 1972 and is currently an adjunct professor in that department and an advisor to engineering schools, business schools, and mathematics departments in major universities. Dr. Bonder is the founder and former chairman/CEO of Vector Research, Incorporated, which employed over 400 professionals providing analysis and information technology services to national security, health care delivery, and financial enterprises in the public and private sectors. In recent years he has focused some of his efforts on improving the planning and operations of health care delivery enterprises. Dr. Bonder and his colleagues have developed models of health care delivery enterprises and have used them in prospective analyses of health care system reengineering issues and chronic disease management. He has participated in a number of National Academy of Engineering/ Institute of Medicine and National Science Foundation workshops on the use of engineering practices to improve the health care delivery system. He was president of the Operations Research Society of America (ORSA) in 1978–1979 and a vice president of the International Federation of Operational Research Societies from 1985 to 1988. He has been the recipient of numerous awards, including ORSA's George E. Kimball Medal for outstanding lifetime contributions to the profession and the INFORMS President's Award. He is a member of the National Academy of Engineering.

Allen Daniels, EdD, is professor of clinical psychiatry and executive vice chair in the Department of Psychiatry at the University of Cincinnati,

College of Medicine. He also is the CEO of University Managed Care, which has two operational units: Alliance Behavioral Care, a regional managed behavioral health care organization, and UC HealthPartners, a medical disease management company. Dr. Daniels also serves as executive director for University Psychiatric Services, a multidisciplinary behavioral group practice. All of these organizations are affiliated with the Department of Psychiatry at the University of Cincinnati. Dr. Daniels is active on a number of boards and professional organizations. In 2002 he chaired the American College of Mental Health Administration's Annual Summit on Translating the Institute of Medicine's Crossing the Quality Chasm Report for Behavioral Healthcare. In 2003 he participated in the Institute of Medicine study, Crossing the Quality Chasm: Priority Areas for Health Care Improvement. Dr. Daniels has published extensively in the areas of managed care and group practice operations, quality improvement and clinical outcomes, and academic health care. He has lectured and consulted both nationally and internationally on these subjects. He is a graduate of the University of Chicago School of Social Services Administration and the University of Cincinnati.

Benjamin Druss, MD, MPH, as the first holder of the Rosalynn Carter chair in mental health at Emory University, is working to build linkages between mental health and broader public health and health policy communities. Prior to serving in this position, he was on the faculty in the Departments of Psychiatry and Public Health at Yale, where he was director of mental health policy studies. Dr. Druss has published more than 50 peer-reviewed articles in journals including the *Journal of the American Medical Association*, the *New England Journal of Medicine*, and the *Lancet*, focusing largely on policy/systems issues related to the interface between primary care and mental health. He has received several national awards for his work, including the 2000 American Psychiatric Association Early Career Health Services Research Award, the 2000 AcademyHealth Article-of-the-Year Award, and the AcademyHealth 2003 Alice S. Hersh New Investigator Award.

Saul Feldman, DPA, at the time of this study, was chairman and CEO of United Behavioral Health (UBH), a subsidiary of United Health Group. UBH arranges for and oversees employee assistance and behavioral health services for more than 23 million people throughout the country. Dr. Feldman is now Chairman Emeritus of UBH. Prior to joining UBH, he was president and CEO of HealthAmerica Corporation of California, a health maintenance organization. Before assuming that position, as an executive at the National Institute of Mental Health, he directed the Staff College, as well as the nation's community mental health and applied services research programs. He has also been a consultant to a number of organizations, including the World Health Organization and Pan American Health Organization. Appointed by the U.S. Secretary of Health and Human Services, he served as a member of the National Advisory Council of the Substance Abuse and Mental Health Services Administration. Currently, he is a member of the MacArthur Foundation Network on Mental Health Policy Research and, as an appointee of the Governor of California, serves as a Commissioner on the State's Mental Health Services Oversight and Accountability Commission. Dr. Feldman has held faculty appointments at a number of universities. He is a founding fellow and former president of the American College of Mental Health Administration and founding editor of *Administration and Policy in Mental Health*, a professional journal for the behavioral health field. His books, many journal articles, and presentations at professional meetings throughout the world have significantly advanced the state of knowledge in behavioral health. Dr. Feldman holds a graduate degree in psychology and a doctorate in public administration, with a specialization in health service policy.

Richard G. Frank, PhD, is Margaret T. Morris professor of health economics in the Department of Health Care Policy at Harvard Medical School, as well as a research associate with the National Bureau of Economic Research. He received his undergraduate degree in economics from Bard College and his PhD in economics from Boston University. He was previously professor of health policy and management at The Johns Hopkins University and served as a commissioner on the Maryland Health Services Cost Review Commission from 1989 to 1994. Dr. Frank is engaged in research in (1) the economics of mental health care, (2) the economics of the pharmaceutical industry, and (3) the organization and financing of physician group practices. He advises several state mental health and substance-abuse agencies on issues related to managed care and financing of care. He also serves as co-editor for the *Journal of Health Economics*. Dr. Frank was awarded the Georgescu-Roegen prize from the Southern Economic Association for his collaborative work on drug pricing, the Carl A. Taube Award from the American Public Health Association for outstanding contributions to mental health services and economics research, and the Emily Mumford Medal from Columbia University's Department of Psychiatry. In 2002 Dr. Frank received the John Eisenberg Mentorship Award from National Research Service Awards. He is a member of the Institute of Medicine.

Thomas L. Garthwaite, MD, in 2002, was appointed director and chief medical officer of the County of Los Angeles Department of Health Services, the second-largest county health system in the United States. With an annual operating budget of $3.3 billion and nearly 24,000 employees, the county's health care delivery system includes five hospitals and numerous clinics. In addition, the department is responsible for public health services including disease control and bioterrorism preparedness. Dr. Garthwaite is the first medical doctor to serve as director since the unified Department of Health Services was formally established in 1972. Prior to this, he served as undersecretary for health in the Department of Veterans Affairs (VA). In that capacity, he was the CEO for the nation's largest integrated health care system and oversaw a dramatic 7-year transformation in which the VA provided demonstrably higher quality of care to 930,000 more veterans with 27,000 fewer employees and with a 24 percent lower cost per veteran served. A graduate of Cornell University, Dr. Garthwaite earned his medical degree from Temple University. He completed his internship and residency at the Medical College of Wisconsin Affiliated Hospitals before joining the VA in 1976, and he is board-certified in internal medicine. His VA career included nearly 20 years of experience as a physician and clinical administrator at the Milwaukee VA Medical Center, where he served as the Center's Chief of Staff for 8 years.

Gary Gottlieb, MD, MBA, is president of Brigham and Women's Hospital; chairman of the Partners Psychiatry and Mental Health System; and a professor of psychiatry at Harvard Medical School, a position he has held since 1998. He also serves as president of Brigham and Women's/Faulkner Hospitals and is a member of both organizations' boards of trustees. Prior to joining Partners, he founded the University of Pennsylvania medical center's first program in geriatric psychiatry and developed it into a nationally recognized research, training, and clinical program, later serving as executive vice chair and interim chair of the Department of Psychiatry and as associate dean for managed care for the University of Pennsylvania Health System. In 1994, Dr. Gottlieb became director and CEO of Friends Hospital in Philadelphia, the nation's oldest independent, freestanding psychiatric hospital. He has conducted extensive research and published numerous papers in the fields of geriatric psychiatry and health care policy. He is a past president of the American Association of Geriatric Psychiatry. Dr. Gottlieb received his BS cum laude from the Rensselaer Polytechnic Institute and his MD from the Albany Medical College of Union University, and completed his internship and residency at New York University/Bellevue Medical Center. He received an MBA with distinction in health care administration from the University of Pennsylvania's Wharton Graduate School of Business Administration while serving as a Robert Wood Johnson Foundation clinical scholar.

Kimberly Hoagwood, PhD, is professor of clinical psychology in psychiatry at Columbia University and director of research on child and adolescent services for the Office of Mental Health in the State of New York. In this capacity, she directs all research programs on youth and family service effectiveness and outcomes and implementation of evidence-based practices for the state. Formerly she served as associate director of child and adolescent mental health research within the Office of the Director at the National Institute of Mental Health (NIMH). Dr. Hoagwood was also chief of the Child and Adolescent Services Research Program at NIMH for 10 years. Prior to her appointment at NIMH, she was research program director and state school psychology consultant with the Texas Education Agency, supervising a statewide, multidisciplinary program of research on community-based mental health and educational services for children with serious emotional, behavioral, and developmental disorders. Dr. Hoagwood earned her doctorate in school psychology in 1987 and practiced clinically for 9 years. She has held academic appointments at Pennsylvania State University and the University of Maryland. She has received numerous grants and awards, including the American Psychological Association's Distinguished Contribution Award and the Outstanding Scholar in Education award from the University of Maryland. Among her many publications are articles and books examining the efficacy and effectiveness of child and adolescent services, evidence-based practices and their implementation in children's service systems, national psychotropic medication practices, research ethics, and genetic epistemology in the work of Gabriel Garcia Marquez.

Jane Knitzer, EdD, is a psychologist whose career has addressed policy research and analysis of issues affecting children and families, encompassing mental health, child welfare, and early childhood. A clinical professor of population and family health, she has produced landmark work on children's mental health, including the ground-breaking policy reports *Unclaimed Children: The Failure of Public Responsibility to Children and Adolescents in Need of Mental Health Services* and *At the School House Door: An Examination of Programs and Policies for Children with Behavioral and Emotional Problems*. Dr. Knitzer became director of the National Center for Children in Poverty in 2004. She has both master's and doctorate degrees from the Harvard Graduate School of Education and did postdoctoral work in community psychology at the Albert Einstein School of Medicine. She was a fellow at the Radcliffe Bunting Institute and has been on the faculty at Cornell University, New York University, and Bank Street College of Education. She is a member of the New York State Permanent Judicial Commission on Justice for Children and serves on the board of Family Support America. She is a past president of Division 37 Child, Youth, and Family Services of the American Psychological Association and of the American Association of Orthopsychiatry. Among her many awards, Dr. Knitzer was recipient of the first Nicolas Hobbs Award for Distinguished Service in the Cause of Child Advocacy from the American Psychological Association.

A. Thomas McLellan, PhD, is a psychologist at the Philadelphia Veterans Affairs Medical Center, professor of psychiatry at the University of Pennsylvania, and scientific director of the Treatment Research Institute. He was educated at Colgate University, Bryn Mawn College, and Oxford University. He has published more than 300 articles and chapters on addiction research. Dr. McLellan and his colleagues have been developing and evaluating treatments for alcohol and drug dependence, as well as evaluation instruments such as the Addiction Severity Index and the Treatment Services Review. They are currently pursuing such questions as "What are the active and inactive ingredients of treatment?" and "What is the appropriate duration and content of treatment for various types of patients?"

Jeanne Miranda, PhD, is a professor in the Department of Psychiatry and Biobehavioral Sciences at the University of California-Los Angeles (UCLA) and a mental health services researcher who has focused her work on providing mental health care to low-income and minority communities. Her major research contributions have addressed the impact of mental health care for ethnic minority communities, including a trial of treatment of depression in impoverished minority patients at San Francisco General Hospital and a study of care for depression in low-income, minority women screened through county entitlement programs. Dr. Miranda is an investigator in two UCLA centers focusing on improving disparities in health care for ethnic minorities. For these centers, she directs an innovative research study focusing on translating diet and exercise interventions for low-income and minority communities. She was the senior scientific editor of *Mental Health: Culture, Race and Ethnicity*, a supplement to *Mental Health: A Report of the Surgeon General*, published August 2001. She holds a PhD in clinical psychology from the University of Kansas and completed postdoctoral training at the University of California-San Francisco. Dr. Miranda was elected to membership in the Institute of Medicine in 2005.

Lisa Mojer-Torres, JD, is an attorney specializing in civil rights and health law, with a subspecialty in representing persons in recovery from substance-use disorders (including stabilized, methadone-maintained patients) who are the victims of employment-related discrimination. She is also an active advocate for consumers of substance-use disorder treatment services, representing this constituency on multiple councils, committees, and boards. Ms. Mojer-Torres is a member of the board of directors of the Alliance Project's Faces and Voices of Recovery Campaign and a member of the editorial board of the *Journal of Maintenance in the Addictions*. Ms. Mojer-Torres recently completed service as a panelist on Discrimination against Individuals in Treatment/Recovery from Addiction, a collaboration between the American Bar Association and JoinTogether. In 2002, she completed a 4-year appointment to SAMHSA's Center for Substance Abuse Treatment's National Advisory Council. She has also served on two committees of the National Academy of Sciences/Institute of Medicine: the Committee on Federal Regulation of Methadone Treatment and the Committee on Community Based Drug Treatment. She has testified before the U.S. Congress, speaks at numerous conferences, and has appeared in the media and in several educational films. She further shares her expertise as a consultant and field reviewer on several projects and grants. She received the first Public Service Award presented by the National Institute of Drug Abuse in 1996. Ms. Mojer-Torres is a graduate of Boston University and New York University School of Law and is admitted to practice law in New York and New Jersey.

Harold Alan Pincus, MD, is professor and executive vice chairman of the Department of Psychiatry at the University of Pittsburgh School of Medicine. He also is Senior Scientist at the RAND Corporation and directs the RAND–University of Pittsburgh Health Institute and The Robert Wood Johnson Foundation's National Program on Depression in Primary Care. Previously, he was deputy medical director of the American Psychiatric Association (APA) and the founding director of APA's Office of Research, executive director of the American Psychiatric Institute for Research and Education, and cochair of the Work Group to Update the Text of DSM-IV (the *Diagnostic and Statistical Manual*, fourth edition). He has edited or coauthored 15 books and over 300 scientific publications in health services research; science policy; research career development; and the diagnosis, classification, and treatment of mental disorders. He has been appointed to the editorial boards of nine major scientific journals and was founder and editor of *Psychiatric Research Report*, a national newsletter on science policy and funding. Dr. Pincus has been a consultant to a variety of federal agencies and private organizations, including the U.S. Secret Service, the John T. and Catherine D. MacArthur Foundation, the Hartford Foundation, the World Health Organization, and the World Psychiatric Association Section on Economics. He graduated from the University of Pennsylvania and received his medical degree from Albert Einstein College of Medicine in New York. He is a recipient of the William C. Menninger Memorial Award of the American College of Physicians for distinguished contributions to the science of mental health, the Health Services Research Senior Scholar Award of the APA, Columbia University's Emily Mumford Award, and the National Institute of Mental Health/APA Vestermark Award for contributions to psychiatric education. Dr. Pincus also maintains a small private practice specializing in major affective disorders and has spent one evening a week for 22 years at a public mental health clinic caring for patients with severe mental illnesses.

Estelle B. Richman's career spans more than 25 years of public service, including her appointment in 2003 as secretary of Pennsylvania's Department of Public Welfare, which provides Medicaid, mental health, and substance-abuse disorder services; child and family services; services to individuals with mental retardation; and numerous other public welfare services. Prior to this she was managing director for the city of Philadelphia, responsible for oversight of 13 city departments. She served as the first director of social services for the city of Philadelphia, leading an initiative to create a more integrated and coordinated health and social services system for children, adults, and families. Philadelphia's Behavioral Health System subsequently was named a winner of the 1999 Innovations in American Government from the Kennedy School of Government, Harvard University. Other positions held by Ms. Richman include the city of Philadelphia's commissioner of public health and deputy commissioner for mental health, mental retardation and substance abuse services; southeast area director for the Office of Mental Health in the Pennsylvania Department of Public Welfare; and assistant director with the Positive Education Program (PEP) in Ohio, a comprehensive day treatment school program for children and adolescents with behavior problems. A nationally recognized expert on issues of behavioral health and children's services, Ms. Richman has been honored for her advocacy efforts by the Alliance for the Mentally Ill, the American Psychiatric Association, and the American Medical Association, among others. She also is the recipient of the 1998 Ford Foundation/Good Housekeeping Award for Women in Government.

Jeffrey H. Samet, MD, MPH, is a graduate of Brandeis University and Baylor College of Medicine and has been a primary care physician in Boston since 1983. He is professor of medicine and social and behavioral sciences at the Boston University Schools of Medicine and Public Health and chief of the Section of General Internal Medicine at the medical school and Boston Medical Center, as well as vice chair for public health of the Department of Medicine. In 1995 he became medical director of the Substance Abuse Prevention and Treatment Services Division of the Boston Public Health Commission. Between 1990 and 2002, he served as director of the HIV Diagnostic Evaluation Unit at Boston City Hospital/Boston Medical Center, a weekly intake clinic for newly diagnosed HIV-infected patients. He was national president (1999–2001) of the Association of Medical Education and Research in Substance Abuse and cochair (1992–2002) of the Society of General Internal Medicine Substance Abuse Task Force, and he is currently program chair of the Annual Medical-Scientific

Conference of the American Society of Addiction Medicine. He has been principal investigator of two National Institute of Drug Abuse (NIDA)–funded studies and four National Institute on Alcohol Abuse and Alcoholism (NIAAA)–funded studies, including *Enhanced Linkage of Drug Abusers to Primary Medical Care* and *Enhanced Linkage of Alcohol Abusers to Primary Care*. He is the primary mentor for two NIDA and one NIAAA career development awardees. He has directed two Center of Substance Abuse Prevention physician faculty development programs and has published over 100 peer-reviewed articles and numerous book chapters.

Tom Trabin, PhD, MSM, is an independent consultant to trade associations, government agencies, organizations, and systems of care within the behavioral health care field. He is the lead organizer of the 2005 National Summit on Defining a Strategy for Behavioral Health Information Management and Its Role in the National Health Information Infrastructure. He organizes and chairs the annual California Information Management Conference for state and county mental health and substance-abuse agencies and treatment provider organizations and for 10 years chaired Behavioral Informatics Tomorrow, the largest trade show of its kind. He helped found and is part-time executive director of SATVA, the trade association of behavioral health software vendors. He leads the adult mental health initiative for SAMHSA's Forum on Performance Measures and the performance measure set and evidence-based practices modules for SAMHSA's Decision Support 2000+. Dr. Trabin represents the behavioral health care field on the Healthcare Information Management and Systems Society's Davies Awards Committee for best implementation of an electronic health record. He has over 60 publications, including several books, book chapters, and articles on performance and outcome measurement and computerization in the behavioral health care field. Previously Dr. Trabin worked in executive positions for U.S. Behavioral Health, Abbott Northwestern Hospital, a behavioral health dot.com, and a conference and publishing company. He has worked as a clinician in diverse settings, including a state mental hospital, Veterans Affairs medical center, county mental health center, hospital-based behavioral medicine clinic, partial hospital program, private group practice, and solo independent practice. He earned masters and doctorate degrees in counseling psychology from the University of Minnesota, a masters degree in management science from Stanford Business School as a Bush Leadership Fellow, and a masters degree in philosophy from Delhi University.

Mark D. Trail is chief of Medical Assistance Plans in the Department of Community Health for the State of Georgia. As director of the state Medicaid agency, he is responsible for all Medicaid functions and services, as well as the State Children's Health Insurance Program, PeachCare for Kids. The combined programs provide health care coverage to over 1.6 million Georgians, with expenditures approaching $6 billion. He has worked for over 27 years in a variety of health care fields, serving in both the public and private sectors. While serving as Medicaid director, Mr. Trail implemented a successful conversion from the outpatient clinic option to the rehabilitation option for people with mental illness and addictive diseases. The conversion provided for the payment and development of assertive community treatment teams, peer support counselors, and certain residential services. Prior to his work with Medicaid, Mr. Trail worked in a variety of positions in the mental health, developmental disability, and addictive disease fields. He has been a member and leader of multiple organizations, including serving as president of the National Association of County Behavioral Health Directors. He currently serves on the executive committee of the National Association of State Medicaid Directors. Mr. Trail received a masters degree in community counseling from Georgia State University.

Sr. Ann Catherine Veierstahler, RN, SCSJA, has had a life-long struggle with mental illness that has been featured in both newspapers and magazines. Although her professional life has included working as a registered nurse in a refugee camp in Cambodia with the Red Cross, serving as a nursing home administrator, starting the first clinics for the homeless in Milwaukee, and creating programs to meet the needs of persons with mental illnesses in boarding homes, her own mental illness of rapid-cycling bipolar disorder, present since age 7, was not correctly diagnosed and treated for decades. On her fiftieth birthday, she was diagnosed with stomach cancer. She has since fully recovered from that illness and devotes much of her time and skills to a website (www.hopetohealing.com). This website contains stories of individuals' successes despite the many challenges of mental illnesses in order to offer hope to persons still struggling with such illnesses and to help overcome the stigma they experience by educating the public. She also is developing and expanding consumer-run Faith in Recovery support programs in several local faith communities. As a member of Al-anon for many years, Sr. Ann Catherine uses the 12-step program in her own life and knows first-hand the challenges of addictive behaviors. She has received many awards for her outstanding programs and innovations in empowering people to meet their needs and lead enriching and meaningful lives. Among her awards are the Mental Health Association Consumer Advocacy Award and several awards from the National Alliance on Mental Illness (NAMI) including the Adult Services Award.

Cynthia Wainscott is chair of the National Mental Health Association and serves on the Governor's Mental Health, Mental Retardation and Substance Abuse Advisory Council and the state's Mental Health Planning and Advisory Council in Georgia. She also is the consumer representative on the Georgia Medicaid agency's Drug Utilization Review Board and has served on the Center for Mental Health Services' National Mental Health Advisory Council. She has 16 years of experience as a leader in mental health education and has directed a pilot site for the National Institute of Mental Health's Depression: Awareness, Recognition and Treatment program, as well as provided training for model education program nationwide. Her passion for mental health advocacy is fueled by the experiences of her mother, daughter, and granddaughter, who have all lived successfully with mental illnesses.

Constance Weisner, MSW, DrPH, is professor, Department of Psychiatry, University of California-San Francisco, and investigator, Division of Research, Northern California Kaiser Permanente. She has an MSW from the University of Minnesota and a doctorate in public health from the University of California-Berkeley. She directs a research program addressing access to, outcomes of, and cost-effectiveness of alcohol and drug treatment and co-occurring disorders in public and private settings. She is a member of the International Expert Advisory Group on Alcohol and Drug Dependence of the World Health Organization, the National Advisory Council of the National Institute on Drug Abuse, and the MacArthur Foundation Research Network on Mental Health and the Law. She has also been a member of the National Advisory Council of the Center for Substance Abuse Treatment. She has participated on several Institute of Medicine committees, including Broadening the Base of Alcohol Treatment and Managing Managed Care. She is a member of the Washington Circle, developing performance indicators for alcohol and drug identification and treatment in health plans. She has received merit awards from the National Institute on Alcohol Abuse and Alcoholism and the National Institute of Drug Abuse, and works closely with chemical dependency programs on policy issues and in developing best practices. Her ongoing work focuses on the changing systems for receiving health, chemical dependency, and mental health services.

Appendix B

Constraints on Sharing Mental Health and Substance-Use Treatment Information Imposed by Federal and State Medical Records Privacy Laws

Timothy Stoltzfus Jost

INTRODUCTION

The privacy regulations issued by the Department of Health and Human Services pursuant to the Health Insurance Portability and Accountability Act (HIPAA) of 1996 (Pub. L. No. 104-191) have had a tremendous impact on health care providers. One of the less studied aspects of this statute, however, is the constraints that exist on the sharing of treatment information among mental health treatment providers when it is applied in tandem with other state and federal medical records confidentiality laws. This paper examines the interaction between these bodies of law, reviewing the federal HIPAA regulations, state statutes that govern mental health medical records privacy, and the federal statute governing confidentiality of substance abuse records.

The study is based primarily on information regarding state privacy statutes obtained from the state law database of the Health Privacy Project, www.healthprivacy.org. In most instances, the information regarding state laws found in this database was confirmed and updated through state-specific Westlaw searches. Like the Health Privacy Project database, this study is limited to state statutes and does not include information on state administrative regulations, attorney general opinions, licensure board opinions, or court decisions, all of which might contain further information on medical records privacy. This report should not be seen, therefore, as a comprehensive legal analysis of all the issues raised by the law of each state. Rather it is intended to identify the major issues raised by the interaction between the laws of the various states and federal law.

THE HIPAA PRIVACY REGULATIONS

Section 264 of HIPAA required the Secretary of Health and Human Services to implement national standards to protect the privacy of individually identifiable health information that was transmitted electronically. The final HIPAA regulation was published in the last minutes of the Clinton Administration on December 28, 2000. That rule was extensively amended in August of 2002 (with further amendments in 2003), and appears at final form at 45 C.F.R. Parts 160 and 164.

Under the final HIPAA rules at 45 C.F.R. § 164.502, covered entities, including health care providers, can disclose protected health information for treatment purposes without patient consent; 45 C.F.R. § 164.506(c) (1) and (2) permit both the use and disclosure of information for treatment purposes. The rules at 45 C.F.R. § 164.501 define treatment to mean:

> . . . the provision, coordination, or management of health care and related services by one or more health care providers, including the coordination or management of health care by a health care provider with a third party; consultation between health care providers relating to a patient; or the referral of a patient for health care from one health care provider to another.

One exception to this general rule of permitting the sharing of treatment information without consent is that "psychotherapy notes" may only be disclosed with authorization (45 C.F.R. § 164.508(a)(2)) except insofar as they are used by the originator of the notes or for a covered entity's supervised mental health education and training purposes. Psychotherapy notes are a special form of treatment information:

> Psychotherapy notes means notes recorded (in any medium) by a health care provider who is a mental health professional documenting or analyzing the contents of conversation during a private counseling session or a group, joint, or family counseling session and that are separated from the rest of the individual's medical record. Psychotherapy notes excludes medication prescription and monitoring, counseling session start and stop times, the modalities and frequencies of treatment furnished, results of clinical tests, and any summary of the following items: diagnosis, functional status, the treatment plan, symptoms, prognosis, and progress to date (45 C.F.R. § 164.501).

Authorization is a special and rigorous form of consent, which must include a description of the information to be disclosed, the identity of the person or class of persons who may disclose the information and to whom it may be disclosed, a description of the purpose of the disclosure, an expiration date for the authorization, and the signature of the person authorizing the disclosure (45 C.F.R. § 164.508(c)). In general, the individual signing the authorization may revoke it at any time, a provider cannot condition treatment on the willingness of an individual to sign an authorization for the release of psychotherapy notes, and an authorization for the release of psychotherapy notes must be a separate and independent document (45 C.F.R. § 164.508(b) and (c)).

THE RELATIONSHIP BETWEEN FEDERAL AND STATE PRIVACY LAWS

The HIPAA statute also provides that:

> A regulation promulgated under paragraph (1) shall not supersede a contrary provision of State law, if the provision of State law imposes requirements, standards, or implementation specifications that are more stringent than the requirements, standards, or implementation specifications imposed under the regulation (42 U.S.C. § 1320d-2(c)(2)).

Accordingly, the HIPAA regulations provide that they preempt state laws that are less stringent than HIPAA, but they are in turn preempted by stricter state laws, which, in the context of information disclosure, are more protective of privacy (45 C.F.R. § 160.203(b)).

Some types of mental health records are also independently governed by the federal substance abuse treatment confidentiality law, 42 U.S.C. § 290dd-2. This statute provides:

> Records of the identity, diagnosis, prognosis, or treatment of any patient which are maintained in connection with the performance of any program or activity relating to substance abuse education, prevention, training, treatment, rehabilitation, or research, which is conducted, regulated, or directly or indirectly assisted by any department or agency of the United States shall, * * * be confidential and be disclosed only for the purposes and under the circumstances expressly authorized under subsection (b) of this section (42 U.S.C. § 290dd-2(a)).

The only statutory exception identified in subsection (b) relevant to treatment information is (b)(2)(A), which authorizes disclosure of information to medical personnel in a "bona fide medical emergency." The regulations recognize further exceptions, however, insofar as they provide:

> (3) . . . The restrictions on disclosure in these regulations do not apply to communications of information between or among personnel having a need for the information in connection with their duties that arise out of

the provision of diagnosis, treatment, or referral for treatment of alcohol or drug abuse if the communications are
(I) Within a program or
(ii) Between a program and an entity that has direct administrative control over the program (42 C.F.R. § 2.12(c)(3)).

The regulations also provide:

> (4) . . . The restrictions on disclosure in these regulations do not apply to communications between a program and a qualified service organization of information needed by the organization to provide services to the program (42 C.F.R. § 2.12(c)(4)).

"Qualified service organizations" are defined to include organizations that provide support services such as billing and data processing, but the definition seems broad enough to include some consultations. Information can also be disclosed with patient consent (42 C.F.R. § 2.33).

With respect to preemption of state law, the substance abuse regulations state at § 2.20:

> The statutes authorizing these regulations do not preempt the field of law which they cover to the exclusion of all State laws in that field. If a disclosure permitted under these regulations is prohibited under State law, neither these regulations nor the authorizing statutes may be construed to authorize any violation of that State law. However, no State law may either authorize or compel any disclosure prohibited by these regulations.

Though the HIPPA privacy regulations do not expressly address their relationship to the substance abuse confidentiality laws, the preamble to the privacy regulations recognizes the constraints of the substance abuse confidentiality law. It states that (1) in general the privacy law and substance abuse law do not conflict, and (2) wherever one is more protective of privacy than the other, the more restrictive should govern (65 Fed. Reg. 82462, 82482–82483).

In summary,

• The HIPPA regulations permit broad sharing of treatment information without consent.

• However, the HIPPA regulations only permit sharing of psychotherapy notes with authorization.

• Moreover, the substance abuse confidentiality law does not permit sharing of records relating to substance abuse treatment or rehabilitation organizations conducted, regulated, or funded by the federal government, without consent, except within a program or with an entity with administrative control over a program.

• Whenever a state law is more protective of privacy than either the federal HIPAA regulations or the federal substance abuse confidentiality statute and regulations, the state law governs.

STATE MEDICAL RECORDS CONFIDENTIALITY LAWS

To understand the actual effect of the HIPAA regulations or federal substance abuse statute or regulations, therefore, one must understand state law. Each of the 50 states (and the District of Columbia) has a number of statutes governing medical record confidentiality. In particular, each has statutes specifically governing some aspect of mental health records, and most have laws governing substance abuse records. The coverage and requirements of these laws vary widely, however.

A number of states have comprehensive medical record statutes that attempt to govern all issues pertaining to medical record confidentiality, much like HIPAA. California is one such state (see Cal. Civil Code D. 1, Part 2.6), although California also has a special statute governing the records of patients in mental facilities (Calif. Welf. and Inst. Code § 5328) and also specifically prohibits the release of information by psychotherapists specifically relating to "the patient's participation in outpatient treatment." Montana has a general health care records statute, which permits disclosure of health information "to a person who is providing health care to the patient" (Mont. Code Ann. § 50-16-529). New York's general medical records statute (N.Y. Pub. Health L. § 18(6)) permits disclosure of general medical records to "practitioners or other personnel employed by or under contract with the facility." Virginia has a general law governing the records of all providers and practitioners. Va. Code Ann. § 32.1-127:03(D) permits disclosure of information when necessary for the care of a patient. Finally, Washington has a comprehensive statute, which permits disclosure "(a) to a person who the provider reasonably believes is providing health care to the patient" (Wash. Rev. Code Ann. § 70.02.050(1)(a)).

STATE LAWS GOVERNING MENTAL HEALTH RECORDS

It is more common for a state to have several specific statutes governing different types of medical records and information. Every state has some form of legislation governing mental health records. These generally take four forms. First, many states have laws governing the records of patients in state mental hospitals or mental health programs. These are in some instances part of general statutes governing state health records (See Idaho

Code § 9-340C(8) and (13)) and are sometimes specific to mental hospitals (see N.Y. Mental Hygiene Law 33.13; N.C. Gen. Stat. § 122C-55).

Second, a number of states have laws governing the records of specific mental health practitioners, most commonly psychologists, social workers, and counselors. Colo. Rev. Stat. Ann. § 12-43-218, for example, requires patient consent for any disclosure by a psychologist or psychotherapist, with no treatment exception. Massachusetts law (Mass. Gen. Laws. ch. 112 § 129A) provides that the records of psychologists are confidential, and makes no exception for sharing of information for treatment. Missouri law (Mo. Rev. Stat. § 337.636) contains similar provisions governing psychologists, social workers, and professional counselors, as does Wyoming (Wyo. Stat. Ann. § 33-38-109). Nebraska law imposes an absolute obligation of confidentiality on "mental health practitioners," but allows the Board of Mental Health Practice to define regulatory exceptions (Neb. Rev. Stat. § 71-1,335(1)). New Mexico law also seems to impose an absolute obligation of confidentiality on any "counselor and therapist practitioner" (N.M. Stat. Ann. § 61-9A27). Utah law permits disclosures "made under a generally recognized professional or ethical standard that authorizes or requires the disclosure" (Utah Code. Ann. 58-61-602(2)(c)). The obligations imposed by these laws may pose the most substantial threat to the broad sharing of treatment information contemplated by HIPAA.

Third, a number of states have specific statutes governing the records of patients who are involuntarily committed to mental institutions (see Idaho Code § 66-348; Neb. Rev. Stat. § 71-961; Wash. Rev. Code Ann. § 71.05.390). These statutes recognize, presumably, that patients who are involuntarily committed to institutions might have a special claim to privacy, though these laws also usually make provision for the use of records in the commitment process. The Tennessee Code, for example, has a special provision for sharing of information for mandatory outpatient treatment in section 33-6-601:

> If (1) a person with mental illness or serious emotional disturbance was committed involuntarily under chapter 6, part 5 of this title, AND (2) the hospital staff determines preliminarily that: (A) the person will need to participate in outpatient treatment on discharge, and (B) there is a likelihood that the discharge will be subject to the outpatient treatment obligation of this part, AND (3) the person refuses to give consent to disclose information which is legally confidential under this title to the proposed outpatient qualified mental health professional, THEN (4) the hospital and qualified mental health professional may exchange information as necessary to carry out this part.

Fourth and finally, most states have statutes that generally govern the records of all mental patients. The Alabama Code, §§ 22-56-4(b)(6) and

22-56-10, provides that mental patients have rights to privacy, but not beyond the rights of other patients. Louisiana law provides that mental patients may not be deprived of their right to privacy, whatever that means (La. Rev. Stat. Ann. § 28.171(A)). The treatment exceptions discussed below are all found in such general mental health confidentiality statutes.

STATE LAWS GOVERNING THE CONFIDENTIALITY OF SUBSTANCE ABUSE RECORDS

Most states also have statutes governing substance abuse records. These in general roughly approximate the federal statute in their terms (see Cal. Health & Safety Code, § 11845.5; Fla. Stat. Ann. § 397.501(7)) and sometimes specifically refer to federal law (e.g., Mass. Gen. Laws. ch. 111E § 18). They may govern facilities not governed by the federal law (because the facilities receive no federal funding) but may also lack the flexibility found in the federal regulations. Some states have specific laws governing substance abuse counselors as a licensed profession and forbid disclosure of records without consent, with no treatment exception (e.g., La. Rev. Stat. Ann. § 37:3390.4).

Several states, on the other hand, permit broader disclosure of substance abuse information than does the federal law. Kansas law provides that disclosure of substance abuse records can be made "upon the sole consent of the head of the treatment facility who has the records if the head of the treatment facility makes a written determination that such disclosure is necessary for the treatment of the patient or former patient" (Kan. Stat. Ann. § 59-2979). Mississippi law (Miss. Code. Ann. § 41-30-33) provides for disclosure without consent "to treatment personnel for use in connection with his treatment." New Hampshire law (N.H. Rev. Stat. Ann. § 172:8-a) provides confidentiality for substance abuse records, but also says they may be used for a rehabilitation or medical purpose without consent. These provisions would presumably be preempted as to facilities governed by the federal statute.

Some state substance abuse statutes, on the other hand, seem to be more narrow. Pennsylvania law, for example, only authorizes disclosure of substance abuse information to medical personnel with consent (see Pa. Cons. Stat. Ann. tit. 71 § 1690.108). Michigan law (Mich. Comp. Laws § 333.6112) only provides disclosure of substance abuse records for treatment with the consent of the patient. New Jersey, on the other hand (N.J. Stat. Ann. § 26:2B-20), only permits disclosure with a court order. Missouri has a special law (Mo. Rev. Stat. § 191.731) governing substance abuse treatment for pregnant women that promises absolute confidentiality.

INFORMATION SHARING FOR TREATMENT
PURPOSES UNDER STATE LAW AND HIPAA

A few state records statutes have no exception to a general confidentiality obligation for sharing records for treatment and only allow it with consent (see Fla. Stat. Ann. § 394.4615 and Wash Rev. Code Ann. § 71.05.630). Michigan law (Mich. Comp. Laws. § 330.1748) provides for disclosure only with consent outside of a treating facility.

Most state laws governing medical records or mental health records, however, make some provision for sharing of information for treatment purposes. The wording of these statutes varies from state to state. Some are quite limited, only permitting sharing within a single facility or among state treatment programs. See 740 Ill. Comp. Stat. § 110/8–110/12.2. The Delaware mental health statute allows disclosure of treatment information to "Departmental contractors to the extent necessary for professional consultation or services" (Del. Code. Ann. tit. 16, § 5161(13)(f)). The District of Columbia mental health law is even more restrictive, only allowing disclosure to other employees within a facility or to participating providers in the organized mental health system, and then only "when and to the extent necessary to facilitate the delivery of professional services to the client" (D.C. Code § 7-1203.01). Some states permit disclosure of mental health information for treatment without consent only in an emergency. Iowa law provides that "mental health information may be transferred at any time to another facility, physician, or mental health professional in cases of a medical emergency or if the individual or the individual's legal representative requests the transfer in writing for the purposes of receipt of medical or mental health professional services" (see Iowa Code § 228.2(3)). The Kansas statute allows for disclosure of mental health records in an emergency, as well as for "communication and information between or among treatment facilities regarding a proposed patient, patient or former patient for purposes of promoting continuity of care between the state psychiatric hospitals and the community mental health centers" (Kan. Stat. Ann. § 65-5603(5) and (13)). Nebraska law provides for disclosure of mental health records to "the department, * * * and any public or private agency under contract to provide facilities, programs, and patient services" (Neb. Rev. Stat. § 83-109(1)).

Ohio permits disclosure for treatment only of limited mental health information and then only to a limited group of providers:

> Hospitals and other institutions and facilities within the department of mental health may exchange psychiatric records and other pertinent information with other hospitals, institutions, and facilities of the department, and with community mental health agencies and boards of alcohol, drug addiction, and mental health services with which the department has a

current agreement for patient care or services. Records and information that may be released pursuant to this division shall be limited to medication history, physical health status and history, financial status, summary of course of treatment in the hospital, summary of treatment needs, and a discharge summary, if any (Ohio Rev. Code Ann. § 5122.31(c)).

The South Carolina statute permits exchange of mental health information among facility staff, but only "on a need to know basis" (S.C. Code Ann. § 44-22-90(A)(1)). South Carolina also permits mental health providers to disclose "in the course of diagnosis, counseling, or treatment, confidences necessary to promote care within the generally recognized and accepted standards, practices, and procedures of the provider's profession" (S.C. Code Ann. § 19-11-95(c)(5)). Texas law only permits the disclosure of information by mental health professionals "to other professionals and personnel under the professionals" direction who participate in the diagnosis, evaluation, or treatment of the patient" (Tex. Health and Safety Code § 611.004(a)(7)). The Illinois statute permits disclosure of therapists records to "the therapist's supervisor, a consulting therapist, members of a staff team participating in the provision of services, a record custodian, or a person acting under the supervision and control of the therapist" (740 Ill. Comp. Stat. § 110/9(1)). The California mental health law requires that "the consent of the patient, or his or her guardian or conservator shall be obtained before information or records may be disclosed by a professional person employed by a facility to a professional person not employed by the facility who does not have the medical or psychological responsibility for the patient's care" (Cal. Welf. and Inst. Code § 5328(a)). Finally, the Oklahoma statute provides that mental health information "shall only be available to persons actively engaged in the treatment of the patient or in related administrative work. The information available to persons actively engaged in the treatment of the consumer or in related administrative work shall be limited to the minimum amount of information necessary for the person or agency to carry out its function" (Okla. Stat. tit. 43A § 109(A)(2)).

Other statutes are more broadly worded. The Alaska Code, for example, allows sharing of the records of mental patients with "a physician or a provider of health, mental health, or social and welfare services involved in caring for, treating, or rehabilitating the patient" (Alaska Stat. § 47.30.845(1)). The Arizona statute similarly permits disclosure of mental health records to "physicians and providers of health, mental health or social and welfare services involved in caring for, treating or rehabilitating the patient" (Ariz. Rev. Stat. § 36-509). The Colorado mental health statue allows disclosure "in communications between qualified professional personnel in the provision of services or appropriate referrals" (Colo. Rev. Stat. Ann. § 27-10-120(1)(a)). Indiana law permits disclosure of mental health records to individuals who "(A) are employed by: (i) the provider at the same facility or agency; (ii) a managed care provider * * *; or (iii) a health care provider or mental health care provider, if the mental health records are needed to provide health care or mental health services to the patient." and "(B) are involved in the planning, provision, and monitoring of services" (Indiana Code § 16-39-2-6). The Minnesota statute, which governs health records generally, provides for disclosure "to other providers within related health care entities when necessary for the current treatment of the patient" (Minn. Stat. Ann. § 144.335 (3a)(b)(2)).

Mississippi provides for disclosure "when necessary for the continued treatment of a patient" (Miss. Code Ann. § 41-21-97). Missouri law provides for disclosure without consent "to persons or agencies responsible for providing health care services to such patients, residents or clients" (Mo. Rev. Stat. § 630.140(3)(2)). Montana law provides for disclosure of records pertaining to "the seriously mentally ill" "in communications between qualified professionals in the provision of services or appropriate referrals" (Mont. Code Ann. 53-21-166(1)). New Jersey law (N.J. Stat. Ann. § 30:4-24.3) provides that the confidentiality requirements that apply in state mental health facilities do not prohibit "the professional staff of a community agency under contract with the Division of Mental Health Services in the Department of Human Services, or of a screening service, short-term care or psychiatric facility * * * from disclosing information that is relevant to a patient's current treatment to the staff of another such agency." The New York Mental Hygiene Code, § 33.16(a)(1) permits disclosure to "practitioners as part of a consultation or referral during the treatment of the patient or client."

The Pennsylvania mental health statute (50 Pa. Cons. Stat. Ann. § 7111) permits disclosure to "those providing treatment to the person." The Rhode Island statute (R.I. Gen. Laws. § 40.1-5-26(b)(2)), on the other hand, permits disclosure "in communications among qualified medical or mental health professionals in the provision of services or appropriate referrals"(though Rhode Island only permits disclosure of mental health treatment in community residences within the same residence (R.I. Gen. Laws § 40.1-24.5-11). Vermont goes even further, allowing for disclosure of information, "upon proper inquiry to the patient's family, clergy, physician or health care agent" (Vt. Stat. Ann. tit 18 § 7103). Finally, Washington permits disclosure of mental health records:

(e) To qualified staff members of the department, to the director of regional support networks, to resource management services responsible for serving a patient, or to service providers designated by resource management services as necessary to determine the progress and adequacy of treatment and to determine whether the person should be transferred to a less restrictive or more appropriate treatment modality or facility. The information shall remain confidential.

(f) Within the treatment facility where the patient is receiving treatment, confidential information may be disclosed to individuals employed, serving in bona fide training programs, or participating in supervised volunteer programs, at the facility when it is necessary to perform their duties.

(g) Within the department as necessary to coordinate treatment for mental illness, developmental disabilities, alcoholism, or drug abuse of individuals who are under the supervision of the department.

(h) To a licensed physician who has determined that the life or health of the individual is in danger and that treatment without the information contained in the treatment records could be injurious to the patient's health. Disclosure shall be limited to the portions of the records necessary to meet the medical emergency.

(i) To a facility that is to receive an individual who is involuntarily committed * * * or upon transfer of the individual from one treatment facility to another. The release of records under this subsection shall be limited to the treatment records required by law, a record or summary of all somatic treatments, and a discharge summary. The discharge summary may include a statement of the patient's problem, the treatment goals, the type of treatment which has been provided, and recommendation for future treatment, but may not include the patient's complete treatment record (Wash. Rev. Code Ann. § 71.05.630).

The North Carolina mental health statute is one of the most comprehensive statutes, providing over a dozen different contexts in which information regarding mental patients may be disclosed (N.C. Gen. Stat. Ann. § 122C-55). It is too complex to summarize here and is attached as an appendix. The Wisconsin statute (Wis. Stat. Ann. § 51.30), not reproduced here, is nearly as complex.

A number of states require some sort of special determination before records can be released to other treatment providers. The Georgia mental health code, for example, states: "When the chief medical officer of the facility where the record is kept deems it essential for continued treatment, a copy of the record or parts thereof may be released to physicians or psychologists when and as necessary for the treatment of the patient" (Ga. Code Ann. § 37-3-166(a)(1)). The Hawaii statute similarly provides for disclosure as it "may be deemed necessary by the director of health or by the administrator of a private psychiatric or special treatment facility to carry out this chapter" (Haw. Rev. Stat. § 334-5. See, similarly, N.D. Cent. Code § 25-03.1-43). The Maryland law provides for disclosure without consent:

(I) To the medical or mental health director of a juvenile or adult detention or correctional facility if: 1. The recipient has been involuntarily committed under State law or a court order to the detention or correctional facility requesting the medical record; and 2. After a review of the medical record, the health care provider who is the custodian of the record is satisfied that disclosure is necessary for the proper care and treatment of the recipient (Md. Code Ann. § 40-307(j)).

Nevada law permits disclosure "to a qualified member of the staff of a division facility, an employee of the Division * * *, when the Administrator deems it necessary for the proper care of the client" (Nev. Rev. Stat. § 433A.360). Nevada law (Nev. Rev. Stat. § 433.482(8)) also provides that a patient may refuse access to his records to persons without a court order or authorization who are not members of facility staff, and permits the sealing of clinical records of patients who are released from a mental health facility as recovered (Nev. Rev. Stat. §§ 433A.703, 433A.711). The Nevada statute further provides, however, "if, after the sealing of the records, the petitioner is being treated by a physician or licensed psychologist, the physician or psychologist may obtain a copy of the petitioner's records from the hospital or facility. Any records so obtained must be used solely for the treatment of the petitioner" (Nev. Rev. Stat. § 433A.711).

At least one state has a provision for obtaining, as opposed to disclosing, the medical records of mental patients. N.H. Rev. Stat. Ann. § 135-C:19-a(II) provides:

> when the medical director or designee determines that obtaining information is essential to the care or treatment of a person admitted pursuant to [the mental health commitment statute] a designated receiving facility may request, and any health care provider which previously provided services to any person involuntarily admitted to the facility may provide, information about such person limited to medications prescribed, known medication allergies or other information essential to the medical or psychiatric care of the person admitted. Prior to requesting such information the facility shall in writing request the person's consent for such request for information. If the consent cannot be obtained, the facility shall inform the person in writing of the care providers who have been requested to provide information to the facility pursuant to this section. The facility may disclose such information as is necessary to identify the person and the facility which is requesting the information.

Several states provide for the transfer of mental health records with a patient. Nevada law provides that when a patient is transferred from a public medical facility, the patient's records must be forwarded to the new facility (Nev. Rev. Stat. §§ 449.705, 433.332). Oregon and Pennsylvania have similar laws (see Or. Rev. Stat. § 179.505(6); Pa. Cons. Stat. Ann. tit. 50, § 4602). Tenn. Code Ann. § 33-3-105 provides for disclosure if "a service recipient moves from one service provider to another and exchange of information is necessary for continuity of service."

New Mexico provides that mental health records can be disclosed without authorization: (1) when the request is from a mental health or developmental disability professional or from an employee or trainee working with mentally disordered or developmentally disabled persons, to the extent their practice, employment or training on behalf of the client requires that they have access to such information; . . . and (3) when the disclosure of such information is to the primary caregiver of the client and the disclosure is only of information necessary for the continuity of the client's treatment in the judgment of the treating physician or certified psychologist who discloses the information (N. M. Stat. Ann. § 43-1-19). See also N.M. Stat. Ann. § 32A-6-15 (making similar provision for child patients).

At least one state permits disclosure for treatment but requires that the patient be notified of the disclosure (Conn. Gen. Stat. § 52-146f). Several others require that an accounting be kept of disclosures (see, e.g., Wash. Rev. Code Ann. § 71.05.420).

Finally, some state statutes contain exceptions that do not clearly cover treatment, but may be construed to do so in some situations. Ky. Rev. Stat. Ann. § 210.235(2), for example, allows disclosure as "necessary to carry out the provisions for the Kentucky Revised Statutes, and the rules and regulations of cabinets and agencies of the Commonwealth of Kentucky." Maine law provides for disclosure of information by the Department of Mental Health "to carry out any of the statutory functions of the Department" (Me. Rev. Stat. Ann. tit. 34B § 1207(1)(B)).

CONCLUSION

In sum, state laws vary widely in terms of authorizing the disclosure of mental health records without consent for treatment purposes. Many of them are, or could be interpreted as being, more restrictive than the HIPAA regulations. A few may even be more restrictive than the substance abuse confidentiality statute. These laws could in many cases stand in the way of coordinated treatment of persons with mental illness. This is an issue that the Department of Health and Human Services should consider in any revision of the HIPAA privacy regulations. State legislatures should also review their state statutes to assure that a proper balance is reached between the need for keeping mental health records confidential, on the one hand, and the need to share information among treatment providers to assure proper treatment on the other.

Appendix: NORTH CAROLINA GENERAL STAT. ANN. § 122C-55

(a) Any area or State facility or the psychiatric service of the University of North Carolina Hospitals at Chapel Hill may share confidential information regarding any client of that facility with any other area or State facility or the psychiatric service of the University of North Carolina Hospitals at Chapel Hill when necessary to coordinate appropriate and effective care, treatment or habilitation of the client. For the purposes of this subsection, coordinate means the provision, coordination, or management of mental health, developmental disabilities, and substance abuse services and related services by one or more facilities and includes the referral of a client from one facility to another.

(a1) Any State or area facility or the psychiatric service of the University of North Carolina Hospitals at Chapel Hill may share confidential information regarding any client of that facility with the Secretary, and the Secretary may share confidential information regarding any client with an area or State facility or the psychiatric service of the University of North Carolina Hospitals at Chapel Hill when the responsible professional or the Secretary determines that disclosure is necessary to coordinate appropriate and effective care, treatment or habilitation of the client.

(a2) Any area or State facility or the psychiatric service of the University of North Carolina Hospitals at Chapel Hill may share confidential information regarding any client of that facility with any other area facility or State facility or the psychiatric service of the University of North Carolina Hospitals at Chapel Hill when necessary to conduct payment activities relating to an individual served by the facility. Payment activities are activities undertaken by a facility to obtain or provide reimbursement for the provision of services and may include, but are not limited to, determinations of eligibility or coverage, coordination of benefits, determinations of cost-sharing amounts, claims management, claims processing, claims adjudication, claims appeals, billing and collection activities, medical necessity reviews, utilization management and review, precertification and preauthorization of services, concurrent and retrospective review of services, and appeals related to utilization management and review.

(a3) Whenever there is reason to believe that a client is eligible for benefits through a Department program, any State or area facility or the psychiatric service of the University of North Carolina Hospitals at Chapel Hill may share confidential information regarding any client of that facility with the Secretary, and the Secretary may share confidential information regarding any client with an area facility or State facility or the psychiatric services of the University of North Carolina Hospitals at Chapel Hill. Disclosure is limited to that information necessary to establish initial eligibility for benefits, determine continued eligibility over time, and obtain reimbursement for the costs of services provided to the client.

(a4) An area authority or county program may share confidential information regarding any client with any area facility, and any area facility may share confidential information regarding any client of that facility with the area authority or county program, when the area authority or county program determines the disclosure is necessary to develop, manage, monitor, or evaluate the area authority's or county program's network of qualified providers as provided in G.S. 122C-115.2(b)(1)b., G.S. 122C-141(a), the State Plan, and rules of the Secretary. For the purposes of this subsection, the purposes or activities for which confidential information may be disclosed include, but are not limited to, quality assessment and improvement activities, provider accreditation and staff credentialing, developing contracts and negotiating rates, investigating and responding to client grievances and complaints, evaluating practitioner and provider performance, auditing functions, on-site monitoring, conducting consumer satisfaction studies, and collecting and analyzing performance data.

(a5) Any area facility may share confidential information with any other area facility regarding an applicant when necessary to determine whether the applicant is eligible for area facility services. For the purpose of this subsection, the "term applicant" means an individual who contacts an area facility for services.

(b) A facility, physician, or other individual responsible for evaluation, management, supervision, or treatment of respondents examined or committed for outpatient treatment under the provisions of Article 5 of this Chapter may request, receive, and disclose confidential information to the extent necessary to enable them to fulfill their responsibilities.

(c) A facility may furnish confidential information in its possession to the Department of Correction when requested by that department regarding any client of that facility when the inmate has been determined by the Department of Correction to be in need of treatment for mental illness, developmental disabilities, or substance abuse. The Department of Correction may furnish to a facility confidential information in its possession about treatment for mental illness, developmental disabilities, or substance abuse that the Department of Correction has provided to any present or former inmate if the inmate is presently seeking treatment from the requesting facility or if the inmate has been involuntarily committed to the requesting facility for inpatient or outpatient treatment. Under the circumstances described in this subsection, the consent of the client or inmate shall not be required in order for this information to be furnished and the information shall be furnished despite objection by the client or inmate. Confidential information disclosed pursuant to this subsection is restricted from further disclosure.

(d) A responsible professional may disclose confidential information when in his opinion there is an imminent danger to the health or safety of the client or another individual or there is a likelihood of the commission of a felony or violent misdemeanor.

(e) A responsible professional may exchange confidential information with a physician or other health care provider who is providing emergency medical services to a client. Disclosure of the information is limited to that necessary to meet the emergency as determined by the responsible professional.

(e1) A State facility may furnish client identifying information to the Department for the purpose of maintaining an index of clients served in State facilities which may be used by State facilities only if that information is necessary for the appropriate and effective evaluation, care and treatment of the client.

(e2) A responsible professional may disclose an advance instruction for mental health treatment or confidential information from an advance instruction to a physician, psychologist, or other qualified professional when the responsible professional determines that disclosure is necessary to give effect to or provide treatment in accordance with the advance instruction.

(f) A facility may disclose confidential information to a provider of support services whenever the facility has entered into a written agreement with a person to provide support services and the agreement includes a provision in which the provider of support services acknowledges that in receiving, storing, processing, or otherwise dealing with any confidential information, he will safeguard and not further disclose the information.

(g) Whenever there is reason to believe that the client is eligible for financial benefits through a governmental agency, a facility may disclose confidential information to State, local, or federal government agencies. Except as provided in G.S. 122C-55(a3), disclosure is limited to that confidential information necessary to establish financial benefits for a client. After establishment of these benefits, the consent of the client or his legally responsible person is required for further release of confidential information under this subsection.

(h) Within a facility, employees, students, consultants or volunteers involved in the care, treatment, or habilitation of a client may exchange confidential information as needed for the purpose of carrying out their responsibility in serving the client.

(i) Upon specific request, a responsible professional may release confidential information to a physician or psychologist who referred the client to the facility.

(j) Upon request of the next of kin or other family member who has a legitimate role in the therapeutic services offered, or other person designated by the client or his legally responsible person, the responsible professional shall provide the next of kin or other family member or the designee with notification of the client's diagnosis, the prognosis, the medications prescribed, the dosage of the medications prescribed, the side effects of the medications prescribed, if any, and the progress of the client, provided that the client or his legally responsible person has consented in writing, or the client has consented orally in the presence of a witness selected by the client, prior to the release of this information. Both the client's or the legally responsible person's consent and the release of this information shall be documented in the client's medical record. This consent shall be valid for a specified length of time only and is subject to revocation by the consenting individual.

(k) Notwithstanding the provisions of G.S. 122C-53(b) or G.S. 122C-206, upon request of the next of kin or other family member who has a legitimate role in the therapeutic services offered, or other person designated by the client or his legally responsible person, the responsible professional shall provide the next of kin, or family member, or the designee, notification of the client's admission to the facility, transfer to another facility, decision to leave the facility against medical advice, discharge from the facility, and referrals and appointment information for treatment after discharge, after notification to the client that this information has been requested.

(l) In response to a written request of the next of kin or other family member who has a legitimate role in the therapeutic services offered, or other person designated by the client, for additional information not provided for in subsections (j) and (k) of this section, and when such written request identifies the intended use for this information, the responsible professional shall, in a timely manner:
(1) Provide the information requested based upon the responsible professional's determination that providing this information will be to the client's therapeutic benefit, and provided that the client or his legally responsible person has consented in writing to the release of the information requested; or
(2) Refuse to provide the information requested based upon the responsible professional's determination that providing this information will be detrimental to the therapeutic relationship between client and professional; or

(3) Refuse to provide the information requested based upon the responsible professional's determination that the next of kin or family member or designee does not have a legitimate need for the information requested.

(m) The Commission for Mental Health, Developmental Disabilities, and Substance Abuse Services shall adopt rules specifically to define the legitimate role referred to in subsections (j), (k), and (l) of this section.

Appendix C

Mental and Substance-Use Health Services for Veterans: Experience with Performance Evaluation in the Department of Veterans Affairs

Robert Rosenheck, MD
Director, VA Northeast Program Evaluation Center (NEPEC),
West Haven, CT
Professor of Psychiatry, Public Health and at the Child Study Center
Yale Medical School, New Haven, CT

August 2004

Prepared for the Institute of Medicine Committee on Crossing the
Quality Chasm: Adaptation to Mental Health and Addictive Disorders

Acknowledgement: Paul Errera MD, Thomas Horvath MD, Laurent Lehmann MD, Mark Shelhorse MD, Mary Jansen PhD, Gay Koerber MA, William Van Stone MD, Robert Gresen PhD and Anthony Campinell PhD and the staff of the Strategic Healthcare Group for Mental Health in VA Central Office have provided invaluable support over many years. The staff of NEPEC is responsible for most of the work reported here (but not for the errors, which are my own), specifically project directors Mayur Desai PhD, Rani Desai PhD, Alan Fontana PhD, Greg Greenberg PhD, Wesley Kasprow PhD, Douglas Leslie PhD, Alvin Mares PhD, James McGuire PhD, Michale Neale PhD, Sandra Resnick PhD. Thanks also to Michael Sernyak MD. Special analyses of the 2001 Survey of Veterans and the Schizophrenia PORT survey for this report were completed by Greg Greenberg and Rani Desai.

Summary

As the largest integrated health and social welfare agency in the United States, the Department of Veterans Affairs is a unique and potentially informative setting in which to examine the challenges of mental health and substance use treatment services quality and performance management.

U.S. Veterans

Of 25 million U.S. veterans, 21% used Veterans Affairs (VA) services in the past year, and 2.7% used VA mental health or substance abuse (MH/SA) services. Although all veterans are now eligible for VA services, those most likely to use VA services receive VA income benefits are older, poorer, and less likely to have health insurance.

Treatment of MH/SA in VA

In 2003, 1.2 million veterans received a MH/SA diagnosis in VA, about 25% of all VA users. While they were a diagnostically mixed, Global Assessment of Functioning scores averaged 53, suggesting poor functioning, and 19% were dually diagnosed.
VA is a cabinet-level agency with many important stakeholders. Concern about war-related Post Traumatic Stress Disorder (PTSD) and homelessness among veterans have given mental health issues greater prominence in the VA community in recent years. In 1995, a major reform was initiated which closed most MH/SA inpatient beds, nearly doubled outpatients treated, and emphasized accountability and performance measurement.

Linkage of VA with the Department of Defense (DoD) and Other Mental Health, Medical, and Social Service Systems

There has been great interest recently in smoothing the transition from DoD to VA, although the integration of information systems has yet to take place. Most VA patients get all of their MH/SA and medical services from VA. Although there has been concern that with extensive recent bed closures, VA patients would be forced to seek care in other health systems and might experience an increased risk of incarceration or suicide, empirical studies conducted thus far have not shown a significant increase in these problems.

Development of MH/SA Quality Measurement and Quality Management in VA

During the past 20 years there have been two notable phases in the development of VA MH/SA services. The first was initiated by the leader of mental health programs in VA central office from 1985–1994 and involved expansion of specialized mental health programs such as Assertive Community Treatment, homeless outreach, and transitional employment. The second was initiated in 1995 by the undersecretary for Health and brought changes in mental health service delivery as part of a major system-wide shift from operating as a hospital-based system of care to a community or population-based system of care. In both phases quality and performance measurement were crucial tools in guiding organizational change. A third phase, characterized by system-wide focus on building MH/SA quality is evolving in response to the recent report of the President's New Freedom Commission on Mental Health.

Quality of VA MH/SA Care

The assessment of quality requires comparison of providers with standards or benchmarks, with risk adjustment for factors that may confound these comparisons. Evaluation of the quality of MH/SA care at VA facilities has been based on comparisons with: (1) VA system average performance, (2) VA performance in prior years, (3) the performance of other systems of care, and (4) comparison of care received by minorities with the majority population. Methods of quality measurement and benchmarking in VA are demonstrated for six aims highlighted in a previous Institute of Medicine (IOM) report: safety, effectiveness, person-centeredness, timeliness, efficiency, and equitability.

Front-Line Experience

Performance management in health care is sometimes experienced ambivalently by front line managers and clinicians. While they often feel empowered by access to data and find it allows them to improve the care they provide, there is also concern that measures are imperfect; that they do not take account of differences across facilities in case mix and in available community resources; that measures can be manipulated or "gamed," resulting in unfair comparisons; and that managerial pressure to improve performance sometimes creates an atmosphere of personal criticism more than joint problem solving.

Conclusion

The complexity and uncertainty of the health care enterprise must be managed through comprehensive quality monitoring systems used by creative and committed leaders in competent organizations. VA has embraced this challenge.

INTRODUCTION: THE DEPARTMENT OF VETERANS AFFAIRS IN AMERICAN MENTAL HEALTH CARE

To bridge a chasm, one needs, at a minimum, a clear view of the terrain surrounding it. One can imagine building a bridge from one side of a chasm to the other, from both sides toward the middle, or even from a scaffolding erected on the floor in the center of the chasm out to both sides. But it is virtually impossible to imagine bridging a chasm if one were blocked from either viewing or accessing even one of its banks. The situation faced by those who would seek to bridge the many quality chasms in mental health care in the United States is in many respects like that of an engineer bridging a complex system of chasms with access to only one of its banks. People with serious mental illness often have needs for diverse services including psychiatric care, substance abuse care, primary and specialty medical care, and numerous social services including income supports, employment, education, and housing assistance, as well as help negotiating with the criminal justice system. And yet each of these needs is addressed by a different set of agencies at different levels of government. The advantage of this decentralized approach is that it increases local control, responsiveness, and flexibility (Peterson, 1995; Smith and Lipsky, 1993). The disadvantage is that agencies tend to compete for sources of funding, carefully guard their independence, and are often wary of sharing information on individual clients, let alone releasing systematic data on their overall operation. Mental health system engineers in America thus often find themselves trying to bridge system chasms while only being able to obtain information on the small patch of ground under their own feet.

The U.S. Department of Veterans Affairs (VA) is a notable exception to this pattern. In most areas of U.S. social or health care policy, programs are operated at state or local levels by private or nonprofit providers, and the role of the federal government is limited. In contrast, the national government takes direct responsibility for providing comprehensive, lifelong, medical and social services to Veterans of the Armed Forces. National defense is the least contested area of federal dominance in the American system of government; as a result, the federal government has been given responsibility for the health and social welfare of military personnel, both on active duty and, for an increasingly large segment of veterans, after their period of military service is over. The VA thus represents the unusual case in which one agency accepts responsibility, at the national level, for providing comprehensive long-term care for a well-defined segment of the population. Mental health care provided by the VA may thus offer a uniquely informative, if atypical, opportunity to examine mental health performance monitoring and management in the American context.

Taking a broad view, this presentation will: (1) describe the veteran population of the United States, compare the mental health needs (including substance use treatment needs) of veterans and those of other Americans, and compare veterans who use VA services with both nonveterans and other veterans who do not. It will then (2) present an overview of the VA health care system, the Veterans Health Administration (VHA)—and specifically its delivery of mental health and substance abuse services, paying special attention to the most prominent needs of the treated population, basic organizational structures, and notable changes in the delivery of those services in the past decade. (3) Next, data on the linkages between VA and non-VA mental health and social welfare systems will be presented to allow evaluation of the level of self-containment of VA mental health care and the nature of its linkages with other systems. The next section (4) describes the organizational processes through which quality management has been developed in VA mental health and substance abuse care in recent years. Having presented the context of mental health performance management, in the next section (5) we present evidence concerning the safety, effectiveness, person-centeredness, timeliness, efficiency and equitability of VA mental health and substance abuse care as it has changed in recent years and as it compares to other health care systems. Finally, (6) we touch on an area that has received virtually no systematic attention, the sometimes ambivalent reactions of front-line health system managers and clinicians to the implementation of performance management systems.

I. AMERICA'S VETERANS: MENTAL HEALTH AND SUBSTANCE ABUSE STATUS AND USE OF VA SERVICES

America's Veterans

In 2001, the national Survey of Veterans (SOV) conducted detailed interviews with a nationally representative sample of 20,000 veterans identified through VA administrative records and random digit dialing (USVA, 2004). Population estimates derived from the survey were based on an overall estimate of 25,196,036 living veterans in 2001, which included 12.4% of all U.S. adults and 24.5% of men 18 years or older (U.S. Census Bureau, 2001) (see column 1 of Table 1). The two most distinctive characteristics of the veteran population is that it is overwhelmingly male (94%) and that its age distribution is shaped by defense manpower needs and particularly wartime recruitment, rather than by the natural rate of population growth.

Veterans are older than other Americans, first, because eligibility for military service begins at 18. In addition, and perhaps more important, World War II, the Korean conflict, and the Vietnam conflict, spanning 34 years from 1941 to 1975, were fought by far larger forces than have served in the 28 years since 1975. Altogether 30 million troops served during the three major war eras from 1941 to 1975 while only 5.7 million living veterans entered military service since 1975 (U.S. Census Bureaus, 2001). Thus 46% of veterans are 60 years old or more as compared to only 16.6% of the general population and 14.5% of men. A detailed characterization of the U.S. veteran population based on the 2001 SOV is presented in the first column of Table 1. Veterans do not differ markedly from the rest of the U.S. population in racial composition, education, or employment although there are somewhat fewer blacks and Hispanics and educational levels are somewhat higher among veterans, most likely due to the availability of specific veterans' educational benefits.

Mental Health and Substance Abuse Disorders Among Veterans and Nonveterans in the General Population

Self-report data from the SOV show that 6.6% of veterans report having received services for a MH/SA problem in the past year, but these data do not allow comparison with the MH/SA status of the general population. The most useful study for comparing MH/SA problems of veteran and nonveteran men is a secondary analysis of data from the Epidemiological Catchment Area (ECA), which surveyed the mental health status of 18,572 Americans, including 10,954 men, and oversampled older Americans, in five locations in 1980 (Norquist et al., 1990).

ECA data reveal no differences in *lifetime* prevalence of mental health disorder among veterans of World War II or either the Korean or Vietnam conflict eras and age-matched nonveteran men. In contrast, veterans of the post-Vietnam era (the initial period of the All Volunteer Force [AVF]) show a *greater* prevalence of lifetime mental disorder (54.6% of veterans vs. 40.9% of nonveterans [p <.0001]). Data on *6-month* prevalence of mental disorder show a similar pattern, although World War II era veterans had a significantly lower overall prevalence of mental disorder than nonveterans (11.8% vs. 17.7%, p <.01).

Examination of specific lifetime disorders shows that World War II era veterans had lower prevalences of any nonsubstance abuse disorder than nonveterans (12.2% vs. 18.5%, p <.01); Vietnam era veterans had lower prevalence of schizophrenic disorders (0.8% vs. 2.2%, p <.05) and affective disorders (4.4% vs. 8.3%, p <.01); and post-Vietnam veterans had *higher* lifetime prevalence of substance abuse disorders (47.4% vs. 30.6%, p <.01, including both alcohol and drug disorders) and antisocial personality disorder (14.9% vs. 5.8%) but lower prevalence of schizophrenic disorder than nonveterans (0.3% vs. 1.5%, p <.01).

Findings of greater rates of mental illness and especially substance abuse among veterans of the AVF are consistent with several studies showing greater substance use among military personnel in the immediate post-

Vietnam era (Rosenheck et al., 1996a) and with studies that have demonstrated a three to four times greater risk of homelessness among post-Vietnam veterans as compared to nonveterans, as well as among female veterans (who have always served on a voluntary basis) (Gamache et al., 2001, 2003). The increased risk of homelessness is completely absent or not statistically significant among veterans of earlier eras in which the draft guaranteed a more representative military force. Thus a major issue in the psychiatric epidemiology of U.S. veterans appears to be the shift from the draft to the AVF. There have been far fewer veterans since the end of the Vietnam conflict, but they appear to have a greater risk of MH/SA problems, not because of the hazards of military service, but because of self-selection processes among those who volunteer.

Findings from the ECA are also consistent with the results of the National Vietnam Veterans Readjustment Study (NVVRS) (Kulka et al., 1990), a major epidemiologic study of representative samples of Vietnam era veterans and a matched sample of nonveterans. While the NVVRS found higher rates of posttraumatic stress disorder (PTSD) among veterans exposed to high levels of combat than among other veterans who were not and civilians; rates of other mental disorders did not differ between veteran and nonveteran populations.

A recent analysis of data from 12,480 male respondents aged 25–60 in the National Household Drug Abuse Surveys from 1994, 1997, and 1998 showed veterans reported greater rates of near-daily alcohol use in the past year (22.9 vs. 19.2%, p <.001) but lower rates of illicit drug use (10.0% vs. 12.9%, p <.001) (Tessler et al., in press). Similarly, an epidemiologic study that compared homeless veteran and nonveteran men in Los Angeles found that veterans were less likely to have nonsubstance abuse mental health disorders (47.5% vs. 65.2%, p <.01) but more likely to meet criteria for alcohol abuse or dependence (72.3% vs. 59.8%, p <.05) (Rosenheck and Koegel, 1993). Both these studies involve representative samples of the veteran population, not those involved in treatment.

MH/SA Status Among Veteran and Nonveteran Users of Mental Health Services

Three studies have compared veteran and nonveteran men who were using MH/SA services (Desai et al., in press-b; Rosenheck et al., 2000a; Tessler et al., 2002). These studies generally have found veterans to be older, less likely to be minorities, better educated, and with higher incomes, and analyses were adjusted for these differences in comparisons of mental health status.

The Schizophrenia Patient Outcomes Research Team (PORT) study of representative samples of patients treated for schizophrenia in Ohio and

Georgia included an over-sampling of VA patients to allow adequate power for comparison of VA–non-VA male service users (N = 466 VA patients and 279 non-VA male patients) (Rosenheck et al., 2000a). After adjusting for age and race differences, no significant differences were found on measures of psychosis, depression, or substance abuse.

A comparison of 1,252 veteran and 3,236 nonveteran men treated at 18 sites in the ACCESS demonstration of service system integration for homeless people with severe mental illness also found no differences between veterans and nonveterans on psychiatric or drug problems, although veterans had somewhat more severe alcohol problems as measured by the Addiction Severity Index (Tessler et al., 2002).

Finally, the Connecticut Outcome Study compared 196 VA patients and 337 non-VA patients treated at nearby state-operated Community Mental Health Centers and also found no significant differences in measures of psychiatric symptoms or substance abuse, after adjustment for age, race and income (Desai et al., in press).

Use of VA Services

Data from the 2001 SOV show that 20.5% of veterans reported using any VA services (i.e., not specifically MH/SA services) in the past year and 34.4% in their lifetimes. These figures are substantially higher than those recorded in a similar national survey conducted in 1987. In that survey, only 5.8% reported VA service use in the past year and 21.2% lifetime (Rosenheck and Massari, 1993). These substantial changes reflect at least three factors. First, eligibility for VA services was vastly expanded in 1996 from those who receive VA compensation or pension benefits or have low incomes, estimated to have represented only 9.4 million veterans (Kizer, 1999), to the entire population of 25 million veterans. In addition, major changes in the configuration of VA facilities have made services far more accessible. In the 1990s major reductions in inpatient beds allowed expansion of outpatient care and the establishment of over 500 accessible community-based outpatient clinics (GAO, 2001). In 2003, the average veteran lived 12.2 miles from the nearest VA facility as compared to 32.0 miles in 1994 (Greenberg and Rosenheck, 2003; Rosenheck and Cicchetti, 1995). In addition, the increasing numbers of uninsured Americans and the growing cost and importance of prescription drugs have also contributed to the growing demand for virtually free VA services.

In spite of the changes in eligibility, veteran characteristics that are associated with use of VA services have changed little since 1987. Columns 2 and 3 in Table 1 show the proportions of veterans in each subgroup who used VA services in the past year and in their lifetimes. Both recent and lifetime VA service use is associated with greater age, minority status, low education and income, lack of private insurance, poor health, mental health service use, and receipt of VA compensation.

Table 2 presents a logistic regression analysis of factors that predict recent and lifetime VA service use to illustrate both the independent and the relative magnitude of the effects of each factor. The fourth and seventh columns rank the absolute value of the magnitude of these effects (both positive and negative) and show the strongest correlates of VA service use to be receipt of VA compensation, low income, lack of private insurance, poor health, age less than 30, African American race, Prisoner of War experience, and mental health service use and related disability. These factors are virtually the same as those identified in the 1987 SOV (Rosenheck and Massari, 1993).

Use of VA Mental Health Services

SOV data further reveal that 6.6% of all veterans used mental health services in the previous year, and 2.7% used VA mental health services (41% of those who used any mental health services) (Columns 4 and 5 of Table 1). Among mental health service users, too, those who used VA services are older, more likely to be minority group members, had less education and lower incomes, lacked private insurance, had poorer health, and received VA compensation (see also Table 3 for logistic regression analysis and ranking). It is notable that veterans who sought services for PTSD were especially likely to have used VA mental health services, replicating a finding from a previous analysis of the NVVRS data (Rosenheck and Fontana, 1995) and showing that, contrary to what was once popular belief, veterans with PTSD related to their military service do not avoid using VA mental health services.

The PORT survey of the treatment of schizophrenia in Ohio and Georgia allows further comparison, with the group of severely mentally ill veterans, of those who used VA services (N = 350) and those who used non-VA services (N = 170) (reanalysis based on data in Rosenheck et al., 2000a). Stepwise logistic regression showed veterans who used VA services to be 2.7 times more likely to be receiving VA compensation, 3.0 times more likely to be living in a supervised residence, 37% less likely to be black, and to have used fewer emergency services and have had less severe symptoms.

A study that focused on administrative data from state mental hospitals in eight states between 1984 and 1989 (Desai and Rosenheck, 2000) found that from 7 to 27% of men in these non-VA facilities were veterans as compared to 29–34% in the general male population, suggesting that veterans are less likely to use non-VA service than other men. In comparison with other state hospital patients, veterans were older, more like to have alcoholism and bipolar disorder, and perhaps of greatest interest: (a) lived further away from VA hospitals than nonveterans; (b) were from states with lower per capita expenditure on VA mental health care; and (c) were from states with higher per capita expenditure on state hospitals. Thus, in addition to personal characteristics, both residential remoteness from a VA facility and scant supply of VA services in relation to non-VA services increased veterans' use of non-VA services.

A study of the proportion of veterans in each U.S. county who use VA MH/SA services similarly found distance from veterans' residences to the nearest VA facility to be the strongest predictor of VA MH/SA services use, along with the relative local supply of VA and non-VA services (Rosenheck and Stolar, 1998). In fact, VA service use among veterans service connected for psychoses was specifically reduced in association with a high supply of state and county mental hospital resources, while VA use among non-psychotic veterans was negatively associated with the supply of non-Federal general hospital resources. The impact of the supply and proximity of VA services has also been demonstrated in a sample of homeless mental health services users (Gamache et al., 2000).

II. TREATMENT OF MENTAL HEALTH AND SUBSTANCE ABUSE IN THE VA: PATIENTS, ADMINISTRATION, RELATIONSHIPS WITH OTHER FEDERAL AGENCIES, STAKEHOLDERS, AND CHANGES SINCE 1995

The VA is a cabinet level federal department that includes two major subdivisions that provide services to people with mental illness: (1) The VHA, which delivered health care services to approximately 5 million veterans in fiscal year (FY) 2003 at 162 medical centers and more than 850 facility and community based clinics; and (2) the Veterans Benefits Administration (VBA), which provided income benefits to over 2.5 million veterans in FY 2003 in addition to rehabilitation and educational support and housing loan guarantees (U.S. Department of Veterans Affairs, 2003). Of the 2.5 million veterans who received compensation from VBA in 2003, 481,000 received compensation for mental illness, and of these 47% used VA mental health services (Greenberg and Rosenheck, 2004a).

VA Patients Diagnosed with Mental Health and Substance Abuse Disorders

Administrative workload data from the VHA show that in FY 2003, 1,218,327 veterans (about 25% of all those who received VA health services) received a mental health or substance abuse (MH/SA) diagnosis (ICD-9 codes 290.00-312.99) during an inpatient, nursing home, residential, or outpatient encounter (Table 4).

The most frequent MH/SA diagnoses (Table 4, numbered column 2) were dysthymia (41%), PTSD (20%), anxiety disorder (20%), and major depressive disorder (20%). Altogether 22% received a substance abuse diagnosis (17% alcohol abuse/dependence and 11% drug abuse/dependence) and 18% were dually diagnosed. Altogether, 38% received VA compensation for medical or psychiatric problems, almost four times that in the general population.

Among veterans who received a MH/SA diagnosis, 930,098 (76%) received a primary diagnosis for MH/SA (Table 4, numbered column 3), meaning that the MH/SA diagnosis was the primary focus of at least one contact during the year; and 705,209 of these received treatment in a MH/SA specialty program (numbered column 4) (76% of those who received a primary MH/SA diagnosis and 57% of those who received any primary or secondary MH/SA diagnosis). An additional 89,372 veterans received services in a specialty mental health program but did not receive a primary mental health diagnosis (not shown on table), for a total of 794,581 or 17% of all VA patients who received mental health services in a specialty clinic setting (Greenberg and Rosenheck, 2004a).

The most frequent MH/SA diagnoses among veterans treated in specialty clinics (Table 4, numbered column 5) were also dysthymia (43%), PTSD (31%), anxiety disorder (22%), and major depressive disorder (24%), with 26% receiving a substance abuse diagnosis (20% alcohol abuse/dependence and 16% drug abuse/dependence), and 18% were dually diagnosed.

Global Assessment of Functioning (GAF) scores based on a single item rating scale ranging from 0 to 100, which is a standard part of the psychiatric diagnosis, average 41.8 (s.d. = 13.1) among inpatients at the time of discharge and 53.3 (s.d. = 11.3) among outpatients (Greenberg and Rosenheck, 2004a). A GAF score of 50 is often used as a cutoff for severe mental illness. Thus although fewer than 15% of VA patients with MH/SA diagnoses have the most severe illnesses such as schizophrenia or bipolar disorder, there is considerable functional impairment among these patients. It is also noteworthy that although only 76% of veterans with a primary MH/SA diagnosis receive care in specialty clinics, 95% or more of those with the most serious illnesses (schizophrenia, major depressive disorder, bipolar disorder, or PTSD) receive care in MH/SA specialty clinics, and 45% receive VA compensation.

Annual surveys conducted from FY 1995 (Rosenheck et al., 1996c) to FY 2000 (Seibyl et al., 2001) showed that almost 30% of VA psychiatric inpatients, and almost 50% of those in inpatient substance abuse programs, had been homeless at the time of admission. Over 100,000 MH/SA outpatients are identified as homeless each year, about 12% of the total, which is most likely a substantial undercount, since coding for homelessness is not uniform in the outpatient files.

Specialized MH/SA Programs

Perhaps the most basic approach to improving the quality of mental health care in VA, as elsewhere, has been through the establishment of specialized programs or treatment units. In the 1950s, VA established a community foster care program that represented one of the early efforts to transfer severely mentally ill patients from the hospital to the community (Linn et al., 1977). In the 1960s and 1970s, day hospitals (Linn et al., 1979) and day treatment centers were established as alternatives to hospitalization along with specialized inpatient and outpatient substance abuse programs and a transitional employment program that offered veterans the opportunity to work, first in workshop settings and subsequently at community jobs. More recently, specialized programs have been established to treat military-related PTSD; to conduct outreach and provide residential treatment for homeless veterans; to provide residential rehabilitation in community settings and to deliver specialized services to veterans with substance abuse problems. Table 5 summarizes workloads in specialized VA inpatient and outpatient MH/SA programs. While it appears that as many as 400,000 may receive treatment in specialized programs, these figures are not unduplicated counts and a substantial number of veterans are treated in more than one program. More will be said about the development, management, and monitoring of specialized VA MH/SA programs, below.

Administrative Organization

The VHA is led by the undersecretary for Health, a presidential appointee approved by the Senate. Line authority for operations devolves through the deputy undersecretary for operations and management to the directors of 21 Veterans Integrated Service Networks (VISNs), the regional unit of administration in VHA. VISN directors are responsible for supervision of the directors of each of the 152 local VA Medical Centers (VAMCs), about 130 of which operate specialty mental health programs. VISNs serve an average of 231,000 veterans per year with an average of 8,671 Full Time Employee Equivalents (FTEE) and consist of 4-8 medical centers, which each serve an average of 37,554 veterans per year with an average of 1,437 FTEE.

The lead mental health expert in VA Central Office (VACO) is the chief consultant of the Strategic Health Care Group for Mental Health, who provides staff support to the chief of Patient Care Services and through that position to the deputy undersecretary for Health. Thus, the national leader of mental health has no direct line or budgetary authority and acts as a staff advisor, several levels below top VHA leadership. The national Office of Quality and Performance (OQP) in VACO is responsible for designing national performance measures and does so with extensive input from the field. The director of OQP reports directly to the deputy undersecretary for Health.

While there is some variability in organization across VISNs and VAMCs, most have a mental health service line manager, most often a psychiatrist or psychologist, who is responsible for coordinating the delivery of mental health care by all the involved professions at that facility. At present, mental health service line managers do not have budgetary authority and appeal to VISN or VAMC leaders for resources in competition with the leadership of other medical specialties. Quality management and preparation for Joint Commission on Accreditation of Health Care Organizations (JCAHO) and Commission on Accreditation of Rehabilitation Facilities (CARF) accreditation are VISN and VAMC responsibilities, in which the mental health service line managers are responsible for the performance of the mental health programs.

Relationships with Other Federal Departments

Collaboration to facilitate the transition from Department of Defense (DoD) to VA care has been of growing interest in recent years. Staff of the VBA counsel military personnel about their VA benefits as they leave military service, but there has been no ongoing sharing of medical records or other information. Specific efforts are now being made to facilitate electronic information exchange between the agencies, especially in response to the concern about the new generation of veterans now returning from Iraq. The position of deputy Secretary for Health for Health Policy Coordination was created 2 years ago to lead interagency program development and to serve as the principle liaison between VA and the Department of Health and Human Services. VA participates actively in joint activities with other federal agencies, as in the Interagency Counsel on Homelessness and the President's New Freedom Commission on Mental Health, and has conducted joint service and evaluation projects with Housing and Urban Development (Rosenheck et al., 2003a) and the Social Security Administration (Rosenheck et al., 1999b, 2000a), among others. VA differs from most other federal agencies in that it is a direct provider of services rather than a channel for funds, and thus collaboration in service delivery is uncommon but may grow with DoD.

Stakeholders

The primary external stakeholders in the operation of VA are the Congress, and especially the Veterans Affairs Committees, and the Veterans Service Organizations (e.g., the Paralyzed Veterans of America, Disabled Veterans of America, the Veterans of Foreign Wars, the American Legion, and Vietnam Veterans of America), which are especially active and influential. Perhaps because issues of PTSD and homelessness among veterans have been prominent in recent years, these stakeholders appear to have shown greater interest in mental health issues over the past 15 years, and particularly in the quality and funding of VA mental health care. Congress also established a committee with VHA, the undersecretary for Health's Special Committee on Treatment of Severely Mentally Ill Veterans (the SMI committee), charged with making recommendations for of improving MH/SA care and monitoring maintenance of MH/SA capacity. The SMI committee is required to submit an annual report to the Congress.

Changes in MH/SA Service Delivery Since 1995

In 1995, Kenneth Kizer, MD MPH, was appointed undersecretary for Health and initiated an extensive reform of VHA. Kizer encouraged a shift to a population-based preventive and primary care focus rather than a hospital, specialty care focus. He vigorously promoted a reduction in inpatient service utilization and championed an expansion of outpatient treatment, in part through the development of community-based outpatient clinics, small satellite clinics located closer to where veterans lived. These goals were reinforced through a capitated system of resource allocation and by placing major emphasis on accountability through the use of performance measures (Kizer, 1999).

Although his focus was not specific to MH/SA, during these years VA mental health underwent a substantial transformation. Between 1995 and 2003, 66% of all general psychiatry inpatient beds and 96% of all inpatient substance abuse beds were closed. The number of long-term psychiatric patients, that is, those hospitalized for more than a year, declined by 81% and the number with psychiatric diagnoses on inpatient medical units declined by 93%. Inpatient length of stay dropped 43%, from an average of 27.8 days to 15.8 days, allowing more patients to use the remaining beds. As a result, the number of episodes of inpatient care declined by only 44%.

With the pressure of a capitated resource allocation system and population-based planning, the total number of mental health outpatients increased by 44.7%, or 5.6% per year, from 545,004 to 788,502. Perhaps to allow time to serve this increasing workload, the average number of annual visits per veteran declined from 15.1 to 12.8 (15%).

Specialized outpatient substance abuse (SA) services initially (FY 1995–FY 1998) followed this general trend, with 3% annual growth in the number of patients treated, but from FY 1998 to FY 2003 the number of veterans who received specialized outpatient substance abuse services *declined* by 19% (3.7%/year). Since there was no reduction in need of SA services in the veteran population (Tessler et al., 2005), this decline may have reflected an unintended decline in supply of VA SA services, which has grown more serious for five consecutive years.

III. LINKAGE OF VETERANS WITH THE DOD AND OTHER MENTAL HEALTH, MEDICAL, AND SOCIAL SERVICE SYSTEMS

As noted in the Introduction, VA is unique in American mental health care as an integrated national system providing comprehensive services to a designated population. There are, however, no restrictions that prevent veterans who use VA services from using other systems of care. In this section we examine the involvement of VA patients with other systems both to better understand the context of VA care and to assess how self-contained VA and its service users actually are.

Issues of confidentiality often complicate examination of service use across systems. While it is occasionally possible to merge data using identifiers such as social security numbers, there are two other approaches that do not require common identifiers. In the first approach, VA patients can be surveyed about their use of non-VA services. In the second, populations can be matched probabilistically on the basis of the degree of overlap in the frequency distribution of birthdates. The greater the overlap in the distribution of birthdates, the greater the likelihood of an overlap in populations (Pandiani et al., 1998).

Transition from DoD to VA

There has been only one study of the flow of mental health patients from DoD to VA. In that study (Mojtabi et al., 2003), records of patients discharged from military service for schizophrenia or bipolar or major affective disorder were merged with VA service use data. Only 52% of discharged veterans had contact with the VA system. Notably, neither women nor minorities were any less likely than other veterans to find their way to the VA. It is unknown whether those who did not contact VA had adequate access to service elsewhere or had been discouraged, somehow, from using VA services.

Cross MH/SA System Use

Several studies have examined use of non-VA MH/SA services by VA patients. First, a number of recent clinical trials have collected detailed cost data on VA and non-VA service use. Data from a study of supported housing for homeless veterans, most of whom had SA problems, found that 23% of all health costs over a three-year period were from non-VA sources

(Rosenheck et al., 2003a). In contrast, two studies of the pharmacologic treatment of schizophrenia found less than 7% of annual health care costs were attributed to non-VA services (Rosenheck et al., 1997a, 2003d).

A study based on merged administrative data from VA and from virtually all public providers of public mental health services in Philadelphia county found that over a six year period from 1988-1993, 17% of VA MH/SA service users used any non-VA MH/SA services in at least 1 year, with 7% using non-VA services in the final year (Desai et al., 2001). In that study there were no differences in cross system use between mental health (MH), SA, and dually diagnosed veterans. Cost data from a related analysis of a subset of Philadelphia veterans suggest that only 4% of total costs among VA MH/SA users were attributable to non-VA service use.

A similar study of 10,950 VA MH/SA users in Colorado from 1995 to 1997 found only 7.7% used services of the state mental health agency over these three years, although annual rates increased from 2.9 to 5.9% over the years (Desai and Rosenheck, 2002). Veterans most likely to use non-VA services had made more extensive use of VA services, resided further away from the nearest VA facility, and lived closer to the nearest non-VA facility.

Finally, two studies examined whether VA inpatient bed closures during the 1990s resulted in greater use of non-VA mental health services. The first study, based on merged data from three large cities in Connecticut with both VA and state mental health agency facilities, found that closure of 80% of VA mental health beds in the state in 1996 resulted in a statistically significant but small increase in the proportion of VA patients who used state mental health services, from 2.7 to 3.6%, but that the proportion of total costs borne by the state ranged from 5.7 to 9.6% over the years studied (1993–1998) and did not increase significantly.

The second study (Rosenheck et al., 2000c) used population probability sampling to compare rates of admission to non-VA inpatient units in northern New York State in association with closure of 37% of VA mental health beds in the region. While finding no significant time trend, the study reported greater risk of admission among VA inpatients than outpatients and greater rates of admission to non-VA hospitals among dually diagnosed and SA patients than among mental health patients.

Primary Care and Specialty Medical Services

It might be expected that in an integrated system that provides both MH/SA and general medical services, access to medical services might be superior. However, two studies that used survey data to compare access to medical services among severely mentally ill patients in VA and non-VA MH systems failed to find any significant differences (Desai et al., in press-b; Rosenheck et al., 2000a). In addition, a randomized controlled trial that compared medical care quality and outcomes in a sample of severely mentally ill veterans when treated in standard VA medical clinics and in an integrated primary care clinic colocated within the mental health clinic area found that both quality and outcomes were significantly increased in the colocated clinic (Druss et al., 2001). Analysis of data on homeless veterans has also identified substantial barriers to accessing primary care services in VA (Desai et al., 2003).

On the other hand, data on quality of preventive services, diabetes care, post-MI care and health and nutrition counseling in VA show that MH/SA veterans who received at least three primary medical care visits had a quality of care that was similar to other veterans but superior to similar measures from non-VA systems (Desai et al., 2002a,b,c; Druss et al., 2002). It seems that some veterans with MH/SA problems have difficulty accessing primary care services, but those who do receive services have access to high-quality care.

Criminal Justice Involvement

There has been considerable concern, and substantial speculation, that VA bed closures have resulted in increased incarceration among former VA patients. Using the population probability matching method (Rosenheck et al., 2000d), incarceration rates among VA patients in northern New York State were not found to have increased over four years during which 37% of mental health beds were closed. Over these years, incarceration among veterans with MH problems alone ranged from 1.3 to 8.0%, as compared 12–15% among substance users, and 8–16% among dually diagnosed veterans. The overall incarceration rate among VA MH/SA patients of 11.6% was quadruple that of the general population (2.5%) but less than that found among general hospital patients (23%) or state hospital populations in northern New York (22%), in part, because veterans were older.

Some VA homeless outreach programs have undertaken active outreach to veterans with MH/SA problems in jails. A study of one such program in Los Angeles (McGuire et al., 2003), showed veterans in the L.A. jail to have substantial health problems, most prominently with drug abuse. Outreach to these veterans did not result in substantially increased service use or costs as compared to outreach to other homeless veterans, although the benefit of this type of intervention has not been evaluated.

Collaborative Relationships with Other Agencies

There has been substantial emphasis on integrating systems of care, especially for homeless people with mental illness. In 1993, VA initiated the Community Homelessness Assessment, Local Education, and Networking

Groups (CHALENG) process at each medical center. Through CHALENG, all agencies concerned with services for homeless veterans are invited to meet at the local VAMC to review the unmet needs of homeless veterans and to plan collaborative interventions to address those needs. Analysis of data gathered at these meetings has suggested that interorganizational relationships are strongest where VA has invested funds in contracts with non-VA providers (McGuire et al., 2002).

As noted previously, VA has conducted successful demonstration projects with demonstrable benefits to veterans in housing and quality of life, in collaboration with HUD (Rosenheck et al., 2003a) and the Social Security Administration (Rosenheck et al., 1999b, 2000b). These specifically targeted interventions stand in notable contrast to more global efforts at organizational integration, which have not demonstrated benefits to clients even though they brought about changes in intraorganizational interactions (Goldman et al., 2002; Rosenheck et al., 2002).

IV. DEVELOPMENT OF MH/SA QUALITY MEASUREMENT AND QUALITY MANAGEMENT IN VA

Discussions of quality and/or outcomes improvement not uncommonly focus on the problem of real-world measurement. Such discussions often seem to assume that the numbers cannot only speak for themselves, but can also change the behavior of people whose efforts they reflect. Performance data, however, have little meaning or usefulness when taken out of their organizational context (Rosenheck, 2001a,b), and any meaningful quality monitoring effort must have a manager or, more abstractly, an agent who wants to use the data to accomplish some goal or goals. In addition, the agent must (1) have adequate authority and must be able to (2) identify appropriate target audiences, (3) communicate with those audiences, (4) generate credibility and legitimacy for the enterprise, and (5) have access to adequate analytic capacity—in short, the agent needs a well-functioning organization.

It is also important to recognize that one cannot assume that the goal of performance measurement is the improvement of performance. In a famous paper, sociologists Meyer and Rowan (1977) pointed out that while the schools and school administrators they studied collected immense amounts of data from their students in the form of test scores, they rarely used those scores to change their educational methods. More generally, they concluded, organizational activities are often maintained less because of their goal-furthering functions than because they become institutionalized, self-legitimating activities in and of themselves. Organizational actors, thus, often do things merely because they are "the thing to do." In the absence of leadership committed to change and development, MH/SA performance data may serve this more limited legitimizing function.

VA is a large and complex organization, with almost 200,000 employees and at least 9 hierarchical levels separating the undersecretary for Health from the veteran. There are active agents concerned about managing quality of care at every level of every organization. Once the bridging of quality chasms is understood as an organizational process, it becomes clearer that it is impossible for any individual to comprehensively grasp the MH/SA quality improvement activities of VA in its entirety. We live in a world that is driven increasingly by networks rather than hierarchies (Castells, 2000), and this account will no doubt overemphasize initiatives in which I have been involved. The goal is thus not to present a comprehensive view of MH/SA quality management in VA, but to present one broad national perspective that will identify informative experiences and perspectives.

Evaluation and Monitoring of Specialized VA MH/SA Programs

As noted above, one of the basic approaches to improving the quality of MH care in VA, as elsewhere, has been through the establishment of specialized programs or treatment units. However, while funds for these programs have typically been distributed from VA Central Office in Washington, through the mid-1980s, there was no systematic monitoring of program performance other than mandatory workload reporting, although some specialized programs had been evaluated by VA researchers (Linn et al., 1977, 1979).

In 1985, Paul Errera, MD, professor of psychiatry at Yale and chief of psychiatry at the West Haven VAMC, was appointed chief of what was then called the Mental Health and Behavioral Sciences Service in VACO (Errera, 1988) (full disclosure: I have worked closely with Dr. Errera for the past 30 years and was involved in the evaluation of many of his initiatives). While applying for this position he read a book on program implementation by two Berkeley political scientists (Pressman and Wildavsky, 1971). Progress in government, they argued, was only possible if plausible initiatives were not assumed to be effective, but rather were taken as learning opportunities, to be evaluated with the tools of science. Errera took this exhortation to heart and in the final negotiations obtained agreement that he would use his Yale colleagues to evaluate new programs he might initiate. The VA's Northeast Program Evaluation Center (NEPEC) grew out of these evaluations.

Errera had two objectives: first, to expand the capacity of VA to deliver community-based MH/SA care, and second, to prevent what he saw as the steady erosion of MH/SA resources (Tomich, 1992). In his experience at a university-affiliated VAMC, resources targeted at MH/SA programs often were diverted to more prestigious medical specialties, and he had been frustrated at his inability to staunch the loss of resources for a highly stigmatized and politically weak group of veterans. His strategy was incremental and opportunistic—he sought any small step forward where an opportunity arose. He also realized that most medical experts thought psychiatry lacked a scientific base and that its outcomes could not be measured. Performance data, he reasoned, could increase the credibility and legitimacy of his initiatives, supporting their preservation and expansion. In part because of the new availability of desk-top computers (the West Haven VA had purchased it first Apple II-E computer the year before Errera went to Washington), it had become possible to monitor the performance and clinical outcomes of hundreds of programs relatively cheaply and flexibly.

The strategy was effective in one additional, unexpected way. Implementing new programs with built-in performance monitoring systems turned out to be a useful approach to training because it clearly communicated to staff and supervisors what the expectations were for both treatment process and outcome. It was also effective in winning legitimacy for the programs in VA and in the Congress, which began to require annual reports on newly funded initiatives. During Errera's nine years in Washington, Congress funded hundreds of new programs for Vietnam veterans with PTSD; outreach and residential treatment for homeless veterans; both inpatient and outpatient substance abuse treatment; and community-oriented work restoration programs. In partnership with one of VA's Regional Directors, he initiated a 10-site pilot program of Assertive Community Treatment, following the model developed by Stein and Test in Wisconsin (Stein and Test, 1980). Ironically, it was not Errera but the Regional Director who wanted and funded an experimental cost-effectiveness evaluation. The evaluation study showed the approach to be cost-effective in the VA setting (Rosenheck and Neale, 1998), and it was expanded during Errera's tenure to 30 sites, and currently operates at almost 80 sites (Neale et al., 2003). Performance data on all of these programs are provided to each site in quarterly installments with a comprehensive Annual Report. Front-line staff find these reports useful in communicating the nature of their activities and accomplishments (most of which take place out of institutional sight in community settings) to their local leadership.

In addition, most of the programs are initiated through training conferences that focus on both clinical concepts and evaluation procedures. These are followed by monthly telephone conference calls at which emergent issues are discussed and clinical experiences are shared. Even with 50 or more program sites on the line, conversational engagement has been achievable, especially when many of the participants have met each other face-to-face at the training conferences. Evaluation reports are reviewed on these calls providing both statistical and administrative guidance to clinicians in how to make use of the data. When a national Outlook-based VA intranet e-mail system was established, conference call communication was supplemented by continuous program-wide e-mail chatter. Through this process participants join in the formation of a nonhierarchical learning community through which local experiences and lessons learned can be widely shared. All reports identify sites by name so that those who were performing poorly could identify and learn from those who were performing well.

While Errera's initiatives were positively received, the "fencing" of funds for new MH/SA programs (i.e., diversion to other uses was prohibited) was experienced as an undue constraint by managers responsible for the full range of VA medical programs, MH/SA and otherwise (Tomich, 1992). After 7 years, fencing was eliminated, with some resultant staff losses and program closures at some sites. Although performance monitoring and management of clinical practice runs counter to norms of professional autonomy, it seems to be accepted. Constraints on the funding decisions of local managers, however, especially over extended periods of time, have been far less acceptable.

In addition, some MH/SA managers complained that the new programs sometimes distanced themselves from other local MH/SA programs because of their special national involvement and followed national practice models too rigidly, as "stovepipes," "chimneys," or "silos." The conflict between adherence to evidence-based practice standards and local flexibility seems to be an intrinsic feature of centrally guided dissemination.

Perhaps the principal lesson of these experiences is that meaningful and effective performance measurement and management are most likely to occur in a well-developed, goal-directed organizational context. The numbers do not speak for themselves.

Expansion of Quality Management in the "New VA" after 1995

When Kenneth W. Kizer, MD, MPH, took over as VA undersecretary for Health in 1995, he considered the future of the agency to be in jeopardy. In response, he initiated what he described as "the most radical redesign since the system was created in 1948." (Kizer, 1999:3), with the overall goal of increasing health care value, defined as quality of care per dollar spent—the return to the taxpayer. He laid out his values, principals and specific plans in explicit detail in a number of widely circulated reports (Kizer, 1995, 1996; Kizer and Garthwaite, 1997) and described a first phase of operational transformation and second phase of quality transformation.

In the first phase, VHA was reorganized into Veterans Integrated Service Networks "premised on funding care for populations rather than facilities, with a concomitant shift in the primary focus of care from hospitals to ambulatory and community-based settings" (Kizer, 1999:6). The restructuring of VHA was thus designed to change basic values and orientations—and it did. Between 1994 and 1998, 52% of all VHA beds were closed, the proportion of patients enrolled in primary care went from 10 to 80%, the proportion of outpatient surgeries increased from 35 to 75%; and 216 community-based outpatient clinics were established to improve access. Kizer also promoted the passage of legislation that would expand eligibility for VA services to *all* veterans, a change that, by FY 2002, would result in vast increases in enrollment, especially among older veterans seeking low-cost prescription drugs that were not available from Medicare.

In the second phase, in addition to these structural changes, an extensive program of national performance measurement was initiated, which systematically assessed patient satisfaction and which resulted in documented improvements in standard indicators reflecting, among other things, the delivery of preventive primary care (including screening for depression), care of chronic disease, and palliative care (Jha et al., 2003). VA also exceeded Medicare on most measures, but data on rates of screening for depression were not available from Medicare for comparison. Data reports were circulated widely, with detailed information on the performance of each VISN and VAMC. The goals for this effort were both internal and external: (1) to improve the quality of care and establish an overall culture of accountability and quality improvement in VHA, and (2) to demonstrate to the taxpaying public that VA health care was a good investment.

Kizer also developed an overall management strategy for fostering quality improvement that consisted of dual systems of: (1) central regulation and (2) competition and rewards. He developed a personal performance contract with each VISN director each year and encouraged them to do likewise with their subordinates. He also established systems of bonuses for high-performance leaders and awards for exceptional accomplishment.

Although MH/SA care was not one of the principal areas of Kizer's initial attention, it was profoundly affected by the emphasis on reducing inpatient care, with substantial reductions in bed capacity. While reductions in general psychiatry inpatient beds were similar to those in non-MH specialties, almost all of the SA inpatient beds were closed. To provide alternative care, residential rehabilitation and domiciliary programs were expanded, and residential treatment for homeless veterans was purchased through contracts with local providers. While Errera's initiatives had been limited, for the most part, to establishing special programs on the periphery of the VA MH/SA system, Kizer's reforms were far more extensive and affected the core.

The new emphasis on local decision making and primary care seemed, to some, to pose a threat to the centrally designed and monitored programs Errera had fostered. In response to such expressions of concern, Kizer issued a directive (VHA Directive 96-051), which established a series of monitors that addressed both the performance of these special emphasis programs as well as service delivery to the broader population they were designed to serve. He also issued a directive (VHA Directive 99-030) stating that no MH/SA program could be substantially altered without approval from VACO—a directive that was inconsistent with the emphasis on local decision making and that was variably adhered to. Similarly, Congress, out of concern that extensive changes might sweep away the special programs it had funded, passed legislation (P.L. 104-262 section 104) requiring VA to maintain its capacity to provide specialized treatment within distinct programs or facilities to disabled veterans with mental illness and several other conditions. VA constructed a definition of capacity with the limited available data that addressed both the number of patients seen and total MH dollars spent on their care. This definition has proved controversial (Mulligan, 2002).

Among his initial proposals in *Vision for Change* (Kizer, 1995), Kizer mandated the development of a National Mental Health Program Performance Monitoring System to be developed by the Northeast Program Evaluation Center, which has continued to monitor the programs begun during Errera's tenure. The "VA mental health report card" (Rosenheck and Cicchetti, 1995; Greenberg and Rosenheck, 2004a) addresses all VA inpatient and outpatient service delivery and, in concept, also includes the reports on the special programs. Many of the performance measures developed initially for these specialized programs have been incorporated into the national performance measurement system as it has evolved under the leadership of the OQP in recent years.

A third phase, characterized by a system-wide emphasis on building MH quality, is emerging in response to the recent report of the President's New Freedom Commission on Mental Health (President's New Freedom Commission on Mental Health, 2003). The deputy secretary for Health for Health Policy Coordination was actively involved in work of the Commission and a national action agenda for implementing the New Freedom commission recommendations has been developed. This document will be the foundation of a national strategic planning initiative for VA MH/SA care that has involved SMI Committee members among others.

Meyer and Rowan describe institutions, at one extreme, in which activities akin to quality management in health care become ritualized formalities with little actual impact on productive behavior. Errera and Kizer represent a quite different pole as leaders with broad-ranging agendas for change for whom quantitative quality management was one of many tools to be used to realize goals that are simultaneously professional (improving patient health) and more broadly political (changing organizational power configurations and values). We began this discussion with the observation that performance information may have little meaning when extracted from its organizational context. We conclude by pushing this thought further in suggesting that such information may play its most important role when used in service of a broad agenda for change. Health care organizations, with their extensive reliance on autonomous professional employees, have never operated as simple top-down hierarchies. Leaders who make the most effective use of performance data are able to facilitate the development of learning communities of peers who can enhance and support each other in pursuit of innovative professional and organizational objectives. Not only do the numbers not speak for themselves, they speak most forcefully when put to the most ambitious of purposes.

V. QUALITY OF VA MH/SA CARE

Even reliable and valid performance measures form an inadequate basis for action in the absence of a standard for comparison. To answer the question, "Is this care good enough?" requires either an absolute criterion of acceptability, based on expert consensus, or a salient reference condition for comparison. Even when there is expert consensus on a standard of practice, 100% compliance is usually not justified, since in clinical practice there are almost always clinical exceptions (Walter et al., 2004). Benchmarking to the actual performance of a relevant comparison program is often the most credible approach. Four types of benchmark that have commonly been used in the evaluation of VA MH/SA programs are:

- *The system average or median*, based on the premise that every program should be able to achieve the current average or some standard above or below it (such as one standard deviation).
- A *historical standard*, on the assumption that even if we don't know what the right level of performance should be, deterioration in quality is unjustifiable.
- The *performance of some other system of care*, on the premise that VA care should be equal to that of other systems.
- A *majority subgroup*, on the assumption that ethnocultural minorities should have equitable care in comparison to the majority subgroup.

A major problem with each of these comparisons is that some of the measured differences in performance may be attributable to uncontrollable differences in either the nature of the populations being compared or to other constraints that are beyond the control of caregivers or health system managers. Numerous studies of VA MH/SA care have shown that risk adjustment can substantially alter the evaluation of performance of clinical units (Busch et al., 2004; Fontana et al., 2003; Greenberg and Rosenheck, 2004a; Hoff et al., 1998; Rosenheck and Cicchetti, 1998; Rosenheck and Stolar, 1998; Rosenheck et al., 1997b; Sernyak and Rosenheck, 2003; Weissman et al., 2002). While statistical methods for evening the playing field and ensuring fair comparison will not be reviewed here, their importance cannot be overemphasized, and perfect risk adjustment is unlikely to be attainable (Walter et al., 2004). Whether "good enough" risk adjustment can be attained probably varies from case to case.

The remaining sections present examples of VA MH/SA measures that address the six aims for health system improvement identified in *Crossing the Quality Chasm* (IOM, 2001), that is, the safety, effectiveness, person-centeredness, timeliness, efficiency, and equitability of VA MH/SA care, using each of the four benchmarks. The Appendix presents a more comprehensive set of program-specific measures used at the Northeast Program Evaluation Center to monitor and evaluate VA MH/SA care.

Safety

Suicide is perhaps the most serious safety risk in MH/SA care and is the eighth leading cause of death among men aged 45-64 nationally in the United States, with 22.4 deaths per 100,000 annually (U.S. Census Bureau, 2001). Suicide is difficult to monitor because it is, fortunately, a rare event and most health care systems do not treat enough patients to make stable or accurate estimates of the suicide rate among their patients. As an integrated national system, VA is among the few large systems of care in the United States in which suicide rates can be meaningfully measured and compared across facilities (Desai et al., 2005). Using mortality records from the National Death Index, all suicides that occurred within 12 month of discharge among 121,000 veterans discharged from VA MH inpatient units between 1994 and 1998 were identified. The suicide rate in this severely ill sample was 445/100,000, (increasing over the years but not significantly), and 13.5% of VAMCs had rates significantly higher than the average across all facilities, after risk adjustment. Time trends were also examined to see if postdischarge suicide rates had increased in association with bed closures or shortened lengths of stay. While there was a trend toward increased suicide in recent years, it was not statistically significant. Although it was impossible to externally benchmark the VA inpatient suicide rate because no comparable data are available from other institutions, it is notable that African Americans had significantly lower rates of suicide than whites. An effort was made to examine the relationship of quality indicators, especially continuity of care, and suicide. While individual patients with poor continuity of care were at greater risk for subsequent suicide, lower continuity of care measured at the facility level was not. Risk adjustment is especially important in comparisons of suicide rates across facilities because risk varies substantially across both sociodemographic and diagnostic characteristics and even with indicators of community social capital (i.e., civic participation, trust, and cooperation) measured at the county level.

Further analyses focusing on gun suicide, an especially important issue among veterans, found that veterans living in states with lower rates of gun ownership, more restrictive gun laws, and higher social capital were less likely to commit suicide with a firearm (Desai et al., in press). Inter-facility comparisons would clearly need to adjust risk for these environmental factors since they are far beyond managerial control.

In a major study of mortality rates among VA patients during the later 1990s, Ashton et al. (2003) found no increase in mortality for several chronic conditions in VA including schizophrenia and major depressive disorder in spite of dramatically reduced inpatient utilization. However, all-cause mortality is an imprecise measure of the quality of MH care.

Another safety issue that has been systematically monitored in VA is the use of excessive doses of antipsychotic medication and antipsychotic polypharmacy, both of which pose increased risk of side effects. An annual report on antipsychotic pharmacotherapy in VA presents risk-adjusted comparison data on each VA facility (Leslie and Rosenheck, 2003a), and comparisons with data from the MarketScan® data base (a compilation of claims from private insurance plans) have shown prescription quality in VA to be similar to that among privately insured patients treated for schizophrenia (Leslie and Rosenheck, 2003b).

Because of the VA's large data bases, its administrators have an unusual capacity to rapidly evaluate safety risks associated with newer medications. VA studies were among the first to demonstrate an increased risk of diabetes with atypical antipsychotics (Sernyak et al., 2002, 2003) and have also been the first to quantify the attributable risk of incident diabetes due to atypicals (about 0.54%) and the additional cost (about $11 per treated patient per year) (Leslie and Rosenheck, 2005).

Effectiveness

Effective care is care that improves health status and health-related quality of life. The effectiveness of treatments is most rigorously determined through formal research, especially randomized clinical trials, but also through clinical experience in the case of treatments that have yet to be studied and direct measurement of outcomes. Since randomized clinical trials and even observational outcome studies cannot be used to evaluate real-world practice in an ongoing way (because of both prohibitive cost and unavailability of control groups), the effectiveness of routine care is typically assessed either by determining whether evidence-based practices are in use and/or by directly measuring outcomes (see, for example, the definition of effectiveness in IOM, 2001). Pharmacologic evidence-based practices that have been monitored across the VA system include use of atypical antipsychotics (Rosenheck et al., 2001a) (see Appendix: section VI, p. 482); antidepressants in both depression (Busch et al., 2004) and alcoholism (Petrakis et al., 2003a); naltrexone in alcoholism (Petrakis et al., 2003b) and methadone in heroin addiction (Rosenheck et al., 2003c). Use of atypicals in schizophrenia and antidepressants in alcoholism is quite extensive, but only 1% of veterans with alcoholism receive naltrexone (in spite of several positive clinical trials, although a large VA trial found no benefit [Krystal et al., 2001]).

Two further studies examined whether more expensive medications (atypical antipsychotics and methadone) were less accessible at fiscally strained facilities and found that they were not (Leslie and Rosenheck, 2001; Rosenheck et al., 2003c). However, in the case of atypical antipsychotics, patients at more fiscally strained facilities were more likely to be prescribed less expensive atypicals. Psychosocial interventions that are used in VA and whose fidelity to evidence based-practices is carefully monitored include Assertive Community Treatment (ACT) (called Mental Health Intensive Case Management in VA) (Neale et al., 2003); Supported Housing (Kasprow et al., 2004); Transitional Employment (Seibyl et al., 2003), and Supported Employment (Rosenheck et al., 2003b). Adherence is somewhat variable but performance is poorest on resource- sensitive measures such as staff:patient ratios.

Many MH/SA interventions and programs have not been subject to rigorous evaluation, and operational criteria for implementing effective practices have yet to be developed. For example, while clinical practice guidelines have been developed within VA for treatment of PTSD, they are broadly worded and not subject to empirical fidelity assessment. Further, while there is broad agreement on the need for case management and residential treatment for homeless people with mental illness (especially if direct placement in permanent housing is not available), operational guidelines for the duration and intensity of such services have not been developed. In addition, in managing costly programs like ACT, administrators may not be satisfied with information showing high levels of fidelity to evidence-based models. In these cases, direct outcome assessments may be needed that demonstrate clinical improvement using psychometrically sound instruments.

There are three substantial challenges to implementing real-world outcomes monitoring. First of all, it is costly, especially if data are to be collected by independent evaluators. Second, since appropriate comparison groups are hard to identify, it is difficult to differentiate improvement that is attributable to effective intervention from improvement that reflects the natural waxing and waning of chronic illness. Third, assessment biases may be introduced if clinicians make ratings on their own patients or programs, and even when patients complete self-report questionnaires, since they may know that the data will be used to evaluate programs that they have come to depend on. As a result of the high cost of high quality data, to paraphrase Abraham Lincoln, "You can get some of the data on all of the people, and all of the data on some of the people, but you can't get all of the data on all of the people."

In VA, outcome assessment of mental health programs is selectively directed at programs that treat high-cost, high-risk patients, for example, those that receive ACT services or intensive PTSD services. Symptom and functional improvements among the more than 3,000 veterans participating in ACT in VA each year have generally improved over the years, and annual reports detail a broad array of outcome measures for each program for each year (Neale et al., 2003) (see Appendix to this paper, section III, p. 479). Measures address symptoms, quality of life, capability for self-care, employment, housing, substance use, inpatient utilization, and satisfaction with services. A system-wide outcomes monitoring evaluation of VA SA treatment similarly showed that veterans who received specialized treatment and more intensive treatment had better outcomes than those who received treatment in general medical or MH clinics (Moos et al., 2000).

PTSD outcome data have proved especially useful in addressing controversies about changes in the intensity of VA care. A study completed in the mid-1990s showed that long-term, intensive inpatient PTSD treatment was no more effective than short-term treatment but cost $18,000 more per patient/year (Fontana and Rosenheck, 1997a). In part, as a result of this study, but also because of wider changes in VA, many long-term inpatient programs were transformed into less costly short-term inpatient or halfway house programs. Stakeholders expressed concern about deterioration in the quality of VA PTSD treatment. To address these concerns, outcome monitoring data from over 6,000 episodes of care between 1993 and 2000 were reanalyzed and showed that outcomes had not changed significantly for PTSD symptoms, SA, violent behavior, and employment (Rosenheck and Fontana, 2001) and that the maintenance of effectiveness applied specifically to blacks and Hispanics as well as to whites (Rosenheck and Fontana, 2002).

The monitoring of outcomes of residential treatment for homeless veterans poses a bigger challenge, since over 10,000 episodes of residential treatment are provided each year, through several different programs, at over 100 VA medical centers. Because of the magnitude and complexity of these services, a simpler system is used to document outcomes—a standardized discharge summary records objective outcomes such as housing (40% are independently housed) and employment status (about 35% in competitive employment) at the time of discharge, as well as linkage with aftercare services, and more subjective (and thus less reliably measured) outcomes such as clinical improvement. These data are risk-adjusted using baseline information obtained at intake, and site-specific reports are circulated quarterly and summarized in an annual report to Congress.

On the largest scale, VA instituted systematic documentation of GAF ratings for all MH/SA patients in 1999. While the reliability and validity of these ratings is uncertain, annual analyses of outcome data for over 250,000 veterans have shown plausible discriminant validity and highly consistent results across medical centers over a 3-year period. The largest improvement over the six month evaluation period is observed for discharged inpatients (6.5 GAF points, s.d. = 14.4) followed by newly admitted outpatients (1.4 GAF points, s.d. = 8.7). Long-term outpatients show little improvement (0.4 GAF points, s.d. = 8.6) (Greenberg and Rosenheck, 2004a).

Three studies have collected virtually the same outcome data from patients treated in VA and in non-VA systems, allowing benchmarking of VA effectiveness against that of other systems. Because the Center for Mental Health Services' ACCESS demonstration, which served homeless people with severe mental illness, was conducted by VA's Northeast Program Evaluation Center, measures were similar to those used in studies of VA homeless programs, thus facilitating comparison of 8–12 month outcomes. These outcomes (addressing psychiatric symptoms, SA, housing, employment, and receipt of benefits, among others) were similar in most domains (Kasprow et al., 2002). Two other studies, the Schizophrenia Care and Outcomes Program and the Connecticut Outcome Study, traced outcomes in symptoms, community adjustment, and medication side effects among severely mentally ill patients treated at the VA Connecticut Healthcare system, and in local community mental health centers. VA and non-VA outcomes and were not substantially different.

Patient-Centered Care

The dimensions of patient-centered care described in *Crossing the Quality Chasm* (IOM, 2001) are well-represented on the inpatient satisfaction measure developed by the Picker Institute, which has been used in VHA since 1995. Subscales address coordination, information, timeliness, courtesy, emotional support, responsiveness to preferences, family contact, physical comfort, and transition to home and are highly intercorrelated, with bivariate coefficients ranging from 0.49 to 0.77 (Greenberg and Rosenheck, 2004a). Absolute satisfaction levels on 0–1 subscales scales, where 0 indicates no satisfaction and 1 indicates complete satisfaction, range from 0.56 for family involvement to 0.75 for respect for personal preferences, with few significant differences across VISNs or VAMCs (Greenberg and Rosenheck, 2004a). Subjective satisfaction and the responsiveness of VA MH/SA care has been the subject of intensive scrutiny since Dr. Kizer initiated systematic satisfaction screening in the VA (Druss and Rosenheck, 1999; Hoff et al., 1998; Kasprow et al., 1999; Rosenheck et al., 1997b). A number of studies have demonstrated that levels of satisfaction bear little relationship to outcomes and seem to be more strongly influenced by the process and intensity of care than by its effectiveness (Fontana and Rosenheck, 2001; Fontana et al., 2003). Risk adjustment is especially important and virtually reversed the results of one study of six-year time trends in satisfaction with VA inpatient MH care (Greenberg and Rosenheck, 2004b).

Recovery orientation has received increasing emphasis in MH care in recent years and can be characterized by general satisfaction with life, hopefulness, knowledge about MH care, and empowerment. A comparison of VA and non-VA patients using PORT data found no differences on these measures except that VA patients felt they knew less about MH care (Resnick et al., 2004a). Peer education groups for mental illness, another emphasis of the recovery movement in MH, have also begun to take hold in the VA setting (Resnick et al., 2004b). Alcoholics Anonymous meetings have been held on VA campuses for many decades.

Timeliness

Although detailed data on waiting times for VA MH/SA care are not available, extensive information is available on contact with outpatient MH/SA services within 30 days of discharge from an inpatient stay. This measure, originally developed for Health Employer Data Information Set (HEDIS) (HEDIS, 1999) was implemented as a national performance measure by the OQP in 1998. Between 1998 and 2003, the percentage of veterans meeting this standard increased from 72 to 77%, well above 61% among Medicare patients and even exceeding the HEDIS performance of 74% from managed care companies. A specific comparison of VA and private sector MarketScan® data showed that VA patients were 10% less likely to receive care within 30 days of discharge but only 2% less likely to have received care by 180 days. A measure of overall continuity of care favored VA, and readmission rates were similar (Leslie and Rosenheck, 2000).

The Mental Health Report Card (Greenberg and Rosenheck, 2004a) presents risk-adjusted data on these measures for each VAMC and VISN each year and also addresses access to general medical care in the 30 days following discharge among those with medical comorbidities (median VISN = 85 % range = 80–90%). While the HEDIS measure has been widely used in VA, and has substantial face-value, efforts to demonstrate its relationship to improved outcomes on clinical measures have shown weak and mixed results (Greenberg et al., 2002, 2003; Rosenheck et al., 1999a).

Efficiency

Dramatic reductions in reliance on inpatient care have yielded substantial efficiencies in VA MH/SA care. Even without adjustment for inflation, per capita costs for all inpatient and outpatient mental health care declined by 28%, from $3,560 in FY 1995 to $2,562 eight years later, in FY 2003. With inflation adjustment, the reduction in per capita cost would approach 70%. A study of the cost of treating dually diagnosed patients from 1993 to 1997 showed VA costs to be about 10% greater than those of a private sector MarketScan® sample, while costs for patients not dually diagnosed were about 35% greater, although diagnostic severity was far greater in the VA sample (Leslie and Rosenheck, 1999).

Efficiency can be a double-edged sword, whose darker side is represented by reduced treatment resources. While 16% of VA medical center dollars were expended on mental health care in FY 1995, only 11.2% of dollars went to mental health care in FY 2003. Although, in the abstract, increased efficiency cannot be distinguished from reduced service delivery, evidence presented above is generally reassuring since outcomes, where measured, have not deteriorated; there has been no increase in suicide or in VA patients seeking services in other health care systems or becoming incarcerated, and some evidence-based services like the use of atypical antipsychotics and ACT have been expanded in VA. A detailed review of how data were used to guide the transformation of PTSD treatment in VA demonstrates a reasoned approach to system change (Rosenheck and Fontana, 1999). However, the steady decline in the number of veterans who receive specialized SA services from VA, accompanied as it has been by reduced expenditures on SA treatment (Chen et al., 2001), in the presence of epidemiologic data showing no reduction in need (Tessler et al., 2005), has generated expressions of concern among stakeholders (Mulligan, 2003).

Equity Minorities

While there has been widespread documentation of inequities in access and quality of health care to minorities in the US, an extensive series of studies has found little evidence of such inequities in VA, perhaps because, by statute, VA provides cost-free care to all veterans who enroll for services (Greenberg and Rosenheck, 2003; Leda and Rosenheck, 1995; Rosenheck and Fontana, 1994, 1996a; Rosenheck and Seibyl, 1988; Rosenheck et al., 1997c). However, a 1995 study of over 5,000 veterans treated for PTSD found that on some measures, when African American patients were treated by African American clinicians, they were less likely to drop out of treatment prematurely than when treated by white clinicians (Rosenheck et al., 1995).

Female Veterans

While there has been growing concern that the increasing number of female veterans are reluctant to use VA services, there is evidence that they use VA service at rates equal to or greater than males (Hoff and Rosenheck, 1997, 1998a,b) (in part because of the generally greater inclination of women to use health services). Female veterans express greater or equal levels of satisfaction with VA services (Hoff et al., 1998).

In recognition of the problems of military sexual trauma (and the possible discomfort of women in the virtually all-male VA setting), VA established four Womens Stress Disorder Treatment Teams, which have documented high levels of trauma among women served by these teams (Fontana and Rosenheck, 1997b, 1998). Outcome evaluation found relatively high levels of comfort with the VA setting among traumatized women and no relationship between levels of comfort in VA and outcomes (Fontana and Rosenheck, 2002). Screening for military sexual trauma has recently been introduced as a system-wide performance indicator by OQP.

VI. FRONT-LINE EXPERIENCE

Although there has been no systematic survey of the experiences of front line VA managers and clinicians with the implementation of performance management for MH/SA programs, this account would be incomplete if it did not include at least a few examples of their sometimes ambivalent reactions.

On the one hand, clinicians and their supervisors often report feeling empowered by access to information on both their clinical interventions and on client outcomes. In the past only top medical center management had access to performance data—and the available data were limited in both detail and in quality. In the absence of good data, as Errera observed (Tomich, 1992), decisions tended to reflect the structure of traditional power hierarchies—hierarchies in which MH/SA programs fall toward the bottom. With the increased availability of higher quality information, MH/SA supervisors and clinicians have direct access to information themselves and can more effectively shape and advocate for their programs on the basis of available factual information.

On the other hand, clinicians sometimes complain that gathering data takes time away from patient care and that many measures: (1) are too crude to reflect the complexity of their work, (2) are applied indiscriminantly to highly variable populations (i.e., without risk adjustment for differences in patient characteristics or differences in service environments); and (3) address outcomes over which clinicians feel they have little control, such as treatment dropouts, housing people who are homeless, or even reducing symptoms. Satisfaction surveys, some have complained, in VA as elsewhere, often have quite low response rates and are typically presented without risk adjustment. A recent study of VA performance measurement in *JAMA* (Walter et al., 2004) presents a set of very sophisticated examples of such problems, elegantly documented by the staff at one VA hospital. While appreciative of the value of performance monitoring, in principle, these investigators identify a number of problems with current practice, largely reflecting application of standards to patients for whom they are clinically inappropriate, (e.g., cancer screening among those who already have terminal illnesses), and it is not hard to imagine that this sophisticated scientific paper had its birth in the discontent of professionals who feel their work has been unfairly judged.

Managers and clinical staff also have observed that many performance measures can be manipulated, and some complain that sites that produce better performance scores have merely been more energetic or inventive in changing various program codes so that patients who do worst are not included in the measure. It is difficult to evaluate these complaints.

Paradoxically, but not surprisingly, it also appears that: (1) the more performance data are used to evaluate high-level managers (and to determine their annual bonuses), (2) the more aggressively middle managers are pressured to get their staffs to improve the scores (often regardless of the availability of new treatments or resources to accomplish these goals), (3) the more likely staff are to feel exploited by their superiors' quest for bonuses and to look for ways to "game" the system, that is, to improve their numbers without actually changing the care that is given. In many situations, it appears, the limitations of the data are appreciated, and clinicians and managers use them, as intended, to identify ways of improving the care they provide, as best they can. In others, however, it seems there may be more browbeating than joint problem solving.

Reports of falsified or fabricated research data are not unheard of, even in well-funded studies conducted by experienced researchers who have a sophisticated understanding of the importance of adhering to established data collection protocols. It would be naïve to imagine that such activities do not occur among clinical staff who are under pressure to produce the desired results by supervisors who are in a position to influence their future careers. Use of objective measures, not subject to manipulation, is the best response to this problem.

It must also be noted that even where data or evidence-based practices are well-measured and credible, they do not necessarily determine which way decisions will go. As Paul Errera observed, resource decisions tend to trump performance data. The intensive PTSD program with the best outcomes in the nation was among the first to be closed because it was judged to be inefficient; and monitoring of intensive case management programs like ACT or supported housing shows that the staff/patient ratio (the most resource sensitive measure) is typically the evidence-based performance criterion with the lowest rate of adherence.

There is no way of knowing how widespread these problems are, or to what extent they affect the integrity of performance management in VA MH/SA programs or elsewhere. It seems important to remind ourselves, however, that performance management is ultimately a human process, and that it is affected by the skills, incentives, and integrity of the those whose behavior it seeks to shape.

CONCLUSION

Health care even for a single family or a small clinic can be characterized by both daunting complexity and uncertainty. In a health care system as large as VA, complexity and uncertainty are increased by many orders of magnitude. Every American deserves the best health care possible each time he or she seeks help, and high-quality health care can only be achieved by creative management of the inherent complexity and uncertainty of both illness and health service delivery. Such management demands comprehensive quality monitoring, used by creative and committed leaders, in competent organizations. It is intrinsic to the challenge posed that this work will never be finished, and we probably cannot even know how far along the way we are toward the ideal of improving health outcomes with data. What can be said is that we have made a beginning and we must continue moving forward.

REFERENCES

Ashton CM, Souchek J, Petersen NJ, Menke TJ, Collins TC, Kizer KW, Wright SM, Wray NP. 2003. Hospital use and survival among Veterans Affairs beneficiaries. *New England Journal of Medicine* 349(17):1637–1646.

Busch S, Leslie D, Rosenheck R. 2004. Measuring quality of pharmacotherapy for depression in a national health care system. *Medical Care* 42(6):532–542.

Castells M. 2000. *The Rise of the Network Society*. 2nd ed. Malden, MA: Blackwell.

Chen S, Wagner TH, Barnett PG. 2001. The effect of reforms on spending for veterans' substance abuse treatment, 1993–1999. *Health Affairs* 20(4):169–175.

Desai MM, Rosenheck RA, Druss BG, Perlin JB. 2002a. Mental disorders and quality of diabetes care. *American Journal of Psychiatry* 159(9):1584–1590.

Desai MM, Rosenheck RA, Druss BG, Perlin JB. 2002b. Mental disorders and quality of care among post-acute myocardial infarction outpatients. *Journal of Nervous and Mental Disease* 190(1):51–53.

Desai MM, Rosenheck RA, Druss BG, Perlin JB. 2002c. Receipt of nutrition and exercise counseling among medical outpatients with psychiatric and substance abuse disorders. *Journal of General Internal Medicine* 17(7):556–560.

Desai MM, Rosenheck RA, Kasprow W. 2003. Determinants of receipt of medical care in a national sample of homeless veterans. *Medical Care* 41(2):275–287.

Desai RA, Rosenheck RA. 2000. The interdependence of mental health service systems: The effects of VA mental health funding on veterans' use of state mental health inpatient facilities. *Journal of Mental Health Policy and Economics* 3(2):61–68.

Desai R, Rosenheck RA. 2002. Service use among VA mental health patients in Colorado: The impact of managed care on cross-system service use. *Psychiatric Services* 53(12): 1599–1605.

Desai RA, Rosenheck RA, Rothbard A. 2001. Cross system service use among VA mental health patients in Philadelphia. *Administration and Policy in Mental Health* 28(4): 299–309.

Desai RA, Dausey D, Rosenheck RA. 2005. Mental health service delivery and suicide risk: The role of individual patient and facility factors. *American Journal of Psychiatry* 162(2):311–318.

Desai RA, Rosenheck RA, Sernyak MJ, Dausey D. (In press-a). A comparison of service delivery by the Department of Veterans Affairs and State providers: The Role of Academic Affiliation. *Administration and Policy in Mental Health*.

Desai RA, Dausey D, Rosenheck RA. (In press-b). Suicide in a national sample of psychiatric patients: The role of gun ownership, legislation, and social capital.

Druss BG, Rosenheck RA. 1999. Patient satisfaction and administrative measures as indicators of the quality of mental health care. *Psychiatric Services* 50(8):1053–1058.

Druss BG, Rohrbaugh RM, Levinson CM, Rosenheck RA. 2001. Integrated medical care for patients with serious psychiatric illness: A randomized trial. *Archives of General Psychiatry* 58(9):861–868.

Druss BG, Rosenheck RA, Desai MM, Perlin JB. 2002. Quality of preventive medical care for patients with mental disorders. *Medical Care* 40(2):129–136.

Errera P. 1988. From Yale professor to Washington bureaucrat: Policy and medicine. *VA Practitioner* 81–93.

Fontana AF, Rosenheck RA. 1997a. Effectiveness and cost of inpatient treatment of posttraumatic stress disorder. *American Journal of Psychiatry* 154(6):758–765.

Fontana AF, Rosenheck RA. 1997b. *Women under Stress: Evaluation of the Women's Stress Disorder Treatment Teams*. West Haven, CT: Northeast Program Evaluation Center.

Fontana AF, Rosenheck RA. 1998. Focus on women: Duty-related and sexual stress in the etiology of PTSD among women veterans who seek treatment. *Psychiatric Services* 49(5):658–662.

Fontana AF, Rosenheck RA. 2001. A model of patient's satisfaction with treatment for posttraumatic stress disorder. *Administration and Policy in Mental Health* 28(6):475–489.

Fontana A, Rosenheck RA. 2002. *Women under Stress II: Evaluation of the Clinical Performance of the Department of Veterans Affairs Women's Stress Disorder Treatment Teams*. West Haven, CT: Northeast Program Evaluation Center.

Fontana AF, Ford JD, Rosenheck RA. 2003. A multivariate model of patients' satisfaction with treatment for posttraumatic stress disorder. *Journal of Traumatic Stress Studies* 16(1):93–106.

Gamache G, Rosenheck RA, Tessler R. 2000. Choice of provider among homeless people with mental illness: Veterans and the VA. *Psychiatric Services* 51(8):1024–1017.

Gamache G, Rosenheck RA, Tessler R. 2001. The proportion of veterans among homeless men: A decade later. *Social Psychiatry and Psychiatric Epidemiology* 36(10):481–485.

Gamache G, Rosenheck RA, Tessler R. 2003. Overrepresentation of women veterans among homeless women. *American Journal of Public Health* 93(7):1132–1136.

GAO (General Accounting Office). 2001. *VA Health Care: Community-Based Clinics Improve Primary Care Access*. GAO-01-678T. Washington, DC.

Goldman HH, Morrissey J, Rosenheck RA, Cocozza J, Randolph F, Blasinsky M, ACCESS National Evaluation Team. 2002. Lessons from the evaluation of the ACCESS program. *Psychiatric Services* 53(8):967–970.

Greenberg GA, Rosenheck R. 2003. Change in mental health service delivery among blacks, whites and Hispanics in the Department of Veterans Affairs. *Administration and Policy in Mental Health* 31(1):31–45.

Greenberg GA, Rosenheck RA. 2004a. *National Mental Health Program Performance Monitoring System: Fiscal Year 2003 Report*, West Haven, CT: Northeast Program Evaluation Center.

Greenberg GA, Rosenheck RA. 2004b. Changes in satisfaction with mental health services among blacks, whites and Hispanics in the Department of Veterans Affairs. *Psychiatric Quarterly* 75(4):375–389.

Greenberg GA, Rosenheck RA, Seibyl CL. 2002. Continuity of care and clinical effectiveness: Outcomes following residential treatment for severe substance abuse. *Medical Care* 40(3):246–259.

Greenberg GA, Rosenheck RA, Fontana A. 2003. Continuity of care and clinical effectiveness: Treatment of posttraumatic stress disorder in the Department of Veterans Affairs. *Journal of Behavioral Health Services and Research* 30(2):202–214.

HEDIS (Health Employer Data and Information Set). 1999. *2000: Health Employer Data and Information Set*. Washington, DC: National Committee on Quality Improvement.

Hoff RA, Rosenheck RA. 1997. Utilization of mental health services by women in a male-dominated environment: The VA experience. *Psychiatric Services* 48(11):1408–1414.

Hoff RA, Rosenheck RA. 1998a. Female veterans use of VA health care services. *Medical Care* 36(7):1114–1119.

Hoff RA, Rosenheck RA. 1998b. The use of VA and non-VA mental health services by female veterans. *Medical Care* 36(11):1524–1533.

Hoff RA, Rosenheck RA, Wilson N, Meterko M. 1998. Quality of VA mental health service delivery. *Administration and Policy in Mental Health* 26(1):214–218.

IOM (Institute of Medicine). 2001. *Crossing the Quality Chasm*. Washington, DC: National Academy Press.

Jha AK, Perlin JB, Kizer KW, Dudly RA. 2003. Effect of the transformation of Veterans Affairs health care system on the quality of care. *New England Journal of Medicine* 348(22):2218–2227.

Kasprow WJ, Rosenheck RA, Frisman LK. 1999. Homeless veterans' satisfaction with residential treatment. *Psychiatric Services* 50(4):540–546.

Kasprow WJ, Rosenheck RA, Dilella D, and Cavallaro L. 2002. *Health Care for Homeless Veterans programs: Fifteenth Progress Report*. West Haven, CT: Northeast Program Evaluation Center.

Kasprow WJ, Rosenheck RA, Dilella D, Cavallaro L, Harelik N. 2004. *Health Care for Homeless Veterans Programs: Seventeenth Progress Report*. West Haven, CT: Northeast Program Evaluation Center [Report to Congress].

Kizer KW. 1995. *Vision for Change: A Plan to Restructure the Veterans Health Administration*. Washington, DC: Department of Veterans Affairs.

Kizer KW. 1996. *Prescription for Change: The Guiding Principals and Strategic Objectives Underlying the Transformation of the Veterans Health Administration.* Washington, DC: Department of Veterans Affairs.

Kizer KW. 1999. The "New VA": A national laboratory for health care quality management. *American Journal of Medical Quality* 14(1):3–20.

Kizer KW, Garthwaite TG. 1997. Vision for change: An integrated service network. In: Kolodner RM, ed. *Computerizing Large Integrated Health Networks: The VA Success.* New York, NY: Springer-Verlag. Pp. 3–13.

Krystal JH, Cramer JA, Krol WF, Kirk GF, Rosenheck RA, and the Veterans Affairs Naltrexone Cooperative Study 425 Group. 2001. Naltrexone in the treatment of alcohol dependence. *New England Journal of Medicine* 345(24):1734–1739.

Kulka R, Schlenger W, Fairbanks J, Hough R, Jordan B, Marmar C, Weiss D. 1990. *Trauma and the Vietnam War Generation: Report of Findings from the National Vietnam Veterans Readjustment Study.* New York: Brunner/Mazel.

Leda C, Rosenheck RA. 1995. Race in the treatment of homeless mentally ill veterans. *Journal of Nervous and Mental Disease* 183(8):529–537.

Leslie DL, Rosenheck RA. 1999. Inpatient treatment of comorbid psychiatric and substance abuse disorders: A comparison of public sector and privately insured populations. *Administration and Policy in Mental Health* 26(4):253–268.

Leslie DL, Rosenheck R. 2000. Comparing quality of mental health care in public sector and privately insured populations: First efforts and methodological challenges. *Psychiatric Services* 51(5):650–655.

Leslie DL, Rosenheck RA. 2001. The effect of institutional fiscal stress on the use of atypical antipsychotic medications in the treatment of schizophrenia. *Journal of Nervous and Mental Disease* 189(6):377–383.

Leslie DL, Rosenheck RA. 2003a. Benchmarking the quality of schizophrenia pharmacotherapy: A comparison of the Department of Veterans Affairs and the private sector. *Journal of Mental Health Policy and Economics* 6(3):113–121.

Leslie DL, Rosenheck RA. 2003b. *Fourth Annual Report on Pharmacotherapy of Schizophrenia in the Department of Veterans Affairs.* West Haven, CT: Northeast Program Evaluation Center.

Leslie DL, Rosenheck RA. 2005. Pharmacotherapy and healthcare costs among patients with schizophrenia and newly diagnosed diabetes. *Psychiatric Services* 56(7):803–810.

Linn MW, Caffey EM, Klett CJ, Hogarty G. 1977. Hospital vs. community (foster) care for psychiatric patients. *Archives of General Psychiatry* 34(1):78–83.

Linn MW, Caffey EM, Klett CJ, Hogarty G, Lamb HR. 1979. Day treatment and psychotropic drugs in the aftercare of schizophrenic patients. *Archives of General Psychiatry* 36(10):1055–1066.

McGuire J, Rosenheck R, Burnette C. 2002. Expanding service delivery: Does it improve relationships among agencies serving homeless people with mental illness? *Administration and Policy in Mental Health* 29(3):243–256.

McGuire J, Rosenheck RA, Kasprow W. 2003. Health status, service use, and costs among veterans receiving outreach services in jails or community settings. *Psychiatric Services* 54(2):201–207.

Meyer J, Rowan B. 1977. Institutionalized organizations: Formal structure as myth and ceremony. *American Journal of Sociology* 83:440–463.

Mojtabi R, Rosenheck R, Wyatt RJ, Susser E. 2003. Transition to VA outpatient mental health services among severely mentally ill patients discharged from the armed services. *Psychiatric Services* 54(3):383–388.

Moos RH, Finney JW, Federman EB, Suchinsky R. 2000. Specialty mental health care improves patients' outcomes: Findings from a nationwide program to monitor the quality of care for patients with substance abuse disorders. *Journal of Studies on Alcohol* 61:704–713.

Mulligan K. 2002. VA allowing mental health care to erode APA charges. *Psychiatric News* 37(7):2.

Mulligan K. 2003. VA Accused of shortchanging substance abuse treatment. *Psychiatric News* 38(9):4.

Neale M, Rosenheck R, Martin A, Morrissey J, Castrodonatti J. 2003. *Mental Health Intensive Case Management (MHICM): The Sixth National Performance Monitoring Report: FY 2002*. West Haven, CT: Northeast Program Evaluation Center.

Norquist GS, Hough RL, Golding JM, Escobar JI. 1990. Psychiatric disorder in male veterans and nonveterans. *Journal of Nervous and Mental Disease* 178(5):328–335.

Pandiani JA, Banks SM, Schacht LM. 1998. Personal privacy versus public accountability: A technological solution to an ethical dilemma. *Journal of Behavioral Health Services and Research* 25(4):456–463.

Peterson PE. 1995. *The Price of Federalism*. Washington, DC: Brookings Institution.

Petrakis I, Leslie D, Rosenheck RA. 2003a. The use of antidepressants in alcohol dependent veterans. *Journal of Clinical Psychiatry* 64(8):865–870.

Petrakis I, Leslie D, Rosenheck RA. 2003b. Use of Naltrexone in the Treatment of Alcoholism Nationally in the Department of Veterans Affairs. *Alcoholism: Clinical and Experimental Research* 27(11):1780–1784.

President's New Freedom Commission on Mental Health. 2003. *Achieving the Promise: Transforming Mental Health Care in America. Subcommittee on Acute Care Report*. DHHS Pub. No. SAM-03-3832. Rockville, MD: U.S. Department of Health and Human Services.

Pressman J, Wildavsky A. 1971. *Implementation: How Great Expectations in Washington are Dashed in Oakland*. Berkeley, CA: University of California Press.

Resnick S, Rosenheck RA, Lehman A. 2004a. An exploratory analysis of correlates of recovery. *Psychiatric Services* 55(5):540–547.

Resnick S, Armstrong M, Sperazza M, Harkness L, Rosenheck RA. 2004b. A model of consumer provider partnership: Vet-to-vet. *Psychiatric Rehabilitation Journal* 28(2):185–187.

Rosenheck RA. 2001a. Organizational process: A missing link between research and practice. *Psychiatric Services* 52(12):1607–1612.

Rosenheck RA. 2001b. Stages in the implementation of innovative clinical programs in complex organizations. *Journal of Nervous and Mental Disease* 189(12):812–821.

Rosenheck RA, Cicchetti D. 1995. *A Mental Health Program Performance Monitoring System for the Department of Veterans Affairs*. West Haven, CT: Northeast Program Evaluation Center.

Rosenheck RA, Cicchetti D. 1998. A mental health program report card: A multidimensional approach to performance monitoring in public sector programs. *Community Mental Health Journal* 34(1):85–106.

Rosenheck RA, Fontana AF. 1994. Utilization of mental health services by minority veterans of the Vietnam era. *Journal of Nervous and Mental Disease* 182:685–691.

Rosenheck RA, Fontana AF. 1995. Do Vietnam era veterans who suffer from posttraumatic stress disorder avoid VA mental health services? *Military Medicine* 160:136–142.

Rosenheck RA, Fontana AF. 1996a. Race and outcome of treatment for veterans suffering from PTSD. *Journal of Traumatic Stress Studies* 9(2):343–351.

Rosenheck RA, Fontana AF. 1996b. Treatment of veterans severely impaired by PTSD. In Ursano RJ, Norwood AE, eds. *Emotional Aftermath of the Persian Gulf War.* Washington, DC: American Psychiatric Press.

Rosenheck RA, Fontana A. 1999. Changing patterns of care for war-related post-traumatic stress disorder at Department of Veterans Affairs medical centers: The use of performance data to guide program development. *Military Medicine* 164(11):795–802.

Rosenheck RA, Fontana A. 2001. Impact of efforts to reduce inpatient costs on clinical effectiveness: Treatment of post traumatic stress disorder in the Department of Veterans Affairs. *Medical Care* 39(2):168–180.

Rosenheck RA, Fontana AF. 2002. African-American and Latino veterans in intensive VA treatment programs for posttraumatic stress disorder. *Medical Care* 40(Supplement 1): I52–I61.

Rosenheck RA, Koegel P. 1993. Characteristics of veterans and nonveterans in three samples of homeless men. *Hospital and Community Psychiatry* 44:858–863.

Rosenheck RA, Massari LA. 1993. Wartime military service and utilization of VA health care services. *Military Medicine* 158:223–228.

Rosenheck RA, Neale MS. 1998. Cost-effectiveness of intensive psychiatric community care for high users of inpatient services. *Archives of General Psychiatry* 55(5):459–466.

Rosenheck RA, Seibyl CL. 1998. The experience of black and white veterans in a residential treatment and work therapy program for substance abuse. *American Journal of Psychiatry* 155(8):1029–1034.

Rosenheck RA, Stolar M. 1998. Access to public mental health services: Determinants of population coverage. *Medical Care* 36(4):503–512.

Rosenheck RA, Fontana AF, Cottrel C. 1995. Effect of clinician-veteran racial pairing in the treatment of posttraumatic stress disorder. *American Journal of Psychiatry* 152(4): 555–563.

Rosenheck RA, Leda C, Frisman LK, Lam J, Chung A. 1996a. Homeless veterans. In: Baumohl J, ed. *Homelessness in America: A Reference Book.* Phoenix, AZ: Oryx Press.

Rosenheck RA, Leda C, Sieffert D, Burnette C. 1996b. *Fiscal Year 1995 End-of-Year Survey of Homeless Veterans in VA Inpatient and Domiciliary Care Programs.* West Haven, CT: Northeast Program Evaluation Center.

Rosenheck RA, Cramer J, Xu W, Thomas J, Henderson W, Frisman LK, Fye C, Charney D. 1997a. A comparison of clozapine and haloperidol in the treatment of hospitalized patients with refractory schizophrenia. *New England Journal of Medicine* 337(12): 809–815.

Rosenheck RA, Wilson N, Meterko M. 1997b. Consumer satisfaction with inpatient mental health treatment: Influence of patient and hospital factors. *Psychiatric Services* 48:1553–1561.

Rosenheck RA, Leda C, Frisman LK, Gallup P. 1997c. Homeless mentally ill veterans: Race, service use and treatment outcome. *American Journal of Orthopsychiatry* 67(4): 632–639.

Rosenheck RA, Fontana A, Stolar M. 1999a. Assessing Quality of Care: Administrative Indicators and Clinical Outcomes in Posttraumatic Stress Disorder. *Medical Care.* 37(2): 180–188.

Rosenheck RA, Frisman LK, Kasprow W. 1999b. Improving access to disability benefits among homeless persons with mental illness: An agency-specific approach to services integration. *American Journal of Public Health* 89(4):524–528.

Rosenheck RA, Hoff RA, Steinwachs D, Lehman A. 2000a. Benchmarking treatment of schizophrenia: A comparison of service delivery by the national government and by state and local providers. *Journal of Nervous and Mental Disease* 188(4):209–216.

Rosenheck RA, Dausey D, Frisman LK, Kasprow W. 2000b. Impact of receipt of social security benefits on homeless veterans with mental illness. *Psychiatric Services* 51(12):1 549–1554.

Rosenheck RA, Banks S, Pandiani J. 2000c. Does closing beds in one public mental health system result in increased use of hospital services in other systems? *Mental Health Services Research* 2(4):183–189.

Rosenheck RA, Banks S, Pandiani J, Hoff R. 2000d. Bed closures and incarceration rates among users of Veterans Affairs mental health services. *Psychiatric Services* 51(10):1282–1287.

Rosenheck RA, Leslie DL, Sernyak M. 2001a. From clinical trials to real-world practice: Use of atypical antipsychotic medication nationally in the Department of Veterans Affairs. *Medical Care* 39(3):302–308.

Rosenheck RA, Frisman LK, Essock S. 2001b. Impact of VA bed closures on use of state mental health services. *Journal of Behavioral Health Services and Research* 28(1):58–66.

Rosenheck RA, Lam J, Morrissey JP, Calloway M, Stolar M, Randolph F, and the ACCESS National Evaluation Team. 2002. Service systems integration and outcomes for mentally ill homeless persons in the ACCESS program. *Psychiatric Services* 53(8):958–966.

Rosenheck RA, Kasprow W, Frisman LK, Liu-Mares W. 2003a. Cost-effectiveness of supported housing for homeless persons with mental illness. *Archives of General Psychiatry* 60(9):940–951.

Rosenheck RA, Desai R, Kasprow, Mares A. 2003b. *Progress report on new initiatives for Homeless Veterans from the Veterans Health Administration.* West Haven, CT: Northeast Program Evaluation Center.

Rosenheck RA, Leslie D, Woody G. 2003c. Fiscal strain and access to opiate substitution therapy at Department of Veterans Affairs Medical Centers. *American Journal on Addictions* 12(3):220–228.

Rosenheck R, Perlick D, Bingham S, Liu-Mares W, Collins J, Warren S, Leslie D, Allan E, Campbell C, Caroff S, Corwin J, Davis L, Douyon R, Dunn L, Evans D, Frecska E, Grabowski J, Graeber D, Herz L, Kwon K, Lawson W, Mena F, Sheikh J, Smelson D, Smith-Gamble V. 2003d. Effectiveness and cost of olanzapine and haloperidol in the treatment of schizophrenia: a randomized controlled trial. *Journal of the American Medical Association* 290(20):2693–2702.

Seibyl CL, Rosenheck RA, Siefert D, Medak S. 2001. *Fiscal Year 2000 End-of-Year Survey of Homeless Veterans in VA Inpatient Programs.* West Haven, CT: Northeast Program Evaluation Center.

Seibyl CL, Rosenheck RA, Corwel L, Medak S. 2003. *Sixth Progress Report on the Compensated Work Therapy/Veterans Industries Program. Fiscal Year 2002.* West Haven, CT: Northeast Program Evaluation Center.

Sernyak MJ, Rosenheck RA. 2003. Risk adjustment in studies using administrative data. *Schizophrenia Bulletin* 29(2):267–271.

Sernyak MJ, Leslie D, Alarcon R, Losonczy M, Rosenheck RA. 2002. Association of diabetes mellitus with use of atypical neuroleptics in the treatment of schizophrenia. *American Journal of Psychiatry* 159(4):561–566.

Sernyak MJ, Gulanski B, Leslie DL, Rosenheck RA. 2003. Undiagnosed hyperglycemia in clozapine-treated patients with schizophrenia. *Journal of Clinical Psychiatry* 64(5):605–608.

Smith SR, Lipsky M. 1993. *Nonprofits for Hire: The Welfare State in the Age of Contracting.* Cambridge, MA: Harvard University Press.

Stein LI, Test MA. 1980. Alternative to mental hospital treatment. I. Conceptual model, treatment program and clinical evaluation. *Archives of General Psychiatry* 37(4):392–397.

Tessler R, Rosenheck RA, Gamache G. 2002. Comparison of homeless veterans with other homeless men in a large clinical outreach program. *Psychiatric Quarterly* 73(2): 109–119.

Tessler R, Rosenheck RA, Gamache G. 2005. Declining access to alcohol and drug abuse services among veterans in the general population. *Military Medicine* 170(3):234–238.

Tomich N. 1992. Paul Errera: "One does have choices." *US Medicine* 28:1.

U.S. Census Bureau. 2001. *Statistical Abstract of the United States.* 121st ed. Washington, DC: U.S. Census Bureau.

U.S. Department of Veterans Affairs. 2003. *FY 2003 Annual performance and Accountability Report.* Washington, DC: U.S. Department of Veterans Affairs.

USVA (U.S. Veterans Affairs). 2004. [Online]: http://www.va.gov/vetdata/SurveyResults [December 5, 2005].

Walter L, Davidowitz N, Heineken P. Kovinsky K. 2004. Pitfalls of converting practice guidelines into quality measures: Lessons learned from a VA performance measure. *Journal of the American Medical Association* 291:2466–2470.

Weissman EM, Rosenheck RA, Essock SM. 2002. Impact of modifying risk adjustment models on rankings of access to care in the VA mental health report card. *Psychiatric Services* 53(9):1153–1158.

TABLE 1 Population Characteristics and Percentage of Veterans Who Used VA Services, 2001

	(1) Total Population Characteristics	(2) Percent Who Used VA Health Services: Past Year	(3) Percent Who Used VA Health Services: Lifetime	(4) Characteristics of Veterans Who Used MH/SA Services: Past Year	(5) % of MH/SA Services Users Who Used VHA MH/SA Services
[Population] Size	25,196,036	5,161,036	8,675,570	1,676,170	681,969
Proportion of All Veterans Who Used Services		20.5%	34.4%	6.6%	2.7% (41.0% of Col 4)
Sociodemographic					
Average Age	57.7	61.7	59.8	50.5	53.4
Age					
<30	3.8%	12.3%	21.2%	5.3%	22.9%
30–49	25.6%	15.0%	31.3%	41.6%	32.3%
50–59	24.6%	18.4%	35.1%	32.8%	48.6%
60–75	29.6%	23.4%	34.0%	14.2%	46.1%
>75	16.4%	29.0%	42.6%	6.2%	52.0%
Race*					
White	83.3%	19.1%	32.4%	76.8%	37.1%
Black	8.8%	30.7%	48.7%	12.2%	51.8%
Hispanic	4.1%	20.1%	35.5%	4.7%	47.1%
Other	3.9%	27.8%	44.4%	6.3%	54.1%
Gender					
Male	94.1%	20.6%	34.6%	87.7%	42.2%
Female	5.9%	17.9%	32.5%	12.3%	28.4%
Education					
<High School Graduate	11.2%	33.9%	46.0%	8.37%	54.0%
High School Graduate	30.0%	21.4%	33.3%	27.8%	45.5%
Post High School Education	35.8%	19.8%	35.0%	42.4%	39.6%
4 Yr College Degree or Higher	23.0%	13.9%	29.3%	21.5%	30.2%

Employment					
Employed	55.1%	12.8%	28.2%	46.8%	25.6%
Retired/Disabled	39.1%	30.3%	42.1%	39.3%	57.7%
Unemployed/Other	5.9%	26.8%	41.2%	13.8%	42.2%
Marital Status					
Married	75.1%	18.6%	32.3%	59.1%	36.2%
Widowed	5.31%	25.5%	40.3%	3.0%	33.2%
Separated/Divorced	12.43%	29.1%	45.5%	25.8%	49.0%
Never Married	7.18%	22.0%	33.6%	12.1%	45.1%
Income					
<$20,000	17.0%	43.8%	56.4%	27.9%	59.6%
$20,000–$40,000	27.9%	25.6%	38.6%	30.5%	48.7%
>$40,000	55.2%	10.2%	25.4%	41.7%	20.7%
Insurance					
Medicaid or Medicare	40.1%	28.7%	41.2%	31.5%	51.0%
Private	63.3%	10.8%	26.0%	49.3%	20.7%
Medigap	18.2%	26.1%	38.7%	6.9%	40.1%
Military Related (for example, CHAMPUS)	7.2%	27.6%	45.7%	8.2%	49.7%
Other Government Insurance (for example, Indian Health Service)	3.5%	27.7%	45.3%	4.0%	58.5%
Military Experience					
Active Duty					
0–2 years	33.2%	20.0%	33.5%	32.1%	39.8%
3–5 years	46.1%	19.1%	33.0%	42.8%	38.2%
5 years or more	20.7%	24.5%	39.5%	25.1%	46.1%
Served in a Combat or War Zone	39.3%	26.2%	42.5%	44.9%	50.4%
Exposed to Dead or Wounded	36.7%	26.0%	42.6%	49.8%	48.9%

(continued on next page)

TABLE 1 continued

	(1) Total Population Characteristics	(2) Percent Who Used VA Health Services: Past Year	(3) Percent Who Used VA Health Services: Lifetime	(4) Characteristics of Veterans Who Used MH/SA Services: Past Year	(5) % of MH/SA Services Users Who Used VHA MH/SA Services
Prisoner of War	.5%	49.3%	64.4%	1.2%	71.6%
Exposed to Environmental Hazards	19.3%	27.3%	45.0%	38.9%	51.1%
Period of Service**					
WWI through WWII	20.5%	28.2%	41.5%	7.5%	50.0%
Btwn WWII & Korean War	2.4%	28.8%	39.9%	1.0%	68.6%
Korean War	12.2%	25.7%	37.5%	5.5%	54.0%
Btwn Korean & Vietnam War	16.3%	19.3%	29.1%	11.8%	46.6%
Vietnam Era	25.6%	18.0%	37.3%	40.3%	45.1%
Post-Vietnam Era	17.7%	13.9%	27.8%	25.2%	29.6%
Persian Gulf War Era (1990–)	4.9%	12.1%	22.3%	8.2%	24.2%
Health Status					
Self-Reported Health Status					
Fair-Poor	24.2%	39.9%	54.0%	45.2%	55.2%
Good	30.2%	19.9%	35.4%	27.3%	38.2%
Excellent-Very Good	45.6%	9.8%	22.7%	27.5%	17.4%
Any Health Service Use For					
Alcohol or Drugs	1.2%	43.1%	59.4%	10.9%	41.6%
PTSD	3.8%	57.3%	73.0%	32.5%	60.3%
Mental Health	6.2%	43.2%	58.1%	52.8%	44.4%
Any	8.9%	45.1%	61.1%	68.9%	46.8%

Service Connected					
Not Service Connected	87.8%	15.9%	28.5%	69.6%	26.1%
<50%	9.6%	43.9%	70.5%	17.3%	63.3%
>50%	2.6%	80.3%	91.2%	13.0%	84.0%
Mental health interferes with work or activities at all	49.9%	29.9%	45.0%	83.0%	43.3%

*Exclusive categories (veterans in more than one category were classified as other).

**Exclusive categories (first period of service used).

TABLE 2 Logistic Regression Analysis of VA Health Service Use: Factors That Predict Recent and Lifetime Use

	Used Service During the Past Year			Ever Used Services		
	Odds Ratio	95% Confidence Interval	Rank Order	Odds Ratio	95% Confidence Interval	Rank Order
Sociodemographic						
Age						
<30	0.58*	0.57-0.58	8	0.63**	0.63-0.64	10
30–49	0.69	0.68-0.69	16	1.11	1.10-1.11	28
50–59	1.01	1.00-1.01	38	1.32	1.31-1.33	17
60–75	1.15	1.14-1.16	24	1.05	1.04-1.05	31
>75	1.00	Reference		1.00	Reference	
Race						
Black	1.57	1.56-1.58	13	1.74	1.73-1.74	7
Hispanic	0.98	0.97-0.99	36	1.13	1.13-1.14	26
Other	1.33	1.32-1.34	19	1.35	1.35-1.36	15
Whites	1.00	Reference		1.00	Reference	
Gender						
Male	1.00	Reference		1.00	Reference	
Female	1.08	1.07-1.08	29	1.08	1.07-1.08	30
Education						
<High School Graduate	1.00	Reference		1.00	Reference	
High School Graduate	0.90	0.90-0.90	28	0.89	0.89-0.90	27
Post High School Education	0.94	0.93-0.94	31	1.04	1.04-1.04	32
4 Yr College Degree or Higher	0.78	0.78-0.78	20	1.00	1.00-1.00	38
Employment						
Employed	1.00	Reference		1.00	Reference	
Retired/Disabled	1.11	1.11-1.12	27	0.99	0.98-0.99	36
Unemployed/Other	1.07	1.06-1.07	33	0.96	0.96-0.97	33

Marital Status						
Married	1.00	Reference		1.00	Reference	
Widowed	0.68	0.68-0.69	15	0.85	0.84-0.85	23
Separated/Divorced	1.07	1.07-1.07	32	1.20	1.20-1.20	21
Never Married	0.96	0.95-0.96	34	0.84	0.84-0.85	22
Income						
<$20,000	1.00	Reference		1.00	Reference	
$20,000–$40,000	0.63	0.63-0.63	10	0.61	0.61-0.61	9
>$40,000	0.34	0.34-0.34	3	0.44	0.44-0.44	3
Income Information Missing	0.57	0.57-0.57	7	0.54	0.54-0.54	5
Insurance						
Medicaid or Medicare	1.01	1.01-1.01	37	1.17	1.16-1.17	24
Private	0.35	0.35-0.35	4	0.57	0.57-0.57	6
Medigap	0.90	0.90-0.90	26	0.97	0.96-0.97	35
Military Related (for example, CHAMPUS)	0.85	0.85-0.86	21	0.96	0.96-0.97	34
Other Government Insurance (for example, Indian Health Service)	1.16	1.16-1.17	23	1.26	1.26-1.27	19
Military Experience						
Active Duty						
0–2 years	1.00	Reference		1.00	Reference	
3–5 years	1.04	1.04-1.04	35	1.00	1.00-1.01	37
5 years or more	1.16	1.16-1.17	22	0.92	0.92-0.92	29
Served in a Combat or War Zone	1.15	1.14-1.15	25	1.26	1.25-1.26	20
Exposed to Dead or Wounded	1.07	1.07-1.07	30	1.15	1.15-1.16	25
Prisoner of War	1.60	1.58-1.63	9	1.52	1.50-1.55	12

(continued on next page)

TABLE 2 continued

	Used Service During the Past Year			Ever Used Services		
	Odds Ratio	95% Confidence Interval	Rank Order	Odds Ratio	95% Confidence Interval	Rank Order
Health Status						
Self-Reported Health Status						
Fair-Poor	1.91	1.92-1.95	5	1.71	1.71-1.72	8
Good	1.40	1.39-1.40	18	1.32	1.32-1.32	18
Excellent-Very Good	1.00	Reference		1.00	Reference	
Any Health Service Use For						
Alcohol or Drugs	1.43	1.41-1.44	17	1.40	1.38-1.41	14
PTSD	1.58	1.57-1.59	12	1.58	1.57-1.59	11
Mental Health	1.58	1.58-1.59	11	1.40	1.40-1.41	13
Service Connected						
Not Service Connected	1.00	Reference		1.00	Reference	
<50%	3.66	3.65-3.68	2	5.21	5.19-5.23	2
>50%	12.10	12.00-12.19	1	14.12	13.98-14.26	1
Mental health interferes with work or activities at all	1.47	1.47-1.48	14	1.33	1.33-1.33	16
Proxy Answered Questions	1.85	1.84-1.87	6	1.91	1.90-1.92	4

*All odds ratios for whether used service in the past year were significant at $p < .0001$ except for age 50–59, which was not significant.

**All odds ratios for whether ever used services were significant at $p < .0001$, except for having a college education or higher and years of service from 3 to 5 years, which were not significant.

TABLE 3   Logistic Regression Analysis of Use of VA MH/SA Services Among Veterans Who Used Any MH/SA Care, 2001

	Odds Ratio	95% Confidence Interval	Rank Order
Sociodemographic			
Age			
<30	0.19*	0.18-0.19	3
30–49	0.38	0.37-0.38	8
50–59	0.86	0.84-0.88	34
60–75	1.21	1.19-1.24	31
>75	1.00	Reference	
Race			
Black	1.68	1.66-1.70	16
Hispanic	1.29	1.27-1.32	24
Other	1.49	1.47-1.52	19
Whites	1.00	Reference	
Gender			
Male	1.00	Reference	
Female	0.83	0.82-0.85	32
Education			
<High School Graduate	1.00	Reference	
High School Graduate	1.26	1.24-1.28	28
Post High School Education	0.79	0.77-0.80	25
4 Yr College Degree or Higher	0.73	0.72-0.75	21
Employment			
Employed	1.00	Reference	
Retired/Disabled	0.90	0.89-0.91	35
Unemployed/Other	1.01	1.00-1.03	37
Marital Status			
Married	1.00	Reference	
Widowed	0.32	0.31-0.33	6
Separated/Divorced	1.41	1.39-1.42	20
Never Married	1.76	1.74-1.79	15
Income			
<$20,000	1.00	Reference	
$20,000–$40,000	0.79	0.78-0.80	27
>$40,000	0.37	0.37-0.38	7
Income Information Missing	0.50	0.49-0.51	10
Insurance			
Medicaid or Medicare	0.79	0.78-0.80	29
Private	0.24	0.24-0.25	4
Medigap	0.53	0.52-0.54	13
Military Related (for example, CHAMPUS)	0.48	0.48-0.49	9
Other Government Insurance (for example, Indian Health Service)	3.43	3.35-3.50	5

(continued on next page)

TABLE 3   continued

	Odds Ratio	95% Confidence Interval	Rank Order
Military Experience			
Active Duty			
0–2 years	1.00	Reference	
3–5 years	1.27	1.26-1.28	26
5 years or more	1.36	1.34-1.38	22
Served in a Combat or War Zone	1.01	1.00-1.02	38
Exposed to Dead or Wounded	1.19	1.18-1.20	33
Prisoner of War	1.34	1.29-1.39	23
Health Status			
Self-Reported Health Status			
Fair-Poor	1.85	1.82-1.87	14
Good	1.95	1.93-1.98	11
Excellent-Very Good	1.00	Reference	
Any Health Service Use For			
Alcohol or Drugs	1.02	1.00-1.03	36
PTSD	1.50	1.48-1.51	18
Mental Health	1.25	1.24-1.26	30
Service Connected			
Not Service Connected	1.00	Reference	
<50%	7.08	6.99-7.16	2
>50%	16.56	16.28-16.85	1
Mental health interferes with work or activities at all	0.64	0.64-0.65	17
Proxy Answered Questions	1.93	1.88-1.99	12

*All odds ratios were significant at p <.0001 except for an employment status of unemployed or other, which was not significant. (Combat p value is .503 and use of mental health services for drugs and alcohol p value is .0325)

TABLE 4 Veterans Treated for Primary or Secondary Mental Health (MH) Diagnosis in the VHA in FY 2003, by Specialty Clinic Treatment

Diagnosis	(1) Total with any MH Dx	(2) Percent of total by Dx/SC	Primary MH Diagnosis*					(8) Secondary MH Dx only	(9) Percent with secondary Dx only
			(3) Total with Primary MH Dx/SC	(4) Treated in Specialty MH Clinic	(5) Percent by Dx/SC	(6) Treated only in non-MH clinic	(7) Percent Treated in Specialty Clinic		
Total	1,218,327	100%	930,098	709,432	100%	220,666	76%	288,229	24%
Dysthymia	495,519	41%	360,511	302,070	43%	58,441	84%	135,008	27%
PTSD	242,850	20%	227,448	216,970	31%	10,478	95%	15,402	6%
Anxiety disorder	238,191	15%	183,062	155,108	22%	27,954	85%	55,129	23%
Major depressive disorder	182,927	15%	177,500	173,010	24%	4,490	97%	5,427	3%
Schizophrenia	100,054	8%	95,733	91,568	13%	4,165	96%	4,321	4%
Adjustment disorder	79,103	6%	73,439	67,674	10%	5,765	92%	5,664	7%
Bipolar disorder	76,702	6%	73,202	70,383	10%	2,819	96%	3,500	5%
Other psychosis	61,985	5%	53,764	39,502	6%	14,262	73%	8,221	13%
Dementia	60,269	5%	38,871	23,047	3%	15,824	59%	21,398	36%
Personality disorder	36,620	3%	35,450	34,427	5%	1,023	97%	1,170	3%
Other psychiatric disorder	274,209	23%	194,649	138,118	19%	56,531	71%	79,560	29%
Substance abuse	266,358	22%	214,251	188,252	27%	25,999	88%	52,107	20%
Alcohol	209,930	17%	166,005	144,854	20%	21,151	87%	43,925	21%
Drug	132,412	11%	121,743	114,994	16%	6,749	94%	10,669	8%
Dually diagnosed (MH and SA)	221,288	18%	211,021	187,808	26%	23,213	89%	10,267	5%
Service connected (1–100%)	462,069	38%	384,133	320,831	45%	63,302	84%	77,936	17%
<=50%	238,690	20%	190,236	150,669	21%	39,567	79%	48,454	20%
>50%<100%	120,818	10%	102,600	88,391	12%	14,209	86%	18,218	15%
100%	102,561	8%	91,297	81,771	12%	9,526	90%	11,264	11%
Total diagnoses/veteran	1.8			2.2		1.0		1.4	

*The primary diagnosis is the principal condition treated during the episode of care.
NOTE: MH = mental health, Dx = diagnosis, SA = substance abuse, SC = service connected, PTSD = posttraumatic stress disorder

TABLE 5 Workload of Specialized VA Mental Health Programs (FY 2003)

Program	Patients Treated	Visits/Pt/Yr.	Total Visits
Outpatient/Community			
Outpatient Substance Abuse[a]	115,954	25.8	2,991,613
Mental Health Intensive Case Management (ACT)	3,961	59.3	234,887
Day Hospital	6,218	27.4	170,373
Day Treatment Center	14,389	39.7	571,243
PTSD Clinical Teams	72,849	8.9	645,895
Community Residential Care	9,436	8.4	79,262
Health Care for Homeless Veterans[b]	61,123	4.1	252,642
Psychosocial Rehabilitation[c]	38,302	33.5	1,283,117
Total	283,930	17.4	4,945,917

Program	Episodes of Care	Days/Ep.	Total Days
Inpatient/Residential			
General Psychiatry Inpatient	87,002	12.8	1,113,626
Psychosocial Residential Rehabilitation and Treatment[d]	12,771	40.1	512,117
Inpatient Substance Abuse	5,763	7.4	42,646
Specialized PTSD Programs	4,302	38.8	166,908
Homeless Veterans Grant and Per Diem Program	10,982	92.6	1,016,933
Health Care for Homeless Veterans Residential Contracts	5,430	52.8	286,599
Domiciliary Care for Homeless Veterans	5,156	110.3	568,707
Total	126,250	24.9	3,138,829

[a]Includes methadone maintenance and substance day treatment
[b]Includes supported housing, homeless outreach, and case management
[c]Includes Compensated Work Therapy, Incentive Therapy, Vocational Assistance
[d]Includes residential programs for PTSD, substance abuse, general psychiatry, and vocational rehabilitation

Appendix

Performance Measures Used by the Northeast Program Evaluation Center in the Evaluation and Monitoring of VA Mental Health Programs (Data from FY 2002)

I. Health Care for Homeless Veterans (HCHV) Program and Domiciliary Care for Homeless Veterans (DCHV) Programs
II. Compensated Work Therapy (CWT) Program and Compensated Work Therapy /Transitional Residence (CWT/TR) Program
III. PTSD Performance Monitors and Outcome Measures
IV. Mental Health Intensive Case Management
V. Performance Measures from the National Mental Health Program Performance Monitoring System
VI. Adherence to PORT Pharmacotherapy Guidelines for Patients with Schizophrenia
VII. Outcomes on the Global Assessment of Functioning (GAF) Scale

I. HEALTH CARE FOR HOMELESS VETERANS (HCHV) PROGRAM AND DOMICILIARY CARE FOR HOMELESS VETERANS (DCHV) PROGRAM

Program Structure

Unique veterans served/stops per clinician (HCHV mean = 147.5 veterans; 619 visits)
Percent of allocated staff slots that are filled (HCHV mean = 96.3%)
Literally homeless veterans seen per clinician (HCHV mean = 90.3)
Per diem cost (HCHV mean = $37.67)
Annual turnover rate[1] (DCHV mean = 3.3)

Process Measures

Patient Characteristics
Percent strictly homeless (living outdoors/shelter) (HCHV mean = 67.8%; DCHV mean = 34.8%)
Percent with no time homeless (HCHV = 8.1%; DCHV mean = 4.1%)
Percent with a psychiatric disorder, substance abuse problem, or medical illness (HCHV mean = 82%; DCHV mean = 99.8%)

---

[1]Annual turnover rate is determined by dividing the total number of discharges in the DCHV Program by the number of DCHV operating beds. Average length of stay and occupancy rates will influence a site's value for annual turnover rate.

Program Participation

Mean days in residential treatment (HCHV mean = 59 days; DCHV mean = 104.1 days)

Percent of successful residential treatment completions (HCHV = 52%; DCHV mean = 69%)

Percent of disciplinary discharges from residential treatment (DCHV mean = 14%)

Percent of premature program departures from residential treatment (DCHV mean = 12%)

Percent contacted through outreach (HCHV = 78%)

Appropriateness for residential treatment (HCHV = 89%)

Outcome Measures

Percent with clinical improvement in alcohol problems (HCHV = 73.1%; DCHV mean = 84% unadjusted)

Percent with clinical improvement in non-substance abuse psychiatric problems (HCHV = 70.7%; DCHV mean = 83% unadjusted)

Percent with clinical improvement with medical problems (HCHV mean = 66.3%, DCHV mean = 88.4%)

Percent discharged to an apartment, room, or house (HCHV mean = 37.9%; DCHV mean = 57.4% unadjusted)

Percent with no housing arrangements after discharge (Supported Housing Program = 21.8%; DCHV mean = 19.3% unadjusted)

Percent discharged with arrangements for full- or part-time employment (HCHV = 49.3%; DCHV mean = 54.5% unadjusted)

II. COMPENSATED WORK THERAPY (CWT) PROGRAM AND COMPENSATED WORK THERAPY/TRANSITIONAL RESIDENCE (CWT/TR) PROGRAM

Process Measures

Program participation

Mean hours worked per week in CWT (CWT mean = 26.1 hr/wk; CWT/TR mean = 33.0)

Mean days in residential treatment (CWT/TR mean = 192 days)

Percent of successful completions (CWT mean = 51.4%; CWT/TR mean = 56.1%)

Percent of disciplinary discharges (CWT mean = 15.4%; CWT/TR mean = 26.8%)

Veteran satisfaction in the residential treatment environment[2] (CWT/ TR Community Oriented Program Evaluation Scale (COPES) index mean = 2.95)

Veteran satisfaction in the therapeutic work environment[3] (CWT/ TR Ward Environment Scale (WES) mean = 6.22)

Outcome Measures

Mean work improvement score[4] (CWT mean = 1.57)

Percent with clinical improvement in alcohol problems (CWT mean = 63.6% unadjusted)

Percent with clinical improvement in drug problems (CWT mean = 63% unadjusted)

Percent with clinical improvement in nonsubstance abuse psychiatric problems (CWT mean = 47.3% unadjusted)

Percent with clinical improvement with medical problems (CWT mean = 35.2% unadjusted)

Percent competitively employed after discharge (CWT mean = 41.3%)

Percent unemployed after discharge (CWT mean = 24.8%)

Percent employment status unknown after discharge (CWT mean = 14.6%)

Percent of veterans relocated and reinterviewed 3 months after discharge (CWT/TR mean = 55.8%)

Mean Addiction Severity Index (ASI) index for alcohol problems 3 months after discharge (CWT/TR mean = 0.08 unadjusted)

Mean ASI index for drug problems 3 months after discharge (CWT/TR mean = 0.03 unadjusted)

Mean ASI index for psychiatric problems 3 months after discharge (CWT/TR mean = 0.18 unadjusted)

Mean days competitively employed past month at 3 months after discharge (CWT/TR mean = 11 days unadjusted)

Mean days housed past 90 days at 3 months after discharge (CWT/TR mean = 71.2 days unadjusted)

III. PTSD PERFORMANCE MONITORS AND OUTCOME MEASURES

Outpatient Programs (Specialized PTSD Outpatient Programs)

Patient Characteristics

War zone service (87%)

DD 214 (Discharge Certification form) service validation (65%)

---

[2]Range equals 0 – 4.
[3]Range equals 0 – 9.
[4]Range equals 0 – 2.

PTSD clinical diagnosis (82%)
Substance abuse diagnosis (41%)
Prior psychiatric treatment (74%)
Prior specialized PTSD treatment (22%)
Workload
Number of visits per filled Full Time Employee Equivalents (FTEE)
(1,160)
Number of veterans treated per filled FTEE (88)
Costs
Direct costs per visit ($73)
Direct costs per capita ($958)

Outpatient Care Measures (All VA PTSD treatment, specialized and non-specialized)

Service Utilization and Continuity of Care Six Months Following Inpatient Index Stay
Any outpatient stop in 6 months after discharge (DC) (92.0%)
Any outpatient stop in 30 days after DC (72.0%)
Days to first outpatient stop in 6 months after discharge (23.7)
Number of stops in 6 months among those with any stops (18.6)
Continuity: Bi-months (2 month intervals) with two stops (2.5)
(Next measure applies only to those with a dual diagnosis (PTSD
and SA)
At least 1 Psychiatric and 1 SA outpatient (OP) stop in 6 months
after DC (14.4%)
Continuity of Care Among Outpatients with PTSD Diagnosis
Number of outpatient stops (15.5)
Number of days with outpatient stops (11.9)
Continuity: bi-months with 2 stops (2.61)
Continuity: months with any MH visit of six months (4.17)
Dropout (6 months with no O/P visit) 13%
Continuity of care index (.57)
Modified Continuity Index (MCI) (.80)

Inpatient/Residential Programs (Specialized PTSD programs)

Patient Characteristics
(Same as for Outpatient programs)
Costs
Direct costs per diem ($136)
Direct costs per capita ($4,662)

Outcomes (4 months after discharge)[5]

PTSD symptoms
Short Mississippi Scale (–5.6%)
NEPEC PTSD Scale (–6.7%)
Substance abuse
ASI Composite for Alcohol problems (–23.5%)
ASI Composite for Drugs problems (–14.3%)
Violence
NVVRS Scale (–38.8%)
Work
Number of days worked for pay (+1.8%)
Satisfaction with treatment
Client Satisfaction Scale (Attkisson et al.) (15.6)

All PTSD Inpatient Care (General and Specialized Programs)

Bed days six months after DC (5.6)
Number of admissions 6 months after DC (.45)
Percentage readmitted within 14 days (5.0%)
Percentage readmitted within 30 days (8.0%)
Percentage readmitted within 180 days (30.0%)
Days to readmission first year after discharge (74.8)

IV. MENTAL HEALTH INTENSIVE CASE MANAGEMENT (MHICM)

Program Structure

Percent allocated FTEE that are filled (84%)
Availability of appropriate medical support (89%)
Availability of appropriate nursing support (96%)
Unfilled FTEE lagged greater than 6 months (43% of teams)
Caseload size (average = 15.4)(should be less than 15)

Appropriateness of Admissions

Hospitalized 30 days or more
Hospitalized more than 30 days in the previous year (82%)
Diagnosis of psychotic illness (78%)
GAF < 50 at admission

---

[5]Negative values on symptom measures represent improvement (i.e., declining symptoms)

Treatment Process

Clients terminated
Intensity (greater than 1 hour per week)(66.7%)
Services provided in the community 60% of the time (87%)
Face-to-face contacts per week (1.45)
Seen for rehabilitation (36.1%)
Improvement in Therapeutic Alliance (10.2%)
ACT Fidelity Score (4.0)

Outcomes[6]

Change in inpatient days (6 months before entry to 6 months after)(–47 days; –73%)
Brief Psychiatric Rating Scale (BPRS, Symptoms)(–3.92; –10%)
Brief Symptom Inventory (BSI, Symptoms)(–.22; –11%)
Global Assessment of Functioning (GAF)(–2.01; –5%)
Instrumental Activities of Daily Living (IADL)(+.95, 2%)
Lehman Quality of Life Question (+2.8, 11%)
Housing Independence (+.43, 15%)
Satisfaction with VA Mental Health Services (+1.54, 17.6%)
Satisfaction with MHICM (+.62, 21%)

V. PERFORMANCE MEASURES FROM THE NATIONAL MENTAL HEALTH PROGRAM PERFORMANCE MONITORING SYSTEM

Population Coverage

Proportion of All U.S. Veterans who received VA MH services (2.5%)
Proportion of Veterans Service Connected for Mental Illness who received VA MH services (42.2%)
Proportion of low-income Non Service Connected Veterans who received VA MH services (7.0%)
Proportion of Female Veterans who received VA MH services (3.1%)

Inpatient Care Measures

Bed days six months after DC (6.47)
Number of admissions 6 months after DC (.55)
Percentage readmitted within 14 days (6.9%)
Percentage readmitted within 30 days (11.5%)

---

[6]Negative values on symptom measures represent improvement (i.e., declining symptoms).

Percentage readmitted within 180 days (32.1%)
Days to readmission first year after discharge (64.7%)

Outpatient Care Measures

Service Utilization and Continuity of Care Six Months Following Inpatient Index Stay

Any outpatient stop in 6 months after DC (82.1%)
Any outpatient stop in 30 days after DC (63.3%)
Days to first outpatient stop in 6 months after discharge (24.9)
Number of stops in 6 months among those with any stops (25.8)
Continuity: Bi-months with two stops (2.16)
Any medical outpatient stop in 6 months after DC (82.8%)
Days to 1st medical OP stop in 6 months after DC (36.6)
Number of OP medical stops in 6 months among those with any stops (10.6)
(Next 4 measures apply to those with a dual diagnosis (Psyc. and SA)
At least 1 Psyc. and 1 SA OP stop in 6 months after DC (21.2%)
At least 3 Psyc. and 3 SA OP stop in 6 months after DC (17.3%)
Continuity: bi-months with two stops (2.17)
Number of Psyc. and SA visits among those with any stops (25.89)

Continuity of Care among Outpatients with Psychotic Diagnoses

Number of outpatient stops (16.8)
Number of days with outpatient stops (12.5)
Continuity: bi-months with 2 stops (2.56)
Continuity: months with any MH visit of 6 months (3.98)
Dropout (6 months with no OP visit) 15%
Continuity of care index (.56)
Modified MCI (.80)

Inpatient Satisfaction Measures

Coordination of Care (.72)
Provision of Information (.66)
Timeliness/Access to Care (.61)
Courtesy (.66)
Emotional Support (.63)
Respect for Patient Preferences (.71)
Family Involvement (.54)
Physical Care (.62)
Transition Home (.62)
General Satisfaction (.53)

VI. ADHERENCE TO PORT PHARMACOTHERAPY GUIDELINES FOR PATIENTS WITH SCHIZOPHRENIA

Percentage of patients receiving oral antipsychotic medication (81%).
Percentage of veterans dosed higher than recommended guidelines (12.3%)
Percentage of veterans dosed lower than recommended guidelines (28.6%)
Percentage of patients receiving polypharmacy (two antipsychotic medications)(8.1%)

VII. OUTCOMES ON THE GLOBAL ASSESSMENT OF FUNCTIONING (GAF) SCALE

Improvement after inpatient discharge

> Change from inpatient GAF to last outpatient GAF in first six months after discharge (4.9)
> Change from inpatient GAF to the last outpatient GAF of the fiscal year (6.4)

Improvement after during outpatient treatment

> Change from first outpatient GAF to last outpatient GAF in the next 6 months (0.46)
> Change from first outpatient GAF to last outpatient GAF of the fiscal year (0.33)
> Change from first outpatient GAF in the second 6 months of the fiscal year to the last outpatient GAF of the fiscal year (0.38)
> Among newly admitted outpatient veterans (those with no outpatient mental health visits in the first 3 months of the fiscal year) the change from first outpatient GAF to last outpatient GAF of the fiscal year (1.9)

Index

S